BASIC
SCIENCE
REVIEW
FOR SURGEONS

BASIC SCIENCE REVIEW FOR SURGEONS

RICHARD L. SIMMONS, M.D.

George V. Foster Professor of Surgery and
Chairman, Department of Surgery,
University of Pittsburgh School of Medicine,
Pittsburgh, Pennsylvania

DAVID L. STEED, M.D.

Associate Professor of Surgery,
University of Pittsburgh School of Medicine
Pittsburgh, Pennsylvania

W.B. SAUNDERS COMPANY

Harcourt Brace Jovanovich, Inc.

Philadelphia, London, Toronto, Montreal, Sydney, Tokyo

W. B. SAUNDERS COMPANY
Harcourt Brace Jovanovich, Inc.

The Curtis Center
Independence Square West
Philadelphia, PA 19106

Library of Congress Cataloging-in-Publication Data
Basic science review for surgeons / [edited by] Richard L. Simmons,
David L. Steed.
   p.   cm.
  ISBN 0-7216-2984-9
  1. Surgery—Physiological aspects.   2. Human physiology.
I. Simmons, Richard L.,   . II. Steed, David L.
  [DNLM: 1. Physiology.   QT 104 B3115]
  RD31.5.B37 1992
  617—dc20
  DNLM/DLC   91-27414

Editor: Lisette Bralow
Developmental Editor: Kitty McCullough

Basic Science Review for Surgeons   ISBN   0-7216-2984-9

Printed in the United States of America.

Last digit is the print number: 9   8   7   6   5   4   3   2

CONTRIBUTORS

ROBERT R. BAHNSON, M.D.
Assistant Professor of Surgery, Division of Urologic Surgery, University of Pittsburgh, Pittsburgh, Pennsylvania
Physiology of the Kidney, Ureters, and Bladder

MORRIS I. BIERMAN, M.D.
Assistant Professor, Anesthesiology and Critical Care Medicine, University of Pittsburgh School of Medicine, Pittsburgh, Pennsylvania
Respiratory Physiology

TIMOTHY R. BILLIAR, M.D.
Research Assistant Professor, Department of Surgery, University of Pittsburgh School of Medicine, Pittsburgh, Pennsylvania
The Liver and Biliary Tree

BRUCE A. BROD, M.D.
Chief Resident in Dermatology, University of Pittsburgh School of Medicine, Pittsburgh, Pennsylvania
The Skin and Its Connective Tissue

MICHAEL C. BRODY, M.D.
Assistant Professor of Anesthesiology, University of Pittsburgh; Medical Director, Pain Evaluation and Treatment Institute, Presbyterian University Hospital, Pittsburgh, Pennsylvania
Pharmacology of Pain Management

JOSEPH M. DARBY, M.D.
Assistant Professor of Anesthesiology/Critical Care Medicine, Internal Medicine, Surgery and Neurologic Surgery; Director, Neurotrauma ICU, Presbyterian University Hospital, Pittsburgh, Pennsylvania
Intracranial Physiology

ROBERT D. DOWLING, M.D.
Resident, Department of Surgery, University of Pittsburgh School of Medicine, Pittsburgh, Pennsylvania
Cardiac Function

SAMUEL J. DURHAM, M.D.
Resident, Division of Cardiothoracic Surgery, University of Pittsburgh School of Medicine, Pittsburgh, Pennsylvania
Physiology of the Exocrine Pancreas

HOWARD D. EDINGTON, M.D.
Assistant Professor, Divisions of Plastic Surgery and Surgical Oncology, University of Pittsburgh School of Medicine, Pittsburgh, Pennsylvania
Wound Healing

PAUL D. FADALE, M.D.
Assistant Clinical Professor, Surgeon-in-Charge, Division of Sports Medicine, Department of Orthopaedic Surgery, Brown University Program in Medicine, The Rhode Island Hospital, Providence, Rhode Island
Skeletal Muscle

CARL R. FUHRMAN, M.D.
Associate Professor of Radiology, University of Pittsburgh School of Medicine, Pittsburgh, Pennsylvania
Radiology

J. BLAKE GOSLEN, M.D.
Associate Professor of Dermatology, University of Pittsburgh School of Medicine, Pittsburgh, Pennsylvania
The Skin and Its Connective Tissue

BARTLEY P. GRIFFITH, M.D.
Professor of Surgery, Chief, Division of Cardiothoracic Surgery, University of Pittsburgh School of Medicine, Pittsburgh, Pennsylvania
Cardiac Function

TODD K. HOWARD, M.D.
Director, Transplantation ICU, Cedars-Sinai Medical Center, Los Angeles, California
The Liver and Biliary Tree

SUZANNE T. ILDSTAD, M.D.
Assistant Professor, Department of Surgery, Division of Transplantation, University of Pittsburgh, Pittsburgh, Pennsylvania
Immunology and Transplantation

RONALD R. JOHNSON, M.D.
Assistant Professor, Department of Surgery, University of Pittsburgh School of Medicine, Pittsburgh, Pennsylvania
Reproductive Physiology; The Breast

PAUL H. KISPERT, M.D.
Assistant Professor of Surgery, University of Pittsburgh School of Medicine, Pittsburgh, Pennsylvania
Infection and Host Defenses; Metabolic Response to Stress

KENNETH K.W. LEE, M.D.
Assistant Professor of Surgery, University of Pittsburgh School of Medicine, Pittsburgh, Pennsylvania
Physiology of the Exocrine Pancreas

ANDREW B. PEITZMAN, M.D.
Associate Professor of Surgery, University of Pittsburgh School of Medicine; Director, Trauma/Emergency Services, Presbyterian University Hospital, Pittsburgh, Pennsylvania
Shock

MITCHELL C. POSNER, M.D.
Assistant Professor of Surgery, University of Pittsburgh School of Medicine, Pittsburgh, Pennsylvania
Tumor Biology

FUAD RAMADAN, M.D.
Assistant Professor of Surgery, University of Pittsburgh School of Medicine, Pittsburgh, Pennsylvania; Assistant Chief of Vascular Surgery, Veterans Administration Medical Center, Pittsburgh, Pennsylvania
Vascular Physiology

GLENN RAMSEY, M.D.
Assistant Professor of Pathology, Northwestern University Medical School; Medical Director, United Blood Services, Chicago, Illinois
Blood Physiology and Transfusion Therapy

JAMES J. REILLY, Jr., M.D.
Clinical Professor of Surgery, University of Pittsburgh School of Medicine, Pittsburgh, Pennsylvania
Principles of Surgical Nutrition

CHARLES H. RICHARDS, M.D.
Assistant Professor of Anesthesiology, Presbyterian University Hospital, University of Pittsburgh; Staff Anesthesiologist, Western Pennsylvania Hospital, Pittsburgh, Pennsylvania
Principles of Anesthesiology

HARRY E. RUBASH, M.D.
Associate Professor of Orthopaedic Surgery, University of Pittsburgh School of Medicine; Director, Joint Replacement Service, Presbyterian/Montefiore University Hospitals; Chief, Orthopaedic Service, Veterans Administration Medical Center, Pittsburgh, Pennsylvania
Bone Physiology

RICHARD L. SIMMONS, M.D.
George V. Foster Professor of Surgery and Chairman, Department of Surgery, University of Pittsburgh School of Medicine; Chief of Surgery, Presbyterian University Hospital, Pittsburgh, Pennsylvania
Molecular Basis of Cell Signaling; Infection and Host Defenses

SAMUEL D. SMITH, M.D.
Associate Professor, Pediatric Surgery, University of Pittsburgh School of Medicine, Pittsburgh, Pennsylvania; Director, Nutritional Support Service, Children's Hospital of Pittsburgh, Pittsburgh, Pennsylvania
Physiology of the Pediatric Patient

K. ERIC SOMMERS, M.D.
Resident, Department of Surgery, University of Pittsburgh School of Medicine, Pittsburgh, Pennsylvania
The Adrenal Gland

JOSEF STADLER, M.D.
Resident, Department of Surgery, University of Pittsburgh School of Medicine, Pittsburgh, Pennsylvania
Molecular Basis of Cell Signaling

DAVID L. STEED, M.D.
Associate Professor of Surgery, University of Pittsburgh School of Medicine, Pittsburgh, Pennsylvania
Mediators of Inflammation; Hemostasis and Coagulation

ANTHONY O. UDEKWU, M.D.
Assistant Professor of Surgery, University of Pittsburgh School of Medicine; Director, General Surgery Residency Program—Pittsburgh; Co-Director, Trauma Service, Presbyterian University Hospital, Pittsburgh, Pennsylvania
Gastrointestinal Physiology

CHARLES G. WATSON, M.D.
Professor of Surgery, University of Pittsburgh School of Medicine, Pittsburgh, Pennsylvania
Physiology of the Thyroid; Calcium Homeostasis: The Parathyroids and Vitamin D; The Adrenal Gland

MARSHALL W. WEBSTER, M.D.
Professor of Surgery, Chief, Section of Vascular Surgery and Wound Healing, University of Pittsburgh School of Medicine, Pittsburgh, Pennsylvania
Vascular Physiology

PREFACE

For surgeons in practice, it has become increasingly difficult to understand the current literature, which refers in a fragmented way to basic biological principles that constantly change. Medical students, residents, and surgeons in practice have major commitments of time to patient care and thus limited time for gathering knowledge. We believe that there is a need for a text that reviews basic science in a clear and concise manner and presents the basic scientific principles pertinent to surgical practice. Our purpose in editing this book therefore was to gather what is known about cell biology, organ function, and basic physiologic principles into a simplified text that could be reviewed both by residents preparing for examinations in basic science and by those actively caring for patients. What is presented here are the basic scientific concepts that are directly relevant to patient care. This book is written at the level of the house officer, because we believe it will be of value to both surgeons in practice and medical students. Our goal was to make it brief enough to be read cover-to-cover yet comprehensive enough to provide an introductory understanding of contemporary basic science. In addition, we hoped to make this book affordable to all surgeons regardless of training level.

We believe you will find the section on cell biology and tissue injury and repair especially valuable. This section is written in such a manner so as to be directly applicable in the daily management of patients.

We acknowledge the support of the surgical faculty and residents at the University of Pittsburgh in completing this book.

DAVID L. STEED, M.D.
RICHARD L. SIMMONS, M.D.

CONTENTS

ix

PART IV   BIOLOGY OF SURGICAL TREATMENTS

Part I

PHYSIOLOGY
AT THE
CELLULAR LEVEL

1

MOLECULAR BASIS OF CELL SIGNALING

JOSEF STADLER *and* RICHARD L. SIMMONS

STRUCTURAL REQUIREMENTS OF CELL SIGNALING

Principle Organization of Biologic Membranes

The plasma membrane, which encloses every cell, has a highly differentiated structure and is capable of various important functions. To guarantee a stable intracellular milieu, the plasma membrane must maintain ionic differentials between the interior and the exterior of the cell. Furthermore, it selectively filters as well as actively transports desirable nutrients and undesirable wastes. A number of mechanisms have been developed that allow the plasma membrane to receive and transduce extracellular signals. These mechanisms, which are the basis for appropriate responses to changes of the extracellular environment and for the organization of a complex multicellular organisms, are also responsible for many pathologic conditions.[1]

All membranes, plasma membranes and membranes of intracellular organelles, are composed of a double layer of lipid molecules in which proteins are embedded (Fig. 1–1). The structure of the membrane allows free movement of the lipids within the layers and of the proteins within the plane of the membrane, and gives the membrane a consistency that can be described as fluid rather than solid. The lipid bilayer is impermeable to water and water-soluble molecules, and basically acts as a barrier of the intracellular against the extracellular space. The membrane proteins serve as specialized structures for (1) molecular transport, (2) enzymatic activities, (3) reception and transduction of environmental signals, and (4) structural connections between the membrane and the interior cytoskeleton or between cells. The lipid and protein composition of membranes differs considerably for various cell types and organelles.

Lipid Bilayer

Although many specific functions of the membrane proteins have been determined, relatively few aspects of the role of membrane lipids are established.[2] Each lipid molecule of the membrane has a hydrophobic and a hydrophilic end. The hydrophilic (polar) end is exposed to the aqueous environment inside and outside the cell so that a bilayer of lipids is formed with the hydrophobic fatty chains sandwiched between the hydrophilic heads (Fig. 1–1). This formation fulfills the most important task of the membrane: it builds up a stable barrier for water-soluble molecules. The self-orienting property and the high degree of translational movement (fluidity) permit biologic membranes to seal spontaneously when damaged. Transverse movements or "flip-flops" between the layers are very rare. Experiments with artificial membranes indicate that the rate of such movements is about 10,000 times slower than lateral diffusion. However, flip-flop exchange occurs in the endoplasmic reticulum, where it is catalyzed by phospholipid translocating enzymes. The lateral and axial movements of membranes, which determine its fluidity or its inverse viscosity, are controlled by its composition. The three major types of lipids in cell membranes are phospholipids, cholesterol, and glycolipids. Long fatty acids chains and unsaturated lipids make the membrane more viscous. The same is true for cholesterol, which is especially abundant in mammalian cell membranes and increases mechanical stability. In contrast to phospholipids, cholesterol has a small polar head that allows movement between lipid layers but decreases permeability to water-soluble molecules. Mitochondrial membranes are basically cholesterol free.

Four groups of phospholipids make up most of the plasma membranes: phosphatidylcholine, phosphatidylethanolamine, phosphatidylserine, and

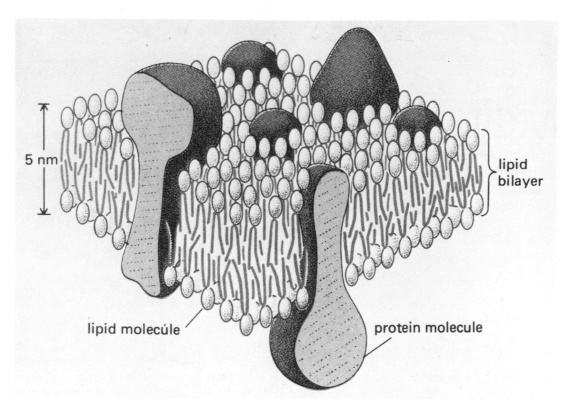

FIGURE 1–1.   Three-dimensional model of a cell membrane. The basic structural units of the membrane are lipid molecules, which aggregate in such a way that their hydrophilic head reagions face the interior and exterior surface of the membrane. The hydrophobic tails form the actual barrier between the aqueous phases of the cytosol and the extracellular environment. The membrane proteins "swim" in the lipid bilayer and perform multiple specific functions. (Reprinted from Alberts, B., Bray, D., Lewis, J., Raff, M., Roberts, K., and Watson, J.D.: Molecular Biology of the Cell, 2nd ed. New York, Garland Publishing, Inc., 1989, p. 275.)

sphingomyelin. Inositol phospholipids play an important role in cell signaling but are present in only small quantities. Glycolipids are found only in the outer layer of the membrane and are derived from ceramide. The ratio of protein to lipid content differs profoundly from cell type to cell type but can be as high as 2 : 1 in some parts of hepatocytic membranes. High protein content decreases the fluidity of the membrane.

Membrane Proteins

Both rotational and lateral movements can be performed by most of the membrane proteins. Therefore, they can be clustered or capped on the cell surface when cross-linked with antibodies or other ligands. Other proteins are immobilized by fixation to the cytoskeleton. The membrane proteins may extend across the entire membrane, which is typical for carrier or receptor proteins, or they may be attached to one side or the other. The parts of proteins that pass through the membrane are usually alpha helices. Proteins can also be anchored in the membrane through binding of lipid chains. The attachment to the inner side of the plasma membrane through prenyl groups, such as farnesyl and geranylgeranyl, which are intermediates of the mevalonate metabolism, has recently been described for subunits of G proteins (see later in this chapter). Binding to phosphatidylinositol has been described for proteins attached to the external side of the membrane. Exterior proteins or the exterior faces of transmembrane proteins are frequently glycosylated. The carbohydrate chain of these glycoproteins or of glycosylated lipids is always oriented to the extracellular space. The carbohydrate chains form a coat around the external cell surface called the glycocalix (Fig. 1–2).

Some cell types have specialized surface areas. In these cases the membrane proteins are distributed asymmetrically over the cell surface. The basal portion of epithelial cells, for example, bears proteins that form the tight junctions between the cells or anchor the cells to the basal membrane, whereas most receptor proteins are found on the apical surface.

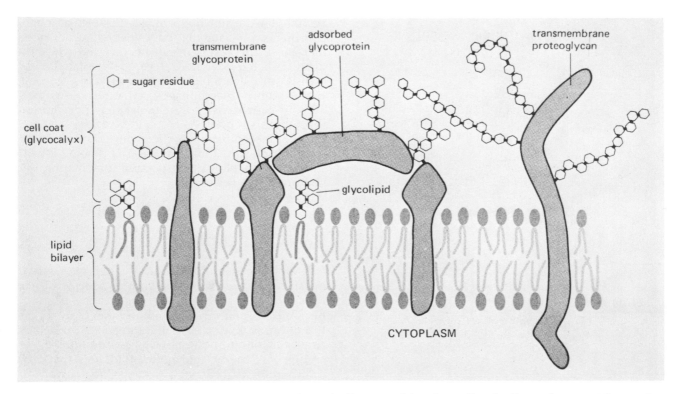

FIGURE 1–2. Schematic diagram of the glycocalix of cell membranes. Oligosaccharide chains bind to the outside of the plasma membrane to form a coat, the glycocalix, around the cell. Note that the glycocalix is comprised by glycosylated proteins as well as by glycolipids. (Reprinted from Alberts, B., Bray, D., Lewis, J., Raff, M., Roberts, K., and Watson, J.D.: Molecular Biology of the Cell, 2nd ed. New York, Garland Publishing, Inc., 1989, p. 300.)

TRANSPORT MECHANISMS ACROSS THE MEMBRANE

Transport of Small Molecules

Some molecules can pass the membrane via diffusion; examples are oxygen, carbon dioxide, ethanol, and urea. However, the lipid bilayer of biologic membranes is practically impermeable to large molecules and ions. To move such molecules across the biologic membranes, transport proteins are employed, each of which is specific for a particular solute. Two classes of such transport proteins exist (Fig. 1–3). *Channel proteins* form pores that allow solutes in aqueous solution to pass through the membrane following their electrochemical gradient. They are usually composed of several homologue subunits that form transmembrane pores with a hydrophilic surface inside the channel. Channel proteins are gated either by receptor proteins, which open the pores in response to specific signals (transmitter gated channels), or by changes in membrane potential (voltage gated channels). This kind of a transport system is not coupled to an energy source. The solutes, mainly ions, always move in the direction of the electrochemical gradient. Ion channels are responsible for electrical excitability of nerve and muscle cells.

Carrier proteins first bind hydrophilic substances, and then undergo conformational changes that carry the solute through the membrane and release it on the other side. Unless the transfer is in the direction of an electrochemical gradient, these processes are energy dependent. Carrier proteins can be uniports or coupled transporters. The uniports move a single solute in a single direction, whereas coupled transporters move cotransfered ions either in the same (symport) or in the opposite (antiport) direction. For example, glucose is absorbed from the intestine utilizing a coupled symportation with sodium ions. On the other hand, most ion exchange pumps work as antiports. A very important example is the export of Na^+ in exchange for K^+. This specific pump, the Na^+/K^+ adenosine triphosphatase pump, uses up one third of the entire energy production of each cell. Other examples for ion exchange carriers are the Na^+/H^+ and the Cl^-/HCO_3^- antiporter pumps, which regulate the intracellular pH.

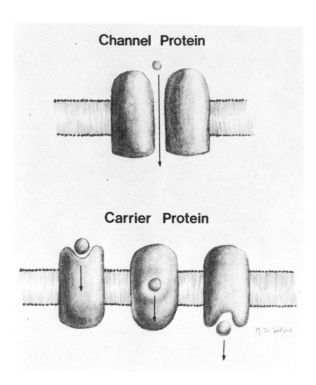

Channel Protein

Carrier Protein

FIGURE 1–3. The principle transport mechanisms provided by transport proteins of biologic membranes. Channel proteins allow passive flux of solutes down an electrochemical gradient. Carrier proteins are capable of actively transporting molecules by conformational changes against such a gradient. This is an energy-consuming process, but carrier proteins also allow passive diffusion in the direction of the gradient without energy consumption.

Transport of Macromolecules and Particles

Macromolecule or particle ingestion or secretion utilizes processes called endocytosis or exocytosis, respectively. Endocytosis involves the formation of membrane vesicles that are pinched off to the cytoplasm and are degraded intracellularly (e.g., in the lysosomes). Exocytosis is performed by fusion of intracellular vesicles with the plasma membrane. Both processes occur spontaneously and continuously (constitutive fashion) or require specific signals (regulated fashion). Similar processes take place when macromolecules are transported between different intracellular compartments. Various secretory proteins, such as insulin, neurotransmitters, or digestive enzymes, are produced within the endoplasmic reticulum. From there they pass to the Golgi apparatus, where they are encapsulated in vesicles. These vesicles migrate to the membrane and release their contents into the extracellular space after they fuse with the lipid bilayer of the membrane. The secretory vesicles can then be retrieved by endocytosis and be reincorporated into membranes of the specific organelles. Receptor-mediated endocytosis has been reported for various ligands such as trans-

ferrin, low-density lipoproteins (LDLs), asialoglycoproteins, or lysosomal enzymes. Following internalization, the receptor can be recycled while the ligand is being degraded. Receptor-mediated endocytosis can reach a high rate of transports per time. For example, macrophages can internalize up to 10,000 α_2-macroglobulin molecules per minute through this route.

Other mechanisms have been developed by evolution that do not transport material objects, but instead are capable of transporting information into and out of the cells.

HOW DO CELLS INTERACT?

A sophisticated information system is necessary to organize the development and to coordinate the functions of multicellular organisms. Communication between various subunits takes place on different levels. For cell-to-cell interactions three basic routes of communication have been defined: (1) secretion of chemicals (hormones, cytokines) that carry information to cells at a distance; (2) surface-to-surface contact, which enables signaling via membrane-bound molecules; and (3) formation of gap junctions allowing exchange of information through a direct communication of the cytoplasms.

Chemical Signaling

Various strategies have been realized in the body to transport information to cells at some distance. Long-range signaling requires the transport of signals via the bloodstream. Specific messenger molecules (hormones) are secreted by specialized cells, which are often but not always organized into glands. *Endocrine* signals reach every cell in the whole body, but only those cells that are able to bind the signal and to "translate" its message will respond. *Paracrine* signals, by contrast, do not normally pass into the circulation in sufficient concentration to affect distant cells, but instead act via mediators that diffuse short distances through the ground substance. Various mechanisms normally keep paracrine signals regionally controlled. For example, substances are released to inactivate the mediators (e.g., proteinases, soluble receptors no longer attached to cells) or immobilize them in the extracellular matrix (e.g., fibronectin, proteoglycans). However, spillover of paracrine signaling molecules may yield profound systemic effects. For example, tumor necrosis factor α regulates wound healing processes by coordinating the action of macrophages, fibroblasts, and other cells; released into the blood stream, it may lead to tissue necrosis and may cause a sepsislike shock syndrome at high concentrations. Therefore, paracrine and endocrine activities may be overlapping, and apparently discordant biologic effects have been demonstrated for the same agent.

In contrast to the endocrine system, the paracrine system is not organized in specific glands. Typical examples for primarily paracrine mediators are cytokines (usually polypeptides), eicosanoids (products of cell wall arachidonic acid), and biologically active amino acid derivatives such as serotonin or histamine. Although *autocrine* stimulation does not belong to the topic of cell-to-cell interaction, it should be mentioned in this context. Autocrine signals act on the secreting cell itself, provided the cell is able to receive its own signals; this provides feedback regulation of cell function. Prostaglandins have been shown to act in this way. They are produced by cells in all tissues and their continuous release is modified through the action of other signals.

The most sophisticated level of communication in multicellular organisms is the nervous system. Highly specialized nerve cells transmit information by electric excitation across long distances to well-defined target cells. The target cells are contacted through *synaptic* signaling by the release of specific neurotransmitters. The nervous system allows coordination of different parts of the body with high speed and precision. It is beyond the scope of this book to discuss its anatomic and physiologic complexity.

The response to chemical signals varies with different cell types and depends on the receptors to which the chemicals bind, how the signals are transduced into the cell, and the intracellular reaction. The interaction of the signals (the ligands) with the receptors follows the same biochemical and kinetic rules as those that govern the interaction of substrates and enzymes. However, the same ligand may have different receptors of differing affinity that transduce their effects in the cell by different mechanisms. The response of the target cell is then at least partially determined by the quantitative presence of the various receptors whose expression is governed by intracellular events. In general, amino acid and peptide ligands each have their own specific protein receptor on the cell surface, whereas lipids such as steroid hormones, or lipid-soluble components, pass through the cell wall and bind to receptors inside the cell. In any case and whether the route of signaling follows an endocrine, paracrine, autocrine, or synaptic fashion, the ligand will bind to a protein receptor that translates the signal into information that leads to a specific reaction of the target cell. Although steroid receptors are probably identical in all cells, different genes are regulated because of other cell-specific gene regulatory proteins in each cell necessary to collaborate with it.

The response of the target cell to the chemical signals may be transient, long lasting, or even irreversible. In some cases the duration of the response depends primarily on the degradation of the ligand. Typical examples are neurotransmitters, which are destroyed very rapidly, thereby limiting the response to a nerve signal to a few milliseconds. Protein signals are usually also eliminated fairly quickly, sometimes by internalization of the whole receptor-ligand complex and intracellular degradation (e.g., insulin-receptor complex), sometimes by being sloughed. In contrast, thyroid hormones and steroids may persist for days.

Signaling Through Surface Contact and Gap Junctions

Permanent adhesion of cells to other cells takes place by connections such as tight junctions, desmosomes, or gap junctions; transient contact is mediated through *adhesion molecules*.[3] Adhesion molecules are proteins that bind to specific receptors on the surface of the target cell. An example is the CD18 complex of neutrophils, which allows adherence to a receptor protein on endothelial cells. This is the first step of neutrophil diapedesis from the venules during acute inflammatory processes. Such a step obviously must be transient; otherwise the neutrophil could not escape the vascular lumen.

Adhesion, however, is not only a process of anchoring cells to other cells; it is also important for intracellular signaling. The CD4 complexes of T lymphocytes are thought to enforce binding of these cells to antigen-presenting cells, thereby enabling the necessary contact of the T cell receptor with the autochthonous MHC-II complex, which in turn presents the antigen within its structure. Other adhesion molecules such as the NCAM (cellular adhesion molecule, which is predominantly found on neurons) have enzymatic activity, in this case as phosphatases.

Gap junctions are pores of 1.5 nm diameter that connect the cytoplasms of contiguous cells and allow free exchange of molecules up to 1000 daltons. This includes small molecules such as inorganic ions, second messenger molecules, and metabolites such as amino acids, peptides, sugars, nucleotides, and others. The structural basis of gap junctions are channel-forming proteins, which allow opening and closing of the channels mediated through physiologic stimuli. Opening of these private transport pathways facilitates metabolic collaboration and endocrine synchronization. This probably optimizes the efficiency of cells with similar biologic function. On hepatocytes, 3 per cent of the whole surface area is occupied by gap junctions. Closing of the channels prevents the passage of toxic material and separates damaged cells from healthy ones (e.g., acidification). Although the structural features of gap junctions have become well understood, the biologic function in terms of their specific role under certain physiologic and pathologic situations still remains to be elucidated.

MECHANISMS OF SIGNAL TRANSDUCTION

In order to effect a change in cell activity or function, ligands such as hormones or cytokines must bind to highly specific receptors either on the cell surface or inside the cell. Water-soluble ligands typically bind to cell surface receptors, whereas lipid-soluble molecules have the capacity to cross biologic membranes and may bind to intracellular receptors in the cytoplasm or in the nucleoplasm.

Intracellular Receptors

Because of their lipophilic nature, both thyroid hormones and steroid hormones pass directly through plasma membranes and bind to receptor proteins inside the cell. The resulting complex is then transported into the nucleus. Changes in their conformation allow the receptors then to bind to certain regions of the DNA, thereby regulating transcription of various genes. It has been proposed that all receptors of the "steroid receptor superfamily," including estrogen, testosterone, thyroid hormone, vitamin A and vitamin D receptors, act in this way. Following this model, the receptors are essentially trivalent, having one set of binding sites for the hormones, another set for DNA, and a third set for the actual activation of the gene. Under unstimulated conditions, binding to the DNA is not possible because the DNA binding region of the receptor is occupied by inhibitory proteins (e.g., heat shock proteins). The binding of the hormone to the receptor leads to the dissociation of the inhibitory proteins from the receptor. This enables binding of the receptor to specific sites on the DNA, called "receptor-dependent transcriptional enhancers." The gene products that are transcribed following induction by steroid hormones may eventually lead to the expression of other genes. Thus a complex cascade of gene activation can be initiated by a single hormone signal.

Cell Surface Receptors

The binding of ligands to cell surface receptors also initiates a cascade of intracellular second messenger systems that regulate cell function directly or change gene expression. There are three major classes of cell surface receptor proteins (Fig. 1–4): (1) channel-linked receptors, which gate ion channels (this kind of receptor is mainly involved in short-term responses to signals such as neurotransmitters); (2) catalytic receptors (these are transmembrane proteins with a cytoplasmic domain that functions as an enzyme with tyrosine-specific protein kinase activity); and (3) G protein-linked receptors, which are indirectly coupled to separate, but membrane bound, enzymes via G proteins.

Channel-linked receptors translate the chemical signal into changes of permeability of the plasma membrane for ions and thus initiate electrical excitation of the cell. They are specifically found in synaptic signaling and will not be further discussed in this chapter.

Catalytic receptors translate specific signals into tyrosine kinase activity. Ligand binding at the extracellular domain leads to the formation of homodimers of the receptor. The enzymatic process that is then activated in the intracellular domain transfers the terminal phosphate group of ATP to the hydroxyl group of a tyrosine residue of selected proteins. The conformational changes that activate this process are not well understood. It has been demonstrated for all receptors of this kind that tyrosine kinase activity phosphorylates not only target protein but also the receptor itself. This mechanism seems to enhance the enzymatic activity of the receptor protein. Tyrosine-specific protein kinase activity has been described for the insulin receptor, for receptors of some growth factors, and for several other receptors. Some of the receptors for growth factors have been identified as products of proto-oncogenes. A certain mutation of the receptor of epidermal growth factor,

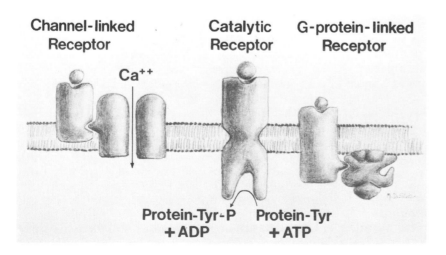

Channel-linked Receptor   **Catalytic Receptor**   **G-protein-linked Receptor**

Ca^{++}

Protein-Tyr~P + ADP   Protein-Tyr + ATP

FIGURE 1–4. The three major classes of cell surface receptor proteins.

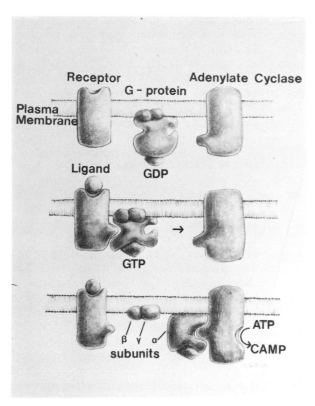

FIGURE 1–5. G protein–linked signal transduction from cell surface receptors to membrane-bound enzymes. Binding of a ligand changes the configuration of its specific receptor, which enables binding of the G protein to the receptor. The GDP of the G protein is then replaced by GTP and the G protein dissociates from the receptor and from its β and γ subunits. This results in a configurational change of the α-subunit of the G protein in such a way that it can now bind to and activate specific enzymes (in this case, adenylate cyclase). This is followed by hydrolysis of the GTP to GDP and reassembling of the G protein. The process can now be repeated as long as the ligand is bound to its receptor.

GDP is displaced by guanosine triphosphate (GTP). The consequence is dissociation of the α subunit from the receptor and from the two other subunits of the GS protein. The α subunit is then free to bind to enzymes such as adenylate cyclase or phospholipase C, which are thereby activated. Finally, hydrolysis of GTP leads to dissociation of the α subunit of the GS protein from the enzyme and to the reassembling of the complete GS protein. This inactivates the enzymes coupled to this process. However, when the receptor is still occupied by its ligand, the whole cycle starts again. The duration of activation of these enzymes therefore depends on two steps. The first is hydrolysis of GTP of the α subunit, which determines the duration of binding of the GS protein to the enzyme. The second is dissociation of the chemical signal from its receptor. Cholera toxin blocks GTP hydrolyzation and leads to an extended binding of the GS protein to the particular enzyme. The inhibitory G_i protein probably acts in a similar fashion, except that binding to the enzyme results in the suppression of its activity. Pertussis toxin prevents binding of the G_i protein to the receptor. G protein coupled receptors have been described for several hundred chemical signals such as catecholamines, parathormone, and many cytokines. Adenylate cyclase, cyclic guanosine monophosphate (GMP) phosphodiesterase, and phospholipases A_2 and C, as well as various ion channels, have been identified as targets of G protein–linked receptors. Oncogene transcripts such as the ras proteins are also involved in G protein–coupled signal transduction. At present it is unknown how they exactly interfere with the process described above.

In many cases the signaling pathway is unknown. Since it seems to be impossible to demonstrate the known receptor types for those signals, it is very likely that new receptor types need to be described in order to understand their mode of action.

for example, is encoded by the *erb*B oncogene. Most of the protein kinase activity of cells, however, is due to serine- and threonine-specific kinases. Some of these enzymes are also anchored in the plasma membrane but they do not have an extracellular receptor domain. Although they are obviously not directly involved in signal transduction, they may be indirectly coupled to such processes.

G proteins function as mediators between *G protein-linked receptors* and membrane-associated enzymes.[4] These proteins can act as stimulators (G_s proteins) or inhibitors (G_i proteins) of signal transduction. The current model of their stimulatory action postulates a conformational change of the specific receptor following binding of its ligand as the initial event (Fig. 1–5). This allows association of the intracellular domain of the receptor with a G_s protein, which has guanosine diphosphate (GDP) bound to its α subunit at that point. In the next step,

INTRACELLULAR PROCESSING OF SIGNALS

Following receptor-ligand interactions, the events occurring in the cell membrane must be translated into messages that can be interpreted within the cell. This is organized through stimulation of second messenger systems. Best characterized are the activities of cyclic adenosine monophosphate (cAMP), Ca^{2+}, and protein kinases.

Second Messenger Function of cAMP

Cyclic adenosine monophosphate is a ubiquitous intracellular messenger in all animal cells (Fig. 1–6). cAMP is produced by adenylate cyclase using ATP, and is broken down by different cAMP phosphodiesterases to 5′-AMP. The activity of adenylate cyclase is

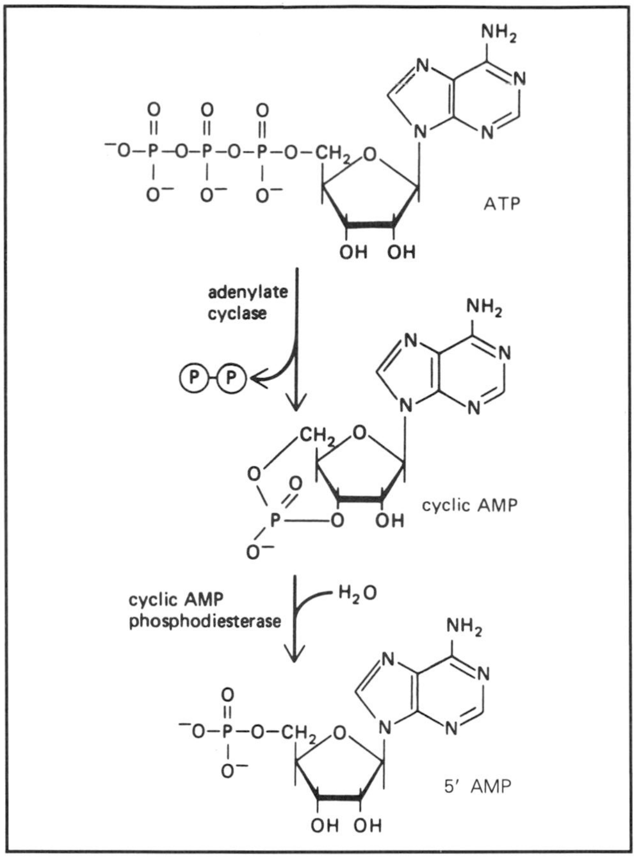

FIGURE 1–6. The synthesis and degradation of cyclic AMP. A pyrophosphatase makes the synthesis of cyclic AMP an irreversible reaction by hydrolyzing the released pyrophosphate. (Reprinted from Alberts, B., Bray, D., Lewis, J., Raff, M., Roberts, K., and Watson, J.D.: Molecular Biology of the Cell, 2nd ed. New York, Garland Publishing, Inc., 1989, p. 695.)

regulated by G_S and G_i protein–coupled cell surface receptors. The interaction of synthesis and degradation makes rapid changes of intracellular concentrations of cAMP in response to external signals possible.[5] The second messenger function of cAMP is mediated through activation of cAMP-dependent cytosolic protein kinases (A kinases). These enzymes in turn activate other enzymes by phosphorylation. In some cases this step initiates a whole cascade of protein phosphorylations, which finally leads to the activation of a metabolic pathway. Many hormone effects are mediated by this pathway (Table 1–1). Besides activating A kinases, cAMP also inactivates inhibitory proteins.

Second Messenger Function of Calcium Ions

Calcium ion concentration regulates many intracellular systems. Under normal conditions the cytosolic Ca^{2+} concentration is extremely low (less than 10^{-7} M). This low concentration is maintained with a high gradient against the extracellular fluid (Ca^{2+} concentration greater than 10^{-3} M) by the ATP-dependent work of various Ca^{2+} pumps. An increase of Ca^{2+} in response to extracellular signals takes place either by influx from the extracellular fluid or by emptying of intracellular storages. Channel-linked receptors enable influx of Ca^{2+} into the cell, whereas G protein–linked receptors lead to sequestration of Ca^{2+} from intracellular compartments. The most important intracellular Ca^{2+} reservoirs are the mitochondria and the endoplasmic reticulum or the sarcoplasmic reticulum, specifically in muscle cells. The release of Ca^{2+} from those compartments is mediated by inositol triphosphate (IP_3), which is synthesized from membrane lipids by a specific phospholipase (C). Activation of this enzyme is coupled to the activation of G protein–linked receptors. The main substrates for this specific phospholipase C are phosphoinositol (PI), phosphoinositol phosphate (PIP), and phosphoinositol biphosphate (PIP_2). The breakdown of PIP_2 produces not only IP_3 but also diacylglycerol, another important second messenger.[6] Diacylglycerol together with Ca^{2+} activates protein kinase C, which transfers the terminal phosphate group of ATP to serine and threonine residues of specific proteins (Fig. 1–7). Most Ca^{2+}-dependent processes are not regulated by the calcium ion directly, but through Ca^{2+} binding proteins

TABLE 1–1. SOME HORMONE-INDUCED CELLULAR RESPONSES MEDIATED BY CYCLIC AMP

TARGET TISSUE	HORMONE	MAJOR RESPONSE
Thyroid	Thyroid-stimulating hormone (TSH)	Thyroid hormone synthesis and secretion
Adrenal cortex	Adrenocorticotropic hormone (ACTH)	Cortisol secretion
Ovary	Luteinizing hormone (LH)	Prostaglandin secretion
Muscle, liver	Epinephrine	Glycogen breakdown
Bone	Parathormone	Bone resorption
Heart	Epinephrine	Increase in heart rate and force of contraction
Kidney	Vasopressin	Water resorption
Fat	Epinephrine, ACTH, glucagon, TSH	Triglyceride breakdown

Reprinted from Alberts, B., Bray, D., Lewis, J., Raff, M., Roberts, K., and Watson, J.D.: Molecular Biology of the Cell, 2nd ed. New York, Garland Publishing, Inc., 1989, p. 696.

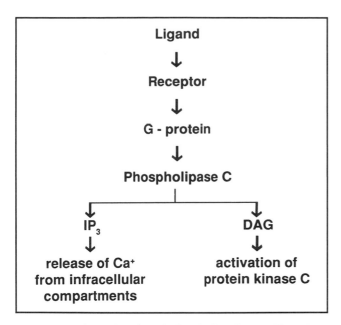

FIGURE 1–7. The phosphoinositol pathway (IP₃ = inositol triphosphate, DAG = diacylglycerol). The breakdown of phosphoinositol from the plasma membrane in response to specific signals results in the release of two second messenger molecules, IP₃ and DAG. The inositol phospholipids comprise only a very small portion (less than 10 per cent) of the total phospholipids of plasma membranes, but play a major role in cellular signaling by providing the substrates for this pathway.

such as calmodulin, which has four binding sites for Ca^{2+}. Ca^{2+}-calmodulin complexes interact with many enzymes and membrane transport proteins.

MODULATION OF THE RESPONSE TO SIGNALS

Cells can change their sensitivity to external signals. For cell surface receptors, various mechanisms for such modulations have been described. The number of receptors can be changed in either direction. Enhanced receptor expression increases the sensitivity, while receptor internalization decreases the response. Receptor expression can be controlled by the signal itself (e.g., interleukin-2) or by secondary signals (e.g., ingerferon γ increases tumor necrosis factor α receptors). Internalization of the receptor by endocytosis may lead to degradation of the receptor and the ligand or to destruction of the ligand alone, followed by reexpression of the receptor. Other mechanisms altering the sensitivity to sig-

nals involve inhibitory proteins that bind to the receptors or to G proteins.

NEW CONCEPTS

The established signaling pathways do not explain all observations in the field of intercellular communication. However, several new pathways of signal generation and transduction utilizing novel biochemical concepts have been described. One of these pathways generates the nitric oxide radical from the amino acid L-arginine. Nitric oxide can readily pass membranes and activates soluble guanylate cyclase by binding to its intrinsic heme group, resulting in an increase in cyclic GMP levels. By doing so, nitric oxide can act as an intra- or intercellular signal. Most unique to this action is the ability to bypass receptors and directly increase the activity of guanylate cyclase. Nitric oxide is very short lived but can diffuse to other cells before it degrades to the inactive end products nitrite and nitrate. A well-established example for the biologic role of this novel signaling pathway is the function of nitric oxide as a endothelium-derived relaxing factor. In this case nitric oxide is released from endothelial cells and leads to relaxation of the smooth muscle cells beneath by activation of their guanylate cyclase and the following increase of cyclic GMP.

Another new concept of signal transduction is also implicated with the generation of cyclic GMP. Some cells possess guanylate cyclases, which are bound to the plasma membrane. These enzymes have been shown to have extracellular domains that serve as receptors for the stimulating ligands, such as atrial natriuretic factor (ANF). This is the only example of receptors that have the capability to generate directly second messengers in response to extracellular signals.

BIBLIOGRAPHY

1. Arbeit, J.M.: Molecules, cancer, and the surgeon. A review of molecular biology and its implications for surgical oncology. Ann. Surg. *212*:313, 1990.
2. Singer, S.J., and Nicolson, G.L.: The fluid mosaic model of the structure of cell membranes. Science *175*:720–731, 1972.
3. Albeda, S.M., and Buck, C.A.: Integrins and other cell adhesion molecules. FASEB J. *4*:2868–2880, 1990
4. Birnbaumer, L.: Transduction of receptor signal into modulation of effector activity by G proteins: The first 20 years or so. FASEB J. *4*:3179–3188, 1990.
5. Lefkowitz, R.J., Stadel, J.M., and Caron, M.G.: Adenylate cyclase-coupled beta-adrenergic receptors: Structure and mechanisms of activation and desensitization. Annu. Rev. Biochem. *52*:159–186, 1983.
6. Berridge, M.J.: Inositol triphosphate and diacylglycerol: Two interacting second messengers. Annu. Rev. Biochem. *56*:159–193, 1987.

2

MEDIATORS OF INFLAMMATION

DAVID L. STEED

IMMUNOGLOBULINS, CASCADES, AND CYTOKINES

Inflammation is a localized response to injury or noxious stimuli that is designed to protect the host. The inflammatory response is mediated through a series of steps designed to recognize a substance as foreign and then to initiate a response. An antigen is recognized by one of two systems: by humoral antibodies or by receptors on T cells. Recognition by either system in turn results in activation of cascades of proinflammatory events that increase vascular permeability and blood flow to allow leukocytes to be brought into the area of injury. The foreign stimulus is then attacked by mononuclear cells or polymorphonuclear leukocytes. The immune response may also occur in response to foreign substances, as cascades of cellular or humoral events can be activated by a variety of foreign stimuli—antigenic or autochthonous. The sequence of events for each inflammatory response (wound healing, graft rejection, infection control) are discussed in each chapter devoted to that subject. Here we review in detail the mediators of the response isolated from the sequence of events.

Immunoglobulins

Immunoglobulins (Ig) or antibodies are a group of glycoproteins that have many similarities in structure and biologic function. Each Ig molecule is made up of two light and two heavy polypeptide chains (Fig. 2–1). The amino acid sequences at the NH-terminal end of the heavy and light chains vary from antibody to antibody depending on their specificity for different antigens. In contrast, the amino acid sequences at the COOH-terminal portions of these chains do not vary. The Igs vary in weight from 150,000 to 900,000 daltons. Each light and heavy chain is composed of units called domains that have over 100 amino acids.

The amino acids in the NH-terminal domains of the light and heavy chains form the antigen-binding sites. The COOH-terminal domains form the Fc (crystallizable) fragment that binds to the Ig receptors and results in activation of the cell. The cellular response can therefore mediate part of the body's reaction to the presence of soluble antigen-antibody complexes. Thus, the NH-terminal is variable whereas the COOH-terminal is constant.

The immunoglobulins are all manufactured by B cells. In most cases, the B cell must interact with a helper T cell for active primary immunization. Although each B cell clone is genetically programmed to synthesize a single light chain and single heavy chain variable region, B cells can produce immunoglobulins of several types, e.g., IgM and IgG. The antigen-specific domain determines the specificity of the antigen, and each variable region is identical in each Ig molecule derived from any given clone. After sensitization, B cells may produce vast quantities of immunoglobulins. Although only one antibody specificity is produced for each clone of B cells, a single antigenic molecule can stimulate many B cell clones because each antigen can bind more or less avidly with the variable portions of the immunoglobulin on the surface of B cells. Thus, many antibodies result from each immunization with a single antigen. This being so, cross-reactivity with a spectrum of related antigens results from immunization with a single antigen.

Antibodies are divided into five classes: IgG, IgA, IgM, IgD, and IgE. There are four subcategories of IgG (called IgG_1, IgG_2, etc.) and two types of IgA. The constant region of the heavy chains accounts for the difference between classes and determines the class-specific properties.

IgG accounts for 85 per cent of all immunoglobulins and has a molecular weight of 150,000. The IgG molecule can be broken down by papain into three fragments—two Fab fragments consisting of a light chain and the NH-terminal domain of a heavy chain,

12

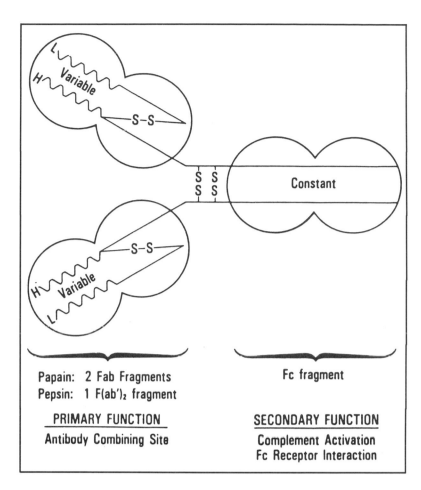

Papain: 2 Fab Fragments
Pepsin: 1 F(ab')₂ fragment

PRIMARY FUNCTION
Antibody Combining Site

Fc fragment

SECONDARY FUNCTION
Complement Activation
Fc Receptor Interaction

FIGURE 2–1. Basic structure of Ig and localization of submolecular sites mediating the primary and secondary or effector functions of antibodies. (Reprinted from Gallin, J.I., Goldstein, I.M., and Snyderman, R. (eds.): Inflammation: Basic Principles and Clinical Correlates. New York, Raven Press, 1988. Chapter 2, Figure 1, p. 12.)

and one Fc fragment containing the COOH-terminal domains of the heavy chain. Each Fab fragment contains a single antigen-combining site. The Fc fragment is identical in antibodies of a given class. It fixes to the cellular receptors, binds to serum complement, and initiates complement activation.

IgG antibodies provide protection against viral and bacterial infections. When the antigen-combining site fragment binds to the antigen, a conformational change is initiated in the molecule that exposes its Fc portion to interact with the Fc receptor (FcR) on the phagocytic cell. The opsonized antigen is thereby fixed to the cell surface and liable to phagocytosis. Two molecules of IgG bound to an antigen are able to activate the classic complement pathway.

IgG levels change throughout life in response to antigenic stimuli. Generally, levels decrease with age. IgG can cross the placenta and is present in the neonate. The Fc fragment determines the biologic half-life of an antibody class. For IgG this is 23 days. Maternal IgG levels decrease in the fourth month of life at a time when the infant is able to produce IgG in adequate quantities.

IgA is the second most common immunoglobulin and is the predominant class in saliva, tears, and bile.

It is produced by B cells residing within lymphoid tissues adjacent to mucosal surfaces and is then secreted onto those surfaces. IgA can bind to viruses and bacteria, but lacking an Fc fragment, it can neither fix complement nor serve as an opsonin for phagocytosis. IgA acts primarily to prevent the adherence of bacteria to epithelium and represents the first line of defense against many mucosal pathogens that invade by adhering to the epithelium before deeper invasion. IgA is not the only mucosal immunoglobulin, since IgG is also produced by mucosal-associated B cells. IgM also is produced in salivary glands and the gastrointestinal tract; IgE is made in the gastrointestinal and respiratory tract mucosa.

A deficiency in IgA is the most commonly identified immunoglobulin deficiency. IgA deficiency is associated with recurrent viral and bacterial infections of the respiratory tract resulting in chronic bronchitis and bronchiectasis.

The largest immunoglobulin is IgM, which has a molecular weight of 900,000 daltons. Because of its large size it is not found in interstitial tissue, but is found mostly in the intravascular space. IgM is the first antibody produced in response to antigen, and its production declines in response to increasing IgG production. IgM is a potent activator of the classic complement sequence.

IgE is present in the lowest plasma concentration of any of the Ig classes, but is an important mediator of acute allergic responses. The Fc portion of the IgE molecule, when exposed to antigen, binds to receptors on mast cells and basophills, which triggers the release of histamine. Thus, IgE is an important mediator of respiratory tract allergies.

IgD is present in a concentration of less than 1 per cent of IgG. Its structure is quite similar to IgG, but it has no known biologic function.

White blood cells and many other cells in the body have receptors on their membrane that bind the Fc fragment of Ig (FcRs). The FcRs generally bind specifically one class of Ig. The affinity with which FcRs bind Ig varies. Low-affinity FcRs generally promote phagocytosis, whereas high affinity FcRs cause the release of mediators of inflammation. Basophils and mast cells have the highest-affinity FcRs of all cells. Cross-linking of cell-bound IgE by antigen induces the release of histamine and other mediators of inflammation. Because IgE antibodies bind with high affinity to these FcRs, only minute amounts of antibody are necessary to trigger mast cells. In contrast, IgE FcRs on eosinophils bind with a low affinity similar to the binding of IgG. This binding of IgG and IgE on eosinophils induces release of the mediators of inflammation, whereas FcRs on neutrophils promote phagocytosis of antibody code of particles. Antigen-antibody complexes can adhere to membranes, such as the glomerular basement membrane, synovial membranes, and endothelium, causing neutrophils to release mediators of inflammation. Monocytes and alveolar and peritoneal macrophages also have FcRs for IgG, as do platelets.

Immunoglobulins act only against pathogens outside cells and play no role in host defense once pathogens have successfully invaded the cell. Thus, they seem to have an opsonization function by which foreign agents are phagocytosed and can also activate the complement system within the circulation. They are important in neutralization of toxins and the inhibition of attachment of bacteria to susceptible host cells.

A detailed discussion of immunology is presented in Chapter 26.

Complement

Antibodies simply bind, thereby identifying foreign antigens. For antibodies to eliminate pathogenic bacteria from the body, phagocytic cells must be present to engulf the bacteria and digest them (Table 2–1). Phagocytes do not, however, have receptors for the ligands on the surfaces of all possible pathogens, and truly efficient phagocytosis requires that the pathogen be opsonized ("buttered up") with agents recognizable to the phagocyte. Antibodies are the most effective opsonin because all phagocytes have receptors for the Fc component of the antibody. IgM is the most efficient opsonin of all. To phagocytose pathogens not previously encountered, a more generalized opsonic system has evolved—the complement system.

The human complement system comprises more than 25 plasma and membrane-bound glycoproteins that interact in a precise manner. The plasma components themselves are inert without known biologic activity. Activity is derived either from proteolytic fragmentation of these plasma components or from fusion of multiple protein molecules into larger units. Interaction of these substances with microbial cell surfaces or antigen-antibody complexes results in the activation of a cascade of proteolytic enzymes that cleave components in sequence. The products of this cascade can interact with either binding sites on the pathogen or with the cell surfaces of a variety of mammalian cells to induce an inflammatory reaction. The normal inactive complement components and their inhibitors are listed in Table 2–1. Note that regulatory proteins are also present and serve to protect host cells from accidental complement attack.

There are two pathways of activation: the classical pathway and the alternative pathway (Fig. 2–2). In the classical pathway, a component of complement, C1, interacts with the Fc fragment of antibody bound to antigen. The Fc fragment of a single molecule of IgM or of two molecules of IgG is involved. C1 is actually a complex molecule composed of three subunits—C1Q, C1R, and C1S. C1 activates C2 which activates C4 which activates C3. The classical and alternative pathways converge on the C3 molecule, and the cascade that follows is common to both pathways. The products of activated C3 are important in phagocytosis: C3a is important as a chemotaxin of phagocytes and is a vasodilator, whereas C3b binds to the targeted microbial cell surface and serves as an opsonin for phagocytes that have C3b receptors. Most important, however, C3b binds plasma factors B and D, forming an enzyme that activates C3 to produce more C3B. This positive feedback limb markedly amplifies the complement cascade.

The alternative pathway serves as a host defense against microbial invaders and operates without antibody intervention. It is triggered by interaction with endotoxin (Gram-negative bacterial lipopolysaccharide), staphylococcal protein A, and numerous other substances so that the degree of specificity of this pathway is low. There are six proteins that initiate, recognize, and activate this pathway (Table 2–2); they correspond to the subunits of C1, C2, and C4, which activate the classical pathway. The alternative pathway was once called the properdin pathway because properdin was the first protein recognized to activate it. Both pathways converge on C3 and produce the opsonin C3b.

TABLE 2–1. PROPERTIES OF THE COMPLEMENT COMPONENTS AND COMPLEMENT REGULATORS

Name	Synonyms	Molecular Weight	Electrophoretic Mobility	Approximate Plasma Concentration (μg/mL)
Classic Pathway				
C1q	C'O, 11S protein	400,000	τ_2	70
C1r	. . .	190,000	β	34
C1s	C̄1 esterase	87,000	α	31
C2	. . .	117,000	β_1	25
C3	β_1C	185,000	β_1	1600
C4	β_1E	206,000	β_1	600
Alternative Pathway				
C3	Factor A, hydrazine-sensitive factor (HSF)	185,000	β_1	1300
Factor B	C3 proactivator (CEPA), glycine-rich β glycoprotein (GBG), β_2-glycoprotein II	93,000	β_2	200
Factor D	C3 proactivator convertase (C3PAse), Glycine-rich β glycoproteinase (GBG)	24,000	α	1
Factor I	C3b inactivator, KAF, C3b INA	88,000	β	34
Factor H	β_1H, C3b inactivator accelerator	150,000	β_1	500
Properdin	. . .	220,000	τ_2	25
Membrane Attack Mechanism				
C5	β_1F	191,000	β_1	70
C6	. . .	120,000	β_2	64
C7	. . .	110,000	β_2	56
C8	. . .	151,000	τ_1	55
C9	. . .	71,000	α	59
Complement Regulators				
C̄1 inhibitor	C̄1 esterase inhibitor, C̄1 inactivator	105,000	α_2	180
C4 binding protein	C4bp	>500,000	β	. . .
Factor I	C3b inactivator, KAF, C3b INA	88,000	β	34
Factor H	β_1H, C3b inactivator accelerator	150,000	β_1	500
Properdin	. . .	220,000	τ_2	25
S protein	Membrane attack complex inhibitor, MAC INH	80,000	α	505
Anaphylatoxin inactivator	A1, SCPB, carboxy-peptidase N	300,000	α	. . .
Abnormal Proteins				
C3 nephritic factor	C3 NeF, NF	160,000	τ	. . .

Reprinted from Cooper, N.R.: The complement system. *In* Stites, D.P., Stobo, J.D., and Wells, J.V. (eds.): Basic and Clinical Immunology, 6th ed. Norwalk, CT, Appleton & Lang, 1987, p. 116.

Opsonization is the process by which ingestion of bacteria by peripheral blood neutrophils is greatly enhanced. Two types of opsonin interact with bacteria and fungi. One is opsonizing antibody (IgM, IgG$_3$, IgG$_2$, IgG$_1$), the Fc region of which is recognized by structurally specific Fc receptors on the surface of the phagocyte. The other opsonin is C3b, which binds to the surface of microbes as a consequence of complement activation by either the classical or alternative pathway. Phagocytic neutrophils and macrophages possesss cell surface receptors for C3b, enabling bacteria to be phagocytized and subsequently killed.

The final common pathway of the complement cascade also depends on C3b. Deposition of C3b on the surface of a bacterium results in cleavage of C5 into C5a and C5b. C5b binds to the cell surface, interacting with C6 and C7 to form a C567 membrane attack complex (MAC) that is physically inserted into the upper layer of the microbial cell membrane. The C567 complex binds to C8 and C9, and the C5-9 complex opens the microbial cell and other cells to osmotic lysis.

Although the complement cascade eliminates pathogens by opsonization and direct lysis, it also activates an acute inflammatory response (Fig. 2–3).

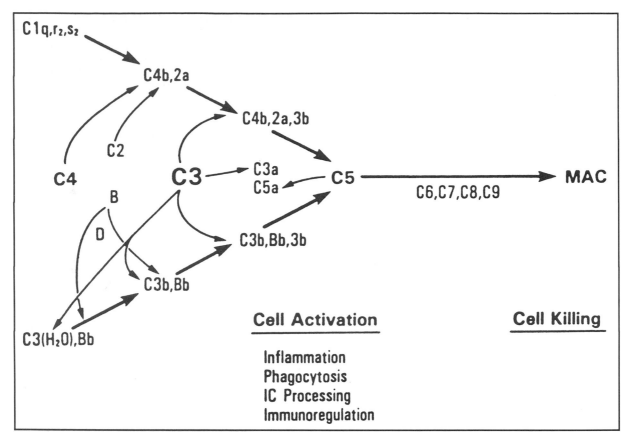

FIGURE 2–2. Molecular organization of the complement pathways. *Upper left,* The classical pathway; *lower left,* the alternative pathway. C3 occupies a central position in both pathways. Regulatory proteins have been omitted. (Reprinted from Gallin, J.I., Goldstein, I.M., and Snyderman, R. (eds.): Inflammation: Basic Principles and Clinical Corrélates. New York, Raven Press, 1988. Chapter 3, Figure 1, p. 22.)

C5a is the most potent chemotactic agent for neutrophils and macrophages. As an anaphylatoxin, C5a activates the release of histamine from basophils and mast cells for increased capillary permeability. C3a and C4a, like C5a, are anaphylatoxins that bind to cell surface receptors on neutrophils, monocytes, macrophages, mast cells, and smooth muscle cells. These cells release histamine, serotonin, and interleukin-1, as well as arachidonic acid metabolites.

The complement cascade is regulated by several mechanisms (listed in Table 2–1). C3b inactivator is the most potent inhibitor of the system; without it, the feedback activation by C3b on C3 would continue indefinitely.

Membrane Attack Complex

The membrane attack complex C5-9 deserves special note. Cell injury by complement occurs as a consequence of activation of the complement system on the surface of the target cell itself. During this set of chemical reactions, a MAC is formed. This is an organization of many molecules of complement from C5 through C9. The C5-7 forms transmembrane channels that vary in size depending on the number of C9 molecules incorporated into the channeled structure. The MAC is a hollow protein cylinder inserted into the target cell membrane. It causes a rapid increase in intracellular free calcium, thereby activating certain cellular functions that result in lethal disruption of cellular membranes (Table 2–3).

Activation of the complement system within the blood can result in a number of damaging effects, such as disseminated intravascular coagulation, peripheral vasodilation (kinins, histamine), and shock. Tissue damage can occur because of the deposition of the antigen-antibody complexes. This occurs in the renal glomeruli, as well as in joints.

The Contact Activation System

This system is of utmost importance to surgeons who deal with wounded tissue. Of the four major plasma protein systems that participate in host defense in the development of the inflammatory re-

TABLE 2–2. MOLECULAR WEIGHTS AND SERUM CONCENTRATIONS OF COMPLEMENT COMPONENTS

COMPONENT	MOLECULAR WEIGHT (DALTONS)	SERUM CONCENTRATION* (μg/mL)
Initiators		
Classical Pathway		
C1q	400,000	180
C1r	180,000	?
C1s	86,000	110
C2	117,000	25
C4	206,000	640
Alternate pathway		
Initiating factor (IF)	150,000	?
Properdin	184,000	25
Properdin factor B	93,000	200
Properdin factor D	24,000	?
Effectors		
C3	180,000	1,600
C5	180,000	80
C6	95,000	75
C7	110,000	55
C8	163,000	80
C9	79,000	230
Inhibitors		
C1	90,000	180
C3b inactivator	100,000	25
C6	?	?
C3a, C5a inactivator	300,000	?

* Serum concentrations given are the means in adults.

Reprinted from Root, R.K. and Ryan, J.L.: *In* Mandell, G.I., Douglas, R.G., Jr., and Bennett, J.E. (eds.): Principles and Practices of Infectious Diseases, 2nd ed. New York, Wiley, 1985, p. 31.

TABLE 2–3. BIOLOGIC EFFECTS OF COMPLEMENT FRAGMENTS RELEASED DURING SEQUENTIAL ACTIVATION OF THE SYSTEM

MEDIATOR	EFFECT
Classical Pathway	
C4a	Release of serotonin
C2b	Kinin-like activity
C4b	Immune adherence
C3a	Anaphylatoxin, vascular effect, chemotaxis, leukocyte mobilization
C3b	Opsonization, immune adherence, release of platelet factor 3
Membrane Attack Mechanism	
C5a	Most potent chemotactic factor; opsonin for *Candida* (?); C5b may attach to platelets, activate distal components, and cause platelet lysis as an innocent bystander
C̄567	Chemotaxis
C̄8	Initiates lytic process, inserted into membrane
C̄9	Completes lytic process

Adapted from Alexander, J.W., and Good, R.A.: Fundamentals of Clinical Immunology. Philadelphia, W.B. Saunders Co. 1977, p. 80.

sponse after tissue injury (the complement system, the coagulation system, the fibrinolytic system, and the contact activation system), the last is the least known, but it is the system that coordinates the other three after tissue injury (Fig. 2–4). The contact activation system comprises four primary proteins: Hageman factor, prekallikrein factor, high molecular weight kininogen, and coagulation factor XI.

Hageman factor (coagulation factor XII) is a beta globulin with a molecular weight of 80,000. For Hageman factor to be active, it must undergo limited proteolysis upon contact with a negatively charged surface, such as a tissue collagen or bacterial lipopolysaccharide. Cleavage results in an active enzyme in a process similar to the mechanism that activates trypsinogen and chymotrypsinogen. Activated Hageman factor then activates two plasma protein proenzymes: prekallikrein and factor XI. In addition, activated Hageman factor feeds back and activates circulating Hageman factor, thus amplifying the response.

Prekallikrein is a gamma globulin with a molecular weight of 88,000. It is activated by limited proteolytic digestion by activated Hageman factor. Kallikrein affects coagulation, fibrinolysis, and kinin release. It cleaves high molecular weight kininogen at two sites, thereby releasing bradykinin; activates plasminogen

to plasmin; and converts latent collagenase to active collagenase in the synovium.

High molecular weight kininogens are alpha globulins that have potent vasoactive peptides, the kinins, within their primary sequence; bradykinin is released by limited proteolytic digestion by plasma and tissue kallikreins.

Factor XI is composed of two polypeptide chains, each of which has a molecular weight of 80,000. It is activated by limited proteolytic cleavage by Hageman factor, and its major function is the proteolytic cleavage and activation of factor IX in the intrinsic clotting cascade (see Chapter 3).

Both activated Hageman factor and plasmin can initiate the complement cascade. Thus, the contact activation system can initiate vasodilation, increased vascular permeability, and an acute inflammatory cellular infiltrate. It is activated by negatively charged surfaces or cellular components. The extravascular space is a prime site for activation of the contact system because the connective tissues are rich in negatively charged molecules. The several proteins of the contact system are brought into opposition with one another on the negative surface, thereby triggering their reciprocal activation. The surface binding not only brings the contact system into opposition but also makes Hageman factor more susceptible to activation.

The contact activation system may be inhibited or blocked by other plasma proteins that are positively

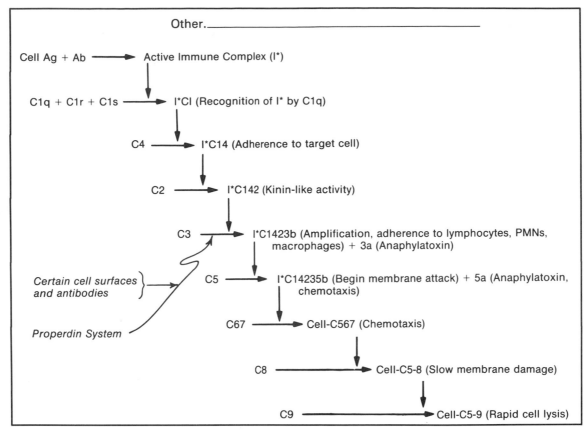

FIGURE 2–3. The complement pathways and the biologic activity released at each step. (Reprinted from Simmons, R.L., Foker, J.E., Lower, R.R., and Najarian, J.S. *In* Schwartz, S.I., Shires, G.T., Spender, F.C., and Storer, E.D. (eds.): Transplantation: Principles of Surgery, 3rd ed. New York, McGraw-Hill, 1979. Howard, Figure 11–17, p. 184).

charged, such as Hageman factor. These cationic molecules compete with Hageman factor or high molecular weight kininogen. The C1 inhibitor of the complement system also inhibits Hageman factor and plasma kallikrein. Antithrombin III and alpha I antitrypsin inhibit kallikrein activity as well. C1 inhibitor also inhibits the active form of factor XI.

The contact activation system produces a number of physiologic changes. Hageman factor is potent in increasing vascular permeability and induces hypotension as well. Bradykinin liberated from high molecular weight kininogen also increases vascular permeability; diminishes arterial resistance, thereby resulting in hypotension; and causes smooth muscle contraction. White blood cell margination and increased intestinal motility have also been reported after bradykinin release.

The contact activation system is active in a number of diseases. Synovial fluid contains components of the contact activation system. Negatively charged particles may activate the contact system in joint fluid and result in rheumatoid arthritis. Bradykinin plays a role in allergic reactions and anaphylaxis. Pre-

kallikrein has been observed to be activated in sepsis. Patients with hereditary angioedema that has been inherited as an autosomal dominant trait have recurrent episodes of abdominal pain and mucocutaneous swelling. They lack C1 inhibitor, an important regulatory protein for control of both complement and the contact activation system. Hageman factor has been identified on the glomerular basement membrane of patients with membranous glomerulonephritis. Diminished Hageman factor and prekallikrein concentrations have been found in patients with nephrotic syndrome. Patients with dumping syndrome have increased plasma kinin levels, as do patients with carcinoid syndrome.

THE PROSTAGLANDINS AND LEUKOTRIENES

All cell membranes are composed largely of phospholipids, which are constantly being metabolized. Arachidonic acid is a 20 carbon fatty acid that is continuously released by the action of phospholipase

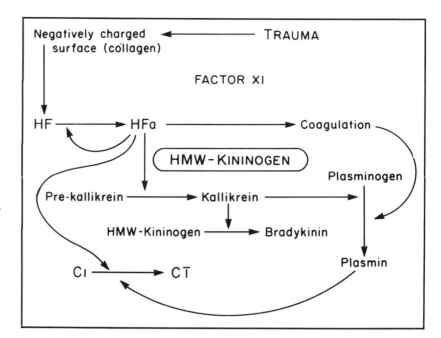

FIGURE 2–4. The interrelationships of the coagulation-kinin, fibrinolytic, and complement systems and their hypothetical activation by trauma. (Reprinted from Burke F.J., and Gelfand, J.A.: Events in early inflammation. *In* Howard, R.J., and Simmons, R.L. (eds.): Surgical Infectious Diseases, 2nd ed. Norwalk, CT, Appleton & Lange, 1988. Figure 12–2, p. 203.)

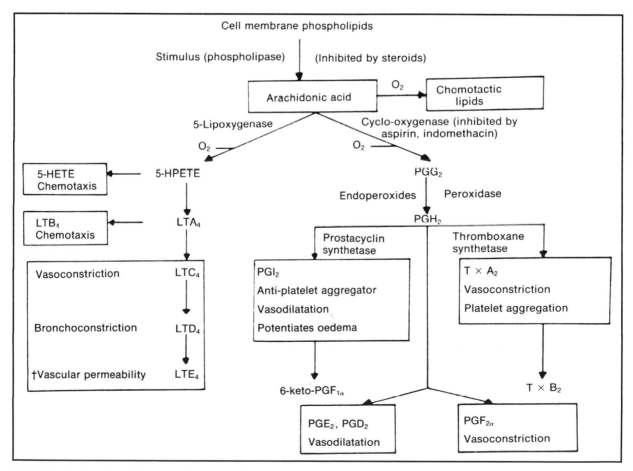

FIGURE 2–5. Arachidonic acid metabolites in inflammation. (Reprinted from Ledingham, I.M., and MacKay, C. (eds.): Jamieson & Kay's Textbook of Surgical Physiology, 4th ed. Edinburgh, Churchill Livingstone, 1988. Figure 28.2, p. 479.)

on these membrane phospolipids. Under some circumstances, this breakdown is accelerated, and further degradation by enzymes converts arachidonic acid into a variety of arachidonic acid metabolites called eicosanoids. There are two types of eicosanolds: leukotrienes and prostaglandins (Fig. 2–5).

Leukotrienes

Arachidonic acid may be metabolized by the 5-lipoxygenase pathway into leukotrienes. This pathway can be activated by a variety of inflammatory cells, including neutrophils, eosinophils, basophils, monocytes, macrophages, mast cells, and some lymphocytes. Leukotrienes are proinflammatory mediators and may participate in homeostatic regulation of the immune system. Arachidonic acid is broken down by 5-lipoxygenase to 5-hydroperoxyeicosatetraeonic acid (5-HPETE). This product is short-lived and spontaneously degrades into 5-hydroxyeicosatetraenoic acid (5-HETE) or leukotriene-A4 (LTA4). LTA4 is then a precursor for other leukotrienes, including LTB4, LTC4, LTD4, and LTE4. Leukotriene synthesis is modulated by the action of cytokines, such as interferon or interleukin-1.

The 5-lipoxygenase pathway can accept other polyunsaturated fatty acids in addition to arachidonic acids, such as the fish oil components: eicosapentaenoic acid and docosahexaenoic acid. These substrates are not metabolized to leukotrienes.

The products of the 5-lipoxygenase pathway are mediators of hypersensitivity reactions and inflammation. These products interact with a target cell by means of a specific receptor. The leukotrienes may act as intracellular regulators in their cell of origin. LTB4, for example, may be involved in leukocyte granule secretion. LTC4, LTD4, and LTE4 are involved in cellular and tissue contractile events, such as airway smooth muscle contraction and arteriolar vasoconstriction. They may also alter vascular permeability by acting on endothelial cells. By changing vascular smooth muscle contraction, they may affect the inotropic state of the heart or glomerular filtration.

The Prostaglandins

Arachidonic acid also may undergo cyclo-oxygenation. This results in the rearrangement of oxygenation of the molecule into endoperoxides (prostaglandin G_2 and H_2). These molecules are modified further and become prostaglandins and thromboxanes (Fig. 2–6).

Within platelets exposed to collagen or thrombin, PgG_2, and PgH_2 are oxidized by cyclo-oxygenase to the endoperoxide thromboxane-A_2, a potent initia-

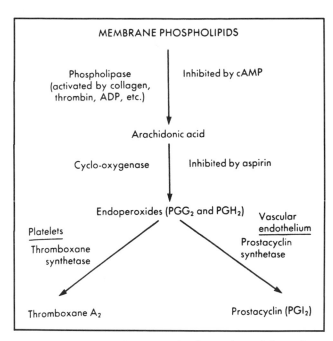

FIGURE 2–6. Pathways to the formation of thromboxane A_2 in platelets and of prostacyclin in vascular endothelial cells. (Reprinted from Ratnoff, O.D.: Blood: Hemostasis and blood coagulation. *In* Berne, R.M., and Levy, M.N. (eds.): Physiology, 2nd ed. St. Louis, C.V. Mosby Co., 1988. Figure 25–12, p. 389.)

tor of platelet aggregation and vasoconstriction. Cyclo-oxygenase can be inactivated by agents that cause acetylation, such as aspirin. Thromboxane-A_2 inhibits platelet adenyl cyclase, resulting in mobilization of calcium from intracellular stores; free cytoplasmic calcium in turn results in platelet activation.

In contrast to human platelets, endothelial cells convert endoperoxides to prostacyclin (PgI_2). Prostacyclin is an inhibitor of platelet aggregation. It stimulates adenylate cyclase, resulting in increased levels of cyclic AMP, and inhibits mobilization of calcium. This results in vasodilation and decreased platelet adhesiveness. Higher doses of aspirin block this cyclo-oxygenase pathway as well.

Arachidonic acid may be oxygenated through a separate enzyme, 12-lipoxygenase. This process results in the formation of 12-hydroxytetraenoic acid (12-HETE). The amount of the 12-HETE synthesized is increased in the presence of aspirin, since increased amounts of arachidonic acid that were not cyclo-oxygenated are available. The function of 12-HETE is not entirely understood.

Eicosanoids can be metabolized by a number of different cells. They are not stored within the cells, but are synthesized in response to stimulation. As a group, these substances are called autocoids and are quite labile. They exert their effects in the immediate environment of the cell. They are important in the regulation of blood flow, smooth muscle contraction, and platelet stimulation. Some cells synthesize their own eicosanoid precursors, whereas others process the precursor if it can be obtained from another stimulated cell in the micro-environment. For example, aspirin-treated platelets can release free arachidonic acid, which can interact with such other cells as neutrophils and serve as a source of proinflammatory eicosanoids, such as leukotriene B4. Various nonsteroidal anti-inflammatory drugs inhibit proinflammatory eicosanoid metabolism.

In summary, injury to the vascular system leads to activation of the coagulation system and inflammatory response. Such cells as platelets, leukocytes, and endothelial cells are involved in these processes and mobilize arachidonic acid, transforming it into eicosanoids with a wide variety of biologic effects. The eicosanoid precursors can be utilized by different cells in the biosynthesis of agents that control inflammation.

Platelet Activating Factor

A number of interacting mediators are involved in the process of inflammation and repair. Autocoids are lipids with pharmacologic activity that work locally to orchestrate the inflammatory process. The most well-characterized autocoids are the eicosanoids and platelet activating factors. These factors are not stored, but are rapidly generated from cell membranes after cell stimulation.

Platelet activating factor (PAF) is an autocoid produced by many different types of cells, including platelets, basophils, neutrophils, eosinophils, mast cells, monocytes, macrophages, natural killer cells, vascular endothelium, and mesangeal cells. It mediates alterations in cardiac, pulmonary, renal, and hepatic function, as well as tumor biology. Although it is called "PAF," its primary function and biologic properties seem to be largely independent and separate from platelets. Nevertheless, platelets release histamine and serotonin in response to PAF that has been released from mast cells by interaction with antigen and IgE. Among stimulants for PAF release are various pathophysiologic insults, such as ischemia, acute allergic reactions, immune complex disease, and endotoxemia. PAF has been found in the heart, lungs, blood, kidney, brain, liver, skin, retina, uterus, and embryo.

PAF's exact chemical structure, cell of origin, and role in the pathogenesis of specific disease states remain to be defined. PAFs are a variety of heterogeneous molecules produced by stimulated cells from cell phospholipids, and many of the biologic activities of PAF are modulated by arachidonic acid metabolites. PAF is probably involved in cell-to-cell communication, as occurs between leukocytes, platelets, and endothelium. It is synthesized after cellular stimulation and requires intracellular calcium.

The overall role of PAF in inflammation remains to be defined. PAFs are known, for example, to be involved in platelet stimulation and smooth muscle contraction. However, the individual molecular species have not yet been structurally defined or synthesized to allow characterization of its biologic activity.

PAFs are potent agonists for inflammatory cells, vascular smooth muscle, and endothelial cells. No other single autocoid is as potent in mediating inflammatory reactions. The most biologically potent member of the PAF family is AGEPC (1-0-alkly-2-acetyl-sn-glycerol-3-phosphocholine), which produces pulmonary vasoconstriction and peripheral vasodilation comparable to anaphylactic shock in animals. This compound is 1000 to 10,000 times more potent than histamine. It both induces vasoconstriction and increases vascular permeability. PAFs have been shown in different species to cause hypotension, pulmonary hypertension, bronchoconstriction, and increased vascular permeability and are important in the pathogenesis of acute inflammation, endotoxin shock, and anaphylaxis. There is evidence that PAFs are important biologic mediators in the pathogenesis of humorally mediated hyperacute allograft rejection. Several PAF antagonists have been reported to block PAF binding to its high-affinity receptor. Although these antagonists may inhibit or reverse PAF-induced hypotension, bronchospasm, anaphylaxis, and neutropenia, they do not appear to prevent humorally mediated hyperacute rejection.

Histamine

Histamine is formed by decarboxylation of the amino acid histidine. It is then stored preformed in mast cells and basophils within the cytoplasmic granules. Mast cells are found in skin, lung, GI tract, and reproductive mucosa. In the lung, they are found in the connective tissue under the basement membrane of the cells lining the airway, which are in close proximity to the submucosal blood vessels. They also are found throughout the bundles of smooth muscle.

Mast cells and histamine release are probably important in a variety of acute inflammatory reactions. In the classical case, mast cells are activated by antigen bridging of membrane-bound IgE. Aggregation of the IgE receptors initiates a cascade of events leading to release of the secretory granules that contain preformed compounds, including histamine. Other agents causing mast cells and basophils to release histamine include the anaphylatoxins of the complement cascade, C3a and C5a; neurohormones, such as substance P and neurotensin; and interleukin-1 and ATP.

The actions of histamine are mediated through two distinct cell membrane receptors: the H-1 and H-2 receptors. These receptors are defined by the actions of their agonists and antagonists. The H-1 receptor is proinflammatory and is stimulated by agonists, such as 2-methylhistamine, and inhibited by the classic H-1 antihistamines: diphenhydramine, chlorpheniramine, mepyramine, and promethazine. The H-2 receptor suppresses inflammation and is stimulated by H-2 agonists, such as 4-methylhistamine, and inhibited by H-2 receptor antagonists, such as cimetidine and ranitidine. Suppressor T cells have the greatest number of H-1 receptors per cell— 3×10^5. Large numbers of H-1 receptors are also found on neutrophils, B cells, helper T cells, and monocytes. Basophils, mast cells, and eosinophils also contain H-1 receptors. H-2 receptors are found on helper (T_4) cells, suppressor T cells, cytotoxic T cells, monocytes, eosinophils, neutrophils, and basophils.

Activation of the H-1 receptor results in intracellular guanosine monophosphate (GMP) release, with resulting smooth muscle contraction and increased vascular permeability as seen in asthma, urticaria, anaphylaxis, and allergic rhinitis. It also results in prostaglandin formation, decrease in conduction time through the AV node, and activation of the vagal afferent nerves in airways. Stimulation of the H-2 receptor produces an increase in gastric acid secretion, esophageal contraction, and airway mucus secretion. Both the H-1 and H-2 receptors, when stimulated, may cause hypotension and tachycardia, as well as headache and flushing. The tachycardia may be due in part to decreased conduction time through the AV node. Local or systemic administration of histamine causes increased vascular permeability with edema formation in connective tissues and mucosa. Wheal formation is an example of this response to histamine. It is thought to occur as a result of contraction of endothelial actin-myosin filaments in postcapillary venules, leading to the formation of intercellular gaps. Proteins leak through these gaps, thus increasing the tissue colloid oncotic pressure and resulting in a fluid shift and edema. This increased vascular permeability is probably H-1 receptor mediated.

Histamine can influence neural reflexes, such as those in the lung. It is capable of stimulating cholinergic discharge, increasing alpha adrenergic responsiveness, and stimulating substance P release. Histamine may cause release of vasoactive intestinal peptide (VIP), which reduces the further release of histamine. It may serve to prime the alpha adrenergic response in the lung. It can also interact with cholinergic and adrenergic nervous systems and with neurotransmitters found in endocrine glands and nerve fibers. Within the lung, airways stimulated by histamine can release prostaglandins E_2 and I_2 from contracting muscle fibers.

Histamine affects a variety of cells. It is capable of enhancing the recruitment of human eosinophils into inflammatory lesions and enhancing the killing efficiency of recruited eosinophils. The eosinophil H-1 receptor has a proinflammatory effect through enhancement of chemotaxis, C3b receptor expression, and cell killing, whereas the H-2 receptor stimulation inhibits complement-directed chemotaxis.

Histamine activation of suppressor T cells results in immunosuppression. In the presence of monocytes or interleukin-1, histamine induces the generation of suppressor T cells, with resultant immunosuppression. Histamine then modulates immunoglobulin synthesis through several different T-cell-dependent mechanisms. It activates suppressor T cells to elaborate histamine-stimulating factor, which interferes with helper T cell maturation, as well as the response of B cells to preformed helper factors.

Histamine causes the release of several lymphokines. The influence of histamine on mononuclear cells at the site of inflammation is dependent on the effects of these lymphokines.

PEPTIDE REGULATORY FACTORS

The cells of the immune system communicate largely through peptides that are secreted locally in response to a variety of stimuli. The cellular interaction is presented in Chapter 26. Here the various peptide regulatory factors are discussed with respect to their role as inflammatory mediators.

Interleukin-1

Interleukin-1 (IL-1) is a key mediator of acute responses to tissue injury and inflammation, the immune response, and bacterial invasion, and its biologic effects are manifested in nearly every tissue. Two forms of IL-1, IL-1-alpha and IL-1-beta, have been identified, but IL-1-beta predominates in humans. Its biologic activity is closely related to tumor necrosis factor (TNF; cachectin). TNF has many properties similar to IL-1, yet the amino acid structure is quite different and TNF receptors are separate from IL-1 receptors.

The major function of IL-1 was once thought to be limited to the upregulation of IL-2 receptors and stimulation of IL-2 release by T helper cells. IL-1 *is* essential to T lymphocyte response (see Chapter 26), and as such it is principally secreted by cells of monocyte/macrophage lineage. Yet, IL-1 is also secreted by endothelial cells, keratinocytes, neutrophils, and B lymphocytes and has multiple systemic biologic properties corresponding to the presence of IL-1 receptors in most cells. IL-1 bound to receptor is internalized and becomes associated with the cell nucleus. Its half-life in the circulation is less than 10 minutes, and unlike TNF it is only occasionally found to be elevated in systemic illness.

Nevertheless, many of the changes occurring acutely after bacterial infection, injury, or chronic inflammatory response—granulocytosis, fever, and the acute phase response—may be mediated by IL-1. IL-1 induces hepatocytes to synthesize a spectrum of acute phase proteins, including C-reactive protein, complement components, various clotting factors, and serum amyloid A. It regulates the synthesis of these proteins at the level of messenger RNA transcription. It depresses the activity of liver cytochrome P-450 dependent drug metabolism, resulting in impaired drug clearance and excretion in patients with infections and fever. IL-1 stimulates the liver to synthesize metalloproteins that bind iron and zinc. Reduction in serum iron and zinc levels may be important in increasing host resistance to infection, since bacteria and tumor cells require large amounts of iron for cell growth.

The effects of IL-1 on endothelial cells serve to localize tissue inflammation, and in fact, IL-1 is produced locally by endothelial cells. IL-1 activates human endothelial cells so that neutrophils, monocytes, and lymphocytes adhere. It also increases the binding of natural killer cells to tumors and is chemotactic for monocytes and lymphocytes. It increases endothelial cell surface procoagulant activity.

IL-1 is also involved in bone and joint disease and local tumor invasion. It is a potent inducer of collagenase production in synovial cells. It increases the production of receptors for endogenous growth factors, such as epidermal growth factor or transforming growth factor β.

Most cells that act as accessory cells to the immune response produce IL-1. These include all cells of monocyte/macrophage lineage, as well as such cells as endothelial cells, keratinocytes, astrocytes, and mesangial cells. However, almost all cells can produce IL-1 when injured.

IL-1 induces a number of systemic changes. In addition to increasing levels of ACTH, cortisone, insulin, and hepatic acute phase proteins and stimulating myelopoiesis, it causes a decrease in the number of circulating neutrophils through the activation of endothelial surfaces and the adherence of leukocytes. It also causes a decrease of blood pressure and systemic vascular resistance.

IL-1-mediated responses may be helpful in the repulsion of invading organisms. Within hours of the onset of infection, fever occurs as a result of the IL-1-induced pyrogen response, which in turn is caused by the release of prostaglandins in the anterior hypothalamus. Those changes may reduce the ability of bacteria and viruses to replicate. There is also evidence that fever may augment T cell and B cell activation, as well as neutrophil phagocytosis. The fact that IL-1 increases the production of hepatic acute phase proteins and metalloproteins suggests its role in host defense, since the absence of these responses is associated with decreased resistance to infection. Metalloproteins bind plasma iron and zinc, both of which are useful to bacteria. Indeed, IL-1 reduces the susceptibility to systemic infection in animal models.

Tumor Necrosis Factor (TNF; Cachectin). TNF is an interleukin to which a number has not been assigned, but it may be the most central mediator of the chemical responses seen in septic shock. Its biologic properties are quite similar to IL-1, but TNF totally lacks IL-1's immunostimulatory effects (Table 2–4). TNF is produced by cells of monocyte/macrophage lineage, including astrocytes and Kupffer cells in response to endotoxin, fungal and parasitic antigens, C5A, and IL-1 and as an autocrine to TNF itself. Mast cells, NK cells, and endothelial cells also can produce TNF. The half-life of injected TNF is about 15 minutes, and it is degraded in many organs. The TNF response to endotoxin infusion peaks in 1 to 2 hours and lasts about 4 hours; thus, its production is tightly regulated. Its biologic effects, like those of endotoxin, last for hours, suggesting that it sets off a series of secondary cascades. Steroid pretreatment downregulates production, and interferon gamma upregulates it. Human TNF is produced as a prohormone of 233 amino acids and is processed to a 157 residue protein (MW = 17KD). A cell surface form also exists.

The cell surface receptors for TNF are distinct from IL-1 receptors, but stimulate similar intracellular messengers and alter cellular metabolism in a similar way. TNF probably functions as an interleukin—that is, as a messenger between cells involved in local response to injury—by increasing the procoagulant activity of endothelial surfaces; increasing vascular permeability; stimulating margination, extravasation, and degranulation of neutrophils; and inhibiting the replication of intracellular pathogens. Through its fibroblast and endothelial production activity, it probably functions in tissue remodeling. At higher concentrations that spill over into the circulation, it causes tissue injury, irreversible shock, and death. Endotoxin or endotoxin-free TNF induces fever, rigors, myalgia, headache, and nausea; higher doses of either form of TNF trigger lethal shock. The tissue injury is due to a procoagulant effect on endothelial tissue that results in disseminated coagulation. Leukocytes are sequestered and stimulated to release superoxides and arachidonic acid metabolites. TNF is probably not responsible for all of the observed phenomena of endotoxin shock, but anti-TNF antibodies do protect against lethal endotoxemia.

TNF is also called cachectin because it induces cachexia in animals. TNF participates in acute phase reactions in liver cells (perhaps via IL-6 production) and downregulates albumin synthesis. Muscle and fat cells become catabolic. Elevated levels of TNF have been found in some cancer patients, in AIDS, and in chronic bacterial infections. Its stimulatory effects on catabolic metabolism are similar to those produced by these severe systemic diseases; namely, an increase in anaerobic glycolysis, an increased breakdown of skeletal muscle protein, and lipolysis in peripheral tissue. In contrast, hepatocyte protein

TABLE 2–4. SOME BIOLOGIC PROPERTIES OF CACHECTIN/TNF IN VARIOUS DISORDERS

PHYSIOLOGIC CONDITION	BIOLOGIC EFFECTS
Acute infection Septic shock, toxic shock syndrome, meningococcal infection, cerebral malaria	Shock; fever; respiratory arrest, capillary leak syndrome, hemorrhagic necrosis, lactic acidosis, stress hormone release, hyperglycemia then hypoglycemia, hyperaminoacidemia; induces reactive oxygen intermediates, platelet activating factor, and eicosanoids
Cachexia Chronic infection, AIDS? malignancy?	Anorexia, weight loss, anemia, fever, increased energy expenditure, hypertriglyceridemia, increased whole-body lipolysis, net protein loss, acute phase protein biosynthesis, suppression of LPL
Inflammation Abscess formation, systemic lupus erythematosus, rheumatoid arthritis, autoimmunity, transplant rejection, graft-versus-host disease	Chemotactic for leucocytes, promotes leucostasis; enhances nonspecific host resistance; leukoctye and endothelial activation; induces expression of MHC antigens, neutrophil degranulation, phagocytosis against pathogens, fibroblast and thymocyte growth factor, reactive oxygen intermediates, collagenase, and eicosanoids
Tissue remodeling Wound healing	Fibroblast growth factor; angiogenesis factor; stimulates TGFs, GM-CSF, and PDGF; induces collagenase and eicosanoids; cell cytotoxicity

LPL-lipoprotein lipase; MHC-major histocompatibility complex; TGF-transforming growth factor; GM-CSF-granulocyte-macrophage colony-stimulating factor; PDGF-platelet-derived growth factor.
Reprinted from Tracey, K.J., Vlassara, H., and Cerami, A.: Cachectin/tumour necrosis factor. Lancet *1*:1123.

synthesis, especially acute phase responses, is enhanced.

Interleukin-2. Interleukin-2 (IL-2) was first identified as a factor capable of promoting growth of human T cells. It exerts its action through binding to specific membrane receptors. However, unlike most other growth factor receptors, IL-2 receptors are not expressed on the surface of resting T cells. Rather, antigen activation is required for IL-2 receptor gene expression and for IL-2 production. IL-1 is a necessary co-stimulant for a subset of T_4 cells, the TH_2 subset (which produces IL-4, 5, 6), but IL-1 is not necessary for IL-2 production by the TH_1 subset that produces IL-2 and interferon (IFN) gamma. Although only TH_1 cells can synthesize IL-2, all T cells express IL-2 receptors. The high-affinity IL-2 receptor on the T cell is unique in that two separate protein chains (alpha and beta) are involved. Binding of IL-2 with newly synthesized, high-affinity membrane receptors stimulates T cell proliferation, producing an expansion of the clone of T cells activated by the antigen. This results in the emergence of effector T cells with helper, suppressor, and cytotoxic functions. The production of IL-2 may also lead to production of other lymphokines, such as IFN gamma, by stimulating TH_1 cells.

IL-2 is a single chain polypeptide, with a molecular weight of 15,000 to 17,000. It is markedly hydrophobic and has no significant homologies with other protein or DNA sequences. Immunosuppressive agents, such as cyclosporine or cortocosteroids, inhibit IL-2 production. Cyclosporine inhibits IL-2 gene transcription.

Although the principal action of IL-2 is to promote the growth of T cells expressing receptors for this lymphokine, IL-2 has other activities as well. It may promote the proliferation of certain B cells and may be implicated in the activation of lymphokine-activated killer (LAK) cells that kill tumor cells in vitro. IL-2, with or without LAK cells, is undergoing trials as a immunotherapeutic agent in human cancer; responses have been seen in melanoma, renal cell carcinoma, and colon cancer.

Interleukin-3. IL-3 is a colony-stimulation factor made by antigen-stimulated T_4 cells. It functions as a growth and differentiation factor for many types of hemopoietic progenitor cells (perhaps including the B cell line).

Interleukin-4. IL-4 is a product of T helper type 2 (TH_2) cells, which also produce IL-5 and IL-6. Although its primary function is B cell maturation, which induces MHC class II expression, IgE receptor expression, immunoglobulin isotype regulation, and proliferation, it also acts to mature both T_4 and T_8 cells and may influence thymus maturation of T cells.

Interleukin-5. IL-5 is made by T cells and induces cellular proliferation and immunoglobulin (IgM, IgG, and IgA) production by B cells.

Interleukin-6. IL-6, like IL-4 and IL-5, was once thought to be solely a product of T cells that was important in B cell differentiation and proliferation.

However, IL-6 has actions that are important in the development and maturation of T cells and has multiple systemic functions as well.

Many cells produce IL-6, especially fibroblasts and macrophages, keratinocytes, and endothelial cells in response to LPS, as well as to IL-1, TNF, and platelet-derived growth factor. IL-6 is not a single protein, but is a mixture of six phosphoglycoproteins. It is elevated after surgical trauma and infection, as is TNF. Like IL-1 and TNF, it is an endogenous pyrogen. It was once named hepatocyte-stimulating factor, and its ability to stimulate acute phase protein response by hepatocytes may be more important than that of IL-1 or TNF. Yet, unlike IL-1 and TNF, it does not seem to play a role in the adverse consequences of sepsis.

Interleukin-7. IL-7 is also a B cell differentiation factor that operates on later stages of B cell development. It may act on thymocytes as well. Its cell of origin is unknown. IL1-8, IL-9, and IL-10 have tentatively been identified, but their various functions have not been worked out.

The Interferons. Interferons (IFN) are a family of proteins and glycoproteins produced by nucleated cells in response to infection with viruses. They were thought to induce an antiviral state in other host cells. Initially, IFN alpha and IFN beta were described. Both are made during bacterial and viral infection: IFN alpha by mononuclear cells and IFN beta by fibroblasts and epithelial cells. Both are secreted in response to various cytokines: IL-1, IL-2, TNF, and the colony-stimulating factors. IFN gamma is made by T cells and is a more effective immunomodulator than IFN alpha or IFN beta.

The predominant effects of IFN are antiviral and antiproliferative activity. Cells treated with IFN do not affect the adsorption of viruses to cells, their penetration into cells, or uncoding of the virions. However, accumulation of virus-specific messenger RNAs, double-stranded RNAs, and proteins is impaired. There appears to be no single mechanism responsible for the antiviral action of IFN. In general, the antiviral activity of IFN gamma is weaker than that of IFN alpha and beta.

IFN alpha and beta are strong inhibitors of cell growth, both normal and malignant. They may be natural regulators of cell growth, and IFN alpha is useful in selected human tumors as a cytostatic agent, e.g., hairy cell leukemia, chronic myeloid leukemia, multiple myeloma, AIDS-related Karposi sarcoma, and several solid tumors. Cures are rare. Surprisingly, IFN alpha has minimal effect in viral infection.

IFN gamma, like IL-1, TNF, and IL-6, seems most intimately involved with host defense against infection. T helper cells, especially TH_1 subsets, produce IFN alpha in response to IL-2 and microbial stimuli. The anti-infectious role of IFN gamma involves not just viruses but also other microbes. IFN gamma primarily upregulates monocyte/macrophage function; INF alpha macrophages can produce more IL-1, TNF, IL-6, and prostaglandins when stimulated with lipopolysaccharide (LPS). INF-alpha-primed macrophages express class II MHC antigens on their surface. Since MHC expression is essential for microbial antigen recognition by T cells, this function is probably very important for antimicrobial defenses against pathogens sequestered in such phagocytes. Furthermore, IFN gamma induces immunoglobulin secretion by B cells, activates macrophages to increased phagocytosis and tumor cytostasis, and activates cytotoxic T cells. IFN gamma enhances production of reactive oxygen intermediates, reactive nitrogen intermediates, hydrogen ions, and tryptophane-degrading enzyme. The growth-inhibiting action of IFN gamma appears to be less important.

GROWTH FACTORS

Growth factors are polypeptide cytokines that regulate the growth, differentiation, and metabolism of cells. They are present throughout the body in nanogram amounts. In general, growth factors are mitogens, some of which operate alone and others of which work in combination with other chemically different growth factors. Growth factors bind to specific membrane receptors that in turn initiate a cascade of intracellular biochemical alterations in the cell known as the pleiotypic response, which results in cell growth. This response includes an increase in the transport of ions and small molecules across the membrane, arachidonic acid release with prostaglandin synthesis, and a number of cytoplasmic phosphorylation reactions. Many of the specific receptors for growth factors have intrinsic tyrosine kinase activity, i.e., they act in the ligand-bound conformation to phosphorylate the tyrosine residues on cytoplasmic proteins. These events eventually result in DNA synthesis and cell division. Growth factors, in addition, may enhance the synthesis of extracellular matrix proteins, such as collagen, proteoglycans, and laminin, again resulting in cellular proliferation, which depends on cellular attachment to these matrix proteins.

Although growth factors have been named from the tissues from which they were first isolated, they are often found in greater amounts elsewhere in the body. Growth factors often have amino acid sequences in common with other growth factors and other polypeptides, such as insulin and viral DNAs. The study of growth factors has been made possible by the ability to produce them through recombinant DNA technology. A few of the relatively well-studied growth factors are listed in Table 2–5. Almost certainly, there are modulating factors that control growth factor activity, but these are less well understood. One such factor is the anchorage dependence

TABLE 2–5. SOME GROWTH FACTORS AND THEIR ACTIONS

FACTOR	COMPOSITION	REPRESENTATIVE ACTIVITIES
Platelet-derived growth factor (PDGF)	AA, AB, or BB	Stimulates proliferation of connective tissue cells and neuroglial cells
Epidermal growth factor (EGF)	53 aa	Stimulates proliferation of many cell types
Insulin-like growth factor I (IGF-I) and insulin-like growth factor II (IGF-II)	70 aa 73 aa	Collaborate with PDGF and EGF, stimulate proliferation of fat cells and connective tissue cells
Transforming growth factor β (TGF-β)	Two chains, each 112 aa	Potentiates or inhibits response of most cells to other growth factors, depending on the cell type, regulates differentiation of some cell types
Fibroblast growth factor (FGF)	Acidic: 140 aa Basic: 146 aa	Stimulates proliferation of many cell types, including fibroblasts, endothelial cells, and myoblasts; induces mesoderm in *Xenopus* embryo
Interleukin-2 (IL-2)	153 aa	Stimulates proliferation of T lymphocytes
Nerve growth factor (NGF)	Two chains, each 118 aa	Promotes axon growth and survival of sympathetic and some sensory and CNS neurons
Hemopoietic cell growth factors (IL-3, GM-CSF, M-CSF, G-CSF, erythropoietin)		

Adapted from Alberts, B., Bray, D., Lewis, J., Raff, M., Roberts, K., and Watson, J.D.: Molecular Biology of the Cell, 2nd ed. New York, Garland Publishing, Inc., 1989, p. 747.

of cells, i.e., the fact that cells that are not attached cannot divide. This characteristic limits the cellular response to a discrete area. Another controlling factor is the acid composition of many cellular receptors for a few growth factor molecules, which causes rapid dilution or depletion of the factor. In addition, a number of factors bind growth factors, both limiting their availability and prolonging their half-life.

Platelet-Derived Growth Factor

Platelet-derived growth factor (PDGF) is a mitogen for connective tissue cells. It is a polypeptide with a molecular weight of about 31,000 and is composed of two chains, A and B, held together by disulfide bonds. The B chain shows about 60 per cent amino acid homology with the A chain. PDGF is a potent mitogen for fibroblasts and smooth muscle cells. It is released by platelets from their alpha granules and is found in thrombus at the site of tissue injury. Release of PDGF at a site of vascular injury is important in wound healing and tissue repair; however, it may also play a role in the pathology of atherosclerosis by stimulating smooth muscle proliferation.

The half-life of PDGF in blood is only minutes. It acts as a potent mitogen and is not normally present in plasma because it is concentrated in the α granules of platelets. However, PDGF is rapidly produced in response to injury as the platelet degranulates. Thus, PDGF is present in serum.

The B chain of PDGF is nearly identical to the transforming gene of the simian sarcoma virus, which is an acute transforming retrovirus. The human proto-oncogene, C-sis, is similar to the viral oncogene, V-sis, and codes for the B chain of PDGF.

Although originally described as a platelet factor, PDGF-like molecules are found in a variety of cells, including vascular endothelium, aorta smooth muscle, activated macrophages, atherosclerotic proliferative lesions, and the placenta in the first trimester. As do most other growth factors, PDGF binds to receptors that change their conformation and act as tyrosine-specific kinases that phosphorylate cell membrane and cellular proteins at the tyrosine residue. A number of cells can secrete a PDGF-like substance, which in turn binds to the PDGF receptor. This results in an autocrine mechanism whereby dividing cells stimulate their own growth.

Growth control in response to PDGF is mediated in several ways. PDGF binds to proteins that block the ligand PDGF for its receptor on cell surfaces. PDGF is bound predominantly by an alpha-2-macroglobulin that is itself a protease inhibitor. In general, plasma-binding proteins both increase the circulating half-life of the growth factors and also inhibit their biologic effects. Modulation of growth factor binding by these proteins regulates the amount of bound and unbound growth factor. This may protect the growth factor against degradation or other mechanisms of inactivation and ultimately may result in prolongation of the potential activity of the growth factor.

Fibroblast-derived growth factor (FDGF) is quite similar to PDGF. It is a potent fibroblast mitogen as well.

Angiogenesis, Endothelial, and Fibroblast Growth Factors

Growth factors responsible for endothelial cell proliferation have been found in a variety of tissues, including the brain, retina, cartilage, and tumors. These types of growth factors have a strong affinity for heparin, which plays a regulatory role in their function. Heparin may play an active role in protecting these growth factors from inactivation by proteases. It can also compete with the growth factors and inhibit their function by a direct effect on many target cells responsive to these growth factors. Heparin-like molecules have been shown to localize and concentrate these growth factors extracellularly. Binding to heparin results in other molecules that interact with heparin, such as heparinase or protamine, which exert a regulatory effect on these growth factors.

Fibroblast growth factor (FGF) is a single polypeptide chain that is a mitogen for endothelial cells. As do other growth factors, it binds to a specific high-affinity cell surface receptor. There are two forms of FGF, acidic FGF (aFGF) and basic FGF (bFGF). Although aFGF and bFGF are two separate entities, both are mitogens for endothelial-, mesodermal-, and neuroectodermal-derived cells, and both have a strong affinity for heparin. They interact with the same cell surface receptors and can displace each other. aFGF and bFGF have 53 per cent amino acid homology. aFGF is the same or quite similar to a number of other factors described, including endothelial cell growth factor, retina-derived growth factor, eye-derived growth factor II, heparin-binding growth factor alpha, astroglial growth factor I, anionic endothelial growth factor I, brain-derived growth factor, and prostatropin. bFGF is also the same or quite similar to cartilage-derived growth factor, chondrosarcoma-derived growth factor, hepatoma growth factor, endothelial cell growth factor II, eye-derived growth factor I, astroglial growth factor II, human prostatic growth factor, and heparin-binding growth factor B. aFGF is present in high quantities in neural tissues, whereas bFGF has been found in the adrenal glands, kidney, placenta, and macrophages. aFGF has some amino acid sequence homology with interleukin-1.

These angiogenesis factors result in the growth of new blood vessels through the proliferation of the capillary endothelial cell. This growth occurs in a developing embryo, wound healing, immune reactions, and the inflammatory response. It also occurs in the pathologic settings of atherosclerosis, diabetes, tumor growth, and arthritis.

Transforming Growth Factors

Transforming growth factors (TGF) are a group of peptide growth factors that result in a trans-formed phenotype in stimulated cells. They were first discovered in retroviral transformed cells that induce anchorage-independent growth of fibroblasts. Two different TGFs have been described, TGF alpha and TGF beta.

TGF-alpha is produced from a large 160 amino acid precursor that may occur as a protein found in cell membranes. The amino acid sequence of TGF-alpha shows a 40 per cent homology with epidermal growth factor (EGF). TGF-alpha and EGF interact with a common receptor on the cell surface. TGF-alpha activates the tyrosine kinase receptor and transforms normal fibroblasts into cells capable of anchorage-independent growth.

TGF-beta is found in human platelets and in the human placenta. Like TGF-alpha, it can be produced by virally transformed cells. However, it bears no structural relationship to TGF-alpha or EGF. TGF-beta-stimulated anchorage-independent growth of fibroblasts occurs in cells that have previously been stimulated by other growth factors, including TGF-alpha, insulin-like growth factors (IGF), or PDGF. TGF-beta has also been found in malignant cells. Unlike TGF-alpha, TGF-beta has no similar amino acid homology with any other growth factor or protein.

Tumor cells manufacture growth factors that are TGFs. These factors serve an autocrine function in stimulating the cell itself to grow. TGFs initially were known as sarcoma growth factor (SGF) because of their ability to stimulate growth of malignant cells in soft agar. Although neither TGF-alpha nor TGF-beta can support fibroblast growth in soft agar independently, together they can induce anchorage-independent growth. TGF-beta can also inhibit rather than promote growth of some cell lines.

Melanoma-stimulating growth factor (MSGF) is a polypeptide similar to TGF alpha and is produced by melanoma cells. Like TGF alpha, it stimulates anchorage-independent growth of these malignant cells.

Epidermal Growth Factor

Epidermal growth factor (EGF) is a single chain polypeptide with an amino acid homology quite similar to TGF alpha. It is a potent mitogen with activity occurring through a receptor that is a transmembrane phosphorylated glycoprotein. This EGF receptor is regulated not only by binding of EGF and TGF alpha but also by phosphorylation by the protein kinase C receptor, which is known to promote tumor growth. EGF is known to be the same as urogastrone.

Somatomedins

Somatomedin (SM) is a polypeptide that is found in blood tightly bound to a specific carrier protein.

The most common somatomedin is somatomedin C (SMC), which is identical to insulin-like growth factor (IGF-1). SMC and IGF have a structural similarity to another compound, multiplication stimulating activity (MSA). IGF-1 is a single chain protein that has a 50 per cent homology in amino acid structure with SMC and a 62 per cent amino acid sequence homology with IGF-2. Both IGF-1 and IGF-2 circulate tightly bound to a carrier protein.

The blood levels of SMC/IGF depend upon the patient's age and sex, and hormonal and nutritional status. Levels rise from birth to adolescence, but then decrease and remain constant in adulthood. Women have higher levels than men. Growth hormone (GH) is an important regulator of some SMC/IGF levels. SMC/IGF levels are increased in patients with acromegaly, and elevated SMC/IGF levels have been used to establish the diagnosis of GH-related disorders. Other hormones, including prolactin, placental lactogen, thyroid hormone, and sex hormones, also influence SMC/IGF levels. Thyroid hormones and sex hormones affect SMC/IGF levels through their effect on GH. Starvation induces resistance of SMC/IGF to GH. In starvation, GH levels are elevated, whereas SMC/IGF levels are low.

As do other growth factors, somatomedins act in an autocrine or paracrine manner. Serum levels of these hormones may be low, in spite of potent effects from increased tissue levels.

MSA, like other somatomedins, has an amino acid sequence homology with IGF-2 and differs from it by only five amino acids. Like IGF-2, it is more insulin-like and has less growth-hormone-dependent actions. It shares with other somatomedins the unique property of circulating in the blood associated with a high molecular weight carrier protein. The role of the carrier proteins has yet to be defined.

Bone and Cartilage Growth Factors

Ten per cent of bone is composed of cells, whereas 90 per cent or more constitutes its matrix. Calciotrophic hormones, including parathormone and vitamin D, determine bone formation and resorption. However, local factors are also important and are called into play in pathologic situations, such as fracture healing. Bone morphogenic protein (BMP) and bone-derived growth factor (BDGF) are known to stimulate bone growth. BMP can cause bone formation in soft tissues. BDGF stimulates osteoblast proliferation and collagen synthesis. Human skeletal growth factor (HSGF) also causes collagen synthesis.

The growth of cartilage is also under hormonal control. Cartilage-derived factor (CDF), which is closely related to the somatodomedins, stimulates the formation of proteoglycans of cartilage. DNA synthesis and cell division of condrasites, however, are not stimulated by CDF, but can occur when stimulated by FGF or EGF, which do not stimulate proteoglycan synthesis. MSA has similar effects as CDF.

Nerve and Glial Factors

Nerve growth factor (NGF) is a neuronotropic protein that causes neural crest tissue to differentiate and develop. It is also required for the maintenance of sympathetic and sensory neurons and stimulates neurite growth and neurotransmitter biosynthesis. Unlike other growth factors, it is not a mitogen; however, it is similar to other growth factors, including EGF and insulin, in its membrane receptor interaction. Glial growth factor (GGF) is a mitogen for Schwann cells. It also stimulates division of astrocytes and fibroblasts. Glial maturation factor (GMF) is a mitogen for astroblasts and may be important in promoting the recovery of brain tissue after injury.

Erythropoietin and Myeloid Growth Factors

All blood cells, including lymphocytes, originate from a common pleuripotential stem cell. Once these stem cells differentiate, their maturation is controlled by specific humoral factors that are different for each line of cells. Erythropoietin (EPO) promotes the maturation of erythroblasts. It is the hormone primarily responsible for erythropoiesis. It is produced in the liver in the fetus, but in the kidney as an adult. Oxygen concentration is important in regulating EPO production, with hypoxia and anemia causing increased blood levels of EPO. EPO has been cloned and is available as a purified agent made by recombinant DNA techniques.

Myeloid Growth Factors. The production of granulocytes and mononuclear phagocytes from the bone marrow cells is tightly controlled to maintain a constant level of cells circulating in the blood. However, with diseases and infection, dramatic increases in the number of circulating granulocytes may occur. The process of granulocyte formation begins with a multipotential stem cell that is capable of reproducing itself, as well as differentiating into several lineages. A myeloid stem cell can become a granulocyte, monocyte, erythrocyte, or platelet. It has no ability to differentiate in the lymphoid line. Conversely, a lymphoid stem cell can become a T cell or B cell, but not a granulocyte, monocyte, erythrocyte, or platelet. Granulocytes and monocytes are regulated by specific growth hormones called colony-stimulating factors, or hemopoietins. Four distinct colony-stimulating factors (CSFs) have been identified: granulocyte-macrophage colony-stimulating factor, granulocyte colony-stimulating factor, macrophage colony-stimulating factor, and multicolony-stimulating factor (interleukin-3). These CSFs are important in host defense. Their major action is to modulate the functional state of mature effector cells, including their motility, metabolism, and cytotoxic capacity. CSF production may occur in response to endotoxin-activated components of the complement system, inflammatory mediators, or bacterial chemoattractants.

BIBLIOGRAPHY

1. Fong, Y., Moldawer, L.L. et al.: The biological characteristics of cytokines and their implications in surgical injury. Surg. Gynecol. Obstet.,*170*:363–378, 1990.
2. Barnes, D., and Sirbaskin, D.A. (eds.): Methods in Enzymology: Peptide Growth Factors, Vol. 146 and 147. London, Academic Press, 1987.
3. Gallin, J.I., Goldstein, I.M., and Snyderman, R. (eds.): Inflammation: Basic Principles and Clinical Correlates. New York, Raven Press, 1988.
4. Braquet, P., Touqui, L., Shen, T., and Vargaftig, B.: Perspectives in platelet-activating factor research. Pharmacol. Rev., *39*(2):97–145, 1987.
5. Metcalf, D.: Peptide regulatory factors: Haemopoietic growth factors I. Lancet, *1*:825–827, 1989.
6. Metcalf, D.: Peptide regulatory factors: Haemopoietic growth factors II: Clinical applications. Lancet, *1*:885–887, 1989.
7. O'Garra, A.: Peptide regulatory factors: Interleukin and the immune system I. Lancet, *1*:943–946, 1989.
8. O'Garra, A.: Peptide regulatory factors: Interleukins and the immune system II. Lancet, *1*:1003–1005, 1989.
9. Balkwill, F.R.: Peptide regulatory factors: Interferons. Lancet, *1*:1060–1063, 1989.
10. Tracey, K., Vlassara, H., and Cerami, A.: Peptide regulatory factors: Cachectin/tumor necrosis factor. Lancet, *1*:1122–1125, 1989.

3

HEMOSTASIS AND COAGULATION

David L. Steed

Normal hemostasis and coagulation rely on a delicate balance among locally responsive mechanisms operative at the site of a vascular injury, the coagulation cascades, and a series of events that terminate clotting and keep it localized. The system fails when local clot formation is impaired, when coagulation spreads beyond the site of injury, or when those mechanisms that keep coagulation in check overrespond and permit rebleeding.

The hemostatic mechanism is a surface-activated system in which the first rapid and highly localized step is the formation of a platelet plug at the site of injured vascular endothelium. Concurrently, there is activation of the extrinsic coagulation pathway and, more slowly thereafter, activation of the intrinsic pathway resulting in a stable clot with fibrin cross-linking. Finally, fibrinolysis occurs to prevent the propagation of the clot beyond what is needed to control hemorrhage and to break down the fibrin polymers to smaller degradable forms. These processes result in both the control of hemorrhage and the subsequent re-establishment of flow through the injured vessel.

Hemostasis after an injury occurs in three phases: (1) reflex vasoconstriction, (2) platelet aggregation and plug formation, and (3) coagulation and clot retraction.

VASOCONSTRICTION

Immediately after injury, the first response designed to control hemorrhage is contraction of the blood vessel wall, which reduces the diameter of the vessel and thus the size of the opening. This spasm is the result of direct damage to the vessel, which causes transmission of action potentials along the wall, resulting in vasoconstriction. This spasm serves to reduce the bleeding while platelets gather in the wound and the coagulation process is initiated. Vaso-

constriction also occurs in response to thromboxane A_2, a product of arachidonic acid metabolism in platelet membranes. Thromboxane A_2 also activates platelets and aggregates them. The principal mechanism of aspirin's anticoagulant action at low dosage is the inhibition of thromboxane A_2 production.

THE PLATELET

Platelets are non-nucleated elements in the blood that bud off from polynuclear megakaryocytes in the marrow; their maturation is controlled by thrombopoietin. They are 2 to 4 μm in diameter and have a lifespan of 8 to 10 days. A normal blood platelet count is 150,000 to 400,000/mL; a further 30 to 40 per cent are stored in the spleen. The surface, granule, and cytoplasmic contents of platelets are listed in Table 3–1.

Endothelial damage exposes blood to collagen and other tissue to which platelets are prone to adhere. The mechanism of adhesion is complex. Plasma von Willebrand factor binds specifically to exposed collagen in the subendothelial tissue. The platelet has a receptor (glycoprotein Ib) for the bound von Willebrand factor that then serves as the bridge between subendothelial tissue and the platelet. Receptor engagement activates the platelet.

Activation results not only in a flattening of the adherent platelet on the damaged tissue but also degranulation, which releases many of the factors listed in Table 3–1. New receptors on the platelet surface called IIb and IIIa are then expressed. These bind fibrinogen, which in turn acts to bind other activated platelets together in an aggregate, thereby plugging the defect. No aggregation of platelets occurs in the absence of fibrinogen.

Thus, platelets carry a number of procoagulants that are released after activation. The release is concentrated at the site of injury to which the platelets

TABLE 3–1. SURFACE, GRANULE, AND CYTOPLASMIC CONTENTS OF PLATELETS WITH PUTATIVE FUNCTION

Receptors on platelet surface
  Ib
  IIb
  IIIa
  Thrombin
  ADP
  Catecholamines
Contents of platelets
  Dense granules
    Serotonin
    Catecholamines
    Nonmetabolic "storage pool" of ATP, ADP
    Ca^{++} ions
    Pyrophosphate
  α-Granules
    Albumin
    Platelet factor 4
    β-thromboglobulin
    Fibronectin
    Plasminogen
    Platelet fibrinogen
    Platelet-derived growth factor (PDGF)
    High molecular weight kininogen
    α₂-plasmin inhibitor
    Proaccelerin (factor V)
    Antihemophilic factor-related antigen (factor VIIR:Ag; von Willebrand factor; factor VIII:VWF)
    Thrombospondin
    C1-esterase inhibitor
  Cytosol
    Actin
    Myosin
  Membrane
    Phospholipids—arachidonic acid

adhere. Furthermore, degranulation initiates the release of thromboxane, a potent smooth muscle constrictor.

The surface of the activated platelet plug is a major substrate for the intrinsic coagulation cascade. Platelet phospholipids interact with factors X_a and V_a and CA^{++} in the production of prothrombinase so that the platelet itself serves as a site for the conversion of prothrombin to thrombin and fibrinogen to fibrin. Then, receptors (IIb, IIIa) for fibrin on the platelet surface yield a platelet aggregate with fibrin glue. The cytoplasm of the platelet also contains the microtubular apparatus that, by altering platelet morphology, serves to retract and localize the clot (Table 3–1).

Regulation of the platelet activation process is probably mediated by the normal endothelial cell at the boundary of the platelet plug. The endothelial cell produces prostacyclin from arachidonic acid. Prostacyclin activates adenyl cyclase in the platelet membrane, thereby raising cyclic AMP levels, which prohibits further platelet aggregation and granule release. Tissue plasminogen activator is also released by the endothelial cell after injury; the resulting fibrinolytic activity reduces excessive fibrin deposition, thus limiting the platelet plug size and increasing the likelihood that the injured vessel will remain patent.

COAGULATION CASCADES

Within the blood are circulating procoagulants (Table 3–2) that, when activated by a preceding event in the clotting cascade, promote fibrin forma-

TABLE 3–2. SUBSTANCES IN THE BLOOD

FACTOR	NAME	SYNONYM	ACTIVATED FORM
I	Fibrinogen	Fibrin	
II	Prothrombin	Thrombin	
III	Tissue thromboplastin	Tissue factor	
IV	Calcium ions		
V	Proaccelerin	Labile factor, Ac globulin	V^a
VI			
VII	Proconnectin	Serum prothrombin conversion accelerator	VII_a
VIII	Antihemophilic factor	Antihemophilic globulin Antihemophilic factor A	
	VIII:C	Coagulant subcomponent of AHF	$VIII:C_a$
	VIII:VWF	von Willebrand factor	
IX	Christmas factor	Plasma thromboplastin component	IX_a
X	Stuart-Prower factor		X_a
XI	Plasma thromboplastin antecedent	Antihemophilic factor C	XI_a
XII	Hageman factor		XII_a
XIII	Fibrin stabilizing factor		XIII_a

TABLE 3–3.   INHIBITORS OF COAGULATION

Blood flow
Endothelial factors
Circulating anticoagulants
  Antithrombin III
  Protein C
  Protein S
  Heparin co-factor II
  Alpha-1 antitrypsin
Fibrinolytic systems
  Tissue plasminogen activator
  Prourinokinase

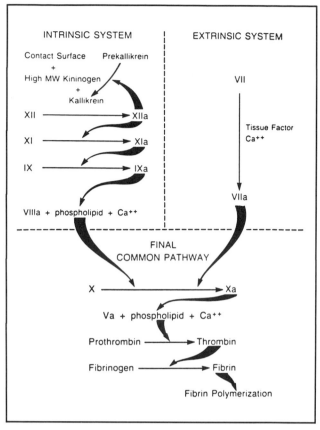

FIGURE 3–1.   The intrinsic system, the extrinsic system, and the final common pathway of all coagulation cascades. (Reprinted from Farmer, J.C., and Parker, R.I.: Coagulation: Essential physiologic concerns. *In* Civetta, J.M., Taylor, R.W., and Kirby, R.R. (eds.): Critical Care. Philadelphia, J.B. Lippincott Co., 1988, pp. 1461–1468. Figure 128.1, p. 1463.)

tion. Other substances in the blood (Table 3–3 act as anticoagulants. Whether or not blood clotting occurs depends on a delicate balance between these two groups of substances. Under normal circumstances, anticoagulants predominate and blood does not clot. However, coagulation of the blood begins within seconds of an injury to the vascular endothelium.

The Final Common Pathway of all Coagulation Cascades (Fig. 3–1).

The traditional clotting cascade culminates in the formation of fibrin, a polymer of fibrinogen, under the influence of thrombin. Thrombin has been activated in turn from its inactive plasma precursor, prothrombin, by the enzymatic action of a prothrombinase complex composed of factors X_a and V_a, calcium, and platelets plus endothelial membrane lipoprotein. These three steps are the final common pathway of all coagulation systems.

The final common pathway has some permutations. Activated factor X is the protease that splits prothrombin to thrombin. Activated factor V accelerates the protease activity, and the tissue and platelet phospholipids act as the assembly mechanism.

Fibrin is initially formed from fibrinogen (MW 340,000) by the splitting off of fibrinopeptide A, which permits polymerization to begin by electrostatic forces. Thrombin acts as the enzyme for this step and also for the splitting off of fibrinopeptide B. Fibrin polymerizes both end-to-end and side-to-side, resulting in a network. The cross-linking of fibrin polymer is catalyzed by activated factor XIII, a fibrin-stabilizing factor, which itself is activated by thrombin. Activated factor XIII also serves as a stimulant to fibroblast growth.

Clot retraction depends on fibrin binding to receptors on activated platelets, the actinomycin microfilaments of which contract.

The Extrinsic Pathway to Prothrombinase (Fig. 3–1).   Two pathways lead to prothrombinase complex, the extrinsic and intrinsic pathways. In the extrinsic system, the phospholipids come from traumatized tissues extrinsic to the blood, whereas in the

intrinsic system, phospholipids come from traumatized platelets intrinsic to the blood. The extrinsic pathway to prothrombinase is activated when blood comes into contact with traumatized tissue, resulting in the release of phospholipids and glycoproteins, which together are called tissue thromboplastin. This substance forms a complex with blood coagulation factor VII and, in the presence of calcium ions, results in activated factor VII, which activates factor X. Activated factor X, the catalytic component of prothrombinase, is critical to the final common pathway. Since the assembly mechanism for prothrombinase requires platelets, platelets are obviously activated as well. Although factor VII is a part of the extrinsic pathway, it can activate factor IX of the intrinsic pathway to a limited degree.

The Intrinsic Pathway to Prothrombinase (Fig. 3–1).   The intrinsic pathway also terminates with activation of prothrombinase, but begins with trauma to the cellular elements of the blood most readily by exposure to collagen. When factor XII (Hageman factor) comes into contact with collagen, a negatively charged surface, its configuration undergoes a conformational change and it becomes activated. Activated factor XII then activates factor XI in the presence of high molecular weight kininogen, a precursor of bradykinin, and of prekallikrein. Activated factor XII cleaves prekallikrein to kallikrein, which in turn activates still more factor XII. Activated factor XI acts enzymatically to activate factor IX. Activated factor IX acts with factor VIII and phospholipids from the injured platelets to activate factor X and the final common pathway.

Factor VIII is composed of two separate glycoprotein moieties. the smaller of the two (VII:C) is the procoagulant glycoprotein, normally made by the liver, that is absent in hemophilia A. It is also the factor influenced by thrombin to form activated factor VIII. Activated factor VIII is inactivated by protein C. The other portion of factor VIII is factor VIII:R or von Willebrand factor (VWF), which is synthesized by endothelial cells and megakaryocytes. It is necessary for normal platelet adherence to subendothelial structures when endothelial damage occurs.

The intrinsic pathway can be amplified at two major points. The first occurs as factor XII and prekallikrein are activated and stimulate further activation of factor XII. The second occurs via the feedback of activated factor VIII on factor IX. Activated factor IX activates factor VIII, which increases the activation of factor IX.

Calcium ions are required for all but the first two steps in the intrinsic pathway. Calcium levels in the body rarely fall to levels low enough to interfere with clotting. Blood can be prevented from clotting in a tube by reducing the calcium ion concentration with citrate or EDTA.

In the body, clotting is initiated by both the intrinsic and extrinsic pathways after injury, with tissue thromboplastin initiating the extrinsic pathway and contact of factor XII and platelets with collagen activating the intrinsic pathway. In a test tube, the intrinsic pathway alone initiates clotting as factor XII, and platelets are activated by contact with a foreign substance.

The extrinsic pathway causes large amounts of clot to be formed in seconds and is limited only by the amount of tissue thromboplastin released and the amounts of factor VII, X, and V available. The intrinsic pathway requires several minutes to form a clot and can be blocked by a number of inhibitors. In clinical practice, the extrinsic pathway is monitored by measuring the prothrombin time (PT), whereas the intrinsic pathway is monitored by the partial thromboplastin time or accelerated partial thromboplastin time (aPTT). The rate-limiting step in hemostasis is the formation of the prothrombinase complex. The subsequent formation of thrombin and fibrin occurs very rapidly. Prothrombin is a plasma protein with a molecular weight of 68,700. It is an unstable protein that splits into two smaller molecules, one of which is thrombin. Prothrombin, like all the procoagulants except VWF, is produced by the liver and requires vitamin K for its production, as does factors VII, IX, and X. In hepatic failure, levels of prothrombin fall below that required for coagulation in about 24 hours.

Thrombin is a proteolytic enzyme that cleaves four low molecular weight peptides from fibrinogen. Thrombin acts on other clotting factors, in addition to fibrinogen. It acts on prothrombin to split it into more thrombin. It also increases the activity of factors XII, XI, X, IX, and VIII and platelet aggregation.

Thus, thrombin is critically important in normal coagulation. It is released almost immediately after injury to an endothelial surface. Thrombin then stimulates platelet aggregation and granule release and modifies factor V to increase its binding affinity, thereby increasing the rate of factor X activation. It also plays a role in activating factor XIII to stabilize the fibrin monomer.

A number of clotting factors are vitamin K dependent, including factors II, VII, IX, and X. They share the unique characteristic of having gamma-carboxyl glutamic acid in the amino acid sequence. Without vitamin K, these proteins do not undergo gamma-carboxylation and are thus inactive in coagulation. Calcium ion is required for the functioning of all these factors. A reciprocal relationship exists between a number of clotting factors, such as factors VII and IX, wherein activation of one results in amplification of the other. Thus, activation of vitamin K-dependent factors occurs through proteolytic cleavage of the proteins in the presence of calcium ions. Generally, there are positive feedback loops between the four vitamin K-dependent factors.

CONTROL OF COAGULATION (TABLE 3–3)

Blood Flow

Formation of the blood clot does not go unchecked. Perhaps the most important control is the continued rapid flow of blood, which carries away thrombin, the other procoagulants, and products of platelet activation. The diluted circulating procoagulants are then removed within minutes by the reticuloendothelial system.

The clotting system is modulated in many other ways to prevent clotting in normal vessels, as well as to ensure that clotting initiated with vessel injury does not propagate beyond the immediate site of injury. In the absence of a regulatory system, 1 mL of blood could activate all the fibrinogen in 3 L of blood.

Role of the Endothelium

An intact endothelium is the most important mechanism to maintain liquid blood. The endothelium is covered with a single layer of a negatively charged protein that repels clotting factors and platelets and thus is thrombus resistant. If neither factor XII nor platelets are activated, coagulation cannot be initiated. The intact endothelium around a growing clot has additional mechanisms to minimize clot propagation. Thrombomodulin on endothelial surfaces binds thrombin, thus removing it; furthermore the thrombin:thrombomodulin complex activates protein C. Intact endothelium synthesizes prostacyclin (prostaglandin I_2), which inhibits platelet aggregation. In fact, endothelium is stimulated by thrombin to make prostacyclin and can use the endoperoxides of platelets for this synthesis.

Role of the Fibrin Clot

When thrombin is formed from prothrombin, most of it becomes attached and inactivated by the strands of fibrin as they polymerize. Thus, the fibrin strands themselves serve an anticoagulant function. Furthermore, tissue plasminogen activator is released by damaged endothelial cells, ensuring lysis at the periphery of the damaged tissue. Tissue plasminogen activator activity is amplified many times by its binding to fibrin so that lysis is concentrated near the clot itself.

Circulating Anticoagulants

A number of circulating anticoagulants also exist in blood (Table 3–3). The most important of them act within the final common pathway to reduce the activity of thrombin or are activated by thrombin and inhibit a component of the prothrombinase complex. Antithrombin III (AT III) is an alpha globulin that, when combined with thrombin, blocks the enzymatic effect of thrombin on fibrinogen, as well as on the prothrombinase complex. To a lesser degree it blocks all of the proteases in the coagulation cascade except factor XIII (fibrin-stabilizing factor). Antithrombin III is so important that its deficiency is associated with abnormal coagulation, in part because it inhibits fibrinolysis as well.

The activity of antithrombin III is increased dramatically by heparin. Heparin is a circulating anticoagulant found in small concentrations. It is a conjugated, highly negatively charged polysaccharide. The AT III-heparin complex also removes factors XII, XI, IX, and X (the intrinsic pathway factors), further increasing its effect as an anticoagulant.

Though heparin is produced by many different cells in the body, it is predominantly made by basophilic mast cells found in the pericapillary connective tissue, especially in the lung and to a lesser extent in the liver—sites where thrombus in the venous circulation commonly lodge. A small amount is also secreted by circulating basophils. Heparin co-factor II aids heparin's antithrombin effect.

Other anticoagulant factors also counteract the final common pathway. Protein C is a naturally occurring anticoagulant that is activated by thrombin. It reduces thrombin formation by inactivating activated factor V and VIII, both of which are important in forming the prothrombinase complex. Activation of protein C is greatly accelerated on the surface of endothelial cells that produce thrombomodulin that binds thrombin to the vascular wall. Protein C also activates plasminogen, but only in the presence of protein S. Both protein C and S are vitamin-K-dependent proteins, as are proteins M and Z, whose role in coagulation is not yet clearly defined. Protein M appears to be a procoagulant enzyme involved in the activation of prothrombin to thrombin. The exact function of protein Z is unknown.

Fibrinolysis (Table 3–4)

Plasminogen is a plasma glycoprotein made primarily in the liver, which when activated becomes plasmin or fibrinolysin. Plasminogen levels in plasma tend to parallel fibrinogen levels and are thus increased after trauma and inflammation. Plasmin is a proteolytic enzyme that breaks down many of the clotting factors found in blood, including fibrin, fibrinogen, and prothrombin, as well as factors V, VIII, and XII. Plasminogen can be converted to plasmin by a component of the clotting cascade, thrombin, as well as by activated factor XII and lysosomal enzymes from damaged tissues.

Tissue plasminogen activator (tPA) is produced by vascular (especially venous) endothelial cells. The production of tPA is increased by such drugs as vasopressin and epinephrine and also by anoxia or damage to the endothelium, so that vessels with stagnant flow do not clot. Another important stimulator of tPA production by endothelium is protein C, a plasma protein enzymatically activated by thrombin, which thus plays an additional important role in modulating clot formation. tPA fibrinolytic activity is limited to the site of fibrin formation because it activates plasminogen only in the presence of fibrin. Thus, tPA does not produce widespread generalized systemic fibrinolysis.

TABLE 3–4. INHIBITORS OF FIBRINOLYSIS

α-2 Plasmin inhibitor
Histidine-rich glycoprotein
α-2 Macroglobulin
C-1 esterase inhibitor
Activated protein C inhibitor

Plasmin destroys not only fibrin but also fibrinogen. Plasmin activity is itself controlled by two additional plasma inhibitors, alpha-2-antiplasmin and alpha-2-macroglobulin (Table 3–4). These compounds serve to inactivate plasmin that may enter the systemic circulation. Therefore, their absence produces bleeding tendencies.

Other enzymes capable of activating plasminogen to plasmin are found in various bodily fluids, tears, colostrum, and semen. Urokinase, found in renal tubular cells and urine, acts directly as a proteolytic enzyme on plasminogen so that, unlike tPA, it does not require fibrin. Streptokinase is a compound formed by beta-hemolytic strains of streptococci that is able to convert plasminogen to plasmin. It activates plasminogen by binding with the plasminogen molecule. This streptokinase/plasminogen complex cleaves a second molecule of plasminogen into plasmin.

Plasmin digests fibrinogen and fibrin at multiple sites on the fibrin molecule, resulting in a variety of compounds known as fibrin degradation products. When fibrin monomers are acted upon by activated factor XIII, they form stable cross-linkages between their strands. When plasmin digests this stable form of fibrin, a unique product called the D-dimer is formed. Increased amounts of D-dimer in the serum indicate active fibrinolysis. Fibrinolysis can be blocked by the drug, epsilon-aminocaproic acid.

Plasmin is not a very specific protease. In addition to its effect on procoagulants, it activates the complement cascade, converts C_5 to C_{5a}, fragments factor XII, and releases kinins from kininogens.

CLINICAL TESTS OF COAGULATION AND HEMOSTASIS

Measurement of the prothrombin time (PT) assesses the functional capacity of the extrinsic system. To perform this test, plasma is incubated with thromboplastin (rabbit brain tissue), which serves to initiate the extrinsic cascade. Factor VII is then activated and subsequently activates the prothrombinase complexes of X_a, V_a, Ca^{++}, and phospolipids, permitting thrombin and fibrinogen formation. Thus, PT is prolonged by deficient levels of factors VII, X, V, II, or I. Because factors VII, X, and II are vitamin K dependent, PT is prolonged in patients receiving coumarin anticoagulants.

The activated partial thromboplastin time (aPTT) measures the functional capabilities of the intrinsic system. In this test plasma is incubated with a substance with a negatively charged surface to activate the "contact factors." A partial thromboplastin and calcium ion are also added so that the vitamin-K-dependent factors in the final common pathway will be stimulated. Thus, the aPTT assesses factors XII, XI, IX, and VIII of the intrinsic pathway, as well as factors X, V, II, and I in the final common pathway. It does not measure factor VII.

Heparin, a naturally occurring anticoagulant, stimulates AT III, which inactivates thrombin, as well as factors XII, XI, X, and IX. Thus, heparin administration blocks the intrinsic system and results in prolongation of the aPTT.

Patients with hemophilia A are deficient in factor VIII. Hemophilia B, a much rarer problem, occurs in patients deficient in factor IX. Both diseases result in prolongation of the aPTT. In patients with hemophilia A or B, the prolonged aPTT can be corrected by the addition of normal serum to their serum, thus supplying the missing clotting factors. If the aPTT is still prolonged and is not corrected by the addition of normal serum, the likely cause is not hemophilia, but rather the presence of a circulating anticoagulant, such as the lupus anticoagulant. A subcomponent of the antihemophilic factor enhances the adherence of platelets to subendothelium exposed in vascular injury. This factor, known as von Willebrand's factor, is not deficient in classic hemophilia. When deficient in Von Willebrand's disease, patients have symptoms of mildly increased bleeding tendency.

The thrombin time measures the conversion of fibrinogen to fibrin. In this test, thrombin is incubated with plasma, and the time to appearance of a fibrin clot is measured. This test is thus abnormal in the presence of heparin, as well as fibrin degradation product and dysfibrinogens. Direct immunoassays for most clotting factors are now available.

COMMON DRUGS AFFECTING CLOTTING

Heparin is a naturally occurring glucosaminoglycan, which inhibits the coagulation process by forming a complex with AT III. This complex inactivates thrombin and factors VII, IX, X, and XI. The half-life of heparin at the usual systemic dose of 100 units/kg is about 1 hour. The half-life is dose related; with increasing doses, it is prolonged. The effect of heparin is best determined by the a PTT. Generally, its effect is reversed by the administration of protamine. One milligram of protamine generally neutralizes 100 units (or 1 mg) of heparin.

Warfarin affects the vitamin-K-dependent factors (II, VII, IX, and X) by competitive binding at the vitamin K receptor site in the liver. It does so because of its similar chemical structure to the 4-hydroxycoumarin nucleus and the naphthoquine ring. In the presence of warfarin, the factors are made, but are inactive. Although all vitamin-K-dependent factors are depleted, factor VII has a half-life of only 2 to 4 hours, and factor VII function is the most sensitive indicator of warfarin effect. The PT is prolonged by warfarin.

Warfarin is metabolized by the liver. Chronic liver failure with decreased production of clotting factors and decreased breakdown of warfarin can result in a significant anticoagulant effect from even small amounts of warfarin. Overtreatment with warfarin is corrected by the administration of fresh-frozen plasma, which provides the missing clotting factors. Vitamin K may be administered, but will not correct the coagulopathy until it has been processed by the liver. This processing generally requires 12 to 24 hours, but may take longer in patients with hepatic dysfunction.

Protein C and S are both vitamin-K-dependent, naturally occurring anticoagulants. warfarin treatment has been reported in certain patients to produce lowered protein C levels to a greater degree than do vitamin-K-dependent clotting factors, resulting in a hypercoagulable state and small vessel thrombosis.

DISORDERS OF CLOTTING IN STRESS, TRAUMA, AND SURGERY

Disseminated intravascular coagulation (DIC) occurs most commonly in patients who are critically ill with a variety of disorders. In this pathologic process, activation of the clotting system results in excess thrombin formation, subsequent fibrin thrombi scattered throughout the body, and consumption of clotting factors and platelets. DIC may be caused either by disease processes that enzymatically activate procoagulant proteins or that cause the release of tissue factors that initiate the coagulation process. Fibrinolysis occurs subsequent to thrombin formation. Plasmin is formed, and fibrin clot is then lysed. Therefore, DIC occurs as an imbalance between (1) thrombin activity leading to thrombus formation and consumption of clotting factors and (2) plasmin, which degrades the fibrin clot. Tissue injury and ischemia often accompany DIC. The products of fibrinogen degradation, fibrinopeptides A and B, are vasoconstrictors that can result in worsening of the tissue ischemia. DIC can be suspected in patients with the proper clinical setting and with prolonged PT and aPTT, low platelet counts, and decreased fibrinogen levels. The presence of fibrin degradation products, specifically D-dimer into serum, supports the diagnosis. Factors II, V, and VIII may be decreased in DIC.

Since nearly all clotting factors are synthesized in the liver, hepatic failure is commonly associated with bleeding disorders. In liver failure, factors II, VII, IX, and X—the vitamin-K-dependent factors—are commonly reduced. In addition, factor V is usually low.

Fibrinogen synthesis is usually maintained until terminal liver failure is imminent. Only a portion of the factor VIII molecule is synthesized by the liver, another portion of the molecule is synthesized by the vascular endothelium. Factors that control coagulation, such as proteins C and AT III, are also produced by the liver, and low levels of these agents in failing livers may account for a hypercoagulable state.

Factor VII has a half-life of only 4 to 6 hours. For this reason, the PT is prolonged in patients with liver failure and is an accurate measure of hepatic function. As the vitamin-K-dependent factors begin to fall, factor V falls also.

Vitamin K is necessary for the gamma-carboxylation of factors II, VII, IX, and X. Without vitamin K, these factors are formed, but are inactive. Vitamin K deficiency most commonly occurs as a result of inhibition by broad-spectrum antibiotics of bacteria that produce vitamin K within the gut. Malnutrition is a less common cause of vitamin K deficiency, as it takes about 2 weeks for vitamin K levels to fall low enough to be significant in the absence of vitamin K intake. For this reason, vitamin K should be given to patients on parenteral alimentation. Since vitamin K is fat soluble, fat malabsorption may be associated with vitamin K deficiency, as in pancreatic or biliary tract disease.

Patients requiring massive blood transfusion may develop a coagulopathy. Factors V and VIII have a short half-life in banked blood and are usually absent by 48 hours. In addition, platelets lose their function quickly in banked blood so that dilutional thrombocytopenia is common after massive transfusion. Although calcium ion is required for activation of the vitamin-K-dependent clotting factors, coagulopathy secondary to low ionized calcium levels is rare. Ionized calcium concentration in the blood can be lowered by the citrate used in the storage of banked blood, but it rarely becomes a problem unless blood is transfused at a rate of greater than 100 cc/min for more than 5 minutes.

Hypercoagulable states

A number of conditions exist that result in hypercoagulable states. One such condition is AT III deficiency, an inherited disorder. Patients with this condition commonly present with recurrent arterial or venous thrombosis and emboli. Because its mechanism of action requires AT III, herparin is not an effective anticoagulant in these patients.

The lupus anticoagulant was first described in patients with systemic lupus erythematosus (SLE), but is more commonly found in other conditions. Blood from such patients does not clot because of the circulating anticoagulant. In contrast with patients with hemophilia, in whom the aPTT returns to normal with the addition of normal plasma that supplies the missing clotting factor, addition or normal plasma to blood from patients with a lupus anticoagulant does not correct the aPTT. The lupus anticoagulant is an anticardiolipin antibody that interferes with phospholipids and lipoproteins, which interact with the coagulation factors when the aPTT or PT is measured. The aPTT is usually affected more than the PT. Although it is called a lupus anticoagulant, in clinical practice these patients are hypercoagulable, and many thrombotic events have been described in them.

Decreased plasminogen levels may be associated with the hypercoagulable state, since plasminogen in clots is activated by tPA, a naturally occurring fibrinolytic promoter. If the plasminogen level in a blood clot is low, the clot cannot be lysed, and thrombosis may go unchecked.

Dysfibrinogenemia has been associated with the hypercoagulable state, although excessive bleeding can occur. Patients may also have hyperfibrinogenemia. When there is an excess of fibrinogen, clotting may be incomplete, and fibrin fragments that inhibit further clot formation may be present, thus resulting in bleeding.

BIBLIOGRAPHY

1. Guyton, A.C.: Hemostasis and blood coagulation. Textbook of Medical Physiology, 7th ed. Philadelphia, W.B. Saunders Co., 1986, pp. 76–87.
2. Farmer, J.C., and Parker, R.I. Coagulation: Essential physiologic concerns. *In* Civetta, J.M., Taylor, R.W., and Kirby, R.R. (eds.): Critical Care. Philadelphia, J.B. Lippincott Co., 1988, pp. 1461–1468.
3. Rutledge, R., and Sheldon, G.: Bleeding and coagulation. *In* Davis, J. (ed.). Clinical Surgery. St. Louis, C.V. Mosby Co., 1987, pp. 635–646.
4. Ratnoff, O.D.: Hemostasis and coagulation. *In* Berne, R.M., and Levy, M.N. (eds.). Physiology, 2nd ed. St. Louis, C.V. Mosby Co. 1988, pp. 371–394.
5. Mosher, D.F.: Disorders of blood coagulation. *In* Wyngaarden, J.B., and Smith, L.H. (eds.): Cecil Textbook of Medicine. Philadelphia, W.B. Saunders Co., 1988, pp. 1060–1081.
6. West, J.B. (ed.): Blood coagulation. *In* Best and Taylors Physiological Basis of Medical Practice, 11th ed. Baltimore, Williams & Wilkins, 1985, pp. 417–425.
7. Bithell, T.C.: Normal hemostasis and coagulation. *In* Thorup, O.A. (ed.): Leavell and Thorup's Fundamentals of Clinical Hematology, 5th ed. Philadelphia, W.B. Saunders 1987, pp. 126–162.

Part II

RESPONSE TO INJURY

4

WOUND HEALING

HOWARD D. EDINGTON

The process of wound healing concerns the tissue response to injury. An understanding of both normal and pathological wound-healing responses as well as their regulation enables a rational clinical approach to a number of diverse disease processes which may be caused by an abnormal or undesirable response to injury. Examples include pulmonary fibrosis, hepatic cirrhosis, keloid scar formation, and burns, as well as poorly defined wound-healing problems in immunosuppressed and diabetic patients. Despite dramatic advances in cellular and molecular biology which have generated a large body of information about wound healing, an understanding of the critical regulatory phenomena in wound healing remains limited.

Neoplasia, embryogenesis, and regeneration seem to share common themes with wound healing and may differ from each other solely in key regulatory steps—perhaps gene expression and translation. For example, neoplastic transformation involves the transcription and expression of oncogene products. Similar proteins are also involved in normal human wound healing.

Platelet-derived growth factor (PDGF), which plays an integral role in normal wound healing, has a striking 93 per cent amino acid homology with an oncogene protein product ($p28^{V-sis}$) derived from simian sarcoma virus, a transforming retrovirus. This suggests a more than casual mechanistic relationship between processes of normal wound healing and neoplastic transformation.

Regeneration involves cellular dedifferentiation, migration, proliferation, and subsequent redifferentiation. Similar cellular processes occur both during embryogenesis and wound healing. Epimorphic regeneration describes the complete regeneration of amputated limbs—a process best studied in amphibians. The same amputation in a more advanced vertebrate would heal by scar formation (fibrosis) and cicatricial closure of the wound with minimal regeneration of form and function. Fibrosis is minimal in regeneration and fetal wound healing. The apparent similarities between fetal wound healing and regeneration and the clinical observation that newborn or premature infants may occasionally regenerate traumatically amputated digits suggests that in adult humans, the regenerative process may be suppressed rather than irretrievably lost. This suppression presumably occurs at the level of gene expression. Exploration of these regulatory phenomena has obvious clinical implications.

In humans, the wound-healing response is traditionally divided into three phases: inflammation, fibroplasia, and maturation (Fig. 4–1), but the later phases of inflammation and the early phases of fibroplasia are better described in terms of the cellular events, namely stages of cell migration and proliferation. The steps overlap broadly with each other, and the process is a continuum rather than a series of discrete steps.

DESCRIPTIVE OVERVIEW

A disturbance of blood vessel integrity exposing the blood to collagen and subendothelial parenchyma is generally considered the initiating factor in wound healing. Even this initial phase is complex: Blood extravasates, contorts tissue surfaces, and initiates an acute inflammatory response; concurrently a hemostatic response is initiated. Hemostasis consists of three components: vasoconstriction, platelet activation, and coagulation. An initial period of intense vasoconstriction follows direct vascular trauma. Platelets are activated, they aggregate, and the clotting cascade is initiated (Chapter 3, Hemostasis and Coagulation). Both the kininogen and complement cascades are activated, leading to vasodilation and increased capillary permeability. Injury activates local factors which lead to an orderly and predictable migration of cells into the wound. A cascade of cell activation and cytokine release ensues which orchestrates mitotic and synthetic events of the immigrating cells. The migratory phase is initiated within hours.

41

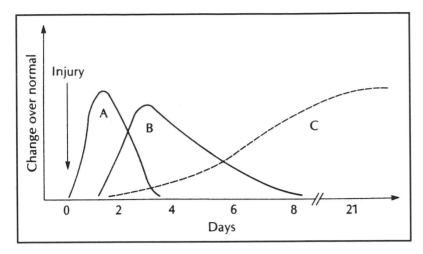

FIGURE 4–1. Schematic diagram of the three phases of wound healing. **A:** Inflammation. **B:** Fibroplasia. **C:** Maturation. (Reprinted from Mathes, S.J. and Abouljoud, M.: Wound healing. *In* Davis, J.H. (ed.): Clinical Surgery. St. Louis, C.V. Mosby Co., Fig. 16–3, p. 475, 1987.)

An efflux of polymorphonuclear leukocytes from the vascular space rapidly follows, with phagocytic elimination of bacteria from the wound. Although neutrophils decrease infection, they are not essential to normal healing of sterile wounds. The second cell to make its appearance, the blood monocyte or tissue macrophage, is not only phagocytic, but is of central importance in regulating subsequent cellular activities in the wound-healing process.

Fibroblasts migrate into the wound during the first week and the proliferative phase of fibroplasia begins. Fibroblasts not only multiply and migrate, but elaborate both interstitial matrix and collagen. During this phase endothelial proliferation and migration take place with the formation of new blood vessels—angiogenesis. The migratory and synthetic activities of the fibroblast are orchestrated by cytokines released by both macrophages and fibroblasts themselves. Additional processes characterizing the fibroplasia stage of wound repair include wound contraction and reepithelialization. Each process represents an interplay of cell division and migration, cell-to-cell interactions, and cell-matrix interactions, modulated presumably by growth factors and possibly by inhibitory factors or chalones.

The final—or maturation—phase is one of indeterminant duration. Fibroblasts and macrophages, whose presence dominated the fibroblastic phase of wound healing, gradually disappear, and the wound becomes relatively acellular. The nature of the ground matrix elaborated during fibroplasia changes, and its structure undergoes prolonged remodeling. Our present understanding of this phase revolves around an interplay between collagen synthesis and collagen degradation. While a good deal is known about activation steps, less is known about processes that control, regulate, or delimit the observed sequence of events.

INFLAMMATION

The acute inflammatory response is actually composed of events which can be separated for descriptive purposes; a vascular response; a platelet response; coagulation and complement cascade activation; then neutrophilic infiltration which blends with the next phase of cellular migration into the wound (Fig. 4–2). Concurrent processes include cytokine factor elaboration, monocyte migration and activation, and wound matrix formation.

Vascular and Platelet Response

The vascular response is biphasic. Vasoconstriction of the arterioles is rapid but transient, seldom lasting more than minutes. The significant mediators are products of platelets activated by contact with exposed collagen. The platelets not only aggregate and initiate coagulation, but also release serotonin and thromboxane—potent vasoconstrictors. Table 4–1 lists platelet products which play a role in other aspects of wound repair.

Vasoconstriction serves a hemostatic function but is followed promptly by vasodilation that permits blood-borne factors to enter the wound. The initial phase of vasodilation is mediated by histamine.

Histamine is the histidine decarboxylase product of L-histidine metabolism and is packaged in vesicles contained by mast cells, platelets, and basophils. The action of histamine is mediated via H1 and H2 cell surface receptors. H1 receptors are found on the endothelial cells, while H2 receptors are found on vascular smooth muscle cells. In humans, vasodilatation appears to be mediated by both H1 and H2 receptors functioning on different cells. This immediate increase in vascular permeability is followed by

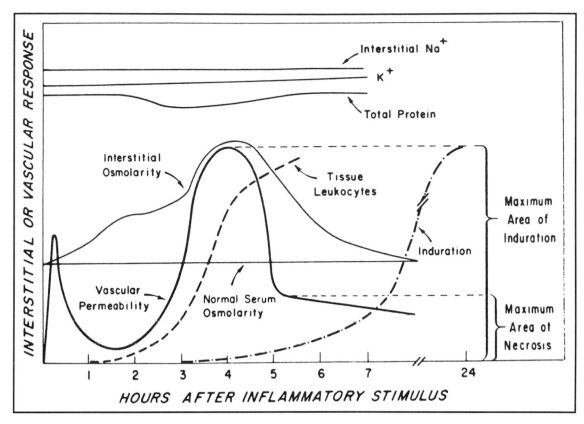

FIGURE 4–2. A comparison of the time of occurrence of events in early inflammation. Changes in interstitial composition (osmolarity; electrolyte and protein concentration) are compared with changes in vascular permeability and development of induration and tissue leukocytosis. (Reprinted from Burke, F.J. and Gelfand, J.A.: Events in early inflammation. *In* Howard, R.J. and Simmons, R.L. (eds.): Surgical Infectious Diseases, 2nd ed. Norwalk CT, Appleton & Lange, Fig. 12–1, p. 202, 1988.)

a delayed but more prolonged increase in permeability involving both capillaries and larger vessels. The junctions between epithelial cells are widened. Although the chemical mediators are unknown, direct neutrophil: endothelial cell interactions are associated with increased vascular permeability. The increased permeability and consequent edema formation probably represent an interplay of multiple systems. For example, prostaglandin E_1 and E_2 are poor edema producers themselves but augment the edema induced by histamine and bradykinin (see below).

Coagulation Response

Direct vascular disruption and increased vascular permeability result in plasma and platelet extravasation and contact with collagen and ground substance. This extravasation initiates a number of chain reactions which generate active factors that perpetuate the inflammatory response by attracting and activating inflammatory cells (neutrophils and monocytes).

Coagulation and Kinin Cascades

The two coagulation cascades—intrinsic and extrinsic—serve both a hemostatic and inflammatory function. Stimulation of the intrinsic coagulation cascade is initiated by Haageman factor activation. Activated Haageman factor (HFa) catalyzes, in turn, the formation of kallikrein from prekallikrein (Fig. 4–3). Kallikrein is a serine protease aminopeptide that liberates bradykinin by cleaving high molecular weight kininogen twice. In addition to catalyzing the formation of bradykinin, kallikrein is also active in stimulating neutrophil activation, aggregation, and secretion. Bradykinin is a very potent vasodilator that increases vascular permeability, an effect that is augmented by PGE1 and PGE2. Its effects are receptor mediated.

Activation of the extrinsic coagulation system is initiated by tissue factor (thromboplastin or pro-

TABLE 4–1.   ROLE OF PLATELET PRODUCTS IN WOUNDS

FUNCTION	MEDIATOR	SOURCE
Vasoconstruction	Thromboxane A_2 Serotonin Epinephrine	Arachidonic acid Dense bodies Dense bodies
Vasodilation	Histamine	Dense bodies
Aggregation	Thromboxane A_2	Arachidonic acid
Activates intrinsic coagulation cascade	Platelet factor 3	
Leukocyte chemotaxis	Platelet factor 4	α-granules
Fibroblast proliferation	Platelet-derived growth factor (PDGF) Serotonin	α-granules Dense bodies
Collagen synthesis	Serotonin	Dense bodies

Adapted from Mathes, S.J. and Abouljoud, M.: Wound healing. *In* Davis, J.H. (ed.): Clinical Surgery. St. Louis, C.V. Mosby Co., pp. 461–508, 1987.

coagulant activity) (see Chapter 3, Hemostasis and Coagulation). Tissue factor is expressed by activated endothelial cells, smooth muscle cells, fibroblasts, and activated neutrophils and monocytes. In addition to cell surface expression of tissue factor, activated monocytes may shed additional tissue factor in vesicles, thus increasing local concentrations of procoagulant activity. Platelet activation occurs at the Xa step (Fig. 4–3). Activation of the coagulation pathways, as well as platelet activation, serve to amplify and localize the inflammatory response.

Arachidonic Acid Metabolites

Numerous stimuli, including direct injury and C5a, activate cellular phospholipases, resulting in the production of arachidonic acid. Arachidonic acid may then serve as an intermediate for the production of prostaglandins, thromboxane A2, leukotrienes, or chemotactic lipids.

Thromboxane A2 is an unstable product of the cyclooxygenase pathway. It is released by activated platelets and causes platelet aggregation and vasoconstriction.

PGE-type prostaglandins, specifically PGE_1 and PGE_2, are intense vasodilators and act in synergy with bradykinin, histamine, and C5a to effect a marked increase in vascular permeability. Prostacy-clin (PGI_2) inhibits platelet aggregation and may induce some vasodilation.

Complement Cascade

A third set of plasma protein cascades are activated when vascular integrity is disrupted. Activation of the cascade can take place via several of the events described earlier as well as by the following:

1. Activated Hageman factor can trigger the intrinsic pathway.
2. Dead tissue can trigger the alternate cascade.
3. The complement system may be activated by platelets via C5 cleavage by platelet-bound thrombin.
4. Neutral proteases generated in response to tissue injury by leukocytes may result in the activation of C5 and C3.

All pathways lead to the generation of the two powerful anaphylatoxins, C5a and C3a. C5a is 100 to 1000 times more powerful than C3a, but C3a is much more abundant. Both C3a and C5a can degranulate mast cells and cause histamine release. In addition C5a is a powerful vasodilator whose effects are magnified by PGE_1, PGE_2, and PGI_2.

C5a is probably the most important factor leading to the margination and intravascular aggregation of neutrophils and their adhesion to vascular endothelium. Furthermore, C5a is probably the most important chemotactic substance inducing neutrophil migration into the area of injury (Fig. 4–4). The carboxyl terminal arginine of C5a is cleaved in the extravascular space by the carboxypeptidase to form C5a-DES-ARG. This C5a breakdown product maintains a somewhat reduced chemoattraction potential, but is ineffective in histamine release.

Other chemoattractants in damaged tissue that might induce neutrophil influx are platelet-derived eicosanoids of the 5-lipooxygenase pathway, including 12-HETE and 5-HETE, the vasodilator leukotriene LTB4, and platelet factor. In addition, substances with chemotactic activity have also been isolated from bacterial culture supernatants, specifically formyl-methionyl-leucyl-phenylalanine (FMLP). Neutrophils have a receptor that recognizes FMLP, and the effects of FMLP appear to be similar to those of C5a. Fibrin degradation products also attract both monocytes and neutrophils.

Growth Factors

While the exact role of growth factors in normal wound healing is not certain, in vitro growth factor activities are compelling and a physiological activity is likely. Platelet-derived growth factor (PDGF) has been studied intensively and is probably most important during the inflammatory phase. Platelet-

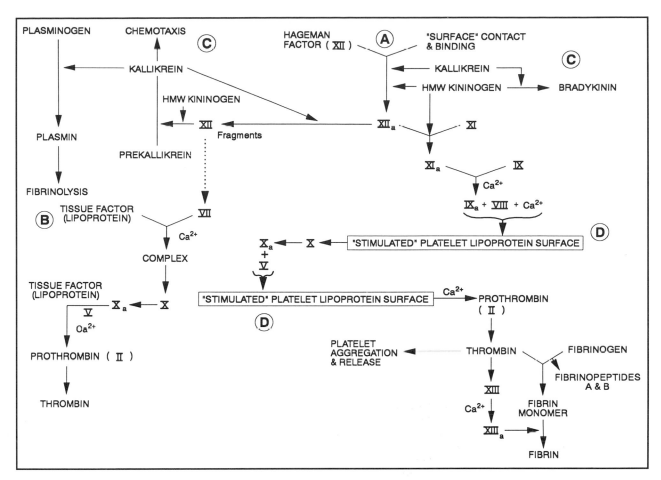

FIGURE 4–3. Outline of interactions between the intrinsic (**A**) and extrinsic (**B**) coagulation pathways with the kinin system (**C**) and activated platelets (**D**). (Modified from Schwartz, S.L.: Hemostasis, surgical bleeding, and transfusion. *In* Swartz, S.L., Shives, G.T., Spencer, F.C. (eds.): Principles of Surgery, 5th ed. New York, McGraw Hill Book Co., Fig. 3.3, p. 108, 1989.)

derived growth factor is elaborated by platelets, activated endothelial cells, activated monocytes, or macrophages, and, interestingly, by neoplastic transformed cells. PDGF is mitogenic and chemotactic for a variety of mesenchymal-type cells. Effects are receptor mediated and cell surface receptors are found on a variety of cell surfaces, including fibroblasts, some endothelial cells, chondroblasts, some embryonic cell types, osteoblasts, smooth muscle cells, and glial cells. PDGF initiates DNA synthesis and mitosis, and activates a number of genes, including the gene for beta interferon and proto-oncogenes c-myc and c-fos. PDGF also induces a reorganization of intracellular actin fibers, resulting in cell shape changes, which may be a prerequisite for cell division and perhaps locomotion and migration. PDGF stimulates the elaboration of ground matrix and collagen in the healing wound. Abnormal PDGF activity has been implicated in a number of pathological processes, including atherosclerosis,

neoplasia, and the desmoplastic response to tumors.

NEUTROPHILS AND CELL MIGRATION

Although platelets are important in setting the stage, the neutrophil is the first nucleated cell to leave the extravascular space. Its primary function appears to be phagocytic and microbicidal. The cell is not necessary for wound healing. Wound healing continues when neutrophils are depleted; however, there is less edema and an increased rate of infection. The neutrophil migrates in response to the chemotactic factors released during injury and inflammation. Vessel binding and diapedesis occur primarily in the postcapillary venule and proceed by poorly understood mechanisms which seem to represent an interplay of hemodynamic factors, includ-

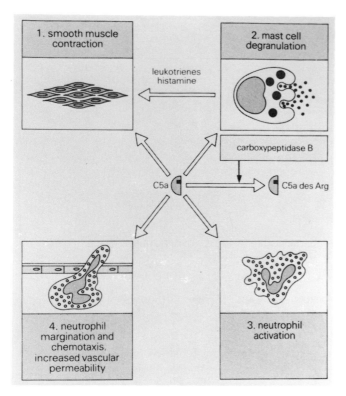

FIGURE 4–4. Biological effects of C5a and C5a des Arg. C5a causes (1) smooth muscle contraction, (2) mast cell degranulation, (3) neutrophil activation, and (4) margination and chemotaxis of neutrophils. Smooth muscle is further affected by histamine and leukotrienes released following mast cell degranulation or activation. Loss of the C-terminal arginine residue, following cleavage by carboxypeptidase B, produces C5a des Arg, which possesses weak cell-activating properties. (Reprinted from Roitt, I., Brostoff, J., and Male, D.: Immunology. St. Louis, C.V. Mosby Co., Fig. 13.20, p. 1311, 1989.)

ing sheer stress and active cellular participation by neutrophil and endothelium. Many of the chemotactic factors (C5a, FMLP, PAF) also increase the adhesion of neutrophils to the vessel wall. These substances may act by upregulation of surface adhesive glycoproteins (SAG) by the neutrophil. The endothelium itself can be stimulated to increase neutrophil binding by interleukin-1 and tumor necrosis factor, both of which are found in sterile wounds.

Neutrophil activation by various stimuli, including bacterial LPS primes release of O_2 radicals and lysosomal enzymes, including neutral proteases, elastase, and collagenases (see Chapter 5, Host Defenses). These enzymes may aid interstitial migration. Neutrophils do not return to the vascular system, but are removed by activated monocytes (macrophages). Their persistence, and in particular, the persistence of lysosomal enzyme activity, has been implicated in the pathogenesis of various pathological states, including adult respiratory distress syndrome, ulcerative colitis, emphysema, and other collagen vascular

disorders. Table 4–2 lists some of the functions of neutrophils.

Monocyte-Macrophage Migration

The monocyte-macrophage replaces the neutrophil as the dominant cell in the wound by the third or fourth day. Monocytes also migrate into the wound from the vascular system, even though macrophages are present in all tissues. Once the monocyte has left the vascular system, it is referred to as a macrophage. Unlike the neutrophil, the macrophage is essential for normal wound healing and is probably the central cell regulating the proliferative phases of wound healing. In animals depleted of macrophages (and monocytes), wounds heal poorly with minimal debridement and significantly impaired fibroplasia. The signals which induce macrophages to accumulate have been less well studied than those signals which attract neutrophils. Chemotactic stimuli may include matrix components (collagen, fibronectin, elastin), products of the coagulation cascade (C5a, thrombin, fibrinopeptides), and cell and bacterial products (platelet factor IV, FMLP).

After leaving the vascular space, the monocyte must differentiate into the inflammatory or responsive macrophage. This differentiation or activation step is triggered by components of the wound matrix including fibronectin.

Some of the roles of macrophages in wounds are listed in Table 4–3. The process of debridement includes not only removal of microbes and cellular debris, but also degradation of the extracellular connective tissue matrix by enzyme secretion and

TABLE 4–2. NEUTROPHIL PRODUCTS WITH A ROLE IN INFLAMMATION

1. **Free radicals:** damage to endothelium, increase in vascular permeability, production of chemotactic lipids from arachidonic acid.
2. **Cyclooxygenase products of arachidonic acid:** platelet aggregation, contraction of vascular smooth muscle.
3. **Lipo-oxygenase products of arachidonic acid:** leukocyte chemotaxis, increased vascular permeability.
4. **Proteases (collagenase, elastase):** tissue destruction, release of kinin-line peptide from kininogen (kininogen-activating factor), complement activation.
5. **Antiproteases (alpha-1-antitrypsin, alpha-2-macroglobulin):** modulation and control of extracellular degradation of structural proteins.
6. **Band 2 protein (arginine-rich-polypeptide):** mast cell rupture, increased vascular permeability.

Reprinted from Mathes, S.J. and Abouljoud, M.: Wound healing. *In* Davis, J.H. (ed.): Clinical Surgery. St. Louis, C.V. Mosby Co., p. 463, 1987.

TABLE 4–3. MACROPHAGE PRODUCTS MEDIATING INFLAMMATION AND REPAIR

1. Neutral proteases: plasminogen activator, collagenase, and elastase
2. Complement factors
3. Reactive oxygen metabolites
4. Growth-promoting factors for fibroblasts and microvessels
5. Arachidonic acid metabolites with vasoactive and chemotactic properties
6. Fibronectin: structural and functional roles
7. Interleukin-1: lymphocyte activator, stimulates collagenase synthesis by fibroblasts
8. Enzyme inhibitors: plasmin and alpha-2-macroglobulin

Reprinted from Mathes, S.J. and Abouljoud, M.: Wound healing. *In* Davis, J.H. (ed.). Clinical Surgery. St. Louis, C.V. Mosby Co., p. 464, 1987.

phagocytosis. The macrophage further regulates matrix remodeling by elaborating one or more cytokines (macrophage-derived growth factors—MDGF). It is likely that MDGF represents a number of regulatory substances whose identities are yet to be defined. Activities consistent with platelet-derived growth factor, transforming growth factors (TGFα, TGFβ), IL-1, tumor necrosis factor (TNF), and IL-6 have been identified. Some of these factors have systemic effects: IL-1 and IL-6 induce fever; TNF functions to induce malaise; IL-6 stimulates production of acute phase proteins by the liver. IL-1 stimulates collagenase production by fibroblasts, while other macrophage-derived growth factors increase fibroblast collagen production. The regulatory steps balancing these activities are not yet clear.

TGF-β is released by platelets and activated lymphocytes, as well as macrophages. It is a very potent chemoattractant for macrophages. TNF-α is also elaborated by activated macrophages. In addition to its well-publicized tumorlytic activity, TNF-α stimulates angiogenesis. In summary, the macrophage plays an active role in the wound debridement and matrix remodeling. The macrophage regulates other cellular activities via cytokine elaboration, and plays a major role in stimulating angiogenesis and fibroplasia.

Formation of the Wound Matrix

The wounded tissue is composed not only of cells but also extracellular space which is filled with macromolecules forming an extracellular matrix. This matrix is composed of fibrous proteins embedded in a hydrated polysaccharide gel, both of which are secreted by fibroblasts. The fibrous proteins have two functions: some are important to the structure (collagen, elastin), and others are adhesive (fibronectin, laminin). The gel is composed of polysaccharide glycosaminoglycans (GAGs) linked to proteins (proteoglycans). The hydrated gel permits diffusion of nutrients to cells; the fibers hold it together; the adhesive proteins attach the cells to the matrix; fibronectin anchors the fibroblast and laminin is part of the basal lamina that promotes the attachment of epithelial cells.

Four main groups of glycosaminoglycans have been chemically differentiated: (1) hyaluronic acid, (2) chondroitin sulfate and dermatan sulfate, (3) heparin sulfate, and (4) keratan sulfate (Table 4–4). Hyaluronic acid is not bound to protein and seems to facilitate cellular migration during repair, after which it is degraded by hyaluronidase. The role of proteoglycans in wound repair is not clear.

Fibronectin seems to play a very important role in wound repair. Fibronectins are linear glycoproteins (molecular weight 440–500 kD) with a modular cell/matrix-binding structure. This structure encourages cell-to-cell and cell-to-substrate interactions. Fibronectin is one of the most intensively studied members of the integrin cell surface adhesive molecule family which also includes thrombospondin, von

TABLE 4–4. MUCOPOLYSACCHARIDES OF CONNECTIVE TISSUE AND THEIR LOCATION IN THE BODY

	SYNONYMS	DISACCHARIDE REPEATING UNIT	LOCATION
Chondroitin	—	Glucuronic acid + galactosamine	Cornea
Chondroitin-4-sulfate	Chondroitin sulfate A	Glucuronic acid + 4 sulfo-galactosamine	Aorta, cornea, bone
Chondroitin-6-sulfate	Chondroitin sulfate C	Glucuronic acid + 6 sulfo-galactosamine	Tendon, costal cartilage, umbilical cord, nucleus pulposus
Dermatan sulfate	Chondroitin sulfate B	Iduronic acid + 4 sulfo-galactosamine	Skin, heart valves, aorta
Heparin sulfate	Heparitin sulfate	Glucuronic acid + glucosamine	Aorta
Keratan sulfate	Keratosulfate	Galactose + sulfo-glucosamine	Cornea, fetal skeleton
Hyaluronic acid	—	Glucuronic acid + glucosamine	Cartilage

Reprinted from Mathes, S.J. and Abouljoud, M.: Wound healing. *In* Davis, J.H. (ed.): Clinical Surgery. St. Louis, C.V. Mosby Co., Table 16-4, p. 474, 1987.

Willebrand factor, and laminin. Plasma fibronectin is synthesized by hepatocytes and reaches the wound site by extravascular extravasation. It is closely associated with the fibrin clot. Tissue fibronectin is synthesized by macrophages, endothelial cells, and fibroblasts and is the characteristic fibronectin of mature wound matrix.

Fibronectin is a dimer consisting of two protein monomers joined by a disulfide bond. The molecule is composed of modules or domains of binding sites (Fig. 4–5). There are two binding sites for fibrinogen-fibrin, and heparin-heparin sulfate. Collagen-gelatin domains are near the amino terminal, and a cell-binding domain is toward the carboxyl terminal. Cell binding is via a family of cell-binding receptors or cytoadhesion molecules that interact with the RGD amino acid sequence (arginine-glycine-asparagine) on the fibronectin molecule. RGD sequences are also found in fibrin, von Willebrand factor, thrombospondin, and vitronectin. Initial fibroblast migration, in association with fibronectin, is mediated via this RGD binding. Fibronectin and its degradation products are strong chemoattractants for monocytes and macrophages and probably act to stimulate differentiation of the monocyte to the activated macrophage.

Fibronectin has both direct and indirect opsonin activity. A number of microbes are opsonized by fibronectin facilitating their phagocytosis. Products of matrix débridement, are also opsonized. Fibronectin binding to macrophages, fibroblasts, and epidermal cells stimulates phagocytosis.

FIBROPLASTIC PHASE

Regulation of the Inflammatory and Cell Migratory Phase

The transition to the stage of fibroplasia is marked histologically by a predominance of macrophages followed by fibroblasts with a decrease in the number of neutrophils. Processes characterizing the fibroplastic phase include fibroblast migration, matrix formation (including collagen synthesis), wound contraction, angiogenesis, and epithelialization.

The first step is to turn off the inflammatory response. This is achieved by decreasing the production of inflammatory mediators and inactivation of those already present. Production decreases when the inflammatory stimulus is removed. Disappearance of mediators may be due to the short half-life of a mediator (e.g., thromboxane A2), diffusion, or a result of active and specific enzymes (e.g., products of the complement and clotting cascades). Inflammatory factors may be disabled and removed by wound macrophages. The disappearance of tissue neutrophils in the wound appears to be due to their short lifespan, as well as decreased extravascular migration. The mechanism of decreased extravascular migration is unclear and may be influenced both passively and actively by endothelial cells.

Fibroblast Migration and Proliferation

The fibroplastic phase is usually established by the 5th day after wounding. The duration is variable, usually 1–2 weeks. This stage involves fibroblast proliferation and migration, extracellular matrix elaboration, wound contraction, angiogenesis, and epithelialization. By the 5th day, the dominant cell in the wound is now the fibroblast. This is the result of increased migration and replication in response to soluble mediators released during the inflammatory phase. Mediators of fibroblast migration and proliferation include C5A, fibronectin, and growth factors—specifically PDGF, fibroblast growth factor (FGF), and possibly TGF-β. Elaboration of enzymes such as collagenase and plasminogen activators by both the differentiating fibroblast and the macrophage facilitates cellular migration into the wound.

The early extracellular matrix is rich in hyaluronate as well as fibronectin, and both facilitate cellu-

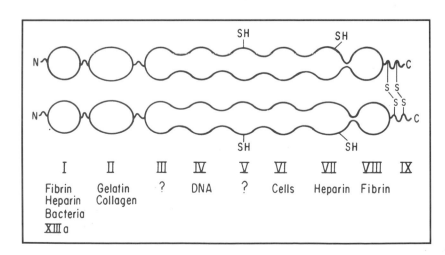

FIGURE 4–5. The fibronectin molecule consists of two subunits linked by two disulfide bonds. Each subunit is composed of domains that are able to bond to cell surfaces and wound matrix components. The structure suggests a scaffold-like function facilitating cell-cell matrix interactions in the healing wound. (Reprinted from Hynes, R.: Molecular biology of fibronectin. Ann. Rev. Cell. Biol. *1*:67–90, Fig. 1, p. 68, 1985.)

lar migration. Hyaluronate is hydrophilic and permits the formation of interstitial chemical gradients. Fibroblast migration is governed by the gradient of the chemotactic factors in the wound. Although a cause and effect relationship is not established, high levels of matrix hyaluronate are associated with cellular migration in both wound healing and embryogenesis. When hyaluronate levels drop, migration ceases.

Fibronectin, by virtue of its ability to bind specifically to both the matrix and the fibroblast, provides a physical pathway along which the fibroblast can migrate—as if climbing a rope. The fibroblast binds to the RGD sequence on fibronectin via its receptor. The fibronectin receptor is a member of the integrin family of transmembrane cell adhesion molecules. Other integrins include the white cell receptor LFA-1 (leukocyte function associated), the macrophage receptor MAC-1, and the platelet receptor glycoprotein IIb-IIIa that binds fibrinogen.

The fibronectin receptors on the fibroblast are proteins which pass through the entire cell membrane. Intracellular domains bind to cytoskeleton actin filaments. These filaments, in turn, are the very molecules on which the cell depends for motion. An intracellular-extracellular continuum is established that aligns the cells with the orientation of the fibronectin and with each other. Thus, the cells march in

linear array down the fibronectin strand and along the chemotactic gradient of growth factors in the wound. The dynamic fibronectin-fibroblast coupling is called the *fibronexus* and the interaction between fiber orientation and cell movement is termed *traction morphogenesis*. Fibronectin is found whenever cell migration occurs and is linked to processes of epithelialization, migration, matrix contraction, and angiogenesis. Fibronectin disappears after cellular migration is accomplished by processes that are incompletely understood.

Both fibroblast migration (chemotaxis) and subsequent proliferation are stimulated by growth factors (Table 4–5). Platelet-derived growth factor is released during the inflammatory phase and is an extremely potent mitogen and chemotactic agent for fibroblasts. Mitosis is correlated with tyrosine kinase activity, which is stimulated by the binding of PDGF to its 18,000-molecular weight glycoprotein receptor on the fibroblast cell surface receptor.

Transforming growth factor-β is released by platelets and may also be active in stimulating proliferation and synthesis of fibronectin and collagen by fibroblasts. Epidermal growth factor (EGF) is mitogenic and may stimulate collagen production by fibroblasts and osteoblasts. Fibroblast growth factor appears to enhance proliferation and collagen deposition by fibroblasts.

TABLE 4–5. FIBROBLAST STIMULATION

Factor	Source	Effect
Serotonin	Platelets	Proliferation Collagen Synthesis
Interleukin-1	Macrophage	Collagenase synthesis
Collagen Collagen degradation products Fibronectin Fibronectin fragments	Wound matrix	Chemotaxis
Macrophage-derived growth factor (MDGF)*	Macrophage	Proliferation
Platelet-derived growth factor (PDGF)	Platelets Endothelial cells ? Activated macrophages	Chemotaxis Proliferation Collagenase secretion
Epidermal growth factor (EGF)	Submaxillary glands Urine Small intestine ? other sources	Proliferation ? Collagen synthesis
Fibroblast growth factors	Endothelial cells Macrophages Numerous other cell types	Proliferation ? Collagen synthesis
Transforming growth factor β (TGF-β)	Platelets	Proliferation Fibronectin synthesis Collagen synthesis

* May represent multiple factors.

Matrix Formation

As the fibroblasts invade the wound, they manufacture additional new matrix including the glycoproteins, structural proteins, and adhesive proteins.

Proteoglycans

The proteoglycans are composed of a protein core to which polysaccharides (glycosaminoglycans) are covalently attached. The preponderance of sulfate and/or carboxyl groups is responsible for the polyanionic nature of glycosaminoglycans and proteoglycans.

Regulation of hyaluronic acid and proteoglycan biosynthesis and the exact role of these substances in wound healing remains incompletely understood. High levels of hyaluronic acid dominate the early wound matrix, and cellular proliferation, migration, and an undifferentiated state are associated with this environment. Interestingly, high levels of hyaluronic acid seem to characterize the matrix of healing fetal wounds, which are characterized by minimal if any fibrosis and scar formation. Later, sulfated proteoglycans predominate, and cellular activity is marked by differentiation and decreased proliferation. Experimental evidence suggests that a role may be played by GAGs in stimulating angiogenesis, however the details are unclear and the results conflicting. Heparin seems to augment angiogenesis, and heparin sulfate proteoglycans may facilitate cell adhesions or fibronexus formation during wound contraction.

Structural Proteins

The collagens compose a family of fibrous proteins secreted by the fibroblast. Collagens are the most abundant proteins in mammals. At least ten types have been described. Of these, types I–IV are the most common (Table 4–6). Types I, II, and III are fibrillar proteins (type I is most common). Type IV collagen is a major constituent of basal laminae and differs structurally from the fibrillar collagens (Fig. 4–6). Collagens are rich in glycine and proline—the proline being responsible for a tight alpha helical structure.

The steps leading to collagen fiber formation are outlined in Fig. 4–7. Pro-α chains undergo post-translation hydroxylation and glycosylation. Three pro-α chains form a triple helical procollagen fibril. Thus, α helical chains are packed together like a cable and their orientation is influenced by the cytoskeletons of the fibroblast (traction morphogenesis); procollagen fibrils are then secured. Nonhelical residues are cleaved from each end of the procollagen molecule by procollagen peptidase to form tropocollagen. Tropocollagen molecules then spontaneously aggregate into fibrils. Cross-linking occurs between the triple helical strands in the matrix to form fibrils and the fibrils are aggregated to form collagen fibers.

The biosynthesis of type IV collagen differs significantly from that of fibrillar collagens I–III, and the secreted collagen assembles into sheets rather than fibrils (Fig. 4–6). Type IV collagen forms an integral part of the regenerating basement membrane.

TABLE 4–6. FOUR MAJOR TYPES OF COLLAGEN AND THEIR PROPERTIES

Type	Molecular Formula	Polymerized Form	Distinctive Features	Tissue Distribution
I	$[\alpha(I)]_2\alpha2(I)$	Fibril	Low hydroxylysine; low carbohydrate; broad fibrils	Skin; tendon; bone; ligaments; cornea; internal organs (accounts for 90% of body collagen)
II	$[\alpha1(II)]_3$	Fibril	High hydroxylysine; high carbohydrate; usually thinner fibrils than type I	Cartilage; intervertebral disc; notochord; vitreous body of eye
III	$[\alpha1(III)]_3$	Fibril	High hydroxyproline, low hydroxylysine, low carbohydrate	Skin; blood vessels; internal organs
IV	$[\alpha1(IV)]_2\alpha2(IV)$	Basal lamina	Very high hydroxylysine; high carbohydrate; retains procollagen extension peptides	Basal laminae

Note that types I and IV are each composed of two types of α chain, whereas types II and III are composed of only one type of α chain each. Only the four major types of collagen are shown, but more than 10 types of collagen and about 20 types of α chain have been defined to date.

Reprinted from Alberts, B., Bray, D., Lewis, J., Raff, M., Roberts, K., and Watson, J.D.: The Molecular Biology of the Cell. New York, Garland Publishing, Inc., p. 810, 1989.

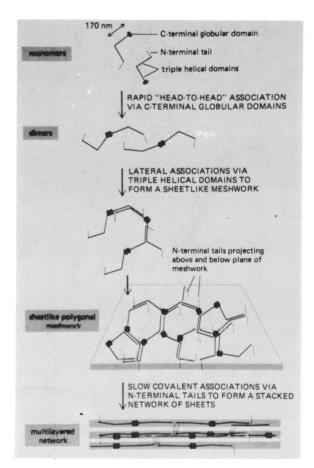

FIGURE 4–6. How type IV collagen molecules are thought to assemble into a multilayered network which forms the core of all basal laminae. Note sheet-like structure as opposed to rope-like structure of fibrillar collagen. (Reprinted from Alberts, B., Bray, D., Lewis, J., Raff, M., Roberts, K., and Watson, J.D.: The Molecular Biology of the Cell. New York, Garland Publishing, Inc., Fig. 14–42, p. 816, 1989.)

Elastin

Elastin is a nonglycosolated protein rich in proline and lysine; it is secreted into the extracellular matrix, not as a tight regular helix like collagen, but as random coils. This allows the network to stretch and recoil. There is limited regeneration of elastin during wound healing.

Regulation of Collagen Metabolism

During the inflammatory and early fibroblastic phase, growth factors including PDGF, EGF, TGF-β, and FGF are elaborated by monocytes, macrophages and other inflammatory cells. These factors stimulate fibroblasts to secrete collagen and ground matrix components (Table 4–5). Initially, type III collagen is secreted in higher concentrations than type I (30 per cent), but by 48-60 hours, the ratio of type I to type III is returning to that found in normal skin (90 : 10 per cent). This relative increase in type III collagen is also seen during embryogenesis.

The macrophage appears to be the key cell in regulating collagen elaboration by fibroblasts. Experiments using antimacrophage serum depletion techniques showed a marked decrease in wound collagen and defective healing in wounds depleted of macrophages. Conversely, when macrophages were injected into wounds, increased collagen deposition and better healing occurred. Presumably, the macro-

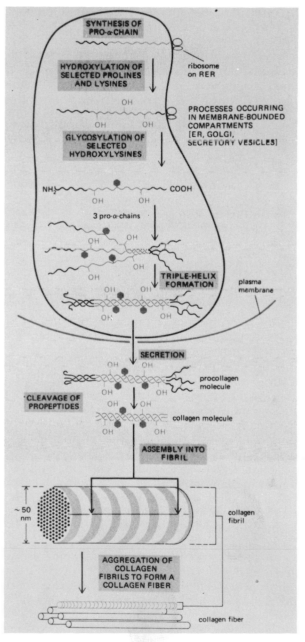

FIGURE 4–7. The intracellular and extracellular events involved in the formation of a collagen fibril. (Reprinted from Alberts, B., Bray, D., Lewis, J., Raff, M., Roberts, K., and Watson, J.D.: The Molecular Biology of the Cell. New York, Garland Publishing, Inc., Fig. 14–40, p. 814, 1989.)

phage exerts its effects by secreting growth factors. Hunt, Knighton, and others have studied in vivo wound healing using transparent wound chambers. Macrophages form a leading edge of cells migrating into the wound; these are followed by young fibroblasts, which are followed by replicating fibroblasts enmeshed in growing endothelial buds emerging from mature vessels. The authors propose a regulatory model for wound healing, where: A decreased PO_2 in the metabolically active healing wound leads to lactate production, which in turn stimulates both collagen deposition and angiogenesis. As the wound heals, interstitial PO_2 increases, and the stimulus favoring fibroplasia is downregulated.

Collagen degradation occurs concurrently with collagen synthesis. Initially, collagen lysis occurs at a slow rate but increases as the wound matures. Total wound collagen content obviously represents a summation of both of these processes. Further understanding of factors regulating this process would have great clinical relevance to diseases marked by excess fibrosis, including cirrhosis, pulmonary fibrosis, and hypertrophic or keloid scars. Therapy of excessive collagenolytic states such as rheumatoid arthritis might also be advanced.

Contraction

Contraction describes a gradual decrease in wound area caused by retraction of the central granulation tissue mass. Complete wound closure by contraction may occur. How a wound contracts is still not clear; however an understanding of the mechanism involved would have an impact on the treatment of unwanted contraction (i.e., burn contractures).

One of the central arguments regarding contraction revolves around the role—and even existence—of the myofibroblast. The myofibroblast is the cell found in granulation tissue that appears morphologically and physiologically to be intermediate between smooth muscle and fibroblast. The cell appears at the onset of wound contraction and disappears when contraction is complete. The cell contains both actin and myosin filaments, and a matrix contractile function is postulated. This is supported by the observation that granulation tissue strips contract or relax in a manner directly analogous to smooth muscle when exposed to pharmacological agents known to contract or relax smooth muscle (i.e., epinephrine). When added to in vitro collagen lattice preparations, myofibroblasts effect a marked contraction of the lattice. However, other experiments have shown that in vitro lattice contraction may be induced in the absence of myofibroblasts, emphasizing that collagen remodelling may also play at least a partial role in wound contraction.

It is likely that the in vivo response is multifactorial. Obviously a great deal of effort has been devoted to attempting to control or halt contraction. Skin grafting appears to be one of the most effective methods of controlling contraction. The effect is most pronounced when full-thickness skin grafts are used, suggesting that an activity lies within the grafted dermis. Glucocorticoids may also inhibit contraction.

Angiogenesis

Additional migrating, proliferating cells involved in filling the fibrin-fibronectin matrix are the endothelial cells needed to build vessels to supply nutrients. Angiogenesis refers to the process by which vessels grow into a previously avascular space. All angiogenesis begins with the endothelial cell, and capillary ingrowth precedes maturation into larger vessels. Endothelial cells retain the ability to migrate and proliferate even though normally cell turnover is very slow. The process of angiogenesis describes the sequence of inflammation, endothelial cell migration, proliferation, capillary formation, and eventual remodeling. New vessels always originate as capillaries which sprout from the sides of small vessels in response to local angiogenic factors. The stimulated endothelial cell first sends out a pseudopod through the basal lamina into the perivascular space. Then it divides, vacuoles form in the contiguous cells, and the vacuoles fuse to create a capillary lumen. The process then repeats itself. The sprout connects itself with other new capillaries so that a circulating network is established. Of the three steps, digesting the basal lamina requires proteases; migration and proliferation do not. Each step is regulated by a different combination of signals collectively called angiogenic factors.

Numerous angiogenic factors have been identified, and angiogenesis can be stimulated in vitro in the absence of flowing blood. Angiogenic factors have been isolated from diverse tissue sources such as kidney, salivary glands, corpus luteum, thyroid, and lymphoid cells. The latter source is the most pertinent to wound healing. Lymphocytes, macrophages, neutrophils, and mast cells have demonstrated angiogenic activity. Angiogenic factors may directly affect endothelial cell migration or division, or they may act by stimulating intermediary cells (i.e. the macrophage or mast cell) to elaborate other soluble mediators (Table 4–7).

Among the earliest angiogenic factors identified were the heparin-binding fibroblast growth factors (basic and acidic). Numerous angiogenic factors were identified subsequently; which seen to have structural homology to either acidic or basic FGF. FGF-like factors have been isolated from macrophages, brain, ovary, adrenal, bone, and cartilage, as well as other tissues. Receptors for FGF have been demonstrated on endothelial cells from various vas-

TABLE 4–7. BIOLOGICAL ACTIVITIES OF ANGIOGENIC FACTORS

| | | ENDOTHELIAL CELL | |
FACTOR	ANGIOGENESIS	*Proliferation*	*Motility*
Acidic FGF	Yes	Yes	Yes
Basic FGF	Yes	Yes	Yes
Angiogenin	Yes	No	ND*
TGF-α	Yes	Yes	ND
TGF-β	Yes	Inhibition	ND
Wound fluid	Yes	No	Yes
Prostaglandins	Yes	No	ND
Adipocyte lipids	Yes	No	Yes

* ND, Not done.

Reprinted from Folkman, T., and Klagsbrun, M.: Angiogenic factors. Science *235*:445, 1987.

cular sources. Acidic and basic FGF initiate in vitro endothelial cell proliferation and cell migration both in vivo and in vitro.

Transforming Growth Factors originally isolated from virally transformed cells and subsequently identified in normal tissues have in vivo angiogenic potential. TGF-α has a 35 per cent amino acid homology to epidermal growth factor and directly stimulates endothelial cell proliferation. TGF-β is released by platelets and activated lymphocytes. TGF-β stimulates granulation tissue formation and neovascularization in vivo; however, it inhibits in vitro endothelial cell proliferation. This apparent paradox may be explained by the action of TGF-β on the macrophage. TGF-β is a potent chemoattractant for macrophages and seems to induce angiogenic activity in part via macrophage-secreted TNF-α. TNF-α activates endothelial cells and their migration into collagen gel matrices and subsequent capillary tube formation. Although TNF-α, like TGF-β, is non mitogenic, it is likely that other macrophage products do stimulate endothelial proliferation.

The exact role of ground substance heparin and related heparin sulfate in angiogenesis remains unclear. The interaction between heparin and angiogenic factors is confusing. Heparin and heparin sulfate have both positive and negative effects on cell growth. Heparin augments in vivo endothelial migration and tumor angiogenesis in the chick embryo model. While heparin appears to favor angiogenesis, when combined with steroids an inhibitory effect is noted. A satisfactory unifying hypothesis for the physiologic role of heparin remains to be developed.

Migration

Mast cells have been observed in high concentrations in tissues undergoing angiogenesis. They may facilitate endothelial cell migration by releasing neutral proteases and heparin. Matrix products, including thrombin, fibrin, and fibronectin, all have been implicated in stimulating endothelial cell migration. Fibronectin, by its cell and substrate binding domains, facilitates adhesion gradient-related migration (haptotaxis). A change in cell polarity and matrix composition are other factors that favor in vitro migration; however the in vivo correlates are still speculative.

Proliferation

Proliferation follows migration. Proliferative stimuli include leukocyte-derived angiogenic mediators (i.e. FGF, TGF α) and matrix products. The loss of cell-cell and/or cell-matrix contact are associated with cell proliferation in both in vitro preparations and embryogenesis. A similar mechanism in wound angiogenesis is inferred. The elaboration of basal lamina is associated with a decrease in replication.

Cell matrix interactions seem to play an important role directing capillary formation. Endothelial cells grown in vitro on type IV collagen (basal lamina) will form tubes. However, when growth is on type I or III collagen, no tube formation occurs.

Regulation

Factors halting angiogenesis are not clear but may involve a combination of effects from matrix binding and soluble factors such as TGF-β. It has been proposed that the angiogenic process may be controlled by macrophages responding to tissue oxygen concentrations. Manipulation of O_2 tension in a rabbit ear chamber model directly affected angiogenesis. Hypoxia stimulated angiogenesis, while increasing oxygen tension in the chamber halted or reversed angiogenesis. Supernatants from hypoxic macrophage cultures showed increased angiogenic activity in vivo, and in vitro increased plasminogen activator and fibroblast mitogenic activity, when compared to supernatants from normal macrophage cultures.

Remodeling

Following wound repair and withdrawal of angiogenic stimulus-stimuli, a period of remodeling occurs which is morphologically associated with vascular stasis followed by coagulation, endothelial cell death, and macrophage phagocytosis of debris. The clinical appearance of a scar over time, with decreasing hyperemia, reflects a gradual decrease in vascularity and progressive organization and maturation of fibrotic tissue.

Epithelialization

Within 12 hours of epidermal wounding, epithelial changes occur with loosening of cell-cell and cell-matrix contacts. Epithelial cells begin to migrate over the collagen-fibronectin wound surface. Migration into the wound occurs as a sheet progressing from either wound edges or skin adnexae. It appears that the mechanism of epithelial regeneration involves a rolling sheet-type migration in which successive parabasal cells roll over attached basal cells and themselves become attached to the basal lamina. Initially, migration is facilitated by the presence of fibrin-fibronectin collagen matrix. However, as migration proceeds, epithelial cells themselves produce their own matrix, and are less dependent on the wound surface. The epithelial cells elaborate proteases and develop intracellular contractile actin proteins, changes that presumably aid their migration over the wound surface.

The leading cells of the migrating sheet do not proliferate; rather, proliferation occurs behind the wound edge by division of stem cells. Contact with the basal lamina appears to be necessary for stem cell division. Proliferation and migration normally occur until epidermis of the appropriate thickness is replaced. The regulatory processes controlling proliferation, migration, and differentiation are unclear. It was originally assumed that loss of contact inhibition caused by the injury was the major stimulus for replication and migration; however this concept is currently being reviewed.

Wound Maturation

Cell and matrix changes in the wound continue long after completion of epithelialization. Figure 4–8 demonstrates changes in the wound's breaking strength as a function of collagen content. Wound strength increases without further collagen deposition, suggesting ongoing wound remodeling. The remodeling process represents an interplay between matrix synthesis and degradation. Enzymes active in early degradation include hyaluronidase, plasminogen activators, collagenases, and elastases. Little is known about late wound remodeling, although it appears that collagenase activity is the most important activity in late remodeling.

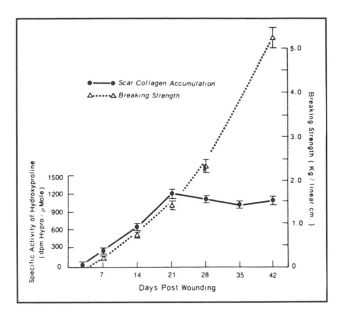

FIGURE 4–8. Comparison of scar collagen accumulation and breaking strength of rat skin wounds. After 21 days, strength increases with no change in wound collagen, reflecting scar remodeling. (Reprinted from Madden, J.W. and Peacock, E.E., Jr.: Biology of collagen during wound healing. Ann. Surg. *174*:511, Fig. 5, p. 517, 1971.)

Hyaluronidase

During the second week of wound healing, the matrix changes from a hyaluronate-rich environment to one characterized by dermatan sulfate and chondroitin sulfate. This change is associated with elevated wound hyaluronidase levels. The environment which previously favored cellular migration and division now favors differentiation. Whether the hyaluronidase itself effects these changes is unclear. Although leukocytes elaborate hyaluronidase, it is unclear whether this is the major source of wound hyaluronidase.

Plasminogen Activators

Plasminogen activators convert plasminogen to plasmin. Plasmin degrades many proteins including fibrin, but cannot directly degrade elastin or collagen. Plasminogen activators include urokinase and tissue-type plasminogen activator. Urokinase is produced by keratinocytes, fibroblasts, leukocytes, and endothelial cells, and appears to be more important physiologically in wound repair. In the wound, plasmin is produced, and matrix components such as fibrin, fibronectin, and laminin are degraded. Plasminogen activators also activate macrophage-secreted procollagenases and elastases. Matrix degradation products appear to be chemotactic for wound inflammatory cells and fibroblasts and appear to stimulate angiogenesis. The activity of the plasminogen activators is in turn influenced by a diverse group of stimulatory and inhibitory factors including cytokines, cyclic AMP, glucocorticoids, retinoids, and others. In the early wound-healing phase, plasminogen activators are responsible for matrix turnover and degradation of fibrin, fibronectin, and laminin. They also actively stimulate in angiogenesis and chemotaxis. Later roles include regulation of collagen and elastin turnover via the activation of macrophage enzymes.

Collagenases

Collagenases are secreted by granulocytes, macrophages, fibroblasts, and epithelial cells. The specificity is dependent on the cell of origin. Dermal fibroblast collagenase is specific for collagen types I–III, whereas monocyte collagenase is specific for type IV collagen. Collagenase is a zinc-containing neutral metalloproteinase which cleaves the collagen triple helix.

Collagenases are secreted in an inactive form which is then activated extracellularly by a variety of proteases, including plasmin. Collagenase activity is downregulated by serum and tissue inhibitors such as serum alpha-2 macroglobulin.

Interleukin-1 and other growth factors, including PDGF, TGF-β, and EGF, stimulate zymogen synthesis by fibroblast. Glucocorticoids, phenytoin and retinoids downregulate collagenase synthesis. A number of pathological processes may be related to disorders of collagen lysis, including rheumatoid arthritis, keloid, and hypertrophic scar formation and, possibly, vascular aneurysm formation.

Collagen Maturation

With time, collagen fibers become more linearly organized along stress lines with increased intra- and interfibril cross-linking. Hyaluronate is replaced with sulfated proteoglycans, with loss of water. With time the collagen becomes stronger and more resistant to proteolysis.

SUMMARY

The process of wound healing starts with an inflammatory response to injury. A predictable, orderly efflux of cells from the vascular compartment ensues, starting with the neutrophil and monocyte, followed by the fibroblast. Normally, wound matrix deposition, angiogenesis, contraction, and epithelialization result in a healed wound.

The similarity between processes of wound healing, regeneration, embryogenesis, and neoplasia is striking. While much is left to be learned about the regulatory steps that differentiate these phenomena, the potential clinical benefit derived from such understanding is substantial.

BIBLIOGRAPHY

1. Clark, R.A.F. and Henson, P.M. (eds.): The Molecular and Cellular Biology of Wound Repair. New York, Plenum Press, 1988.
2. Mathes, S.J. and Abouljord, M.: Wound healing. In Davis, J.H. (ed.): Clinical Surgery. St. Louis, C.V. Mosby Co., 1987, pp. 401–508.
3. Alberts, B., Bray, D., Lewis, J., Raff, M., Roberts, K., and Watson, J.D.: The Molecular Biology of the Cell. New York, Garland Publishing, Inc., 1989, pp. 792–839.
4. Folkman, T. and Klagsbrun, M.: Angiogenic factors. Science 235:442–447, 1987.
5. Gospodarowicz, X., Neufeld, G., and Sweigerer, L.: Fibroblast growth factor. Mol. Cell. Endocrinol. 46:187–204, 1986.
6. Hynes, R.: Molecular biology of fibronectin. Ann. Rev. Cell. Biol. 1:67-90, 1985.
7. Hunt, T.K., Knighton, D.R., Thakral, K.K., Goodson, W.H., and Andrews, W.S.: Studies on inflammation and wound healing: Angiogenesis and collagen synthesis stimulated in vivo by resident and activated wound macrophages. Surgery 96:48–54, 1984.
8. Leibovich, S.J. and Ross, R.: The role of the macrophage in wound repair. A study with hydrocortisone and antimacrophage serum. Am. J. Pathol. 78:71–100, 1975.

5

INFECTION AND HOST DEFENSES

RICHARD L. SIMMONS *and* PAUL H. KISPERT

MICROBIOLOGY OF SURGICAL INFECTION

An understanding of the structure and unique characteristics of commonly encountered organisms in surgical practice is vitally important in order to understand the principles of the prevention, recognition, and treatment of disease produced by microorganisms. The goals of this chapter are (1) to briefly review the structure and unique characteristics of bacteria, fungi, and viruses; (2) to discuss pathogens commonly encountered in surgical illness and their relevance; and (3) to discuss the implications of treatment of surgical infection.

Microbiology of Bacteria, Fungi, and Viruses

Bacteria

Bacteria are prokaryotic organisms by definition because they lack a true nucleus, chromosomes, and a mitotic apparatus. They are classified by morphology as rods (*Escherichia coli*, *Bacteroides fragilis*), spheres (*Staphylococcus* and *Streptococcus*), and spirals (*Treponema pallidum*). Bacterial DNA lies in a single circular chromosome. In addition, bacteria may possess additional small autonomously replicating strands of DNA called plasmids. Plasmids carry particular significance because they often carry genes for resistance to single or multiple antibiotics that may be transferred between bacteria of the same or another species by conjugation. These transferrable resistance genes are called R factors. Bacteria possess no mitochondria and produce energy through the electron transport chain and oxidative phosphorylation on their cell membranes. Bacterial cytoplasm also contains many ribosomes that are structurally different from those of human cells. These bacterial ribosomes are the targets of several types of antibiotics (gentamicin and chloramphenicol), while human ribosomes are not affected by these antibiotics.

The cytoplasm of bacteria is enclosed by a plasma membrane which is used for many functions, including energy generation, secretion, and DNA and protein synthesis. External to the cell membrane, bacteria have a cell wall that is much thicker in gram-positive than in gram-negative organisms (Fig. 5–1). Many antibiotics (penicillins, cephalosporins) work by inhibiting cell wall synthesis. This thick cell wall allows bacteria to withstand osmotic stress without

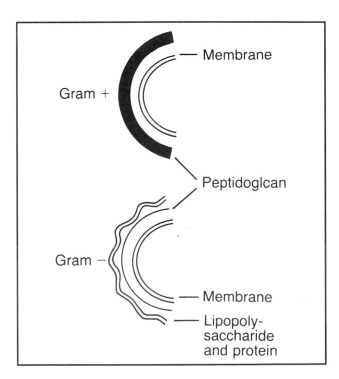

FIGURE 5–1. Comparison of cell wall of gram-positive and gram-negative bacteria. (Reprinted from Howard, R.J. and Simmons, R.L. (eds.): Surgical Infectious Diseases. 2nd ed. Norwalk, CT, Appleton & Lang, Fig. 1–5, p. 4, 1988.)

56

bursting. The gram-positive cell wall is composed of peptidoglycan, a complex of polysaccharides and protein. Teichoic acid serves as a major surface antigen. The presence of circulating teichoic acid antibodies has been implicated in deep-seated gram-positive infections. Gram-negative bacteria, in addition to their cell wall, have an outer membrane containing lipopolysaccharide (LPS or endotoxin). Lipopolysaccharide has a lipid A core, but the polysaccharide structure determines the antigen strain of the bacteria (O antigen) (Fig. 5–2). Recently, it has been shown that administration of antibodies to endotoxin improves survival in gram-negative sepsis.

Surrounding the cell wall in some bacteria is a capsule, a thick gel-like structure that can be seen on India ink stains and is responsible for the mucoid appearance of some bacterial colonies. Capsules appear to function by protecting the bacteria from phagocytosis—thereby acting as a virulence factor.

Short, hairlike structures called pili and long, thin, hairlike structures called flagella are present on some bacteria. Pili are often responsible for bacterial adherence to mucosal surfaces, which is an essential property for invasion. Flagella are responsible for motility and are rarely virulence factors.

When living conditions are harsh, particularly those related to nutritional deficiency, some gram-positive bacteria form spores that are resistant to heat and freezing. The spore wall is composed of peptidoglycan.

Rickettsia, Chlamydia, and *Mycoplasma* are all bacteria which can cause disease. Rickettsiae are obligate intracellular pathogens and are transferred between hosts by an arthropod vector. Chlamydiae are bacteria which cannot synthesize ATP. Mycoplasmas are the smallest bacteria known and lack a cell wall.

Fungi

In contrast to bacteria, fungi are eukaryotic cells (DNA separates into chromosomes during division) with nuclear structures. In addition, unlike bacteria, fungi possess mitochondria and endoplasmic reticula. The fungal cell wall is external to the plasma membrane and is rigid, being composed of a polysaccharide termed chitin. Fungi, like some bacteria, have a capsule that inhibits phagocytosis.

Yeasts are unicellular fungi and molds are multicellular fungi. Molds usually grow as branching hyphae with septal divisions and reproduce by spore formation (conidia).

Of the 80,000 species of fungi, only about 100 cause human disease. The diseases caused by fungi can be classified as deep (systemic) or superficial (cutaneous). Systemic mycosis leads to granuloma formation in the host, with abscess formation. Fungi can be classified as those that occur as endemic infections (histoplasmosis, blastomycosis, coccidiomycosis, cryptococcosis) and those that are opportunists (*Candida* and *Aspergillus*).

Protozoa

Protozoa are eukaryotes with nuclei, mitochondria, and mitotic structures similar to human cells. Organisms commonly causing infection include *Pneumocystis carinii* and *Trichomonas vaginalis*.

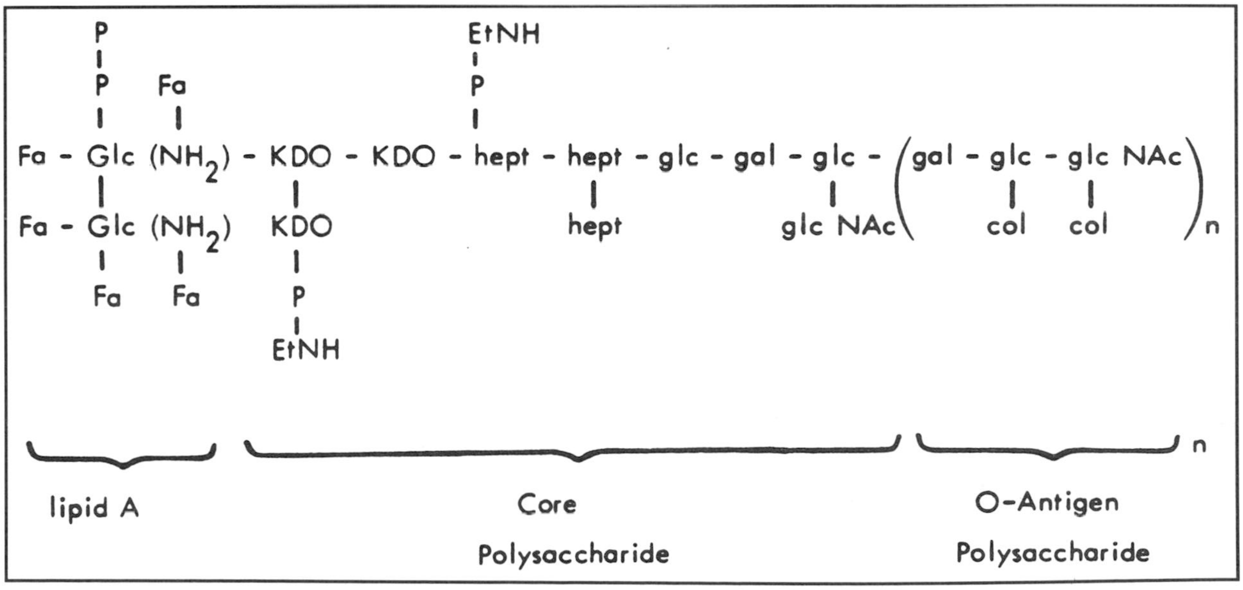

FIGURE 5–2. Chemical structure of *Escherichia coli* lipopolysaccharide (endotoxin). Fa, fatty acid; P, phosphage; Glc (NH₂), glycosamine; KDO, 2-keto 2-deoxyoctulosonate; EtNH, ethanolamine; hept, L-galactose; glcNAc, N-acetylglucosamine; col, colitose. (Reprinted from Howard, R.J. and Simmons, R.L. (eds.): Surgical Infectious Diseases. 2nd ed. Norwalk, CT, Appleton & Lang, p. 11, 1988.)

Viruses

Viruses are the smallest of the pathogenic organisms. They are obligate intracellular pathogens which use host biosynthetic and energy-generating mechanisms to synthesize their individual molecular components within the host cell. These individual components are reassembled into the intact viral particle (virion). Each particle consists of a central core of DNA or RNA surrounded by a protein coat (capsid). Viruses possess an outer coat (envelope) of glyco- or lipoprotein derived from the cell or nuclear membrane of the host. The envelope or capsid acts to invade the host cell by penetration or cell fusion, inserting its genetic material into host cells. Viruses are not capable of independent existence.

Viral reproduction requires several steps. Viruses are initially absorbed into the host cell and the viral envelope is removed by host enzymes, thereby exposing the viral DNA or RNA to the host cytoplasm. Replication of viral RNA occurs in the cytoplasm and DNA replication occurs in the host cell nucleus. The protein capsid is reproduced by transcription of the RNA with reassembly of the nucleocapsid and release of new viral particles by cell lysis or budding from the cell surface.

Viruses can cause disease as the result of host cell lysis, inflammation, teratogenesis, and mutagenesis. An excellent example is the human immunodeficiency virus (HIV), which can infect, cause malfunction, or kill T lymphocytes, which in turn predisposes the host to opportunistic infections and malignancy. Viruses can cause local, disseminated, or inapparent infection with a long latent period between infection and the development of symptoms. In general, surgeons deal with the local complications caused by the viral infections and less often with the generalized infections themselves. For example, generalized cytomegalovirus infection occasionally causes gastrointestinal ulcers which perforate and bleed. Surgeons encounter viral infections most often as a complication of immunosuppression. For example, opportunistic herpes viruses (simplex, varicella zoster, cytomegalovirus [CMV], Epstein-Barr virus [EBV]) are seen in immunosuppressed transplant patients, while hepatitis B or C is most often a complication of transfusion.

Prevention of Microbial Illnesses

Vaccines are preparations of live attenuated or killed virus that elicit a protective immune response. Live attenuated vaccines are made by viral passage in tissue culture, selecting less pathogenic strains. Although attenuated vaccines elicit prolonged vigorous responses and can be given orally or intramuscularly, there is risk of disease transmission. Killed viruses or inert viral components cannot transmit disease. Viral vaccines are effective in hepatitis A, hepatitis B, zoster, rabies, and CMV, but the protection is short lived. Bacterial vaccines are of generally low immunogenicity and relatively ineffective, because they tend to be made of polysaccharide capsules (e.g., pneumococcal vaccine). The most effective bacterial vaccines are those directed against exotoxins (i.e., diphtheria and tetanus).

Passive immunizations utilize infusion of monoclonal or polyclonal immunoglobulins and are most effective against toxins (antitetanus toxin, anti-LPS) and hepatitis, but passive immunization has not been widely exploited. Monoclonal antibodies to the endogenous mediators of disease (anti-TNF) are also under development.

Chemoprophylaxis of viral infection is limited to a few viruses. Amantadine and rimantadine are useful for Asian influenza prophylaxis. Both have been replaced by acyclovir, which is effective orally in the prophylaxis of herpes simplex and CMV. Intravenous acyclovir is useful treatment of herpes simplex, varicella zoster, and perhaps EBV. The topical drug may be helpful in simplex. Gancyclovir is an effective prophylactic of CMV in transplant patients. Chemoprophylaxis of bacterial infections is widely practiced and highly effective in all types of surgery.

The interferons have been extensively studied as antiviral agents. Their properties are discussed in Chapter 2 (Mediators of Inflammation).

Pathogenesis of Infection

We are all normally colonized with a multitude of microbes—bacteria, viruses, and fungi. Normally, neither the host nor the organism harm one another, and a commensal relationship exists. These bacteria are saprophytes; they colonize the skin and mucosal surfaces. Beneficial effects may be derived from this relationship. Intestinal bacteria may produce vitamin K and B_{12} that may be used by the host. Infection can be considered to be one form of parasitism—a situation in which the microorganism lives at the expense of the host—but it is difficult to predict the manifestations of a given pathogen in an individual host. There is great variation in the ability of a microbe to cause disease.

Of critical importance is what enables microbes, particularly bacteria, to be virulent and cause disease in the host. Some bacteria possess specific characteristics that make them virulent. These characteristics are the exception rather than the rule and include factors associated with virulence on the surface of the bacteria (capsules, pili for attachment, and flagella for motility) and the elaboration of exotoxins such as those commonly associated with diphtheria, shigella, cholera, botulism, and tetanus. Perhaps as important as virulence factors are a failure of host defenses that allows normally nonvirulent bacteria (opportunists) to invade the host and induce tissue injury.

In general, organisms which cause surgical infections are residents of the skin or mucosal surfaces and have little intrinsic power to invade normal tissues. They are instead inoculated into wounds created by the surgeon, trauma, or disease. The surgeon may induce an iatrogenic failure of host defenses by breaching the skin, resulting in failure of the skin to act as a barrier to bacterial invasion. Thus, the organisms are opportunistic in that they invade tissue when host defenses are already compromised. Organisms which are intrinsically nonvirulent may invade when there is a failure of host defense.

Polymicrobial infections with both anaerobes and aerobes are common in surgery, although there are many monomicrobial infections. The very heterogeneous inoculum in breached barriers becomes simplified because of competition between bacterial species within a new environment. The more virulent organisms which survive do so because they find nutrients within tissues (iron from hematomas), they can avoid phagocytosis and intracellular killing (encapsulation), and they can produce toxins which permit their invasion. Almost all common surgical pathogens are those that divide and grow extracellularly.

To avoid phagocytosis, pathogenic microbes have evolved several identifiable virulence mechanisms: (1) thick capsules which are poor activators of the alternative complement cascade (therefore, specific immunity with immunoglobulin G (IgG) binding to the capsule is required for complement activation and phagocytosis); (2) *Staphylococcus aureus* has a protein A which binds the Fc portion of the IgG molecule so that it is not available for binding the Fc receptors of phagocytes; (3) *Mycobacterium tuberculosis* is easily phagocytized, but somehow fusion of the lysosome (containing proteolytic enzymes) with the phagocytosed bacterium is prevented. *Toxoplasma, Aspergillus,* and *S. aureus* also show this characteristic; (4) *S. aureus* produces catalase, which degrades hydrogen peroxide.

Table 5–1 compares the properties of exotoxins and endotoxins produced by bacteria, and Table 5–2 lists the principle exotoxins. In general, exotoxins that are important to surgeons are those produced by invading gram-positive organisms, i.e., diphtheria, toxic shock syndrome, and gas gangrene.

Endotoxins

Most facultative gram-negative bacteria have outer cell walls composed of LPS protein complexes (Figs. 5–1 to 5–3). This LPS has three layers: outer, middle, and inner.

I. The outer layer is itself composed of three layers (Fig. 5–3)
   A. O-specific polysaccharides which are repetitive units of specific sugars that convey the serologic specificity of an organism. This region is responsible for agglutination reaction in response to specific antisera to the bacteria and helps in identification.
   B. The O-specific region is linked to a core polysaccharide. Of clinical significance is the fact that the core polysaccharide (middle) is widely shared among gram-negative bacteria, and antibodies to this region are broadly cross reactive. Therefore, clinically effective antibodies against gram-negative bacterial infection have been developed.

TABLE 5–1. COMPARISON OF EXOTOXINS AND ENDOTOXINS

EXOTOXINS	ENDOTOXINS
Excreted by living cells; found in high concentrations in fluid medium	Integral part of microbial cell walls of gram-negative organisms liberated upon their disintegration
Polypeptides, molecular weight 10,000–900,000	Lipopolysaccharide complexes. Lipid A portion probably responsible for toxicity
Relatively unstable; toxicity often destroyed rapidly by heat over 60°C	Relatively stable; withstand heat over 60°C for hours without loss of toxicity
Highly antigenic; stimulate the formation of high-titer antitoxin. Antitoxin neutralizes toxin	Do not stimulate formation of antitoxin; stimulate formation of antibodies to polysaccharide moiety
Converted into antigenic, nontoxic toxoids by formalin, acid, heat, etc.	Not converted into toxoids
Highly toxic; fatal for laboratory animals in micrograms or less	Weakly toxic; fatal for laboratory animals in hundreds of micrograms
Do not produce fever in host	Often produce fever in host

Reprinted from Howard, R.J.: Microbes and their pathogenicity. *In* Howard, R.J. and Simmons, R.L. (eds.): Surgical Infectious Diseases. 2nd ed. Norwalk, CT, Appleton & Lang, p. 10, 1988.

TABLE 5–2.   SELECTED EXOTOXINS PRODUCED BY SOME TOXIGENIC BACTERIA

Bacterium	Diseaes	Toxin	Action
Streptococcus pyogenes	Pyogenic infections	Streptolysin O	Hemolytic
	Scarlet fever	Streptolysin S	Hemolytic
		Erythrogenic	Causes scarlet fever rash
		Streptokinase	Deoxyribonuclease
		Streptodornase	Fibrinolytic
		Streptococcal DPNase	Cardiotoxic, leukotoxic (?)
Straphylococcus aureus	Pyogenic infections	α-toxin	Necrotizing, hemolytic, leukocytolytic
		β-toxin	Hemolytic, lethal
		γ-toxin	Hemolytic, necrotizing, lethal
		TSST-1	Toxic shock syndrome
		Enterotoxin	Emetic
		Leukocidin	Kills leukocytes
		Hyaluronidase	Spreading factor
		Coagulase	Coagulates plasma
Clostridium tetani	Tetanus	Tetanospasm	Muscle spasms
		Tetanolysin	Hemolytic cardiotoxin
Clostridium perfringens	Gas gangrene	α-toxin	Lecithinase: necrotizing, hemolytic
		β-toxin	Necrotizing, lethal
		γ-toxin	Lethality
		δ-toxin	Hemolysis
		ϵ-toxin	Necrotizing
		^{n}-toxin	Lethality
		ϕ-toxin	Hemolytic cardiotoxin
		μ-toxin	Hyaluronidase, spreading factor
Clostridium botulinum	Botulism	Neurotoxin (6 types)	Paralytic
Clostridium difficile	Enterocolitis	Cytotoxin A	Lethal to cells
		Cytotoxin B	
Corynebacterium diphtheriae	Diphtheria	Diphtheritic toxin	Necrotizing
Shigella dysenteriae	Dysentery	Neurotoxin	Paralytic, hemorrhagic
Haemophilus pertussis	Whooping cough	Whopping cough toxin	Necrotizing

Modified from Howard, R.J. and Simmons, R.L. (eds.): Surgical Infectious Diseases. 2nd ed. Norwalk, CT, Appleton & Lang, Table 1–3, p. 9, 1988.

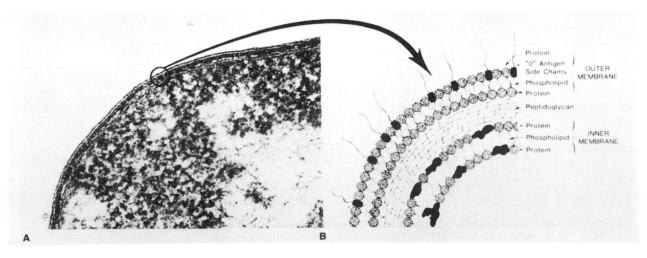

FIGURE 5–3.   A: *Escherichia coli* showing cell wall (× 200,000). (Courtesy of R.G.E. Murray.) **B:** Schema of *E. coli* cell envelope. (Reprinted from Howard, R.J. and Simmons, R.L. (eds.): Surgical Infectious Diseases. 2nd ed. Norwalk, CT, Appleton & Lang, Fig. 1–4A and B, p. 4, 1988.)

C. The core is linked to lipid A, which is the toxic portion of LPS. Minute quantities of endotoxin cause gelatination of an extract from the horseshoe crab, *Limulus polyphemus*, forming the basis for the limulus lysate assay for endotoxin.

II. The middle (intermediate or solid membrane) is composed of mucopeptide, and it is at this level that β-lactim antibiotics such as penicillin act to disrupt cell wall synthesis.

III. The inner cytoplasmic membrane.

Lipopolysaccharide is the toxic moiety (Fig. 5–2) and lipid A is responsible for the toxic effect (Table 5–3). The febrile response is probably due to LPS-induced release of tumor necrosis factor (TNF), IL-1, and IL-6 from macrophages. In addition, LPS can activate the alternative complement pathway of the complement cascade with release of anaphylatoxins, vasodilators, and kinins. The coagulation cascade can be activated by Factor XII or its effects on polymorphonuclear leukocytes and macrophages. Hageman factor activates the kinin system and causes the degranulation of platelets with the release of serotonin. Macrophages stimulated with LPS produce an array of over 100 products (including cytokines such as TNF, IL-1, IL-6, and prostaglandins) and become activated to kill tumor cells and intracellular organisms. Tumor necrosis factor release seems to be a major final common pathway of many of the systemic effects.

Indigenous Microflora

Since most surgical infections arise by the invasion of surface organisms into tissues, we have listed here the most common organisms on the skin and mucosal surfaces of the body. A knowledge of the normal flora will guide the surgeon in the treatment of likely surgical infections. The skin is a relatively harsh environment, and only *Staphylococcus epidermidis* and diptheroids successfully colonize the skin. Other contaminating flora, such as fecal flora in the lower abdomen, survive only transiently unless a constant supply of moisture is available. Shortly after birth, the oral cavity becomes colonized with bacteria. Because of constant swallowing and the flow of saliva,

TABLE 5–3. SOME PHYSIOLOGIC CONSEQUENCES OF ENDOTOXIN IN VIVO

SITE	COMMENT
Thermoregulatory center	Causes fever; releases pyrogens from WBC
Blood	
Leukocytes	Induces luekopenia followed by leukocytosis
Platelets	Thrombocytopenia; platelet aggregation; release of platelet constituents
Coagulation system	Activates extrinsic coagulation pathway and intrinsic coagulation pathway; causes disseminated intravascular coagulation
Complement	Activates complement via the alternative pathway
Vascular system	
Shock	Mechanism works partially by releasing TNF (tumor necrosis factor) from macrophages; hypotension, decreased cardiac output, decreased venous return, increased peripheral resistance, pooling of blood
Vasoactive substances	Causes release of activation of histamine, serotonin, kinins
Endocrine system	Causes release of ACTH and growth hormone, increases plasma cortisol
Immune system	
Endotoxin is immunogen; adjuvant	Antibodies can be detected 7-10 days after endotoxin administration; Endoxin is an adjuvent for a variety of antigens
Adjuvent	
B cell mitogen	
Metabolism	
Carbohydrate	Initial hyperglycemia followed by hypoglycemia with concomitant decrease in liver glycogen
Lipid	Hyperlipidemia; increases free fatty acids, serum cholesterol, serum phospholipids, and plasma triglycerides
Proteins	Stimulates liver protein synthesis; increases serum hepatocyte enzymes
Minerals	Decreases serum iron and iron-binding capacity
Gastrointestinal system	Decreases gastric emptying; diarrhea
Reticuloendothelial system	Activates macrophages to release IL-1, TNF, IL-6, prostaglandins, etc.

Modified from Howard, R.J. and Simmons, R.L. (eds.): Surgical Infectious Diseases. 2nd ed. Norwalk, CT, Appleton & Lang, Table 1–5, p. 12, 1988.

only those bacteria with the ability to adhere to mucosa or dentition remain as the predominent organisms. Anaerobes flourish in the gingival clefts, where the oxygen tension is low. The remainder of the gastrointestinal tract is sterile at birth but rapidly becomes populated with organisms. The acidic stomach acts an effective barrier to normal bacteria, but the constant passage of food raises the pH and allows bacteria to gain access to the lower gastrointestinal tract. Gastric achlorhydria, as occurs in pernicious anemia or gastric cancer, obviously permits overgrowth of bacteria in the normally sterile stomach. Bacteria resident in the small bowel must adhere to the mucosa to survive or they will be washed away by the rapidly moving enteric stream. Adherence is therefore a property important for small bowel disease; for example, the *E. coli* causing traveler's diarrhea is caused by an adherent enterotoxigenic strain.

Bacterial adherence is less important in the colon because of the reduced transit time. Aerobes in the colon rapidly utilize available oxygen, favoring the growth of anaerobes as reflected by the ratio of anaerobic to aerobic bacteria in the colon (1000 : 1). The most common components of the fecal flora are listed in Table 5–4. It is important to note that no important pathogenic species is found among the most common 25 organisms.

Viable bacteria can escape the normal intestine in small numbers. Such bacterial translocation is increased in stress, when the mucosa is damaged, or when bacterial overgrowth occurs within the gut lumen. Most translocating bacteria are eliminated by phagocytes, but the enteric flora is probably a source for sepsis in patients with compromised host defenses.

TABLE 5–4. RELATIVE FREQUENCY OF BACTERIAL SPECIES IN FECAL FLORA

RANK	PER CENT	ORGANISM(S)
1	12	*Bacteroides vulgatus*
2	7	*Fusobacterium prausnitzii*
3	6.5	*Bifidobacterium adolescentis*
4	6	*Eubacterium aerofaciens*
5	6	*Peptostreptococcus productus II*
6	4.5	*Bacteroides thetaiotaomicron*
7	3.6	*Eubacterium eligens*
8	3.3	*Peptostreptococcus productus I*
9	3.2	*Eubacterium biforme*
10	2.5	*E. aerofaciens III*
11	2.3	*Bacteroides distasonis*
28	0.7	*B. ovatus*
29	0.6	*B. fragilis*
59–75	0.13	*Streptococcus faecalis*
76–113	0.06	*Escherichia coli, Klebsiella pneumoniae,* and 37 other bacterial species

Adapted from Moore, W.E.C. and Holdeman, L.V.: Appl. Microbiol. 27:961, 1974.

COMMON SURGICAL INFECTIONS

The Pyogenic Cocci

Staphylococci

The pyogenic cocci includes the genuses *Staphylococcus, Streptococcus,* and *Neisseria. S. aureus* and *S. epidermidis* are the most common cause of nosocomial infection in surgical patients. *S. aureus* is a truly invasive organism which possesses virulence factors which permit it to invade normal tissues (Fig. 5–4). *S. epidermidis,* by contrast, is an opportunist which causes infection in the context of indwelling or intravascular devices. Both are facultative anaerobes, which can grow either in the presence or absence of air. All staphylococci producing coagulase are termed *S. aureus.*

S. epidermidis is a normal resident of the skin, whereas *S. aureus* is a transient skin organism found in the anterior nares and areas of moist skin of up to 40 per cent of healthy people, where it serves as a reservoir for person-to-person spread. What factors enhance the virulence of the staphylococci? One of the most important factors is the environment of the wound and the presence of foreign bodies in the form of sutures. It takes 7.5×10^6 staphylococci injected intradermally to produce an abscess. This number is decreased 500 times in the presence of skin sutures.

Most people have evidence of staphylococcal antibodies, but the presence of these antibodies does not provide production against subsequent infection. There is no evidence that effective immunity develops.

Other pathogenic factors responsible for the infectivity of *S. aureus* are illustrated in Fig. 5–4. No single staphylococcal species possesses all of these factors. Each of the cell wall components—peptidoglycan, teichoic acid, and protein A—contributes to the pathogenicity of the organism. The peptidoglycan component is capable of inhibiting leukocyte migration, thereby allowing bacterial proliferation. The peptidoglycan also has endotoxin like properties and can activate complement and elicit a cell-mediated immune response as well as conferring rigidity on the cell, allowing the organism to grow under unfavorable osmotic conditions. Teichoic acid also activates complement. The cell surface properties of protein A facilitates binding to the Fc component of IgG and the Fc receptor on phagocytes. Protein A can act as a blocking factor, inactivating IgG as an opsonin and thereby inhibiting phagocytosis. Furthermore, the IgG-protein A complex can activate the complement cascade and initiate neutrophil influx responsible for the ability of these organisms to elicit abscess formation. Some strains of staphylococcus have the ability to survive within phagocytes, a factor related to antibiotic resistance

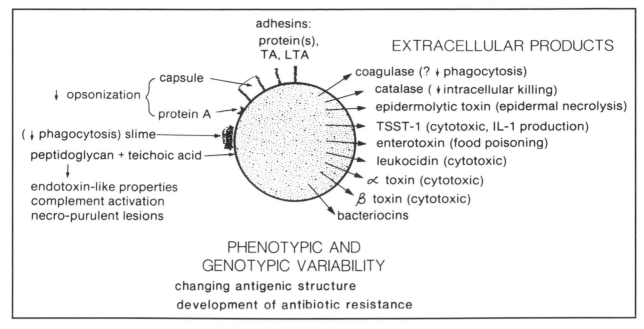

FIGURE 5–4. Virulence factors of *Staphylococcus aureus* and their proposed biologic effects. (Reprinted from Howard, R.J. and Simmons, R.L. (eds.): Surgical Infectious Diseases. 2nd ed. Norwalk, CT, Appleton & Lang, Fig. 3–1, p. 24, 1988.)

and recrudescent infection. Some strains of *S. aureus* are encapsulated. *S. aureus* possesses receptors for laminin, the major glycoprotein in the basement membrane of blood vessels. Binding may promote metastatic infection. Production of hyaluronidase, a major ground substance in connective tissue, may favor spreading of the infection.

In addition to these virulence factors, staphylococci produce enzymatically active agents that may be important for invasion and proliferation of bacteria (Table 5–5). For example, coagulase production is associated with virulence, but the mechanism is unknown. Catalase, an enzyme responsible for the destruction of hydrogen peroxide produced by phagocytic cells in the respiratory burst, may protect the bacteria from attack by oxygen radicals. About 30 per cent of isolates produce an enterotoxin capable of producing food poisoning. Epidermolytic toxins cause the diffuse exfoliative bullae and skin sloughing seen in childhood staphylococcal scalded skin syndrome. Toxic shock syndrome (TSS), most commonly associated with tampon use by menstruating women, but also seen in early postoperative wound infections, is caused by another exotoxin (TSST-1) produced by some species. This TSST-1 can directly activate macrophages and lymphocytes to produce lymphokines. Several other exotoxins listed in Table 5–2 and Figure 5–4 also contribute to the pathogenicity of *Staphylococcus* organisms.

Staphylococci have variable phenotypic characteristics and can therefore adapt to changing environments. For example, L-forms lack cell walls and can exhibit resistance to antibiotics that inhibit cell wall formation. The clinical importance of L-forms remains unknown. Many hospital strains of Staphylococcus produce a β-lactamase which renders drugs with β-lactim rings (e.g., penicillin, cephalosporins) ineffective as antimicrobial therapy. This is so common that penicillinase-resistant antibiotics are routinely recommended in the treatment of *S. aureus* infections.

Staphylococcus saprophyticus is the second most common cause of urinary tract infections in healthy

TABLE 5–5. VIRULENCE FACTORS OF GROUP A STREPTOCOCCI

BACTERIAL FACTORS	BIOLOGIC EFFECTS
Cell surface components	
M Protein	Antiphagocytic (decreased opsonization)
Hyaluronic capsule	Antiphagocytic
Peptidoglycan	Endotoxinlike properties, necropurulent lesions
Lipoteichoic acid	Attachment to epithelial cells
Extracellular products	
Streptolysins O and S	Cytotoxic
Proteinase	Cytotoxic
Hyaluronidase, streptokinase	Promote spread of infection
Pyrogenic exotoxins	Endotoxinlike properties

Reprinted from Peterson, P.K.: The pyogenic cocci. *In* Howard, R.J. and Simmons, R.L. (eds.): Surgical Infectious Diseases. 2nd ed. Norwalk, CT, Appleton & Lang, p. 28, 1988.

women. It has factors favoring adherence to the urothelium and also produces urease, favoring struvite stone formation.

Streptococci

Streptococci, which are facultatively anaerobic, are gram-positive cells in chains or pairs. Streptococci may be classified based on their ability to hemolyze blood agar or on their serologic classification (Lancefield) based on the presence of cell surface carbohydrates and teichoic acid. A single species comprises Group A streptococci; *Streptococcus pyogenes* is always β-hemolytic, is spread by droplets, and is a common cause of rapidly spreading skin and soft tissue infection. Group B streptococci (*Streptococcus agalactiae*) are harbored in the female genital tract and are largely responsible for neonatal meningitis and bacteremia. Group D contains five species. Three of the five, *Streptococcus faecalis*, *Streptococcus faecium*, and *Streptococcus durans*, are collectively referred to as enterococci. Bacteremia or endocarditis with a nonenterococcal Group D streptococcus, *Streptococcus bovis*, has been associated with colon carcinoma. The enterococci, which are normal residents of the bowel and vagina, serve as opportunists in polymicrobial infections originating at those sites, but enterococci are true pathogens in endocarditis and urinary tract infections. Pneumococci are common residents of the normal nasopharynx and a common cause of pneumonia. There are at least 80 pneumococcal types. Overwhelming postsplenectomy sepsis is the principal late septic complication of pneumococcal infection of importance to surgeons.

The virulence factors for Group A streptococci are listed in Table 5–5. Both bacterial surface components and extracellular products play a role in the pathogenesis of disease. The surface components can be divided into hyaluronic acid (potentially antiphagocytic), surface proteins (M, T, and R), Lancefield group carbohydrates, and peptidoglycan. The M surface protein is a major virulence factor. The M proteins seem to inhibit phagocytosis by PMNs by masking a cell surface component responsible for the activation of complement and they block bacterial recognition by opsonic complement molecules. Lipoteichoic acid present on the cell surface binds to fibronectin in ground substance. Like staphylococci, the streptococci may secrete a number of extracellular products favoring virulence. Scarlet fever in children is caused by a strain of Group A streptococci producing erythrogenic toxin.

Pneumococci produce no exotoxin but possess a polysaccharide capsule with antiphagocytic properties. An antipneumococcal capsular vaccine is available against 23 strains that account for nearly 90 per cent of infections, but its efficacy in preventing infection is only 65 to 70 per cent. Because of the importance of antibody-mediated opsonization of pneumococci, those patients with abnormalities in immunoglobulin production such as hypogammaglobulinemias and multiple myeloma seem more susceptible to pneumococci. Viral infections which disrupt the respiratory epithelium often immediately precede an episode of pneumococcal pneumonia.

Streptococcus viridans organisms remain the most common cause of infective subacute endocarditis. All of the viridens streptococci are sensitive to penicillin.

Neisseria

Morphologically, neisseria are gram-negative, spherical or oval cocci found in pairs with flattened adjacent sides. Human disease is caused predominantly by two species, *Neisseria gonorrhoeae* and *N. meningitidis*. They have special growth requirements and their isolation requires special culture media (chocolate agar or Thayer-Martin media) and the presence of carbon dioxide. *N. gonorrhoeae* is harbored in the urethra, endocervix, pharynx, and conjunctiva. Transmission is usually by sexual contact. Infection is not necessarily accompanied by symptoms, and asymptomatic carriers are the primary reservoir for gonoccal infection. Contiguous spread from the endocervix can result in pelvic inflammatory disease (PID).

Several bacterial factors enhance the virulence of *Neisseria*. Its surface contains pili and other protein components that facilitate attachment to epithelial surfaces and inhibit phagocytosis. Most of the *meningitidis* species are encapsulated and thereby strongly inhibit phagocytosis. These species can acquire iron from the host, an important virulence factor. Also unique to *Neisseria* is an extracellular enzyme, IgA protease, which breaks down IgA that normally facilitates clearance of bacteria from mucosal surfaces.

Pelvic inflammatory disease is the best known infectious outcome caused by *N. gonorrhoeae*. About 20 per cent of women exposed to *Neisseria* develop PID and about 50 per cent of all cases are caused alone or in combination with gonococci. Anorectal infection, skin lesions, tenosynovitis, and septic arthritis are also seen. The spread of gonococci into the upper abdomen can result in gonococcal perihepatitis (FitzHugh-Curtis syndrome).

Facultative Enteric Gram-Negative Bacteria and Pseudomonads

The Enterobacteriaceae are facultative aerobes—i.e., they grow best in air, but can survive in anaerobic conditions. These species, normally commensal in the gastrointestinal tract and vagina, are now the most common etiologic agents in surgical infections. Table 5–6 lists species of greatest surgical importance. The cell structure of these organisms (Fig. 5–5) is of importance. Many organisms, such as *Klebsiella* and *E. coli*, possess a capsule (K antigen) which

TABLE 5–6. AEROBIC (OR FACULTATIVE GRAM-NEGATIVE BACTERIA OF SURGICAL SIGNIFICANCE

IMPORTANT	OCCASIONALLY IMPORTANT	RARELY SIGNIFICANT
Enterobacteriaceae	Enterobacteriaceae	
Escherichia coli	*Citrobacter*	*Achrombacter*
Enterobacter	*Edwardsiella*	*Alcaligenes*
Klebsiella	*Providencia*	*Flavobacterium*
Proteus	*Salmonella*	*Moraxella*
Serratia	*Shigella*	*Eikenella*
Pseudomonas	*Yersinia*	*Kingella*
aeruginosa	*Acinetobacter*	
	calcoaceticus	
	Acinetobacter lwoffi	
	Aeromonas	
	Legionella	
	Pasteurella	
	Pseudomonas, not	
	aeruginosa	
	Vibrio	

Reprinted from Martin, W.J. and Young, L.S.: Enteric gram-negative bacteria and pseudomonads. *In* Howard, R.J. and Simmons, R.L. (eds.): Surgical Infectious Diseases. 2nd ed. Norwalk, CT, Appleton & Lang, p. 36, 1988.

acts to inhibit phagocytosis and is an important virulence factor. The flagella (H antigen) on some organisms may be essential for motility and for ascending in urinary tract infections. Pili are thought to act by attaching organisms to normal mucosal cells, the initial step prior to invasive infection. Endotoxin (O antigens) are lipopolysaccharides which form part of the cell coat (Figs. 5–2 and 5–3), and its role in the pathogenesis of the many clinical aspects of infections are hinted at in Table 5–3. Endotoxins probably bind to an acute-phase protein made by the liver, called LPS binding protein (LBP protein). The LPS-LBP protein complex in turn, binds more avidly to cells and initiates the release of cytokines (IL-1, IL-6, TNF) and other mediators of the physiologic phenomena observed. The most well-studied mediator is TNF, which is released by macrophages that bind LPS-LBP and which is seemingly responsible for many of the manifestations of endotoxin shock.

Many of these organisms also produce exotoxins useful for invasion. For example, *pseudomonas*, which is not a true member of the Enterobacteriaceae, re-

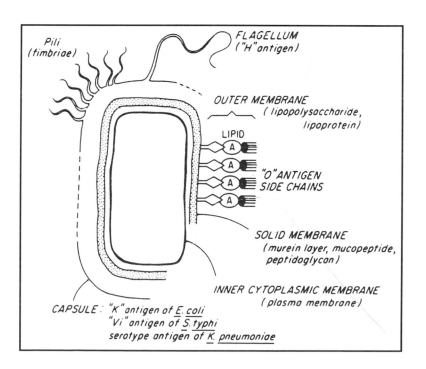

FIGURE 5–5. The major cell wall antigens of the gram-negative bacillus. Some are flagellated (H antigen) and may have capsules (K antigen). The O, or heat-stable somatic antigen, is part of the outer of three membranes and contains lipid A, which is responsible for endotoxicity. (Reprinted from Howard, R.J. and Simmons, R.L. (eds.): Surgical Infectious Diseases. 2nd ed. Norwalk, CT, Appleton & Lang, 1988.)

lease exotoxin A which inhibits protein synthesis. Antibodies to exotoxin A are protective against infection. The principle host defense against these organisms is opsonization and phagocytosis. Specific antibodies to LPS have proven to be protective if administered in gram negative sepsis.

E. coli is the most common facultative gram-negative aerobe in the gastrointestinal tract and in biliary, urinary, and intra-abdominal infections. The ascending course of these organisms from feces to urethra and the upper GU tract is thought to account for their importance in urinary infections and bacteremia. *E. coli* are important causes of wound, bone, and central nervous system (CNS) infection. They are often found in mixed infections in combination with *Bacteroides* species. Some strains produce an enterotoxin-like cholera toxin and tenaciously adhere to and invade normal intestinal mucosa; such strains are responsible for most cases of traveler's diarrhea. Most *E. coli* are sensitive to a wide array of antibiotics, including broad-spectrum penicillins, cephalosporins, aminoglycosides, and trimethoprim-sulfamethoxazole.

Klebsiella, Enterobacter, and *Serratia* species are commonly present in nosocomial pneumonias and biliary tract and intra-abdominal infection. *Klebsiella* is an encapsulated organism commonly associated with necrotizing pneumonias in alcoholic patients. *Klebsiella* pneumonia may account for up to 10 per cent of all hospital-acquired pneumonias and multiple-drug-resistant strains have appeared in many institutions. *Enterobacter* infections are now one of the commonest causes of nosocomial infections in surgical patients because of their capacity to become resistant to the cephalosporins. *Serratia* species have only recently been recognized as significant human pathogens and are seen as bacteremias associated with indwelling catheters and urinary tract instrumentation. They often occur as superinfecting pathogens in patients receiving broad-spectrum antibiotics.

Proteus species are not part of the normal enteric flora, but may be seen in the gastrointestinal tracts of antibiotic treated patients. They commonly cause urinary infections because of their ability to split urea and alkalinize the urine, potentiating the formation of stones. In addition, many species possess pili that allow attachment to the urothelium. The indole-positive strain of proteus is resistant even to aminoglycosides. *Shigella* and *Salmonella* species are important causes of diarrheal syndromes, which may mimic an acute surgical abdomen. *Yersinia enterocolitica* is a common isolate in appendicitis and mesenteric adenitis. *Campylobacter* infections of the gastrointestinal tract sometimes simulate acute abdominal infections.

The pseudomonads are not members of the enteric gram-negative family. They do possess endotoxin and secrete exotoxins, but they owe their ubiq-uity to an ability to survive in water almost without other nutrients. Because they are strict aerobes, they do not contribute much to the normal fecal flora, which is relatively anaerobic. Normal individuals cannot be colonized with pseudomonads because normal host defenses are highly effective. Colonization, however, occurs in debilitated hosts whose own flora has been depleted by antibiotics. Thus, pseudomonads flourish in intensive care units when they contaminate wet equipment and are spread by the personnel from patient to patient. *Pseudomonas* may simply contaminate the tracheobronchial tree of such patients or cause a fulminating infection with rapid progression to shock and death. Pseudomonal infection has a predilection to form necrotizing vasculitis that may lead to the rapid development of a condition similar to acute respiratory distress syndrome in the lungs. Vasculitis lesions, termed *ecthyma gangrenosum,* are characterized by vesicle formation with erythema followed by ulceration and are secondary to venular invasion of the vascular tree; their presence implies systemic pseudomonas infection with bacteremia. Mucoid encapsulated *Pseudomonas aeruginosa* strains cause a particularly aggressive pneumonia.

Anaerobic Bacteria

Anaerobes are bacteria that require reduced oxygen tension for growth, but most anaerobes associated with human disease are relatively aerotolerant. As many as 500 species of anaerobes have been isolated from the stool, but relatively few are isolated from human infection. Aerotolerance implies that they can survive up to 72 hours in the presence of oxygen, although they will not multiply. All morphologic types contribute to the pathogenic anaerobic flora, but the gram-negative rods (*Bacteroides, Fusobacterium,* and pigmented *Fusobacterium*) and gram-positive cocci (*Peptostreptococcus*) predominate. Gram-positive spore-forming rods (Clostridial species) produce potent toxemias and necrotizing infections of great clinical significance.

Of the gram-negative rods, *Bacteroides* and *Fusobacterium* are commensals in the flora of the mouth, distal gut, and female genital tract. These organisms do not produce endogenous bacterial endotoxin. Thus, they are of low virulence. They contribute to mixed infections within the peritoneum by extension or perforation from the colon, appendix, pelvic organs, and biliary tract. They may also lead to localized pneumonias and brain abscesses. In infections, they produce gas and a foul odor as a result of breakdown products of anaerobic metabolism, but they are almost always copathogens with aerobes. Their slow growth (up to a week) in culture may delay their diagnosis and make empiric anaerobic antibiotic treatment important in the absence of immediate culture positivity for anaerobes. The most frequent mixture found in man is *B. Fragilis* and *E. coli*.

Peptococcus and *Peptostreptococcus* are normally commensal in the mouth, gut, and vagina and are found with facultative organisms and *B. fragilis* in mixed infection.

The clostridia are gram-positive spore-forming rods. The most common, *Clostridium perfringens* does not form spores in infected tissue. They are the only spore-forming anaerobic organisms. All are soil organisms and are found in the gut as normal flora. The pathogenic strains are toxigenic and *Clostridium tetani* and *Clostridium botulinum* cause intoxications more than infections. Myonecrosis is most often caused by *C. perfringens*, *Clostridium novyi*, and *Clostridium speticum*. *Clostridium difficile* causes pseudomembranous colitis.

Actinomyces species and *Propionibacterium* are gram-positive non-spore-forming rods. *Propionibacterium acnes* is commensal on the skin and is implicated in acne. Actinomycosis is characterized by the presence of "sulfur granules" in purulent material.

Cultural identification of these organisms requires growth of inoculated plates under anaerobic conditions in a Gas Pak (BB2) jar which liberates hydrogen and carbon dioxide in response to addition of water to the jar. This creates anaerobic conditions inside the jar. Oxygen is removed and anaerobic conditions are produced.

All mucosal surfaces are heavily colonized with anaerobes and the ratio of anaerobes to aerobes varies from 10 to 1 in the mouth and upper respiratory tract to 1000 to 1 in the colon (Table 5–4). Therefore, *E. coli* makes up only 0.1 per cent of the total colonic flora, and *Bacteroides* species are numerically dominant (Table 5–4). Because virtually all anaerobic infections are derived from endogenous flora, and because the sites normally colonized by anaerobes are also colonized by numerous other species, anaerobic infections usually are polymicrobial. Thus, almost all anaerobic infections arise from damaged mucosa, except infections from clostridia, which are soil organisms inoculated into tissue as a result of trauma.

The predisposing conditions for anaerobic infections include a poor vascular supply, tissue necrosis, or a foreign body—any condition which reduces the redox potential and the pH, creating an environment favorable to the growth of anaerobes. Phagocytes depend on molecular oxygen for their full microbicidal activity, with the result that host defenses are seriously impaired in ischemic tissue; this permits organisms of low virulence to survive and grow. Except for clostridial infections, death rarely results from pure anaerobic infections—instead, anaerobes act to facilitate the growth of facultative aerobes by several mechanisms: (1) the mixed organisms supply each other with essential nutrients; (2) anaerobic metabolism produce certain products (succinic acid) which inhibit neutrophil function; (3) the capsules of certain bacteroid species are abscessogenic.

B. fragilis is the most common anaerobe found in mixed infections and possesses several mechanisms to heighten its synergistic potential, including a capsule that induces abscess production.

Although most gram-negative anaerobes do not have potent endotoxins, a few do (*Fusobacterium*). On the other hand, exotoxins of clostridial species (prototype *C. perfringens*) are numerous (Table 5–2). Lecithinases can destroy cell membranes, rupture capillaries, and lyse red cells (alpha toxin); the collagenases impair localizing defenses; and hyaluronases facilitate spread through tissue. In addition, DNAase, lipases, proteases, fibrinolysins, hemolysins, elastase, and leukocidins are produced. *C. difficile* and *C. perfringens* both produce enterotoxins.

The neurotoxicity of tetanus is a manifestation of toxemia. *C. tetani* is a gram-positive rod that forms a spore resembling a tennis racket. *C. tetani* produces two exotoxins—tetanospasmin and tetanolysin. Tetanospasmin is under plasmid control and is a single polypeptide chain. The organism itself cannot invade, but its ability to form spores permits prolonged survival despite extremely harsh environmental conditions. Tetanus occurs almost exclusively in nonimmunized or partially immunized individuals who have contaminated wounds. Toxin production occurs only under conditions of low redox potential. Tetanospasmin released into the wound binds to peripheral motor neuron terminals and is transported to the CNS both by the blood and along nerve trunks. It then enters the synapse, where it acts on the inhibitory interneurons to block neurotransmitter release, resulting in heightened reflex motor activity. By a similar mechanism the toxin causes heightened sympathetic activity. Its action thus mimics strychnine, resulting in convulsions and spasticity in response to external stimuli. Because the autonomic system is involved, hypertension, tachycardia, and cardiac arrhythmias occur. Therapy involves penicillin to eradicate the source of the toxin and tetanus immune globulin (TIG), to neutralize circulating and unbound toxin. The antibody in the immune globulin has no effect on toxin already bound to neural tissue.

C. perfringens is also inoculated into wounds where it proliferates in ischemic tissues aided by heme pigments and a high-calcium environment around fractures. All clostridial infections do not lead to gas gangrene, which is an infection in traumatized muscle or soft tissue with invasion of normal muscle. Thus, débridement of all devitalized tissues is the best prophylaxis. *C. perfringens* secretes many toxins (Table 5–2), the most important of which may be phospholipase C (lecithinase or alpha toxin). This toxin is hemolytic, destroys platelets, neutrophils, and capillary membranes. Treatment with débridement or amputation, penicillin and clindamycin, polyvalent antitoxin, and hyperbaric oxygen is usually too little, too late.

Pseudomembranous colitis is caused by the toxins elaborated by *C. difficile* with the manifestations of mild to sever colitis in recently hospitalized patients who have received antibiotics. Only sporadic cases are seen outside this context. It is an opportunistic nosocomial infection. Toxin A is most important in the pathogenesis of the syndrome, and toxin B is the cytopathic toxin used for laboratory diagnosis. *C. difficile* toxin has been found in less than 50 per cent of patients with antibiotic-associated colitis, suggesting the presence of other mechanisms. The mere presence of the toxin and bacteria without evidence of infection does not mean that the patient has colitis. Oral vancomycin or metronidizole are equally effective treatments. Cholestyramine binds the toxin but does not eliminate the etiologic agent.

Mixed and Synergistic Infections

Surgical infections most often result from a break in the skin or mucosal barrier that permits endogenous mixed flora on these surfaces to penetrate and infect the surrounding tissue. One would expect that tissue exposed to a multitude of species would be infected with unpredictable combinations of bacteria. However, a profound simplification of the flora contaminating the wound occurs, so that only several organisms predominate. Mixed infections usually contain anaerobes because the inocula contain anaerobes and because damaged tissue is ischemic. Aerobic bacteria soon utilize all available oxygen and a combination of facultative organisms and aerotolerant anaerobes take over.

Bacteria compete for available nutrients. As nutrients are depleted, those bacteria possessing the metabolic machinery to utilize alternative energy sources will outcompete other organisms and predominate. *Pseudomonas* is able to use at least 100 different organic substrates for energy, making it an excellent competitor. Furthermore, it is an obligate aerobe, which in the presence of oxygen generates much energy and enjoys explosive growth and outcompetes anaerobes in this setting. In contrast, obligate anaerobes using fermentative processes generate only 5 per cent as much energy as the aerobes, so that their growth is much slower and they rarely cause disease (*Clostridium* species excepted). Anaerobic metabolism produces many byproducts that can be used as energy sources by other bacteria, so that facultative organisms (*E. coli*) tend to dominate the environments that have suboptimal oxygen tensions. Conversely, bacteria may produce end products (lactic acid by lactobacilli) that makes the local environment unsuitable for some competing species which die out. Thus, mixed infections of two to five bacteria evolve from a polymicrobial one as bacteria compete for substrates. Although some bacteria secrete antibiotics favoring their own growth, this factor probably plays little role in mixed surgical infections.

While bacteria compete, they may also have a synergistic relationship. One bacterial species may lower the redox potential in the wound, favoring growth of another pathogen. One pathogen may break down local defenses to facilitate the growth of another species. For example, the nematode *Strongyloides* can carry enteric bacteria from the intestine to various other organs during its migration from the bowel with resulting polymicrobial septicemia. A variety of pathogens are capable of inhibiting systemic defense mechanisms and favor the survival of a second pathogen. As an example, many viruses (i.e., cytomegalovirus, human immunodeficiency virus [HIV]) are capable of suppressing cell- (T4 helper) mediated immunity and have been shown to increase the lethality of opportunistic microbes, e.g., *Mycobacterium* and *Pneumocystis*. Encapsulated bacteria may inhibit phagocytosis of other organisms. Leukocidins, which are exotoxins released by bacteria, are toxic to white cells and may facilitate bystander opportunists.

Not only may one organism provide a growth factor for another, an organism may confer increased virulence on another. The best example is the transmission of antibiotic resistance factors between gram-negative organisms or different species. Multiple drug resistance is usually transferred. This plasmid-mediated R factor differs from selection of drug-resistant organisms, which require multiple sequential mutations, whereas antibiotic resistance can be transmitted in one step during conjugation. Gram-positive organisms do not undergo conjugal transfer but rely on a viral vector. As viral phage particles are formed in a bacterial cell, they sometimes incorporate part of the bacterial genome, including plasmid coding for beta lactamase. These particles can then attach to phage-susceptible strains of bacteria, and the genetic contents are injected into the cell, which is then capable of elaborating β-lactamase. The virally injected DNA can then undergo recombination with the bacterial genome to allow replication and expression of the antibiotic-resistance plasmid. Even in the absence of transmission from one organism to another, bacteria-producing enzymes that inactivate antibiotics can protect otherwise sensitive copathogens from these antibiotics.

Mixed infections are commonly found as a result of gastrointestinal perforation. The 1000 : 1 ratio of anaerobes to aerobes in the colon favors anaerobic growth and abscess formation. Mixed anaerobic bacteremia implies a gastrointestinal source.

Fungi

Fungal infections seem always to surprise the surgeon. The differentiation between invasive infection and colonization can at times be difficult to make and treatment decisions may be complex. Of the thousands of known fungal species, only a few are pathogenic to humans and can be divided into three major groups, based on the mechanism by which they cause disease: (1) Inhalation—histoplasmosis, blastomycosis, coccidioidomycosis, and cryptococcosis; (2) colonization of mucosal surfaces with invasion under certain circumstances—candidiasis, aspergillosis, and mucormycosis; (3) innoculation into the subcutaneous tissue—sporotrichosis or mycetoma.

Diagnosis can be made using several techniques. Serology is rarely diagnostic because patients may have positive serology based on past exposures. Skin tests similarly will be positive if the patient has had infection in the distant past and will often be positive in areas in which the fungus is endemic. Histopathology or culture is probably the best test. Staining secretions with potassium hydroxide (KOH prep) results in dissolution of white blood cells and mucus but leaves the fungi intact. Hematoxylin and eosin stains may reveal granuloma formation suggestive of fungus but rarely demonstrates the fungus. The best available stain is the Gomori methenamine stain to visualize fungi in tissue sections. The Mayer mucicarmine stain stains the mucopolysaccharide capsule of *Cryptococcus neoformans*. Culture on Sabouraud media with maintenance of the culture of up to one month is often necessary for the slower-growing species and some (*Mucor*) are almost impossible to diagnose by culture.

Fungal surgical infections are primarily by the opportunistic fungi. Aspergillosis refers to infection by any of the numerous members of the genus *Aspergillus*. They can colonize the upper airway in healthy individuals and are noninvasive in the absence of abnormalities in host defense. In the compromised host, they may infect the ear, paranasal sinuses, orbit, lung, and brain. Microvascular thrombosis leads to expanding abscess formation with pulmonary cavitation, mimicking tuberculosis.

Mucormycosis is caused by opportunistic fungi of the *Mucor*, *Absidia*, or *Rhizopus* genera and occurs in the context of unregulated diabetes, immunosuppression, and thermal burns. The organisms invade surrounding vascular structures, which causes infarction of tissue and necrosis. The most fulminant infection in humans ifs rhinocerebral mucor, which begins in the nose and can spread contiguously to the orbits, palate, eye, and brain. Pulmonary, cutaneous, and gastrointestinal forms also exist. Successful therapy usually involves aggressive surgical therapy and amphoteracin B.

Candida species are normal inhabitants of the mouth, upper airways, and gastrointestinal tract, thus making definitive diagnosis of the disease difficult. The most common species is *Candida albicans*. Overgrowth occurs when competing bacteria are eliminated by antibiotic therapy, but this must be distinguished from invasive candidiasis. Risk factors for invasive candidiases include overgrowth, malnutrition requiring hyperalimentation, diabetes, systemic steroids, and immunosuppression. Invasion may be self limited or systemic. Cutaneous candidiasis involves moist areas of the skin, particularly skin folds. Mucocutaneous candidiasis consists of oral thrush with patches of white exudate. Esophageal candidiasis with ulceration is a more serious form. Vaginal candidiases is common in pregnancy, diabetes, and during antibiotic therapy. Invasive candidiasis may begin as overgrowth of *Candida* in the mouth, esophagus, bowel, bladder, or skin with deep penetration and intermittent seeding of the bloodstream. Transient fungemias with *Candida* are of little importance in a normal host. In the compromised patient, however, hematogenous spread with the formation of multiple microabscesses may develop. A macronodular skin lesion and enophthalmitis may aid in diagnosis. Endocarditis with bulky vegetations and systemic emboli may occur in drug addicts or on previously damaged or prosthetic heart valves. Intra-abdominal *Candida* often accompany polymicrobial infection. Culture of *Candida* is easy but the significance of a positive culture is difficult to assess. Oral, esophageal, vaginal, or skin candidiasis can be treated with nystatin. Failure to respond may require treatment with amphotericin B or fluconazole.

Viral Diseases of Surgical Significance

Viruses are ubiquitous in nature. Several viruses are especially important for surgeons on the basis of the risks they impose to the surgeon as well as to the patient. We will discuss viral hepatitis, CMV infections, and AIDS.

Hepatitis

At least four types of hepatitis are recognized: A, B, C (formerly non-A non-B), and D or delta. Herpes, CMV, and EBV can also cause hepatitis.

Hepatitis A is an RNA virus spread predominantly by the fecal-oral route and thus rarely effects surgical patients.

Hepatitis B is a DNA virus with numerous circulating markers that help in the assessment of disease. The outer protein coat contains a surface antigen (HB$_s$Ag). This antigen can circulate as the intact virion (Dane particle) or as part of the incomplete virus. It also has an inner core antigen (HB$_C$Ag) expressed on the surface of the nucleocapsid. The core also contains a soluble necleocapsid antigen (HB$_e$Ag) whose presence in the serum indicates the complete infectious virus. Hb$_e$Ag is found only in HB$_s$Ag-positive serum. HB$_s$Ag is made in great excess of the core antigens. Sera containing HB$_e$Ag are one million times more infective than serum containing HB$_s$Ag without detectable HB$_e$Ag. Of clinical importance is the fact that the elevation in the

HB_sAg is transient, and there is a window between the development of antibodies to HB_sAg and the disappearance of the surface antigen. This will suggest that no infection has occurred if markers are obtained in the "window." However, anti-HB_c antibodies are elevated during this period and allow demonstration of hepatitis B infection.

Approximately 5 per cent of adults in the United States have evidence of earlier infection with hepatitis B virus. Of the 200,000 people infected yearly with hepatitis B, 25 per cent become clinically jaundiced and 0.1 per cent die of fulminant hepatitis. Between 6 and 10 per cent of those infected become chronic carriers. Chronic active hepatitis develops in 25 to 50 per cent of carriers and often progresses to cirrhosis and/or liver cancer. Another 25 to 50 per cent of carriers develop chronic persistent hepatitis. Chronic hepatitis B carriers are important in the transmission of disease. The highest concentrations of the virus are in the blood, with lesser amounts in other body fluids. Infection occurs percutaneously through needle sticks, sexual contact, or exposure to blood. With extensive blood bank screening, hepatitis B now accounts only for 5 to 10 per cent of posttransfusion hepatitis.

Hepatitis C virus (formerly non-A non-B) has recently been identified as the major cause of transfusion-related hepatitis. An antibody to hepatitis C has been developed (anti-HCV). There is a long latent period of up to four months between infection and the development of the antibody, which will make detection of early cases more difficult. Units of blood infected with hepatitis C will test negative for the virus during this four-month period. Most patients with hepatitis C are asymptomatic. A large number of infected patients go on to develop chronic liver disease. Hepatitis C accounts for 90 to 95 per cent of posttransfusion hepatitis. The incubation period of hepatitis C varies from one to fifteen weeks. The clinical course tends to be less severe than hepatitis B but progression to chronic persistent and chronic active hepatitis may occur in 40 to 45 per cent and may progress to cirrhosis. Interferon alpha is used in currently evolving therapy for chronic hepatitis C infection.

Hepatitis D (delta virus) is an RNA virus coated with HB_sAg as the surface protein. Infection with hepatitis D can only occur as either co-infection with hepatitis B or superinfection of a hepatitis B carrier. Such infections are frequently fulminant and lead to chronic active hepatitis and cirrhosis in a larger percentage of cases than hepatitis B infection. Hepatitis D is diagnosed with identification of the delta antigen or IgM antibodies to the delta agent. The delta antigen is found only in the serum of patients positive for HB_sAg, so screening for hepatitis B should be effective to eliminate hepatitis D infection.

Both passive and active immunization are available for hepatitis B. Immune globulin (IG) and hepatitis B immune globulin (HBIG) are used for passive immunization in individuals exposed to hepatitis B (postexposure prophylaxis). Immune globulin is prepared from plasma not secreted for its anti-HB_sAg content, while HBIG should be considered under the following circumstances: (1) Perinatal exposure of an infant to an HB_sAg-positive mother; (2) following sexual contact with an HB_sAg-positive person; (3) after accidental percutaneous or permucosal exposure to HB_sAg-positive blood.

Hepatitis B vaccine (Heptavax) is prepared from inactivated surface antigen particles or from recombinant DNA technology (Recombivax). Immunization is 80 to 95 per cent protective and is recommended for individuals who are at substantial risk for acquiring hepatitis B virus, especially those with frequent exposure to blood. Because the risks of infection are often the highest during the period of training of healthcare workers, vaccination should be completed prior to surgical training.

Cytomegalovirus

Cytomegalovirus is a member of the herpes virus family. It can infect virtually any organ, but most commonly infects the kidney, gastrointestinal tract, lung, liver, and brain. It is the most common viral pathogen complicating organ transplantation. It may exist in a latent form in many tissues and be reactivated at a later time. Compromise of T cell-mediated immunity, as occurs in organ transplantation and lymphoid malignancies, is associated with reactivation of latent CMV infection. Potent T cell immunosuppressive agents, such as antithymocyte globulin, are associated with a high rate of CMV disease. It is commonly transmitted with blood product transfusions. High-risk groups for transmission include premature infants, seronegative organ transplant recipients, and immunosuppressed oncology patients. Infection in transplant recipients usually occurs one to four weeks after transplant. Infection may occur either primarily in a seronegative patient, as reactivation in patients with latent virus, or as reinfection with a different strain of virus. Symptoms in immunocompetent patients are usually those of a mononucleosis-like syndrome. Immunosuppressed patients may have a much more virulent form of infection with pneumonia, pancreatitis, and hepatitis. Pneumonia is a common manifestation of CMV infection in the immunocompromised patient. Cytomegalovirus infection of the retina may lead to blindness. Infection of the gastrointestinal tract with CMV may result in ulceration, perforation, or hemorrhage.

Diagnosis is made by demonstrating intranuclear inclusions (owl's eye) in tissue sections. A fourfold rise in antibody titer betwen acute and convalescent titers is needed to make the diagnosis serologically. The virus may be cultured in human fibroblasts, but a positive culture may take weeks to obtain. Monoclonal antibodies against CMV allow overnight diagnosis from tissue cultures. Difficulty in interpretation of results is encountered because patients without symptoms may also shed virus for months, making a cause and effect relationship between symptoms and the presence of the virus difficult.

A large percentage of the population has had past exposure to CMV and are seropositive. In general, transfusion of CMV-seropositive blood to an immunocompetent patient will result in only a mild infection, if any. Immunocompromised oncology patients or transplant recipients who are CMV-seronegative are at the greatest risk of severe infection if they receive seropositive blood products, and in these patients consideration should be given to transfusion of only seronegative units of blood products or blood that has been frozen or deglycerolized, which is associated with a greatly decreased risk of transmission.

In addition to prevention of infection, immunocompromised patients may be treated with ganciclovir, an analogue of acyclovir with much greater anti-CMB activity. Prophylactic acyclovir appears to reduce the risk of CMV in seronegative renal transplant recipients. Ganciclovir appears to be efficacious in transplant patients with CMV infections or patients with CMV retinitis. Leukopenia and marrow suppression may limit the use of ganciclovir.

Acquired Immunodeficiency Syndrome

AIDS refers to the occurrence of constitutional symptoms and/or AIDS-defining diseases such as secondary infection, neoplasms, and neurologic disease in a patient infected with a retrovirus, human immunodeficiency virus. By mid-1990, approximately 120,000 cases in adults and adolescents and 2000 cases in children had been reported in the United States. It is estimated that between 1 to 1.5 million people are infected. Human retroviruses consist of human T cell lymphotrophic (leukemia) viruses (HTLV-I and HTLV-II) and the human immunodeficiency viruses (HIV-I and HIV-II). The retroviruses are distinguished by their DNA polymerase (reverse transcriptase). HTLV-I induces an aggressive form of leukemia/lymphoma and HTLV-II is associated with T cell malignancies. The relationship of HTLV to HIV is not entirely clear, but frequently patients at high risk for HIV infection are infected with the HTLV virus and dual infection may lead to the accelerated emergence of AIDS. The RNA in the viral core is transcribed into a double stranded DNA by reverse transcriptase and becomes incorporated into the host DNA (provirus). Once the transcribed retrovirus DNA is incorporated into the host's genome, it is duplicated with the cell DNA. Therefore, once established, infection of an organism is usually lifelong. AIDS first appeared in 1978 to 1979 and is caused by HIV-I. Although HIV-II has been isolated from some patients—primarily in western Africa—with immunodeficiency, it is a relatively uncommon cause of AIDS. HIV isolates may

have a great deal of heterogeneity in their genome, and a single individual may be infected with a group of closely related viruses. In developed countries, the vast majority of patients are adults, and over 90 per cent are men. The case fatality rate is 75 per cent in patients diagnosed before 1983. Certain high-risk groups have been identified: homosexual men 60 per cent; intravenous drug abusers, 20 per cent; hemophilia patients, 1.0 per cent; heterosexual contacts, 5.0 per cent; and transfusion recipients, 2.0 per cent. The risk of acquiring AIDS through transfusion is approximately 1 in every 100,000 transfusions. The prevalance of HIV in certain groups is alarmingly high: 17 to 67 per cent of homosexuals; 50 to 87 per cent of intravenous drug abusers in New York City, and 72 to 85 per cent of persons with hemophilia A being treated with clotting factor concentrate. Transmission occurs by sexual contact or blood products. All blood donors in the United States are now screened for the presence of the antibody to the HIV virus. The presence of antibodies does not preclude the carrier state, because antibodies are not neutralizing. Most patients develop progressive disease despite the presence of neutralizing antibodies and cytotoxic T cells.

The AIDS virus induces profound depressions in cell-mediated immunity, allowing for the development of opportunistic infections and malignancies such as Kaposi's sarcoma. The cellular receptor for HIV is the CD4 receptor present on mononuclear cells. The immunologic defects detected include lymphopenia, selective CD4 cell subset deficiency, anergy, and elevation in serum immunoglobulins caused by B cell hyperactivity, resulting in hypergammaglobulinemia. This nonspecific activation of B cells interferes with the ability to mount an adequate humoral immune response. The virus exhibits an affinity for the activated T4 helper lymphocyte subset and replicates well in this cell population without being adversely affected by the host's antibody response. The monocyte-macrophage is also a major garget for the HIV-I, particularly the fixed tissue macrophage, which possesses the CD4 receptor. Different isolates of the virus exhibit significant genomic diversity, making the task of developing a vaccine difficult. Once the absolute T4 lymphocyte count drops below 200 cells/μl, the chances of developing an opportunistic infection are high. The T4 helper lymphocyte subset is responsible for the induction or regulation of virtually the entire immune system; therefore, defects in this subset result in global immune suppression.

The occurrence of viral infections in patients with the AIDS virus may be responsible for the development of malignancy. As examples, CMV has been associated with Kaposi's sarcoma, EBV with Burkitt's lymphoma and B cell lymphoproliferative disease, herpes simplex type 2 infection with cloacogenic carcinoma of the rectum, and squamous cell cancers of the anus. Actual HIV infection is not the cause of these malignancies, because viral DNA sequences cannot be demonstrated in the tumor cells.

The clinical manifestations of AIDS are myriad. Most patients exhibit no symptoms at the time of initial infection, but acute infection of seronegative patients can cause a mononucleosis-like syndrome including fever, malaise, generalized lymphadenopathy, a macular rash, and thrombocytopenia lasting one to three weeks occcurring three to six weeks after primary infection. Seroconversion occurs 8 to 12 weeks after initial exposure. The length of time from initial infection to the development of clinical disease varies, but is estimated to be between eight to ten years. A persistent malaise syndrome lasting months has been described in homosexual males. This syndrome of chronic lymphadenopathy has been termed pre-AIDS. AIDS-related complex (ARC) occurs in individuals with nonspecific symptoms with or without depressions in the T4 lymphocyte subset. ARC manifests itself as fatigue, fever, weight loss, rash, leukoplakia, herpes simplex, and oral thrush. Advanced ARC is diagnosed if more than two of these manifestations are present. Other manifestations of AIDS include direct infection of the brain resulting in dementia, enteropathy with malabsorption and diarrhea, glomerular disease, hypercalcemia, and adrenal insufficiency.

Opportunistic infections as a result of HTLV immunosuppression are common. Patients may be infected with a myriad of organisms, but *P. carinii* and *Mycobacterium avium-intracellulare* are most common. *P. carinii* pneumonia can be prevented by co-trimoxazole, dapsone, or aerosolized pentamidine. It is the most common opportunistic infection, occurring in 80 per cent of patients at some point during their illness. *Candida* (thrush, esophagitis) and CMV are common.

Approximately 30 per cent of AIDS patients present with Kaposi's sarcoma, which commonly involves the lymph nodes and visceral organs, in contrast to the cutaneous manifestations of classic Kaposi's sarcoma occurring in elderly patients. The HIV virus likely induces the production of growth factors from infected cells that facilitate the development of Kaposi's sarcoma and B cell non-Hodgkins lymphomas that are aggressive. Other lymphomas are not uncommon.

The diagnosis of AIDS is made in an HIV-positive patient with the occurrence of opportunistic infection, malignancy, constitutional symptoms, or neurologic disease. A positive antibody test using the enzyme-linked immunosorbent assay (ELISA) method does not determine the diagnosis of AIDS, it just confirms exposure to the virus. False positive tests can be problematic, and all positive tests should be repeated and confirmed by a more specific Western blotting technique to specific viral proteins. Conversely, some infected patients fail to make antibody or the antibody may not appear for three to four years after initial infection. The ratios of helper cells to suppress cell (CD4/CD8) are reduced in AIDS patients from normal values of 1.2 to 0.9, reflective of the cytotoxic effect on the T4 helper lymphocytes. At seven years after infection, only 20 per cent of HIV-positive homosexual men were free of symptoms. It is currently believed that virtually all infected individuals will ultimately develop progressive disease.

The implications for surgeons are significant. Patients who are HIV-positive may be totally asymptomatic for long periods, yet remain infective. It is vitally important to adhere to universal precautions in every patient seen, in order to minimize the risk to the surgeon. Similarly, careful disposal of needles and sharp instruments is crucial to prevent inadvertent injury and infection to those individuals responsible for cleaning these instruments. The risk of developing seropositivity from an isolated needle stick contaminated with the HIV virus is less than 0.5 per cent. Seroprevalence studies of emergency room patients in Baltimore revealed that 5 per cent of all ER admissions were HIV-seropositive. In non-high-risk patients, the incidence of seropositivity is less than 0.04 per cent. Screening of the blood supply for antibodies to HIV has nearly eliminated infections among transfusion recipients and hemophiliacs. The risk of transmitting HIV-I by transfusion of blood products is approximately 1 : 150,000 units. Of significance for screening of the blood supply is the latent period of 8 to 12 weeks before a patient will seroconvert. If they donate blood during this interval, the blood may contain HIV-I but test negative because the antibodies to HIV have not yet reached detectable levels.

Current drug therapy involves the use of attempts to inhibit the viral reverse transcriptase with zidovudine (AZT), dideoxycytodine (ddC) and dideoxyinosine (ddl). Zidovudine seems to be indicated in patients with symptoms of AIDS and depressed levels of T4 helper cells; it delays the progression to advanced ARC and AIDS. The principle toxicity of AZT is marrow suppression.

Miscellaneous Infections

Legionella

Legionella species are fastidious and ubiquitously present gram-negative aerobic bacilli that in humans behave as facultative intracellular bacteria. They are transmitted through inhalation with resultant pulmonary infection. The most common pathogen is caused by *Legionella pneumophila*. Growth is facilitated in hot water and heat exchange units that frequently contain stagnant water. Airborne transmission occurs. *Legionella* organisms are ingested by phagocyte, but the organisms inhibit fusion of the phagosome to the lysozone, protecting the organisms from destruction by lysozomal enzymes. Infection is controlled with the appearance of cell-mediated immunity, similar to that seen with other intracellular pathogens. Diagnosis is by culture or serologic methods. *Legionella* may be visualized in clinical specimens by direct fluorescent antibody staining. The test has a low specificity for *Legionella* (50 per cent). The urine may be examined for *Legionella* antigens, but they may persist for months after infection. Serum antibody is measured using the indirect fluorescent antibody test. Erythromycin and tetracycline are effective antibiotics. Patients with severe disease should receive rifampin.

Antimicrobial Therapy

The knowledge of bacterial and fungal morphology may seem far removed from the treatment of patients. Recent developments in antibiotic therapy have demonstrated the importance of a basic knowledge of bacterial structure and how this relates to the mechanism of the action of antibiotics—and similarly to the mechanisms by which microbes become resistant to antibiotics.

It should be readily realized from the preceding sections that antibiotics alone are not sufficient to cure many surgical infections. A continuous source of contamination from leaking viscera must be eliminated. Necrotizing infections with devitalized tissues that provide a low oxygen tension favor the continued growth of facultative and strict anaerobes. Without surgical debridement of these areas or drainage of abscesses, antibiotic therapy will be ineffective and the patient will not improve. The ischemic nature of many wounds may also prevent antibiotics from reaching the infected areas. One should look at antimicrobial agents as an adjunct to surgical drainage and debridement.

In this section, we will review the currently available antimicrobial agents with regard to their mechanism of activity and their spectrum of activity.

Antibacterial agents can be divided into four groups, based on their mechanisms of action.

1. Inhibitors of cell wall synthesis.
2. Inhibitors of the ribosomal component of protein synthesis.
3. Inhibitors of the pathway for folic acid synthesis leading to the inhibition of purine nucleotide synthesis.
4. Inhibitors of nucleic acid synthesis and packaging.

It is important to be aware of the mechanisms of action of various antibiotics. In general, combinations of antibiotics acting by different mechanisms (gentamicin, ribosomal inhibition; and piperacillin, cell wall synthesis) will be more effective than the use of several drugs that compete for the same mechanism.

The selection of antibiotics depends on the consideration of several factors. These include the spectrum of the antibiotics, the suspected or proven pathogens, the ability to achieve appropriate levels of drug in specific tissues, allergies or underlying organ dysfunction in the host, and cost.

Inhibitors of Cell Wall Synthesis

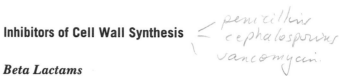

penicillins
cephalosporins
vancomycin.

Beta Lactams

Penicillins. All penicillins have the same basic structure; a β-lactam ring fused to a five-member sulfur-containing ring. (Fig. 5–6). Classes of penicillins vary in their side chain substitutions. β-Lactam antibiotics act by inhibiting cross linking in the bacterial cell wall. Cell wall cross linking requires the function of an enzyme (penicillin binding protein [PCP]) present on the bacterial cytoplasmic membrane. β-Lactam antibiotics bind covalently to this protein, inhibiting cell wall synthesis, leading to microbial killing. Penicillin is the prototypical β-lactam antibiotic. It remains effective against gram-positive aerobic and anaerobic streptococci and some gram-negative organisms, including *N. meningitidis*, *Eikenella corrodens*, and *Pasteurella multocida*. Penicillin is the treatment of choice for clostridial infections and many anaerobes other than *B. fragilis*. Resistance to penicillin has increased. Up to 90 per cent of *S. aureus* is resistant, resulting in the need to develop penicillins resistant to β-lactamases produced by resistant organisms. Extended-spectrum penicillins (ampicillin and amoxicillin) can kill many gram-negative organisms, including *Haemophilus influenzae*, but are destroyed by β-lactamases.

Antipseudomonal penicillins include the ureidopenicillins (piperacillin, azlocillin, and mezlocillin) and the carboxypenicillins (carbenicillin and ticarcillin) and are effective against pseudomonads. These drugs are also destroyed by β-lactamases.

Antistaphylococcal penicillins are resistant to bacterial β-lactamases and include cloxacillin, methicillin, nafcillin, and fluoxacillin.

Cephalosporins. Cephalosporins are a complicated group of antibiotics that have been divided into first, second, and third generation, depending on their spectrum of activity. Their mechanism of action is similar to that of the penicillins. In general, first-generation drugs kill gram-positive organisms better than they kill gram-negative organisms; later-generation drugs have extended activity against gram-negative organisms and against *B. fragilis*—but they lose some activity against gram-positive organisms. First-generation drugs (cefazolin and cephalothin) are very effective against streptococci and staphylococci but less effective against gram-negative organisms. They are not effective against the enterococci or methicillin-resistant staphylococcus. Second-generation drugs are divided into two

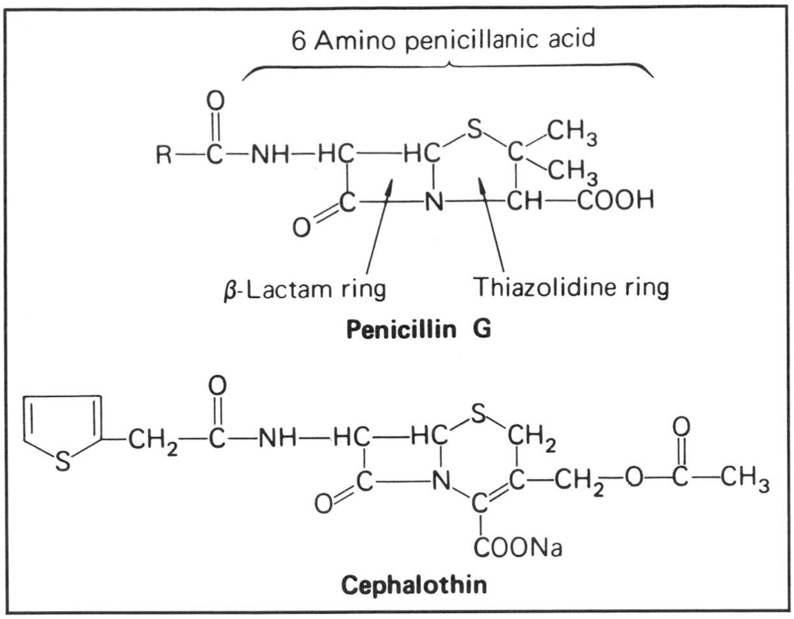

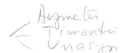

FIGURE 5–6. Structure of β-lactam antibi-
otics. (Reprinted from Howard, R.J. and
Simmons, R.L. (eds.): Surgical Infectious
Diseases. 2nd ed. Norwalk, CT, Appleton &
Lang, p. 276, 1988.)

groups. The first group (cefamandole, cefuroxime, cefonicid, and ceforanide) are effective against *H. influenzae* but are less effective against gram-positive organisms. The second group of the second-generation cephalosporins (cefoxitin and cefotetan) are highly effective against *B. fragilis*. They again are less effective than the first generations against gram-positive organisms, but they are more effective against gram-negative enteric organisms. Third generations can similarly be divided into two groups. The first group (cefotaxime, ceftizoxime, ceftriaxone, and moxalactam) is most effective against gram-negative enterics and some anaerobes. This group is not very effective against *Pseudomonas* organisms. The second group of the third-generation drugs (cefoperazone and ceftazidime) have a spectrum similar to the first group but have relatively good activity against *Pseudomonas*.

Carbapenems. Imipenem is the representative drug in this class. It is metabolized by a renal tubular enzyme (transpeptidase). Therefore, it is marketed with cilistatin, an inhibitor of this renal tubular enzyme, to slow urinary excretion and prolong the drug's half-life. Imipenem has the broadest parenteral antimicrobial spectrum of any antibiotic, encompassing gram-positive organisms; gram-negative organisms, including *Pseudomonas;* and anaerobes, including *B. fragilis*. Several species, including *Pseudomonas cepacia, Pseudomonas maltophilia,* methicillin-resistant *S. aureus* and *S. epidermidis* are usually resistant to imipenum.

Monobactams. Aztreonam is the prototypic drug in this class. It has a very broad spectrum against gram-negative bacilli including *Pseudomonas.* It is ineffective against gram-positive cocci or anaerobes. Its spectrum is similar to that of the aminoglycosides, but it is neither nephrotoxic nor ototoxic.

β-Lactam Inhibitors

Clavulanic acid and sulbactam inhibit β-lactamases produced by bacteria, thereby allowing antibiotics susceptible to hydrolysis by β-lactamases to reach their target and be effective. Several commercially available preparations (amoxicillin-clavulanic acid, ticarcillin-clavulanic acid, and ampicillin-sulbactam) are available that greatly expand the spectrum of the antibiotic.

Vancomycin

Vancomycin inhibits bacterial cell wall synthesis at an earlier step than the β-lactam antibiotics. Vancomycin is effective primarily against both facultative and anaerobic gram-positive organisms, including all streptococci (including enterococci) and staphylococci. It is the treatment of choice for methicillin-resistant *S. aureus* and *S. pidermidis*. It is sometimes used as gram-positive prophylaxis in surgical patients allergic to penicillin. Oral vancomycin, which is not absorbed, is used in the treatment of *C. difficile* colitis.

Inhibitors of Ribosomal Protein Synthesis

Aminoglycosides

Aminoglycosides function by inhibiting bacterial protein synthesis at the 30s ribosomal subunit. They therefore require active bacterial metabolism for their optimal effects and are less effective under conditions of hypoxia and low pH—i.e., conditions which exist in areas of necrosis. Their spectrum is primarily against gram-negative aerobic bacilli. Gentamicin, tobramycin, netilmicin, and amikacin have excellent activity against *Pseudomonas aeruginosa.*

Aminoglycosides alone are not effective against staphylococci or streptococci, but are highly effective when combined with a β-lactam-resistant penicillin or vancomycin. Streptomycin is used in the treatment of tuberculosis.

Chloramphenicol

Cloramphenicol inhibits bacterial protein synthesis at the 50s ribosomal subunit. It is bacteriostatic rather than bactericidal and is highly effective against most gram-negative bacilli and anaerobes, including B. fragilis. It is ineffective against P. aeruginosa and staphylococci but may be effective against other pseudomonads. It is rarely used for the treatment of gram-positive infections because of the availability of effective less toxic alternatives.

Clindamycin

Clindamycin inhibits protein synthesis at the 50s ribosomal subunit and is most effective against gram-positive anaerobic organisms. Nearly all anaerobic bacteria are susceptible not including C. difficile. Clindamycin is effective against streptococci and staphylococci, but not against methicillin-resistant staphylococci.

Erythromycin

Erythromycin binds to the 50s ribosomal subunit in a position similar to clindamycin and is bacteriostatic, not bacteriocidal. It is active mainly against gram-positive organisms, including S. aureus (nonmethicillin resistant), S. epidermidis, and streptococci. Of particular importance is that erythromycin is effective in the treatment of Legionella, Mycoplasma, and Chlamydia species.

Tetracycline never give to children < 7y

Tetracyclines are bacteriostatic agents that bind to the 30s ribosomal subunit. It is quite effective in the treatment of streptococcal, staphylococcal, and Neisseria infections, but resistant strains have emerged. The tetracyclines are the therapies of choice in several situations including rickettsial, mycoplasmal, and chamylidial infections, Lyme disease (Borrella burgdorferi), and syphilis.

Inhibitors of Folic Acid Synthesis

Sulfonamides

All sulfonamides inhibit the enzyme tetrahydropteric acid synthetase in the folic acid pathway to purine metabolism. Sensitive organisms are unable to use folic acid of the host and must synthesize their own supply. They have a broad activity against gram-positive and gram-negative organisms, including enteric gram-negative organisms. They have no activity against staphylococci, enterococci, Serratia, or Pseudomonas. They are used in combination with trimethoprim in the therapy of protozoal infections such as P. carinii.

Trimethoprim

Trimethoprim is a folic acid antagonist that inhibits dihydrofolate reductase and purine synthesis. It is commonly used in combination with the sulfonamides for synergy, acting at two different sites in the same metabolic pathway. It is active against most aerobic gram-negative bacilli except P. aeruginosa.

The combination of trimethoprim-sulfamethoxazole is synergistic in inhibiting purine synthesis and has a broad spectrum of activity. It is effective against staphylococci, streptococci, the Enterobacteriaceae, and Shigella and Salmonella. It is ineffective against P. aeruginosa.

Inhibitors of DNA Synthesis

Metronidazole

The actual mechanism of action of metronidazole is uncertain, but is believed to act through disruption of DNA transcription and microbial replication. Its spectrum of activity is limited to anaerobes, including all Bacteroides species. It is also effective against protozoal infections such as trichomoniasis and amebiasis. It has become the treatment of choice for C. difficile colitis because of low cost, the low incidence of side effects, and low resistance to treatment.

Quinolones

The quinolones act by inhibiting the DNA gyrase enzyme needed to package DNA into dividing bacteria. Norfloxacin and ciprofloxacin are currently available. They have a very broad antimicrobial spectrum including gram-negative and gram-positive aerobes. They are ineffective against anaerobes. They are effective against P. aeruginosa, enterococci, and S. aureus and S. epidermidis. Ciprofloxacin is the only oral drug effective against Pseudomonas.

Rifampin

Rifampin blocks RNA synthesis is inhibiting DNA-dependent RNA-polymerase. It has a broad spectrum of activity but resistance emerges rapidly if rifampin is used as a single agent. It may be used with a penicillinase-resistant penicillin to treat S. aureus or S. epidermidis.

Antifungal Agents

Amphotericin B.   Amphotericin B is a polyene macrolide antifungal that combines with fungal membrane sterols to increase porosity of the membrane leading to death of the fungus. It is the most effective antifungal agent available.

Nystatin.   Nystatin is an oral antifungal agent related to amphotericin B. It is used for prophylaxis of ill patients receiving broad spectrum antibiotics, to prevent fungal overgrowth in the gut.

Ketoconazole.   Ketoconazole interferes with the formation of membrane sterols. It has excellent activity against *Candida* and is effective for the treatment of mucocutaneous and mucosal *Candida* infections.

Fluconazole.   Fluconazole is a promising new antifungal agent to be used instead of amphoteracin B in systemic fungemias. It is significantly less toxic than amphotericin B.

Antimicrobial Resistance

Resistance to antimicrobials has become an increasingly important problem in the treatment of infections. Bacteria have a limited number of mechanisms available through which resistance can develop. These include the following:

1. Change in the drug target. Alterations in ribosomal proteins, the enzymes of bacterial folic acid metabolism, penicillin-binding proteins, and DNA gyrase may modify the antibiotic site to such an extent that binding cannot occur, rendering the antibiotic ineffective.
2. Production of detoxifying enzymes. β-lactamases and aminoglycoside-modifying enzymes (AME) break down penicillins and aminoglycosides, rendering them ineffective.
3. Decreased antibiotic uptake. To be effective, antibiotics need to be taken up by the microbe. Failure to take up the drug will prevent its action.

Bacteria have successfully adapted to our high-technology environment and have overcome our attempts to eradicate them. Some of the mechanisms involved in their defeat of modern antibiotic technology are discussed below.

Nearly all gram-negative organisms possess a chromosomal gene for β-lactamase production, usually mediated by a plasmid. Some bacteria possess promoters, which facilitate increased production of a β-lactamase that is normally produced at a low level. In addition, several different types of β-lactamase are produced by bacteria. Strategies used to deal with this problem include the use of different antibiotics or the use of a β-lactamase inhibitor such as clavulanic acid or sulbactam, thereby allowing the β-lactam antibiotic to be effective.

Methicillin-resistant staphylococcal infections have become a major problem in hospitals. These staphylococci are able to produce a new enzyme to maintain cell wall integrity during growth and division when their native enzymes needed for cell wall synthesis are inactivated by a β-lactam antibiotic. They have essentially found a way to bypass the inactivated enzyme.

Enterococci have become resistant to many penicillins because they possess a low-affinity penicillin-binding protein, thereby preventing or diminishing binding of the drug to this cytoplasmic membrane enzyme needed for cell wall synthesis.

Resistance to vancomycin has begun to emerge. Vancomycin acts by blocking cell wall synthesis by binding to peptidoglycan. Resistance has developed because the bacteria are capable of synthesizing a protein that can selectively inhibit the binding of vancomycin to peptidoglycan.

Aminoglycoside resistance has emerged through several mechanisms. Many aminoglycoside-resistant organisms are able to synthesize an AME, which is transmissible through plasmids. The AME results in phosphorylation, adenylation, or acetylation of the drug, preventing its binding to ribosomes. Different aminoglycosides are more or less difficult to modify through this mechanism. Some pseudomonads exhibit diminished aminoglycoside uptake as a resistance mechanism. Resistance has also emerged because some gram-negative bacteria have modified their 30s ribosomes such that they fail to effectively bind to the aminoglycoside.

Resistance to ciprofloxacin has emerged as bacteria have modified the antibiotic target, DNA gyrase, to diminish inhibition by the antibiotic. In addition, outer membrane porosity can decrease and depress the accumulation of the antibiotic.

These represent the general adaptations bacteria have made in developing antibiotic resistance to single drugs. Increasingly today, resistance to multiple antibiotics is developing. Multiple resistance occurs when a mechanism confers resistance to several agents. Many antibiotics enter the bacterium through a common porosity pathway or have a common target that can be modified. In addition, it appears that resistance genes to individual antibiotics cluster on the bacterial chromosome or plasmid. Plasmids may be single or multiple and carry resistance for as many as ten antibiotics. Under these circumstances, resistance to any one antibiotic will perpetuate the existence of that kind of bacteria, which is simultaneously resistant to many other antimicrobials and can pass on these factors to other bacteria.

HOST DEFENSES AGAINST INFECTION

The host defenses against infection are of three types: those that prevent lodgment of the potential pathogen, those that serve to localize the infection, and those that defend against systemic spread once such infection occurs.

Prevention of Lodgment. There are generally four components of any host's defenses against the requirement that microbial organisms adhere to bodily surfaces, proliferate, and invade: (1) Physical barriers such as skin or mucous membrane; (2) surface functional modifications like cilia; (3) local secretions such as mucus or immunoglobulin; and (4) the indigenous microbial flora which compete for available nutrients.

Skin. The skin consists of an outer epidermis and a deeper dermis firmly cemented together. Epidermal appendages (sweat glands, hair follicles, sebaceous glands, apocrine gland, and nails) extend into the dermis. The principle defenses of the skin against lodgment of microbes are dryness and desquamation. The keratin constantly sloughs and the sparse flora are desquamated as well. Because bacteria need moisture they grow poorly on normal exposed skin, which has a low moisture content. Whenever skin becomes moist, bacterial populations increase; therefore, the skin adjacent to wet wounds, the perineum, and the backs of bedridden patients frequently develop infective dermatitis. Of lesser importance are the secretions of sebaceous glands, consisting of lipids inhibitory to most pathogens but stimulatory to diphtheroids (*Corynebacterium* species). Most bacteria adhere to the openings of hair follicles, which are the exit points for sebaceous glands. Of least importance seems to be the low pH, a result of lactate, aspartate, and glutamate secretion, and a low temperature.

Colonization by bacteria is sparse on normal skin except in intertriginous areas where moisture accumulates. The most common organisms are the diphtheroids and *S. epidermidis* (plus related micrococci). Gram-negative bacteria are found in the moist areas of the groin, perineum, and axillae where *Candida* species are also found. These organisms are considered to be residents; other organisms are traditionally called transients. Any damage to skin (by shaving, abrasion, hair plucking, etc.) increases the transient flora.

Intact skin is difficult to infect and an intact corneal barrier cannot be penetrated by any organism unless it is damaged and moisture is present.

Eye. A tear film continually moistens the eye. Although *S. epidermidis* and *Lactobacillus* are resident organisms, bacterial infections of the undamaged eye are uncommon because tears contain lysozyme, which lyses bacteria, plus IgA (and lesser amounts of IgG and IgE). Immunoglobulin A acts to bind bacteria and prevent their adherence to conjunctival epithelium. Immunoglobulin G may play an antiviral role. The chemical (lysozyme), mechanical (tears and blinking), and immunologic properties (IgA) make eye infections unusual.

Respiratory Tract Barriers. The respiratory tract provides a variety of physical barriers to infection. Because of the gross physical configuration and the changes in gas velocity during inhalation, most inhaled particles, including microbes, never reach the alveoli. Large particles are filtered out by nasal vibrissae, moist nasal septum, and turbinates. Those that escape collide with the posterior pharyngeal wall, carina, or early bronchial septum. As the respiratory tree branches, it increases in cross-sectional area and velocity slows so that particles settle by gravity on the distal bronchial wall.

Retained microbes are excluded or expelled by two reflexes: reflex bronchoconstriction (vagal response to noxious particles) and coughing, which propels mucous plugs toward the mouth. A third mechanism of clearance utilizes mucociliary transport, which itself has two components—namely, mucous secretions and the cilia. Two mucous layers, a superficial gel-like layer and a deeper layer in solution (sol), enable the cilia that sweep through the sol to move the gel layer toward the mouth. The gel contains a number of defenses—IgA, α-1-antitrypsin, lactoferrin (to bind iron needed by bacteria), lysozyme (which lyses bacterial walls), and complement.

The cilia (about 200 per respiratory cell) beat at 1000 to 1500 times per minute and touch the mucous gel only at the apex of the respiratory epithelial cells. This asynchronous motion is not under nervous control but responds to serotonin; the cilia's function is impaired by carbon monoxide, cigarette smoke, pentobarbital, atropine, and alcohol.

There are no cilia distal to the terminal bronchioles. The alveolus contains alveolar macrophages which can become activated, as can any macrophage (see below). Macrophages provide the major bactericidal function in the normal lung.

Alimentary Tract. The squamous epithelium of the oropharynx is a potent mechanical barrier, and saliva possesses lysozyme and IgA which kill bacteria and prevent their adherence, respectively. The normal mixed flora of the mouth prevent colonization by more pathogenic organisms.

The esophagus is covered with saliva, and the rapidity of transit prevents microbial lodgment.

The stomach when empty has such a low pH that it is sterile. Some bacteria (i.e., *Camphylobacter pylori*) may survive, but are different to culture. Food, antacids, and histamine receptor blockers permit bacteria to flourish, however, by neutralizing the normal acidic pH. Gastric achlorhydria, such as occurs in gastric carcinoma and pernicious anemia, will also permit bacterial overgrowth.

The small intestine is lined with a mucosal epithelial barrier and has such powerful propulsive motion that bacteria without special ligands cannot adhere. IgA also inhibits adherence, which is the first step to invasion. In stagnant areas such as the ileum, the bacteria count increases exponentially. Intestinal epithelial cells can endocytose bacteria and transport them into the submucosal tissues in amounts proportional to their number in the lumen, but phagocytes (usually macrophages) ingest them and can transport them to local nodes (bacterial translocation). Sometimes such bacteria can escape killing, enter venules, and can cause infection.

The urinary tract is protected from pathogenic infection by means of periodic flushing of urine, which is somewhat bacteriostatic by virtue of its high urea content, high osmolarity, high ammonia concentration, the presence of IgA, and acid pH. The long urethra in the male limits—but the short female urethra facilitates—microbial access. The prostate and semen contain poorly characterized microbicidal substances.

The female genital tract offers a mechanical barrier in its thick squamous epithelial covering and the cervical mucous plug. Immunoglobulin A and lysozymes are secreted. In the adult, lactobacilli flourish in the glycogen-rich acidic secretions and tend to compete successfully with nearby fecal pathogens.

The importance of these defenses against lodgment of microbes is clear when one considers by what mechanisms pathogenic microbes produce disease. The initial step in almost all naturally occurring infections is microbial attachment to epithelial surfaces. Bacteria and viruses attach via pairs of complementary receptors on microbe and surface cell. Some of these ligand-receptor systems are well known and others are obscure. Once attached, the organism can invade, can produce local or systemic toxins, or can employ host "defenses" to induce tissue damage.

Tissue Host Defenses

It is useful for conceptual purposes to divide the host defense system into two parts, the nonspecific cellular and humoral components and the truly immunologic components in which antigenic recognition takes place. Certain pathogens are primarily removed by specific portions of the host defense system (Table 5–7). The two interact at multiple points.

The Phagocytes

Once microbes have penetrated the surface skin or mucosa or have been implanted in tissue via trauma, surgery, or disease, the most important host defense against infection is the phagocytic system. There are two components to the phagocytic system: the circulating phagocytes and the fixed phagocytes (reticuloendothelial system). The granulocytes (neutrophils, eosinophils, and basophils) plus the monocytes compose the circulating phagocytes, and the macrophages in all tissues, especially liver, spleen, and lung, are the fixed phagocytes. Most phagocytes are capable of killing the ingested microbes, but they also can contribute to adverse effects of systemic infection and tissue damage.

TABLE 5–7. EFFICACY OF THREE COMPARTMENTS OF HOST DEFENSE IN COUNTERING INFECTIOUS ORGANISMS

HUMORAL	CELL-MEDIATED	PHAGOCYTIC
Bacteria	Bacteria	Bacteria
Pneumococcus	*Mycobacteria*	*Staphylococcus**
Streptococcus	*Listeria*	*Klebsiella*
Haemophilus	*Brucella*	*Aerobacter*
Meningococcus	*Salmonella*	*Serratia*
Pseudomonas	*Staphylococcus**	*Proteus*
		Probably most other enteric and anaerobic bacteria
Toxins	Fungi	Fungi
Diphtheria	*Candida**	*Candida**
Tetanus	*Aspergillus*	
	Histoplasma	
	Mucor	
Viruses	Viruses	
Polio	*Vaccinia*	
Hepatitis	Cytomegalic	
Rubella	inclusion	
Others	disease	
	Most others	
	Parasites:	
	Pneumocystis carinii	

* Many infectious agents are attached by two compartments of host defense; selecting the predominant compartment may not be possible.

Reprinted from Howard, R.J. and Simmons, R.L. (eds.): Surgical Infectious Diseases. 2nd ed. Norwalk, CT, Appleton & Lang, Table 11–1, p. 152, 1988.

Granulocytes

Polymorphonuclear leukocytes (PMN) function in the phagocytosis and killing of microbes and are essential in the localization and containment of infections. The PMN responses occur long before the production of specific antibody and cell-mediated responses. They are the major effector of the nonspecific immune response. Polymorphonuclear cells are produced only in the bone marrow. Normal neutrophil reserves in the marrow contain six to ten times the daily neutrophil requirement. Marrow production and release is stimulated by several colony-stimulating factors (CSF), G-CSF, GM-CSF, M-CSF, and IL-3 (a multicellular CSF). These glycoproteins are released by macrophages and lymphocytes in response to bacterial products such as endotoxin. The total neutrophil pool consists of circulating (40 per cent) and marginated (60 per cent) compartments. Marginated PMNs are transiently sequestered along endothelial surfaces of small veins. They have segmented nuclei and cytoplasmic granules. The function of the segmented nucleus is unknown. Immature neutrophils are called bands or stabs because of their elongated twisted nucleus. The most important phagocytic cell is the neutrophil, which contain two types of granules: azurophil and specific. The azurophilic granules (primary granules) contain a number of hydrolytic enzymes (amylase, α- and β-glucosidase, β-glucomonidase, elastase, neutral proteases, collagenase, cathepsin D with a optimum ph of 5). Such enzymes can digest almost any organic molecule. Lysozyme and myeloperoxidose are present in azurophilic granules and can kill bacteria. Azurophilic granules also contain cationic proteins which can induce inflammation (Table 5–8).

Specific granules contain lysozyme and lactoferrin, which binds up the free iron that bacteria need to proliferate. Specific granule contents also can activate the alternate pathway of complement. The specific granule may play a role in the modulation of cellular membrane receptors. Plasma membrane receptors for C3b and methonine-leucine-phenylalanine (FMLP) exist intracellularly, probably on the inner surface of the specific granule. Exocytosis of the specific granule not only discharges the granule's contents into the extracellular space, but also results in increased receptor expression for C3b and FMLP. Resisting PMNs have receptors for FMLP, C5a, and C3b homogeneously distributed over their cell membrane surface. In response to chemoattractants, some receptors cluster at the leading edge of the cells in the direction of the chemoattractant.

Granulocytes are end cells which do not proliferate and have a life span of only one to two days. However, RNA is present and such cells can make protein. Mitrochondria are scarce and energy for movement and phagocytosis is derived almost totally from anaerobic glycolysis of the glycogen reserves. Energy for bacterial killing after phacogytosis relies on the hexose monophosphage shunt and requires molecular oxygen. Granulopoiesis takes about 14 days. Once released into the circulation, the PMNs have a half-life of approximately six hours and can maintain function in the tissues for one to two days. In the face of infection, large numbers of preformed PMNs can be rapidly released into the circulation from preformed pools in the bone marrow and on endothelial cells.

Of utmost importance for host defense is the ability of the neutrophil to deform itself and migrate. Half the neutrophils are sequestered in the spleen and lung and are released in response to adrenocortical steroids or catecholamine stimulation, accounting for the neutrophilia of stress. The ability of neutrophils to adhere to specific endothelial receptors (called homing receptors) are upregulated in the region of an insult. ICAM is the best characterized of these receptors. The adherent marginated PMN must then insinuate themselves between endothelial cells (diapedesis) and migrate toward a stimulus, which depends on chemotaxis—the ability to mi-

TABLE 5–8. NEUTROPHIL GRANULE CONTENTS

CLASS	AZUROPHILIC	SPECIFIC
Microbicidal enzymes	Lysozyme Myeloperoxidase	Lysozyme
Neutral serine proteases	Elastase Cathepsin G Proteinase 3	
Acid hydrolases	N-acetyl-β-glucosaminidase Cathepsins B & D β-glucuronidase β-glycerolphosphatase α-mannosidase	
Metalloproteases		Collagenase
Others	Bactericidal cationic proteins	Lactoferrin Vitamin B$_{12}$-binding proteins Cytochrome b Histaminase FMLP receptors

Adapted from Falloon, J. and Gallin, J.I.: Neutrophil granules in health and disease. J. Allergy. Clin. Immunol. 77:653, 1986.

grate in a suitable chemical gradient. Known chemotaxins include C5a and C3a of the complement cascade and bacterial substances including certain bacterial peptide sequences (e.g., FMLP). See Figure 5–7.

Leukocyte function in response to infection can be divided into three components: chemotaxis, phacogytosis, and intracellular killing.

Chemotaxis

The neutrophil can migrate in anaerobic, acidic environments, but stops migrating in very high concentrations of chemotactic mediator and after phagocytosis. Chemotaxis (the unidirectional migration of neutrophils in response to a chemical gradient) is impaired by steroids and by unknown substances in severely stressed persons. A number of congenital and acquired defects in chemotaxis have been identified. Chemotaxis generally requires ligands for specific chemotactic receptors on the surface of neutrophils. Migration requires adequate chemotactic factors and neutrophils that are competent to migrate.

The receptors for the chemotaxins are somehow tied to the motility apparatus of the PMN, resulting in the PMN moving toward the chemoattractant. Chemotactic factors are derived from the complement and coagulation cascades, cytokines (IL-8) released from injured tissue, bacterial peptides, and cytokines released by antigenically stimulated lymphocytes. Complement is the most important source

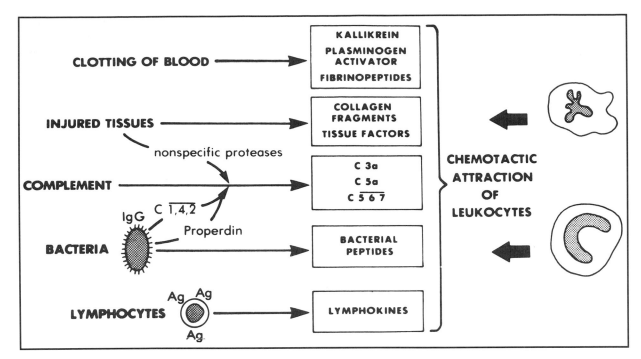

FIGURE 5–7. Major mechanisms for generation of chemotactic factors. (Reprinted from Howard, R.J. and Simmons, R.L. (eds.): Surgical Infectious Disease. 2nd ed. Norwalk, CT, Appleton & Lang, Fig. 11–7, p. 160, 1988.)

of the most powerful endogenous chemotactic agents, C3A and C5A, cleavage products of C3 and C5. The most important chemotaxin is C5A. Lymphokines derived from activated lymphocytes may be more important in chronic infections. Leukocyte migration depends on glycolysis and proceeds normally under anoxic conditions. The hyperglycemia accompanying stress and sepsis may facilitate PMN energy production. Regulators of leukocyte movement are present normally and can be produced by some bacteria (leukocidins).

Chemotactic disorders may be secondary to a congenital or acquired cellular disorder, defects in the production or chemotactic factors, or inhibitors of chemotactic factors or cell migration. Leukocyte motility disorders are usually manifested as protracted and recurrent soft tissue infections. Septicemia is uncommon. Offending pathogens are *S. aureus* (most common), *S. epidermidis,* gram-negative bacilli, and fungi. The acquired cellular defects seen after trauma and infections and accompanying diabetes are of most concern to the surgeon.

Phagocytosis

After leukocytes have migrated down the chemotactin gradient, recognition and ingestion of the offending organism occurs. The phagocyte must first recognize that the organism is "bad." In the first step, opsonins bind first to the microbial surface and then to specific receptors on the phagocytic cell membrane, so that the phagocyte and microbe are stuck together by opsonic glue. In the absence of opsonins, most organisms are not ingested or effectively cleared by phagocytes, because the C3b component of the complement activation pathway is the best opsonin. The phagocyte has receptors for C3b, which in turn is bound to the microbe that activated the complement cascade. Specific Ig binds to the Fc receptors on the phagocyte after engaging the microbe. After attachment, pseudopods are extended around the particle so that cell membrane-lined vacule, the phagosome, is formed. The process requires energy and further requires a linkage between the cell membrane receptor and its contractile protein—actin and myosin. The phagosome then fuses first with the specific granules and then the primary (azurophilic) granules so that the particle becomes exposed to lysozyme—to break down microbial cell walls, lactoferrin—to bind up iron required for microbial growth, and most importantly, cationic proteins, which break up membranes of bacteria.

Phagocytosis of inert particles occurs, but in vivo phagocytosis requires recognition of opsonins bound to the microbial surface. The major opsonic mechanisms involve the Fc protein of IgG and the complement component C3b, which has been activated by either the direct or alternative pathways. Some IgG is necessary for the most efficient phagocytosis, since its binding seems to best activate the process. Normal serum contains little IgG for opsonic activity, while hyperimmune serum possesses large amounts. The effects of IgG are amplified because IgG activates the complement cascade with the generation of C3b, a potent opsonin. Fibronectin (α-2-surface binding glycoprotein) binds weakly to bacteria and nonspecifically opsonizes tissue debris, facilitating its clearance.

Defects in opsonization result in infections with encapsulated organisms, which relay on opsonification for their clearance. These virulent encapsulated organisms include pneumococci, *P. aeruginosa*, streptococci, and *H. influenzae*. Patients with congenital or acquired C3 or immunoglobulin deficiencies are particularly susceptible.

Intracellular Killing

Ingested microorganisms are best killed by the products of molecular oxygen, not by degranulation (Table 5–9). When microbes are phagocytized, there is a large increase in oxygen consumption associated with increased production of hydrogen peroxide (H_2O_2) and superoxide radicals ($\cdot O_2^-$) (see Fig. 5–2). A plasma membrane-associated enzyme, NADPH oxidase, converts O_2 to superoxide with the production of NADP. Superoxide is converted to peroxide by the enzyme superoxide dismutase. The energy for this process is derived from the hexose

TABLE 5–9. LEUKOCYTE MICROBICIDAL MECHANISMS

Oxygen-dependent Killing Mechanisms
  Hydrogen peroxide (H_2O_2)
  H_2O_2 + halide + myeloperoxidase
  Superoxide anion O_2^-
  Hydroxyl radicals ($OH\cdot$)
  Singlet oxygen (O_2^*)
Oxygen-independent Killing Mechanisms
  Acid
  Lactoferrin
  Lysozyme
  Granule cationic proteins

Reprinted from Meakins, J.L., Hohn, D.C., Simmons, R.L., Dunn, D.L., Hunt, T.K., and Knighton, D.R.: Host defenses. *In* Howard, R.J. and Simmons, R.L. (eds.). Surgical Infectious Diseases. 2nd ed. Norwalk, CT, Appleton & Lang, p. 163, 1988.

monophosphate shunt pathway of glucose oxidation. The hexose monophosphate involves the oxidation of glucose-6-phosphate with the production of NADPH (Fig. 5–8).

Peroxide alone kills microbes only at high concentrations. However, in the presence of myeloperoxidase and halide ions, the toxicity of hydrogen peroxide is greatly increased. Myeloperoxidase augments the killing effects of hydrogen peroxide by pro-

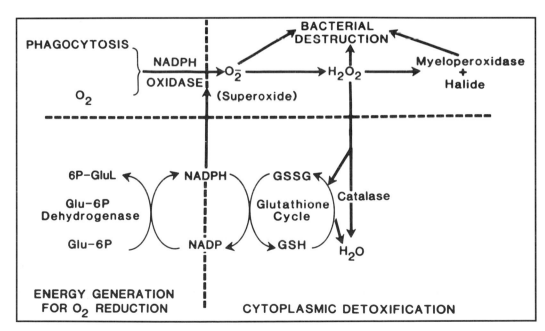

FIGURE 5–8. Metabolic pathway of the leukocyte primary oxidase system. The interaction between phagocytosis and bacterial destruction is schematically outlined. Phagocytosis stimulates the production of superoxide and hydrogen peroxide, which, in conjunction with the myeloperoxidase-halide system, leads to bacterial destruction within the phagosome. Excess hydrogen peroxide, which could damage the cell, is detoxified by catalase and the glutathione cycle. The energy for both H_2O_2 production and detoxification is provided by the hexose monophosphate shunt. (Reprinted from Howard, R.J. and Simmons, R.L. (eds.): Surgical Infectious Diseases. 2nd ed. Norwalk, CT, Appleton & Lang, Fig. 11–10, p. 162, 1988.)

ducing hypochlorous acid from chloride anion and hydrogen peroxide. Singlet oxygen and hydroxyl radicals are highly toxic to microbes and are produced as intermediate steps in the conversion of oxygen to superoxide to hydrogen peroxide. Products of the respiratory burst plus granule contents act within the phagocytic vacuoles to kill and degrade ingested microbes (Table 5–8). The neutrophil is protected from the effects of toxic oxygen radicals by the action of catalase and glutathione peroxidase.

Interestingly, degranulation can be dissociated from the respiratory burst. Suppression of the hexose monophosphate shunt, used to generate NADPH for the production of oxygen radicals, fails to inhibit degranulation. Similarly, inhibition of glycolysis inhibits degranulation but not superoxide formation.

Mechanisms whereby neutrophils kill microbes in an oxygen-independent manner are listed in Table 5–9. Acid present in the phagosome is toxic to microbes. Lactoferrin chelates iron, an essential element for the growth of bacteria. Lysozyme and cationic proteins are also important in bacterial killing.

The consequences of a failure of the respiratory burst is exemplified by the congenital leukocyte disorder known as chronic granulomatous disease. These patients lack the oxidase system and, therefore, the ability to generate superoxide and peroxide. Such patients are susceptible to severe bacterial and fungal infections.

The respiratory burst-degranulation system is extremely toxic to organic molecules. There is considerable evidence that exocytosis of granules and the respiratory burst occur independently of phagocytosis and when the phagosome has not completely closed. Tissue injury can result by such nonspecifically activated PMN.

Monocyte-Macrophage System

Circulating monocytes and the fixed macrophages also act as phagocytic killers of microbes. These cells contain lysosomes and mitochondria and synthesize a vast array of proteins, including many of the inflammatory mediators (tumor necrosis factor, IL-1, and complement C2, C3). Monocytes are capable of producing over 100 different products. The functions of the monocyte-macrophage system are summarized in Table 5–10.

Monocytes circulate for only 8 to 12 hours, whereas fixed macrophages (such as Kupffer's cells, alveolar macrophages) take on properties specific for the tissue in which they reside and may live for months. The vast majority of the total pool of mononuclear phagocytes resides in the tissues as macrophages. The macrophages play a role in cell-mediated immunity as well as in phagocytic host defense.

TABLE 5–10. BIOLOGIC FUNCTIONS OF THE MONOCYTE-MACROPHAGE SYSTEM

Scavenger function
Microbicidal activity
Cooperative immune processing
Cytotoxic activity
Regulation of granulopoiesis
Generation of pyrogen
Synthesis of complement (C2), prostaglandin E2, and plasminogen activator
Generation of mediators of wound repair—collagen synthesis, angiogenesis

Reprinted from Meakins, J.L., Hohn, D.C., Simmons, R.L., Dunn, D.L., Hunt, T.K., and Knighton, D.R.: Host defenses. *In* Howard, R.J. and Simmons, R.L. (eds.): Surgical Infectious Diseases. 2nd ed. Norwalk, CT, Appleton & Lang, p. 164, 1988.

Normal macrophages can act as phagocytes to clear bacteria and other debris from tissue. Like neutrophils, macrophages possess surface receptors for IgG-Fc, for C3a and C3b, and for cell surface glycoproteins. These receptors permit macrophages to ingest their opsonized microbial targets as well as macromolecular materials by both pinocytosis and phagocytosis, as do neutrophils. The internalization of the target particle within a phagosome, the fusion of phagosome with lysosome, and respiratory burst all progress in large part as they do in neutrophils. But the process is slow and relatively ineffective unless the macrophage has been "activated."

Macrophage activation is an adaptive response to stress which is mediated in large part by exposure of the macrophage to IFN-8 or to bacterial products such as lipopolysaccharide of gram-negative bacteria. Interferon-γ, in turn, is a product of antigen or mitogen T 4 (T helper) lymphocytes. Activated macrophages are much more efficient microbicidal cells, not only against pyogenic organisms, but also against obligate intracellular pathogens like *Leshmania, Mycobacterium, Salmonella,* and others. Not only do activated macrophages kill by the respiratory burst, but they also utilize the production of nitric oxide, derived from the metabolism of arginine, to kill these intracellular pathogens. The latter mechanism is very weak—if present at all—in neutrophils.

Activated macrophages not only kill microbes more efficiently, they can kill tumor cells and secrete cytokines (such as IL-1, IL-6, M-CSF, G-CSF, and GM-CSF. Of utmost importance, antigens are more effectively processed by macrophages and class II major histocompatibility complex antigens presented on the cell surface; the antigen is then presented to the responding clone of lymphocyte in combination with the class II self-antigen, and it is only in this context that the antigen can be recognized. In turn, stimulated responding lymphocytes secrete IFN-σ to maintain the activated state of the macrophage, which then can kill the intracellular pathogen to which T cell immunity has been generated.

Many of the systemic responses to infection are mediated by cytokines released by activated macrophages: IL-1 and tumor necrosis factor (TNF) produce fever; procoagulants which help to localize the infection are produced. IL-1 is an important costimulant with antigen in the responses of T 4 cells; TNF is the single most important factor which mediates the complex picture of systemic sepsis; IL-6 induces most of the hepatocyte acute phase proteins.

The role of the spleen in presenting systemic sepsis may derive from its lymphokines, such as IFN-σ, which pass into the liver to maintain a state of priming for activation in the Kupffer's cells. The Kupffer's cells, in turn, are the most active sites for bacterial clearance from the blood.

Although the preceding section discusses the role of cell-mediated immunity in the host defenses against infection, the following chapter describes the structure and function of this system in greater detail.

BIBLIOGRAPHY

1. Howard, R.J. and Simmons, R.L.: Surgical Infectious Disease. Norwalk, Appleton & Lang, 1988.
2. Wilson, J.D., Braunwald, E., Isselbacher, K.J., Petersdorf, R.G., Martin, J.B., Fauci, A.S., and Root, R.J.: Harrison's Principles of Internal Medicine. New York, McGraw-Hill Inc., 1991.
3. Pachulski, R.T.: Internal Medicine Notes. Norwalk, Appleton & Lang, 1991.
4. Davis, J.M. and Shires, G.T.: Principles and Management of Surgical Infections. Philadelphia, J.B. Lippincott, 1991.
5. Davis, J.H., Drucker, W.R., Foster, R.J., Gamelli, R.L., Gann, D.S., Pruitt, B.A., and Sheldon, G.F.: Clinical Surgery. St. Louis, C.V. Mosby Co., 1987.
6. Jacoby, G.A. and Archer, G.L.: Mechanisms of disease: New mechanisms of bacterial resistance to antimicrobial agents. *N. Engl. J. Med. 324:*601–612, 1991.

6

IMMUNOLOGY AND TRANSPLANTATION

Suzanne T. Ildstad

THE BASIC COMPONENTS OF THE IMMUNE SYSTEM

An understanding of the basic cellular interactions involved in the immune response has resulted in great progress in the field of transplantation over the past 30 years. The discovery of the current conventional immunosuppressive agents used to prevent rejection has revolutionized the field of transplantation. Livers, kidneys, lungs, hearts, bone marrow, and pancreases are now transplanted with facility and ever-improving results. However, appropriate management of rejection requires an understanding of the interaction of the components of the immune system which respond to foreign transplanted tissues. This review will focus on the major components of the immune response: *macrophages; T lymphocytes; B lymphocytes; natural killer (NK) cells; and cytokines*, the soluble proteins through which the cells of the immune system communicate. An understanding of the cells and interactions involved in the immune response is critical to understanding the mechanisms through which immunosuppressive agents function.

Although a number of cells are involved in host defenses, the lymphocyte is *the* specifically reactive cell. The fundamental paradigm in immunology is that the lymphocytes involved in the immune response are genetically *preprogrammed* during development to respond to a foreign material (antigen) that induces an immune response by activating specifically reactive *clones* of cells. The antigen does not instruct individual lymphocytes to generate an immune response; only those cells which have been preprogrammed during development (ontogeny) to produce a cell surface receptor of the appropriate specificity for the antigen will respond. Reactive lymphocytes are stimulated through antigen binding to proliferate, resulting in the expansion of specific clones of antigen-specific reactive cells. This process, known as the *clonal* nature of the immune response, has dominated immunology for over 30 years.

Six steps occur in generation of the immune response to foreign tissue or to an invading microbe: *encounter, recognition, activation, deployment, discrimination*, and *regulation*. To initiate the immune response, lymphocytes with antigen-specific receptors must encounter the invading foreign tissue or antigens derived from it. This response is very specific; only those clones of cells which contain antigen-specific receptors on their cell surface can bind to the offending antigenic molecules. When lymphocytes recognize and bind to an antigen, they are activated to respond in one of two forms, depending upon cell type. Activated T lymphocytes produce an inflammatory response through cellular activity, while activated B lymphocytes produce a humoral response in the form of antibody. Antibodies and activated lymphocytes then cooperate in an elaborate deployment response to eliminate foreign antigens. The immune response is simultaneously amplified by cytokines, protein cell regulators secreted by the various activated cells. The cytokines serve as soluble mediators to "spread the word" locally and to recruit additional lymphocytes. Other humoral mediators such as complement, kinin, and coagulation factors also contribute to the total inflammatory response. Theoretically, evolution has ensured discrimination between self and non-self to avoid autoimmune reactivity. To prevent unnecessary damage to the surrounding normal host tissues, regulation of the immune response occurs by which the intensity of the immune response is correlated with the antigenic load imposed. In effect, this is the feedback control for the immune system. When the stimulus is no longer present, the response usually ceases.

Macrophages, or accessory cells, are the scavenger cells that capture and present antigen to lymphocytes. In contrast with lymphocytes, macrophage binding of antigen is nonspecific. This heterogenous group of cells includes macrophages, monocytes, fixed tissue histiocytes, dendritic cells and Langerhans' cells. All are bone marrow-derived and serve to digest antigens into smaller molecular fragments (epitopes). These antigen-presenting cells then bind the epitopes to their cell surfaces to "process" the antigen and present it to specifically reactive lymphocytes that migrate past. For most antigens, this step is critical to lymphocyte activation, since most lymphocytes recognize antigen only in the context of the epitope bound to the macrophages and are blind to the antigen in soluble form independent of the macrophages. The greatest concentration of accessory cells is present in the spleen, lymph nodes, and lymphoid tissues. Binding of antigen to macrophages is nonspecific, while binding to T and B lymphocytes is highly specific. Macrophages that have bound antigen also produce a number of immunoregulatory cytokines that amplify the immune response.

The Ontogeny of the Immune Response

In this complex and elegant system, the immune system does not know in advance which antigens it will encounter. It must, therefore, have in its armamentarium a nearly infinite variety of cell receptors or antibodies in order to recognize virtually every antigen in existence. Most of the diversity of the immune response is believed to be acquired before birth. The cellular components of the immune system are all derived from a pluripotent stem cell in the bone marrow. At least nine cell lineages are provided by this one totipotent cell: B cells, T cells, NK cells, neutrophils, platelets, macrophages, eosinophils, basophils, erythrocytes, mast cells, glial cells, and dendritic cells (Fig. 6–1). Production of the different lineages is under direct regulation by various cytokines, including colony-stimulating factors, which influence differentiation and proliferation of the bone marrow stem cell progeny. The first immature cell lines to be established are the lymphoid and myeloid (Fig. 6–1). After the lymphoid progenitor cells differentiate into mature T and B lymphocytes in the primary lymphoid organs (thymus and bone marrow), they enter the blood stream and migrate to populate the secondary, or peripheral lymphoid tissues (spleen, peripheral lymph nodes, and various tissues including skin) (Fig. 6–2). Two major cell types of the lymphoid lineage participate in the immune response for rejection: B lymphocytes and T lymphocytes. The B cells produce a humoral response in the form of antibody in response to antigen, while T cells are responsible for cell-mediated functions of the immune system. Some mature T cells mediate effector functions such as direct cytotoxic attack to produce graft rejection, while others

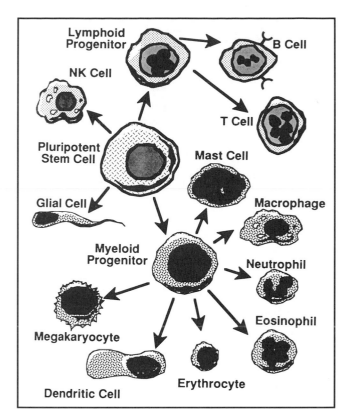

FIGURE 6–1. Components of the immune system. A pluripotent stem cell produces all components of the immune response.

play an immunoregulatory (helper) role through secretion of cytokines to up- or down-regulate nearly all aspects of immune response.

Macrophages and Monocytes: The Accessory Antigen-presenting Cells

Macrophages play a critical role in the immune response. They function as accessory cells to ingest antigen and to present it to lymphocytes, and, by supporting lymphocyte function through the release of *CYTOKINES*, they amplify the immune response. The specific cytokines produced by these mononuclear cells are sometimes referred to as monokines. Macrophages were previously referred to as the reticuloendothelial system, but the term mononuclear-phagocyte system has replaced that term. The macrophage cell line is derived from the bone marrow pluripotent stem cell through a common committed progenitor cell which produces granulocytes, monocytes, and macrophages. Cytokines termed colony-stimulating factors (CSF) induce differentiation of these progenitors into monoblasts, which in turn differentiate into promonocytes. Promonocytes, in turn, migrate randomly throughout

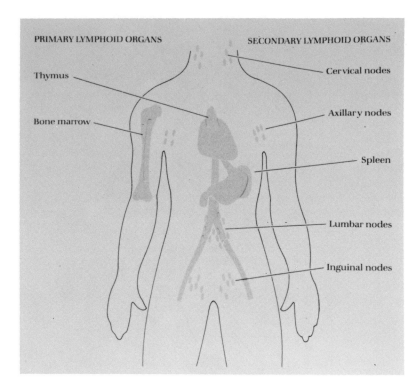

PRIMARY LYMPHOID ORGANS

SECONDARY LYMPHOID ORGANS

Thymus

Cervical nodes

Bone marrow

Axillary nodes

Spleen

Lumbar nodes

Inguinal nodes

FIGURE 6–2. Distribution of human lymphoid tissue. The location of primary and secondary lymphoid tissue in humans. After lymphoid progenitor cells differentiate in the primary lymphoid organs (bone marrow and thymus), they migrate to the spleen, peripheral lymph nodes, and tissues of the secondary lymphoid tissue. (Reprinted from Golub, E.S.: Immunology: A Synthesis. Sunderland, M.A.: Sinauer Associates, Inc., Chapter 11, Fig. 2, p. 182, 1987.)

the body to give rise to the differentiated fixed-tissue macrophages (Fig. 6–3), such as hepatic Kupffer cells and dendritic cells. Migration of the developing monocytes into tissues occurs as a random phenomenon. Upon entering the tissue, monocytes undergo transformation into fixed-tissue macrophages and develop functional and morphologic characteristics specific for the tissue in which they finally reside. In recipients of transplanted bone marrow, host macrophages are replaced by those of the donor phenotype within three months after transplantation. The final maturational step of development in the mononuclear-phagocyte line is the transformation of tissue macrophages into multinucleated giant cells in response to a variety of infections and inflammatory stimuli. Gamma interferon (IFN-γ), a cytokine released by activated T lymphocytes, aids in inducing this transformation. Recent data indicate that these cells may serve as a reservoir for the human immunodeficiency virus (HIV) in individuals with acquired immunodeficiency syndrome (AIDS).

The primary role for macrophages is host defense. These phagocytes ingest and kill intracellular parasites and clear extracellular pathogens from the bloodstream and tissues. A role in surveillance for tumors and tumoricidal capabilities has been suggested, but is most likely mediated by soluble products produced by these cells rather than through direct cellular attack by the macrophage itself. Macrophages process antigen and present it on their cell surface to lymphocytes in a more reactive form, thereby serving as accessory cells in the activation of lymphocytes. A complete absence of cells of macro-

phage lineage has not been described clinically, indicating that this condition is probably not compatible with life. Table 6–1 lists the major activities of macrophages.

The differentiation between the resting and activated macrophage was first suggested by Mackaness in the 1960s. Activated macrophages are larger, have an increased capacity for adherence and spreading on surface, and have increased numbers of vesicles containing cytokines. This activation occurs as a result of response to the release of macrophage-activating lymphokines (especially IFN-γ) secreted by T lymphocytes which have been stimulated by a foreign antigen. This interaction is at the crux of cell-mediated immunity. When macrophages have been exposed to endotoxin on bacterial surface membranes, they release a peptide hormone referred to as tumor necrosis factor (TNF), which in turn can itself activate macrophages. Therefore, macrophages exposed to endotoxin can activate themselves, permitting a more rapid immune response to invading microbes. An increase in receptors specific for fungi and an increase in immunoglobulin G (IgG) Fc receptors which would bind

TABLE 6–1.   MAJOR ACTIVITIES OF MACROPHAGES

Microbicidal activity
Chemotaxis
Pinocytosis
Phagocytosis
Antigen presentation

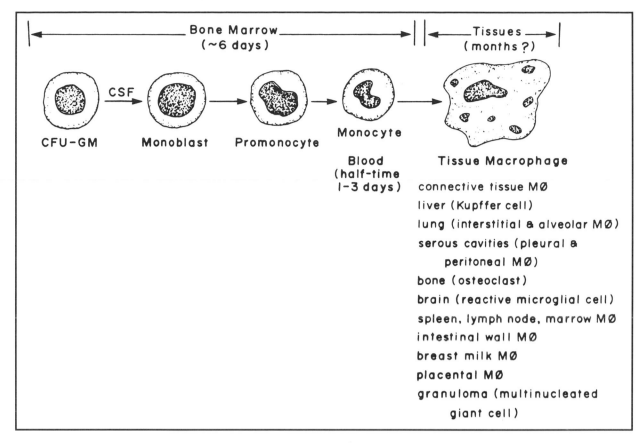

FIGURE 6–3. Development of cells in the mononuclear phagocyte system. CFU-GM denotes colony-forming unit, granulocyte-monocyte, CSF colony-stimulating factors, and MØ macrophage. (Reprinted from Johnson, R.: N. Engl. J. Med. *318*: 747–752, 1988.)

antigen coated with antibody accompanies the macrophage activation.

The macrophage is an extremely active secretory cell. Over one hundred substances produced by these unique cells have been identified (Table 6–2 contains a partial list of these products). Interleukin-1 (IL-1) is probably the most important factor produced by these cells. Interleukin-1 stimulates B lymphocyte proliferation and subsequent antibody production. It also stimulates production of lympho-

kines by T lymphocytes. The increased synthesis of IL-1 by activated macrophages results in an amplification of the immune response (Table 6–2). Synthesis of IL-1 is also induced by endotoxin. Concomitantly, the presence of endotoxin causes release of TNF by macrophages, resulting in increased production of IL-1 by endothelial cells as well as by macrophages. Both TNF and IL-1 can produce the fever and the synthesis of acute phase reactants characteristic of inflammation (see Chapter 2, Mediators of Inflammation).

TABLE 6–2.   PRODUCTS SECRETED BY MACROPHAGES

Tumor necrosis factor (cachectin) (TNF)
Interleukin-1 (IL-1)
Interferon /β
Angiogenesis factor
Fibronectin
Lysozyme
Prostaglandins
Apolipoprotein E
Elastase
Complement components
Arginase

T Lymphocytes: Ontogeny, Function, and Role in Rejection

T lymphocytes, like macrophages, are also derived from the same bone marrow-derived pluripotent stem cell (Fig. 6–1). Committed lymphoid progenitors differentiate into pre-T cells, which migrate to the thymus and mature there. All T lymphocytes express on their cell membrane a specific T cell receptor (TCR) that is the antigen binding site and associated proteins that make up the T cell receptor complex (CD3). Foreign antigens bind to this receptor and activate the immune response (Fig. 6–4).

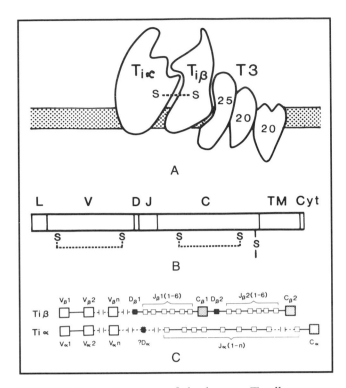

FIGURE 6–4. Structure of the human T cell receptor and its subunits. Part A shows subunit composition of the human T cell receptor. The Tiα and Tiβ subunits are held together by S–S bonds and are most closely associated with the 25-kd γ chain of the T3 molecule. The α and β subunits are anchored in the cell membrane with their transmembrane segments. The T3 complex consists of two additional subunits (δ and ε), with molecular weights of 20,000. Although not shown, a recently described 16-kd homodimer (32-kd nonreduced), termed *zeta*, is also noncovalently associated with the T3-Ti complex. Part B shows the structure of the Ti subunits. The predicted primary structure of the β-chain subunit after translation from the cDNA sequence is depicted, as are the variable region leader (L), V, D, and J segments, a hydrophobic transmembrane segment (TM) and cytoplasmic part (Cyt) in the C region, a potential intrachain sulfhydryl bond with the α subunit. Part C shows a scheme of the genomic organization of human β- and α-chain genes. In the β locus, V indicates the V gene pool located 5', at an unknown distance from the $D^{\beta}1$ element, the $J^{\beta}1$ cluster, and the $C^{\beta1}$ constant-region gene. Further downstream, a second $D^{\beta2}$ element, $J^{\beta2}$ cluster, and $C^{\beta2}$ constant-region gene are indicated. A similar nomenclature is used for the TI α locus, in which only a single constant region is found. ?D indicates the uncertainty about the existence of a putative Ti α-diversity element. (Reprinted from Royer, H. and Reinherz, E.: N. Engl. J. Med. *317*:1136–1142, 1987.)

The T cell receptor complex is acquired in the thymus. At the same time, immature T cells acquire in the thymus additional subset or differentiation receptors. These differentiation antigens are expressed on most lymphocytes and designate various T cell subsets. The most common subsets are the CD8+ cytotoxic/suppressor group, which lyse target cells and kill cells infected with virus, and the CD4+ immunoregulatory cells (helper/inducer), which mediate interactions of T cells, B cells, macrophages, and other cells, primarily through cytokine (lymphokine) production. After maturation in the thymus, T cells of both types migrate to populate the peripheral lymphoid tissues.

Until recently, the T cell differentiation antigens were referred to by different terms in different species. In 1982, an international symposium convened to rename T lymphocytes subsets by clusters of differentiation or CD antigens to allow general application of the same terminology to all species. T lymphocyte cellular subsets are now designated by cellular function. The most frequently encountered CD antigens for each cellular type are listed in Table 6–3.

The T Cell Receptor

The T cell receptor is composed of two polypeptide chains referred to as alpha (α) and beta (β). Each chain has a variable region which makes it antigen-specific plus a constant region. Like most other receptors, the TCR is a heterodimer, with the chains linked by disulfide bonds (Fig. 6–5). Cloning of T cells has allowed characterization of the TCR and a better understanding of how and where it binds antigen. The human T cell receptor is a cell surface complex consisting of a 90-Kd Ti alpha-beta (αβ) heterodimer. It is associated with three invariant polypeptides that are collectively referred to as the T cell receptor complex or CD3 (Fig. 6–4). This is remarkably constant for all species characterized. The majority of T cells acquire the αβ-TCR heterodimer in the thymus as an active process. A second TCR, termed gamma-delta (γδ), which is only expressed in a minority of T cells, has recently been identified. The tissue location of acquisition of the γδ receptor has not yet been determined.

Gene rearrangement of the TCR to give specificity and diversity occurs at the Ti αβ gene loci during intrathymic development. Receptor acquisition is critical, since it is responsible for antigen recognition by both helper (CD4+) and cytotoxic (CD8+) T lymphocytes. At this time, the CD4 and CD8 surface glycoproteins are also acquired in the thymus. Any strongly self-reactive clones are eliminated at this time by an active process of programmed cell death (apoptosis). The CD4+ cell subset contains the majority of helper/inducer T lymphocytes and a small fraction of cytotoxic T cells, while the CD8+ subset includes the majority of cytotoxic and suppressor T cells. Most CD4+ cells demonstrate specificities for antigen plus Class II MHC molecules. CD4 is also the receptor for the Human Immunodeficiency Virus (HIV). Most CD8+ cells specifically recognize antigen associated with Class I major histocompatibility complex (MHC) molecules (Fig. 6–4).

TABLE 6–3. CLUSTERS OF DIFFERENTIATION

Cluster Designation	Distribution Characteristics	Prototype Monoclonal Antibody	Population
CD 1	T cell associated	T6	Cortical thymocytes, dendritic cells.
CD 2		T1	T cells, NK cells.
CD 3		T3	All mature T cells; T cell receptor complex.
CD 4		T4	Helper/inducer T cells.
CD 5		T1	Pan T and subpopulation of B cells.
CD 6		T12	Mature T cells and subpopulation of B cells
CD 7		Leu 9	Pan T, NK cells.
CD 8		T8	Cytotoxic/suppressor T cells, NK cells.
CD 19	B cell associated	Leu 12	B cells.
CD 22		Leu 14	B-lineage cells.
CD 11	Myeloid cell associated	LFA-1	Pan leukocyte.
CD 14		Leu M3	Monocytes.
CD 68			Macrophage specific.

Each T cell is antigen specific and thus must have a chemical receptor capable of recognizing (binding) its antigen. Like other antigen receptors, the TCR is composed of two protein chains (alpha and beta), linked by a disulfide bond, and each chain has a constant region and a variable region. The protein is integral to the cell surface, and the constant region extends into the cytoplasm. The variable region is composed of amino acid sequences that permit each T cell clone to interact with a specific antigen. The alpha chain is encoded on chromosome 14; the beta chain on chromosome 7, and the diversity of the variable region can be explained by the fact that there are multiple gene clusters encoding for the amino acid sequences. More than one million distinct T cell clones exist.

The TCR does not recognize soluble antigen in isolation. It can only recognize the antigen when the antigen is presented in conjunction with the cell surface antigen encoded by its own major histocompatibility complex. Soluble antigens are recognized in the context of Class II MHC molecules by CD4$^+$ T cells. Viral antigens are recognized in the context of Class I MHC molecules by CD8$^+$ T cells. Moreover, antigens must be processed by an accessory cell which expresses the processed antigen in conjunction with the appropriate Class I or Class II MHC molecule. The TCR then recognizes antigen plus MHC complex. This is known as corecognition (Fig. 6–5).

The T cell receptor is physically associated with the CD3 marker on all T cells. Collectively, these are referred to as the TCR complex. This molecule is identical in all T cells, even though the heterodimer of the antigen recognition ($\alpha\beta$) site is hypervariable. The CD3 molecule is probably important either in MHC recognition and/or transduction of the signal of antigen binding to the cellular mechanisms trig-

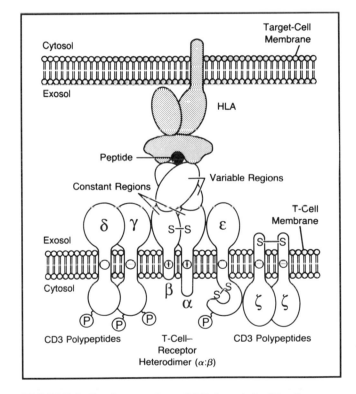

FIGURE 6–5. Interaction of HLA and the T cell receptor complex. The alpha and beta polypeptide chains of the T cell receptor form a heterodimer linked by a disulfide bond (S-S) and anchored in the T cell membrane. The heterodimer recognizes and binds to peptide associated with an HLA molecule on the surface of a presenting cell. The nonpolymorphic DC3 polypeptides (designated gamma, delta, epsilon, and zeta) are assembled together with the T cell antigen receptor and are probably involved in signal transduction. P denotes phosphorylation site. (Reprinted from Krensky, A. and Porhan, P.: N. Engl. J. Med. 322:510–516, 1990.)

gered by such binding. Monoclonal antibodies to the CD3 molecule (OKT3 monoclonal antibody) can block antigen recognition. The CD4 and CD8 complex is important in corecognition of the MHC gene products. Antibody to CD4 or CD8 blocks antigen responses in primary responses, too.

T cell activation occurs through the CD3, IL-2 (previously called T cell growth factors), and the IL-2 receptor (IL-2R). Resting T cells express the T cell receptor but do not express receptors for IL-2 (Fig. 6–6). When TCRs are stimulated by antigen plus MHC gene products, IL-2R appear within hours. At the same time, CD3 expression on the cell surface is down-regulated. T cell activation leads to IL-2 production and secretion by the activated T cells. The IL-2 produced binds to the new IL-2Rs on the same cells, resulting in the initiation of cell mitosis. When the antigenic stimulus is no longer present, the number of cell surface IL-2Rs decreases and the T cell CD3 antigen-receptor complex is again reexpressed on the cell surface. In this way, external antigens influence the magnitude of T cell activation and proliferation through both positive and negative feedback control (Fig. 6–6). T lymphocytes are the primary cells which respond to the transplantation antigens present on virtually all tissues. Those antigens are referred to as the MHC locus. As a result, T cells are the pivotal element in the rejection response, and immunosuppressive therapy is therefore often targeted at these cells.

BIOCHEMICAL EVENTS IN T CELL ACTIVATION

The elegant biochemical events associated with T cell activation are just now being characterized. The TCR does not recognize soluble antigen in isolation. It must see antigen associated with the MHC of an accessory cell which expresses self-type MHC antigens (Fig. 6–5). Four major events take place when a T cell binds an antigen in the presence of the MHC on an accessory cell. First, membrane inositol is converted to inositol triphosphate. This, in turn, increases cytoplasmic free calcium from stores in the endoplasmic reticulum (Fig. 6–7). Concomitantly, diacylglycerol activates protein kinase C. These two steps plus the IL-1 produced by activated accessory cells are required for T cell activation. Finally, when T cell receptors are stimulated, the number of MHC antigen receptors rapidly decreases and IL-2 surface receptors (IL-2R) appear on the cell surface within hours. The CD4 helper T cells are stimulated to produce and secrete IL-2, which binds to the new IL-2Rs on the same cells and on other cells in the vicinity. Only those lymphocytes which have encountered their specifically coded antigen and thus have IL-2Rs expressed on their cell surfaces can respond. Once a critical number of IL-2Rs have bound IL-2, DNA synthesis begins and cell mitosis ensues. When the antigenic stimulus is no longer present, the number of cell surface IL-2Rs decreases and the CD3 is reexpressed on the cell surface. The inverse relationship between TCR expression and IL-2Rs expression on the cell surface suggests a feedback mechanism where external antigens influence the magnitude of T cell activation and proliferation through an IL-2 hormone-receptor system with both positive and negative feedback control.

Although CD8[+] T cells do not secrete IL-2, they require it for activation. Therefore, CD8[+] (effector) lymphocytes also require CD4[+] (helper-inducer) immunoregulatory cell responses. B cells also require "help" through a different set of cytokines produced by the helper CD4[+] cells.

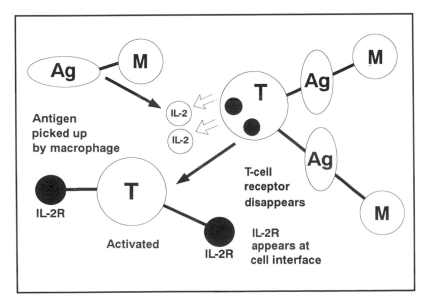

FIGURE 6–6. Steps in T cell activation. T cell activation occurs through the T cell receptor complex, IL-2, and the IL-2 receptor (IL-2R). Resting T cells express CD3 but not the IL-2R. When T cell receptors are stimulated by antigen plus MHC gene products, they manufacture IL-2Rs, which appear at the cell surface. Simultaneously, IL-2 secreted by these cells binds to the new IL-2R to stimulate proliferation and differentiation. When the antigenic stimulus is no longer present, the number of IL-2Rs decrease and the T cell CD3 receptor complex is again reexpressed on the cell surface. In this way, a feedback control mechanism is maintained.

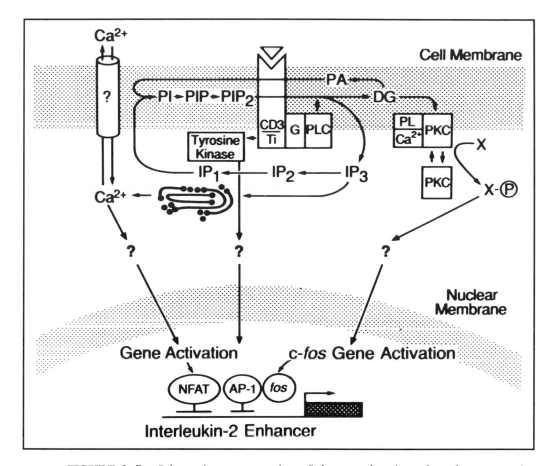

FIGURE 6–7. Schematic representation of the cytoplasmic and nuclear events involved in T cell activation. Ligands (open triangle) that bind to the T cell antigen receptor (CD3/Ti) complex induce the activation of two signal-transduction pathways. The DC3/Ti complex is coupled to phospholipase C (PLC) by a guanine-nucleotide-binding protein (G). Activated PLC hydrolyzes phosphatidylinositol 4, 5-bisphoasphate (PIP$_2$), yielding inositol 1,4,5-triphosphate (IP$_3$) and diacylglycerol (DG). IP$_3$ mobilizes calcium ions from internal stores and may regulate a transmembrane flux of calcium from a putative calcium channel. DG activates the enzyme protein kinase C (PKC), which depends on the presence of calcium ions and phospholipid (PL) and phosphorylates as yet unidentified critical intracellular substrates (X). The second signal-transduction pathway involves the activation of a tyrosine kinase. Through undefined events, these signals-transduction pathways induce the transcription of early-activation genes (such as NFAT and c-fos). The protein products of these genes, together with other transcriptional regulators such as activator protein-1 (AP-1) contribute in turn to the transcriptional activation of a second wave of genes (such as the interleukin-2 gene). Pl denotes phosphatidylinositol; PIP, phosphatidylinositol 4-phosphate; PA, phosphatidic acid; IP$_2$, inositol 1, 4-phosphage; and IP$_1$, inositol 4-phosphate. (Reprinted from Krensky, A. and Porham, P.: N. Engl. J. Med. *322*:510–516, 1990.)

T-Cell Effector Function

CD8$^+$ T cells serve primarily as effector cells to mediate cellular cytotoxicity. Almost all CD8$^+$ T cells have cytotoxic potential. If they recognize antigen bound to a macrophage, they can be activated to kill that cell. This cellular cytotoxicity is critical to the rejection of allografts and the lysis of cells infected with virus.

The CD4$^+$ cells also specifically recognize and bind antigen. However, they mediate their effects in a helper or immunoregulatory fashion by secreting an array of cytokines into the microenvironment. These lymphokines (CD4$^+$ T cells) activate macrophages to secrete their own cytokines, and in addition, enhance the cytolytic activity of macrophages. The activated CD4$^+$ cells thus amplify the immune response and in so doing influence other cells (e.g., CD8$^+$ antigen-sensitive cells) in their vicinity to proliferate and respond. Other cytokines (e.g., IL-4) produced by CD4$^+$ cells are also useful in the maturation of CD8$^+$ cells. The entire cellular and humoral response results in a delayed hypersensitivity response against viruses, foreign tissue, fungi, mycobacteria, and other intracellular organisms.

Two distinct subsets of T helper cells (CD4$^+$) have been characterized in the mouse. They are classified by their functional role as immunoregulatory cells, as T helper 1, and T helper 2 cells (Fig. 6–8). Most of their effects in immunoregulation are mediated through the cytokines they produce. Cross-regulation of the two different cell types by each other through cytokine production has been demonstrated in the mouse. Interleukin-10 is a potent cytokine synthesis inhibitory factor (CSIF) which suppresses cytokine production by TH1 cells, thus inhibiting the function of TH1 cells. Whether a similar phenomenon exists in humans has not yet been determined.

Understanding the process of activation the T cell via its receptor pathway and the role of each lymphocyte subset in the immune response is essential to understanding the techniques currently employed to prevent rejection. This understanding has definitely led to the use of more focused, specific immunotherapy with monoclonal antibodies directed at those specific clones of cells which are responsible for the rejection response. As mechanisms responsible for rejection are further characterized, additional progress can be anticipated. Theoretically, specific targeted antibodies could modify the activation of the subsets of T cells responsible for rejection. As the mechanism of TCR activation is elucidated, potent agonists and antagonists of key intermediates involved in plasma membrane and nuclear communication could be generated. Inhibitors of the triggering events for T cell activation could theoretically serve as potent immunosuppressive agents.

The Natural Killer Cell

The NK cell is a cytotoxic cell capable of killing certain tumor cells. It is probably derived from a T lymphocyte precursor. Natural killer cell morphology is distinctive because the cytoplasm contains large azurophilic granules which probably mediate tumor lysis. The NK cell receptor is unknown but is definitely not the T cell receptor. Natural killer cell lysis of tumor is nonspecific. A "missing self" hypothesis has been proposed to explain NK cell function: NK cells function to recognize and eliminate cells which fail to express normal self MHC Class 2 molecules. Natural killer cells have also been charac-

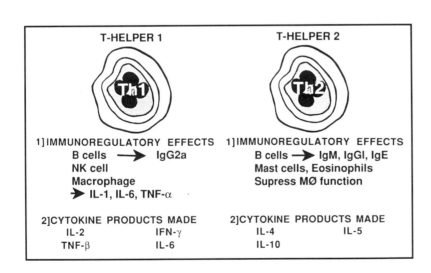

FIGURE 6–8. Heterogeneity of helper T cell function. TH1 cells are believed to play a primary role in alloreactivity while TH2 cells predominate in allergic states and in antibody production.

terized as playing a major role in rejection of non-self bone marrow stem cells in bone marrow transplant recipients.

B Lymphocytes: Development, Differentiation, and Role in the Immune Response

B Lymphocytes (B cells) produce antibody in response to foreign antigens. Each individual antibody is called an idiotype. Nine different immunoglobulin subclasses, or isotypes, have been identified (IgM, IgD, IgG_1, IgG_2, IgG_3, IgG_4, IgA_1, IgA_2, IgE). Like most receptors, each antibody is composed of a heterodimer of two identical heavy chains and two identical light chains (Fig. 6–9). The heavy and light chains both have a constant region (Fc) that is identical for antibodies of that class, plus a recognition or binding part that is highly *VARIABLE*. The antibody binding site for antigen is formed by the association of the variable regions of both the heavy and light chains. The specificity of the variable region occurs during B lymphocyte development. Each B lymphocyte can produce only one highly specific antibody. This is referred to as the *clonal nature of the immune response*. When pre-B cells developing in the bone marrow divide, they produce clones of immature B cells which are each committed to produce only one antibody (Fig. 6–10). The variable region of the immunoglobulin molecule gives each individual antibody its specific binding characteristics (Fig. 6–11)

and is responsible for the tremendous variety of antibody molecules possessed by each of us. Most of the diversity of the immune response occurs during fetal development. However, certain regions of the genome in B lymphocytes are highly susceptible to mutation, which teleologically may favor still more immunoglobulin diversity.

All of the immunoglobulins are glycoprotein products whose functions are best understood in the context of their structure. The variable region of the antibody binds antigen, resulting in a change in conformation of the constant portion. This, in turn, stimulates a number of effects, including complement fixation and histamine release by mast cells. A schematic model of an IgG molecule is shown in Fig. 11 as a prototype for all immunoglobulins. There are four polypeptide chains—two heavy (H) and two light (L). Each chain contains a variable (V) region and a constant (C) region. The antigen binding site resides in hypervariable regions in the V region of both H and L chains. Digestion with papain yields 2 Fab (antigen binding) fragments plus an Fc (crystallizible) fragment. Digestion with pepsin yields 1 F(ab)2 molecule possessing 2 Fab regions. The five classes of immunoglobulin, IgG, IgA, IgM, IgD, and IgE, are designated according to differences in the H chain constant region. There are several subclasses of IgG and two subclasses of IgA. There are two classes of L chains (Kappa and Lambda) and four subtypes of Lambda. Immunoglobulin G normally exists as a dimer and IgM as a pentamer.

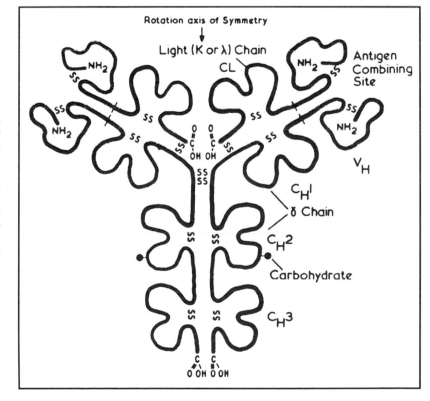

FIGURE 6–9. Schematic diagram of a molecule of human IgG, showing the two light (k or λ) chains and two heavy (H) chains held together by disulfide bonds. The constant regions of the light (CL) and heavy (CH1, CH2, and CH3) chains and the variable region of the heavy chain (VH) are indicated. Loops in the peptide chain formed by intrachain disulfide bonds (CH1, and so forth) make up separate functional domains. (Reprinted from Nossal, G.: N. Engl. J. Med. *316*:1320–1325, 1987.)

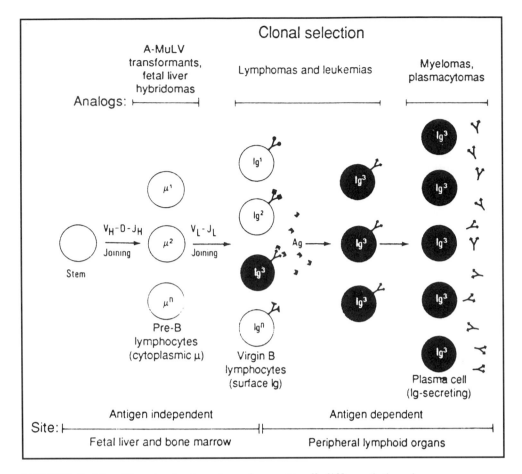

FIGURE 6–10. Clonal selection. In primary B cell differentiation, bone marrow pluripotent stem cells give rise to surface Ig-carrying B cells during the *antigen-independent* phase of B cell differentiation. After migrating to peripheral lymphoid organs (such as the spleen and lymph nodes, such B cells may come into contact with cognate antigen (depicted for shaded B cell), which cause that particular cell to divide and mature into an antibody-secreting cell. Tumor cell analogs of the various stages are indicated at the top of the figure. (Reprinted from Alt, F., Blackwell, T.K., and Yoncopoulus, G.: Science *238*:1079–1087, 1987.)

Each class of antibody has a specific role in immune function. Immunoglobulin M antibodies are the first antibodies made in response to a foreign antigen. They are very efficient at complement fixation, activating a cascade which promotes phagocytosis and the killing of microorganisms. The IgM antibodies bind to receptors on phagocytic cells to facilitate destruction of invading microorganisms. Immunoglobulin G antibodies appear later in the immune response. Levels of IgG rise as the level of IgM antibodies falls. The IgG antibodies also bind to receptors on phagocytic cells. Unlike IgM, IgG can cross the placenta to protect the fetus and give residual protection to the newborn infant. Both IgM and IgG immunoglobulins are primarily involved with internal host defenses within the body. Immunoglobulin D is present in only trace amounts in serum, but is the predominant immunoglobulin (with IgM) on the surface of resting B cells.

In contrast with IgM and IgG, IgA antibodies function in mucosal defenses to protect the body from invasion from external sources. They are made by a special subset of B lymphocytes termed gut and respiratory-associated lymphoid tissue and are actively transported across mucosal barriers in combination with a secretory component added by surface epithelial cells. Secretory IgA antibodies bind antigen to prevent it from crossing mucosal barriers and entering the blood stream. Immunoglobulin A is found in greatest concentration in saliva, tears, bronchial fluid, nasal mucus, and the small intestine. Immunoglobulin E antibodies stimulate mast cells, eosinophils, and basophils, and function primarily in allergy and defense responses against parasites.

Like T lymphocytes, NK cells, and macrophages, B cells are also derived from the pluripotent stem cell. There are two stages in B lymphocyte maturation: the first is antigen-independent; the second is

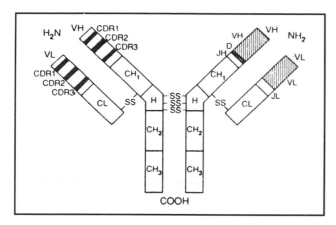

FIGURE 6–11. The immunoglobulin molecule. A typical subunit of an Ig molecule, composed of two identical heavy chains and two identical light chains linked by disulfide bridges. Variable regions are indicated on the right subunit; CDR sequences are indicated on the left subunit. (Reprinted from Alt, F., Blackwell, T.K., and Yoncopoulos, G.: Science *238*:1079–1087, 1987.)

antigen-dependent. The development of individual clones of pre-B cells that will provide the host with a diversity of antibodies to deal with potentially any antigen the immune system will encounter in a lifetime is antigen-independent. The "repertoire" for antibody diversity is, for the most part predetermined; it results from multiple gene mutations in the variable region that encodes antibodies during development of the B cell. Mature B cells then enter the blood stream and migrate to the spleen, lymph nodes, and other peripheral lymphoid tissues. Individual B lymphocytes can produce only one highly specific antibody. Unless stimulated by antigen, B cells become senescent at this antigen-independent stage of development.

B cells are stimulated to differentiate and mature to produce antibody-secreting plasma cells and memory cells only if they encounter antigens which bind to their surface immunoglobulin receptors. Antibody production involves interaction between B cells, CD4$^+$ T helper cells, and accessory cells. The antigen-MHC complex on the macrophage cell surface membrane binds to the receptors of an appropriate T helper (CD4$^+$) cell. This stimulates the accessory cell to produce IL-1. The T helper cell simultaneously begins to secrete lymphokines, (IL-4, IL-5, IL-6) which stimulate B cell and further T cell proliferation. The first immunoglobulin produced by an activated B cell is usually IgM. Subsequently, isotype production switches to IgA, IgG, or IgE, a process referred to as isotype switch. With this, the specificity of the antibody does *NOT* change. The switch from IgM to other isotypes of immunoglobulin is antigen-dependent. Unless stimulated by antigen, the B cells become senescent at this stage of development. B cells are induced by antigen stimulation to mature into both antibody-secreting plasma

cells and memory cells, which are primed cells that remain in reserve, ready for their next encounter with the antigen. During the sojourn within the memory cell pool, the immunoglobulin genes undergo frequent point mutations in their hypervariable region, which may result in production of antibody with a greater affinity for antigen.

The Role of Cytokines in the Immune Response

Cytokines are a group of soluble protein cell regulators produced by a number of cells in the body. They play a pivotal role in many physiological responses, are participants in a number of disease processes, and have therapeutic potential. They are called various terms based upon the cells which produce them. Lymphokines are produced by activated lymphocytes; monokines are produced by macrophages. They all share certain common characteristics: (1) They are low molecular weight proteins (<80 kDa) which are often glycosylated; (2) they serve as regulators of inflammation; (3) they are usually produced and act locally. They are very potent, generally acting at picomolar concentrations, and interact with cell surface receptors specific for that cytokine. They are released in response to antigen by a number of cells and play a major role in the execution and regulation of the cellular immune responses. Table 6–4 lists some sources of cytokines. In effect, cytokines are a way for the cellular components of the immune response to communicate with each other. They may function in an autocrine fashion to act on the same cell type which produces them, or they may exert a paracrine effect to stimulate cells of other types in the vicinity. They rarely exert a systemic endocrine effect except in disease states. Because most cytokines exert more than one effect, they are now assigned an interleukin (IL) number rather than a name for classification (Table 6–5).

Some of these factors play a critical role in rejection of transplanted tissues. The response of a cell to a given cytokine is dependent upon the local concentration of the cytokine, the cell type, and other cell regulators to which it has been or is simultaneously exposed. Binding of the cytokine to a cell surface receptor results in a change in conformation of the

TABLE 6–4. CELLS WHICH PRODUCE CYTOKINES

T-Lymphocyte
B-Lymphocyte
Natural killer cells
Macrophages
Mast cells
Dendritic cells
Keratinocytes
Epithelial cells
Vascular endothelial cells (VEC)

TABLE 6–5.   PROMINENT BIOLOGIC PROPERTIES OF HUMAN CYTOKINES

Cytokine	Biologic Properties
Lymphokine	
IL-1	15,000-kilodalton protein secreted by macrophages. Primary role is to activate helper T lymphocytes.
IL-2	T cell growth factor secreted by some CD4$^+$ helper T cells. It stimulates proliferation and differentiation of various T lymphocytes.
IL-3	Secreted by T helper cells. Target is various hematopoietic cells to stimulate proliferation. Species-specific with major regulatory role in stem cell lineage production.
IL-4	B cell stimulating factor produced by some CD4$^+$ helper T cells. Target is B cells, T cells, and mast cells to activate and promote proliferation. Also => increase in expression of Class II MHC molecules on B cells.
IL-5	B cell growth factor made by some helper T cells that secrete IL-4. Promotes proliferation and maturation of B cells and eosinophils.
IL-6	B cell stimulating factor produced by some helper T cells and macrophages. Promotes B cell maturation into immunoglobulin-secreting cells and helps to activate T cells.
IL-7	Mitogenic for some cells. Stimulates B cell proliferation. Stimulates T cell proliferation.
IL-8	Stimulates granulocyte activity. Induce chemotactic migration of cells.
IL-10 (CSIF)	Suppresses cytokine production by TH1 cells, growth co-stimulator for thymocytes, suppresses antigen presentation by *macrophages*. Growth co-stimulator for mast cells, B cell viability enhancement; thymocyte co-stimulator.
Colony-stimulating factor (CSF)	
Granulocyte-macrophage (GM-CSF)	Promotes neutrophil, eosinophil, and macrophage bone marrow colonies; activates mature granulocytes.
Granulocyte CSF (G-CSF)	Promotes neutrophil lineage maturation.
Macrophage CSF (M-CSF)	Promotes macrophage lineage production and maturation.
Gamma-interferon (IFN-γ)	Induces Class I, Class II (DR), and other surface antigens on a variety of cells; activates macrophages and endothelial cells; augments or inhibits other lymphokine activities; augments natural killer cell activity; exerts antiviral activity.
Interferon (alpha and beta) (IFN-α, IFN-β)	Most important role is to inhibit cell growth or directly kills cells. Exerts antiviral activity; induces Class I antigen expression; augments natural killer cell activity; has fever-inducing and antiproliferative properties.
Tumor necrosis factor (TNF)	Inhibits cell growth and directly kills cells.

receptor, which signals the intracellular cell machinery to undergo a number of changes that results in increased cellular RNA and protein synthesis, with altered cell behavior. Cytokines function as a network (1) to induce each other, (2) to modulate cell surface receptors, and by (3) synergistic, additive, or antagonistic interactions on cell function. All cytokines have more than one effect and may be stimulatory for the same cell types yet inhibitory for other cell types.

A number of cytokine receptors on target cells have been characterized (Table 6–6). Only a few receptors are present on each cell surface (100–10,000 receptors/cell). Two types of receptor exist: single chain receptors and double chain receptors (Table 6–6). The receptors are much more simple than the other receptor complexes characterized for components of the immune system. The receptors for IL-1, IL-4, IL-6 and interferon (IFN), TNF, and M-CSF are all composed of a single chain. The receptors for IL-2, IL-3, IL-5, IL-7, and GM-CSF are composed of two distinct chains. Binding of the specific cytokine to its receptor results in transmission of a signal across the cell membrane (signal transduction) and the cell genetic machinery is put into action to mediate the specific effect.

TABLE 6–6.   CYTOKINE RECEPTORS

Single chain receptor
IL-1R
IL-4R
IL-6R
IFN-R
TNF-R
M-CSF-R
Double chain receptor
IL-2R
IL-3R
IL-5R
IL-7R
GM-CSFR

Cytokines Which Influence T Cell Activation

T cells recognize antigens when they are presented on the surface of a macrophage in association with a Class II MHC molecule of self type. Most T cells are blind to soluble antigen alone. Although all T cells possess the CD3 T cell receptor complex, there are two additional peptides present on the T cell that vary from clone to clone and that make individual T cells unique in antigen recognition patterns. When an antigen is presented to a T lymphocyte by a macrophage, those clones that can bind to the antigen become activated. The activated lymphocytes then secrete a number of proteins (interleukin-1, -2, -3, -4, gamma interferon, B cell growth factor). At the same time, the IL-2 receptor is synthesized for incorporation into the surface of the cell membrane.

During T lymphocyte activation, the IL-1 produced by macrophages stimulates a number of T cell functions including IL-2 receptor expression, the release of IL-2, and production of colony-stimulating factors, B cell growth factors, and IFN-γ. Interleukin-2 will not act alone; antigen plus Class II-expressing accessory cells are also essential to mount a complete immune response.

The lymphokines that are produced act to amplify the immune response in the rejection reaction (Fig. 6–12). Gamma interferon (IFN-γ) released from activated T cells enhances MHC Class II (HLA-DR) molecule expression on macrophages, resulting in an increase in the T cell response to the antigen. Interleukin-2 binds to IL-2 receptors on activated T cells, resulting in an expansion of the activated clones. Interleukin-4 and B cell growth factor stimulate the proliferation and maturation of activated B cell. Interleukin-1 stimulates the synthesis of IL-2, -3, and -4, IFN-γ, and IL-2R. Each of these cytokines play a critical role in amplification and orchestration of the local immune response to foreign antigen.

Interleukin-2 (T cell growth factor). The most important role of IL-2 is to initiate proliferation of activated T cells. Interleukin-2 receptors that are not expressed in the resting state are synthesized and expressed on the cell surface when T cells are activated. Interleukin-2 binds to the IL-2Rs on activated T cells and produces a clonal expansion. When antigen is no longer present, the IL-2Rs on the T cell membranes disappear. In effect, through cytokines a positive and negative feedback system exists to control the strength and duration of the immune response.

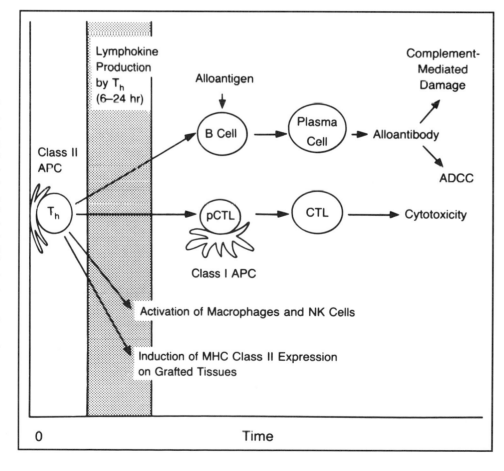

FIGURE 6–12. Cellular interactions in transplant rejection. The diagram outlines the activation of a T helper (T$_h$) cell by an antigen-presenting cell (APC) expression MHC Class II to produce lymphokines. These lymphokines promote the activation, proliferation, and differentiation of numerous effector mechanisms to contribute to transplant rejection. NK denotes natural killer; CTL, cytotoxic T lymphocyte; pCTL, precursor CTL; ADCC, antibody-dependent cell-mediated cytotoxicity. (Reprinted from Krensky, A., Webs, G., Crabtree, M., et al.: N. Engl. J. Med. 322:510–516, 1990.)

Cytokines that Influence B Cell Activation.
Three major steps are required for production of
antibody by B cells in response to foreign tissue.
When a resting B cell is stimulated by binding of a
specific antigen, a number of cytokines are produced. As a result, B cell proliferation occurs. Subsequently, B cell-differentiating factors, especially
IL-4, stimulate the activated B cell to become an
antibody-secreting mature plasma cell. Interleukin-1
stimulates the production of B-cell-differentiating
factor. Interleukin-2, IL-3, and alpha and gamma
interferon enhance the action of the B-cell-
stimulating lymphokines.

Interleukin-1 and Tumor Necrosis Factor. In-
terleukin-1 is produced by a number of cell types,
including T and B lymphocytes, NK cells, skin keratinocytes, brain astrocytes, epithelial cells, and vascular endothelial cells, in response to antigens, toxins,
injury, and inflammation. In turn, IL-1 activates
resting T cells and stimulates the synthesis of lymphokines. Interleukin-1 exerts systemic effects
which are associated with infection or injury and is a
primary mediator of the acute phase response. Some
effects are mediated through nonlymphoid tissues.
The effects of IL-2 are broad, including fever and
the release of hepatic acute phase proteins, neutrophils, ACTH, cortisol, and insulin. Effects on endothelial cells include increased leukocyte adherence,
prostaglandin release, and hypotension. Inter-
leukin-2 is cytotoxic for tumor cells and insulin-
producing B cells.

Tumor necrosis factor shares many of the multiple
systemic properties of IL-1. It is produced by activated macrophages but appears to have no direct
effect upon lymphocyte activation. However, it acts
synergistically with IL-1 to mediate a variety of acute
phase changes including tumor necrosis, hypotension, and inflammatory reactions. The vascular endothelium and several endocrine organs are the primary targets for TNF.

Cytokines are recognized as playing a critical role
in allograft rejection. Both corticosteroids and cyclosporine inhibit lymphokine synthesis and some of
the cellular effects of lymphokines. Targeting of immunotherapy to cytokine/receptor interactions and
the use of inhibitory cytokines to modify cellular
activation are two additional potential methods to
alter graft rejection. The most sensationalized recent
clinical application of lymphokines has been the use
of IL-2 in cancer therapy. Lymphocytes are removed
from cancer patients, transformed by treatment with
IL-2 in vitro into activated "killer cells" or LAK (lymphokine-activated killer cells), which are strongly
nonspecifically tumoricidal, and reinfused into the
patient. Similar studies using tumor-infiltrating lymphocytes (TILs) stimulated by IL-2 treatment have
provided similar activated tumor killer cells which
are specific for the tumor from which they were
harvested.

THE MAJOR HISTOCOMPATIBILITY LOCUS: TRANSPLANTATION ANTIGENS

The MAJOR HISTOCOMPATIBILITY LOCUS
is a gene complex in which virtually every aspect of
the immune response is genetically encoded. The
nomenclature for this complex varies between species. It is referred to as the HLA in humans and as
the H-2 in the mouse. Genes of the MHC encode the
information necessary for antigen recognition and
the cellular interactions involved in the immune response.

When tissue is transplanted into a non-identical
recipient, antigens present on the cell surface of the
transplanted tissues are recognized by the recipient
as foreign. This process of non-self-recognition can
initiate the rejection response and knowledge of it is
critical to understanding solid organ transplantation. In general, the strength of rejection is directly
related to the degree of genetic disparity between
donor and recipient. An allograft is a graft transplanted from one individual to genetically different
individual of the same species. Xenografts (hetero-
grafts) are grafts transplanted between two different
species. Although rejection of tissues transplanted
between allogeneic differences can be controlled
with conventional nonspecific immunosuppressive
agents, the same success has not been achieved for
xenotransplantation. Grafts between identical twins
(syngeneic) or from individuals to themselves (auto-
grafts) are never rejected, because there is no genetic
disparity.

The Genetics of Histocompatibility

The MHC is a large gene complex that controls
traits that influence the entire spectrum of the immune response. Graft rejection is only one aspect of
the response of the host to MHC antigens expressed
on foreign tissues. These genes have been mapped to
chromosome 6 in the human. The MHC genes are
divided into three classes: *Class I, II, and III* (Table
6–7).

The class I genes encode cell surface transplantation antigens, which serve as the primary targets
for cytotoxic T-lymphocytes in graft rejection. Class
I antigens are composed of heavy and light chains.
The highly polymorphic Class I heavy chains (37-45
kDa) are non-covalently associated on the cell sur-

TABLE 6–7.   THE MHC GENES

Class	HLA Region
Class I	B, C, A
Class II	D, DR, DQ, DP
Class III	Complement components

face with the nonpolymorphic β_2-microglobulin light chain (β_2-M). Class I antigen expression is developmentally regulated; it is composed of integral membrane proteins that function in the presentation of antigens to T cells. Class I antigens are hardly detectable until the midsomite stage of embryogenesis. They are expressed on almost all somatic cells of the adult, but level of expression varies from tissue to tissue. Expression is greatest in lymphoid cells (Table 6–8). A number of cancer cells lack Class I expression.

Interferons (IFN-α, IFN-β, IFN-γ) have been noted to induce expression of Class I molecules in a wide variety of cell types through binding to a specific cell surface receptor. IFN-α and IFN-β are produced by fibroblasts while IFN-γ is produced by T lymphocytes. All types of IFNs can increase Class I expression, but IFN-γ is the most potent. This effect may be useful in cancer therapy and in modulation of the response to transplanted tissues.

The CLASS II genes encode virtually all of the genetic material for the immune response. They control the level of the response to some antigens and also encode a series of antigens which are expressed on lymphocytes. They serve as the primary targets for helper T lymphocytes and also control the expression of some components of the complement system. The Class II loci in humans include HLA-DR, -DQ, and -DP. Class II antigenic expression is normally limited to those cells of hematopoietic stem cell origin.

Minor transplantation antigens, located on chromosomes outside of the MHC, also code for weaker histocompatibility loci. They elicit a weaker rejection response but can have a major impact upon the outcome of a transplanted organ. Grafts between HLA-(MHC) identical siblings will still reject if chronic immunosuppression is not utilized after transplantation of a solid organ, because of the presence of these minor transplantation antigens. Identical twins who have the identical major and minor transplantation antigens accept grafts from each other without rejection.

The Genetics of Histocompatibility: Tissue Typing. The application of histocompatibility to the clinical setting has been elegant. A central paradigm has proven true for the transplantation of tissues and organs: the more antigenic the graft, the more vigorous the rejection response. Since the antigenicity of a graft is determined by the degree of genetic disparity, matching to minimize differences in histocompatibility is critical. The presence of HLA antigens on a cell surface can be detected both functionally and serologically. The functional method is most specific for Class II antigens, while the serologic method detects Class I. The functional method measures the reactivity of the lymphocytes from a potential recipient to those of the donor. The responding lymphocytes are cultured with cells of the donor and

TABLE 6–8. TISSUE DISTRIBUTION OF H-2 CLASS I ANTIGENS (HUMAN)

Cells of the endocrine system	
Thyroid	+
Parathyroid glands	+
Pancreatic islets of Langerhans	+
Adrenals	++
Gastrointestinal tract	
Epithelium of	
Esophagus (basal layer)	++
Stomach	+
Small intestine	++
Colon	
Pancreas	
Acinar cells	−
Duct cells	++
Liver	
Kupffer cells	++
Sinusoids, biliary epithelium	+/−
Hepatocytes	+/−
Respiratory and cardiovascular system	
Lungs	
Bronchial and alveolar epithelium	
Interstitial cells	++
Bronchiolar epithelium	
Heart	
Myocardium	+
Endocardium	
Pericardium	
Endothelium	
capillaries and large vessels in all organs	
Nervous system	
Central	
Neurones	−
Astrocytes, microglia and oligodendrocytes	
Peripheral	−
Kidney	
Tubular epithelium	− −
Glomeruli	− −
Testis	
Germline cells	
Spermatozoa	−
Epididymis	
Spermatozoa	− −
Muscle	
Skeletal	− −
Smooth	−
Langerhans cells and interstitial dendritic cells (all organs)	− −
Keratinocytes	−
Placenta	−
Lymphoid organs	

will proliferate in response to transplantation antigens of the donor, if they recognize them as being foreign. Only HLA (MHC) antigens are detected with the functional method. The antigens most effective at generating this response are those of the Class II MHC.

Clinical analyses have demonstrated that Class I antigens also play an important role in transplantation, and alloantisera specific for each of the Class I loci (A, B, or C), is therefore also used for serologic typing of a potential donor and recipient. The serologic method uses antigen-specific antisera which reacts only with cells which express that specific antigen.

As a final analysis, serum from the recipient must also be tested for preformed cytotoxic antibody against the donor cells to exclude the possibility of hyperacute rejection, using a cross-matching test. Hyperacute rejection could otherwise result in the face of an excellent histocompatibility match, if preformed antibodies to that donor were present in the recipient.

The Cellular Basis of Allograft Rejection. The rejection response to a graft is elicited if histocompatibility antigens on the transplanted tissue differ from those of the recipient. A number of antigens can produce this response. In kidney transplantation, ABO blood group antigens will elicit a rapid, violent, and immediate antibody-mediated graft rejection in recipients with preformed cytotoxic natural antibody. This represents *hyperacute rejection*. A similar form of rejection occurs with some xenografts between different species when preformed cytotoxic antibodies are present in the recipient. The most common form of rejection encountered in clinical transplantation is acute rejection. It is mediated almost exclusively by T lymphocytes in response to the MHC or transplantation antigens. During graft rejection, antibodies against the MHC antigens are also produced. However, for the most part, acute rejection is purely T cell mediated. Chronic rejection is observed in solid-organ grafts over months to years and is probably due to the deposition of anti-MHC antibodies. As a result, the graft undergoes a slow gradual loss of function. The genetic differences vary in allografts between members of the same species. The length of time for rejection of a transplanted graft is dependent upon the degree of genetic disparity between the two individuals and may take from 8 to 100 days.

Host versus graft responses to the MHC-encoded alloantigens are mediated by both helper T lymphocytes and cytotoxic T lymphocytes. Through studies of graft rejection and the mixed leukocyte-culture test, it was established that Class I antigens are the primary targets for cytotoxic T lymphocytes and Class II antigens serve as the primary stimulating determinants for helper T lymphocytes. However, helper T lymphocytes and cytotoxic T lymphocytes cooperate in the generation of cytotoxic responses in vivo.

Monoclonal antibodies directed at T cell subpopulations have been helpful in characterizing the sequence of events involved in rejection. Virtually, all T cells express the T cell receptor complex on their membranes. It plays a crucial role in T cell activation and is the receptor to which OKT3 binds in order to inactivate T cells. Anti-CD4 antibodies detect markers on populations of lymphocytes which react primarily with Class II antigens, the T helper lymphocytes. Anti-CD8 antibodies detect antigens on lymphocytes which react with Class I antigens, the cytotoxic T lymphocytes. Cellular infiltrates harvested from rejecting grafts have been shown to contain both CD4 and CD8 cells, implicating a role for both helper and cytotoxic T lymphocytes in graft rejection. The relative importance and participation of each cell varies with the nature of the antigen being recognized. In recipients of grafts with a Class I disparity only, $CD8^+$ cytotoxic lymphocytes predominate. Conversely, rejection of Class II disparate grafts is mediated primarily by $CD4^+$ lymphoid cells. However, both CD8 and CD4 lymphoid cells cooperate in nearly all clinical graft rejection. This cooperation involves the production of lymphokines and other soluble factors, including IL-2, that help cytotoxic T-lymphocytes to proliferate and mature into active function.

When a transplanted organ or tissue contains viable mature T lymphocytes, graft versus host (GVH) reactivity may occur. In this setting, viable and immunocompetent lymphocytes of donor origin recognize the transplantation antigens of the host as foreign and alloreactivity to the host is initiated. Simply, the graft attempts to reject the host. This occurs clinically in transplantation of tissues and organs which contain mature donor lymphocytes and is most common in bone marrow and small bowel transplantation. This GVH reactivity is mediated primarily by T cells and is currently controlled by the same nonspecific immunosuppressive agents used to control host-versus-graft rejection.

Control of Rejection

Specific tolerance to a transplanted organ or tissue does not result after transplantation. The only exception to this is in bone marrow transplant recipients, who become specifically tolerant to the donor. In fact, a chronic state of host-versus-graft, or alloreactivity, ensues after organ transplantation and must be suppressed for the duration of graft survival, using nonspecific immunosuppression, if rejection is to be prevented; if discontinued at any time, rejection will almost always ensue.

A number of methods have been proposed to achieve allograft prolongation. These methods have been developed from an understanding of the body's immune response to foreign antigens and are one of the most elegant demonstrations of how laboratory investigation has been applied directly to the clinical setting. Clinically, most of the agents currently utilized act via nonspecific suppression of lymphocyte activation and proliferation and/or by destruction of immunocompetent cells prior to transplantation.

Two main subclasses of immunosuppressive agents used clinically are the antiproliferative agents (azathioprine, folic acid antagonists, alkylating agents, antibiotics) and agents which cause lymphocyte depletion (adrenal corticosteroids, antilymphocyte globulin, radiation, and monoclonal antibodies to molecules on the T cell surface) or lymphocyte inactivation (cyclosporine, FK506, rapamycin).

Agents Used for Clinical Immunosuppression

The first agents used for clinical immunosuppression were a combination of corticosteroids plus agents with antiproliferative activity. Most were adapted for use in transplantation after development for cancer therapy. This primarily included the antimetabolites (especially azathioprine), alkylating agents, or irradiation. Azathioprine and corticosteroids are still used in most transplant patients in combination with some of the newer agents. Recently, the introduction of agents that specifically influence the T lymphocytes that are responsible for most graft rejection (cyclosporine, OKT3, FK506, and rapamycin) has radically changed both the principles of immunosuppression in the organ allograft recipient and the outcome after transplantation. A combination of agents which each function by a different mechanism has been found to allow maximum immunosuppression with a minimum of side effects, since lower doses of each agent are required. However, at the present time, all methods of immunosuppression currently in use function through nonspecific suppression of most, if not all, aspects of the immune system.

Antiproliferative Agents. Antiproliferative agents inhibit the immune response by preventing the differentiation and proliferation of lymphocytes that are activated by antigen. The two major subclasses include the antimetabolites and the alkylating agents. The antimetabolites, which structurally resemble cell metabolites, function to inhibit enzymes of critical metabolic pathways or are incorporated during synthesis to produce faulty molecules. These agents are most effective against rapidly dividing cells. The most frequently used antimetabolites include purine, pyrimidine, and folic acid analogues. They are effective when given at the time of transplantation, before the rejection response has been initiated.

Purine Analogues. Until recently, azathioprine (Imuran) was the most widely used immunosuppressive drug in clinical organ transplantation. Prior to the availability of this agent, radiation was the only method available to prevent rejection. The immunosuppressive effects of azathioprine were characterized by Elion and Hitchings in their Nobel Prize-winning work. Azathioprine, a purine analog, is 6-mercaptopurine (6-MP) with a side chain to protect the labile sulfhydryl group. This minor modification of 6-MP results in a less toxic compound with excellent immunosuppressive effects. The side chain of azathioprine is cleaved in the liver to form the active compound 6-MP. Full metabolic activity comes with the addition of ribose-5-phosphate from phosphoribosyl pyrophosphate to form 6-MP-ribonucleotide. Because of its structural resemblance to inosine monophosphate, 6-MP ribonucleotide inhibits the enzymes which convert inosine nucleotide to adenosine and guanosine monophosphate, resulting in interference with nucleic acid synthesis. Azathioprine has its greatest effect in rapidly proliferating cells. As a result, it inhibits the development of both humoral and cellular immunity by interfering with the differentiation and proliferation of activated lymphocytes. The toxicity of azathioprine results from the nonspecific nature of its antiproliferative action and includes bone marrow suppression (leukopenia) and liver toxicity. However, virtually all side effects are reversible, and it remains a mainstay in clinic immunosuppressive therapy.

Folic Acid Antagonists. Folic acid antagonists inhibit the enzyme dihydrofolate reductase, preventing the conversion of folic acid to tetrahydrofolic acid, a step necessary for the synthesis of DNA, RNA, and certain coenzymes. Methotrexate is the most commonly used folic acid antagonist. Because the immune reactions that accompany bone marrow transplantation can be difficult to control, methotrexate is sometimes used to control the severe GVH reactions that may occur. However, the toxicity of these agents has not justified their use in clinical solid-organ transplantation because so many other less toxic agents are now available.

Alkylating Agents. The alkylating agents have an important historic role in clinical solid-organ transplantation. These agents have as part of their molecular structure highly reactive rings which combine with electron-rich nucleophilic groups such as the tertiary nitrogens in purines and pyrimidines or with $-NH_2$, $-COOH$, $-SH$, and $-PO_3H_2$ groups on a variety of DNA and RNA molecules. The high-energy rings of the alkylating agents break and combine with these constituents to form stable covalent bonds which interfere with cell function. Although alkylation of DNA and RNA can occur at several locations, the most common site appears to be N-7 of the guanine ring.

The most frequently used alkylating agents include nitrogen mustard, phenylalanine mustard, busulfan, and cyclophosphamide. Their use in transplantation is limited by their toxicity. Cyclophosphamide was used with good results in renal transplantation when hepatic toxicity prohibited the use of azathioprine. However, with the availability of more specific immunosuppressive agents, it is less frequently used. It is now used primarily in clinical bone marrow transplantation to prepare recipients for transplantation, allowing lower doses of radiation to provide space for donor stem cell engraftment.

Cyclosporine. The discovery of cyclosporine in 1972 marked an important advance for the field of transplantation. It is now one of the most frequently used immunosuppressive agents. In combination with modest doses of prednisone, cyclosporine is equal or superior to combinations of other immunosuppressive agents. A cyclic peptide produced by a fungus (Fig. 6–13), cyclosporine represents a completely new class of immunosuppressive agents. Many of its suppressive effects act specifically on T cells and appear to be related to the inhibition of T cell receptor-mediated activation and maturation events (Fig. 6–14). Cyclosporine selectively inhibits activation of resting T lymphocytes by IL-2. In addition, it prevents activated T lymphocytes from manufacturing and/or releasing IL-2. Because IL-2 is necessary for the expansion of activated clones of T cells, cyclosporine effectively inhibits the immune response to antigens without eliminating any of the clonal repertoire. Cyclosporine is virtually insoluble in aqueous solutions and absorption from the gastrointestinal tract is slow and incomplete. Excretion of the drug is primarily through the bile, and there is a well documented enterohepatic cycle (Fig. 6–15). Some of the by-products produced by the enterohepatic cycle may be even more efficient at immunosuppression than cyclosporine itself.

A number of solid-organ transplantation trials have shown that cyclosporine induces potent immunosuppression without the same bone marrow suppression associated with antimetabolite use. Adverse effects of cyclosporine include hirsutism, tremor and other neurotoxicities, hypertension, hyperkalemia, nephrotoxicity, and hepatotoxicity. The most frequent toxic effect is nephrotoxicity.

FK506. FK506 is a potent new immunosuppressive agent which, like cyclosporine, is produced by a fungus. It is classified as a macrolide antibiotic. The immunosuppressive potency of FK506 is approximately 500 times greater than that for cyclosporine

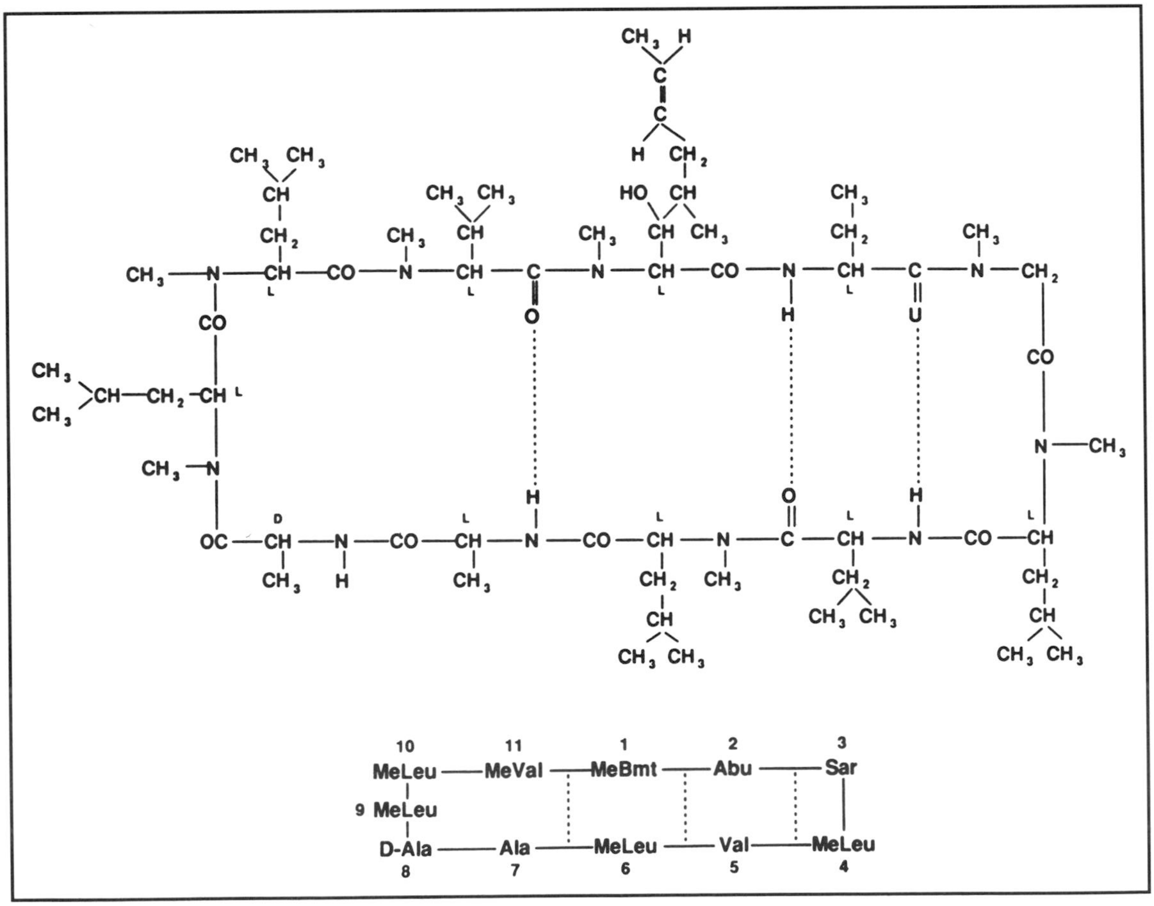

FIGURE 6–13. Atomic structure (top) and alignment of amino acids (bottom) of cyclosporine. The unique structure at position 1 is MeBmt, a novel β-hydroxy, unsaturated, 9-carbon amino acid ((4R)-4-[(E)-2-butenyl)]-4, N-dimethyl-L-threonine). Abu denotes α-amino-butyric acid; Sar, sarcosine; MeLeu, N-methyl-L-Leucine; Val, valine; Ala, L-alanine; D-Ala, alanine; and MeVal, N-methyl-L-valine. (Reprinted from Kahan, B.: N. Engl. J. Med. *321*:1725–1738, 1989.)

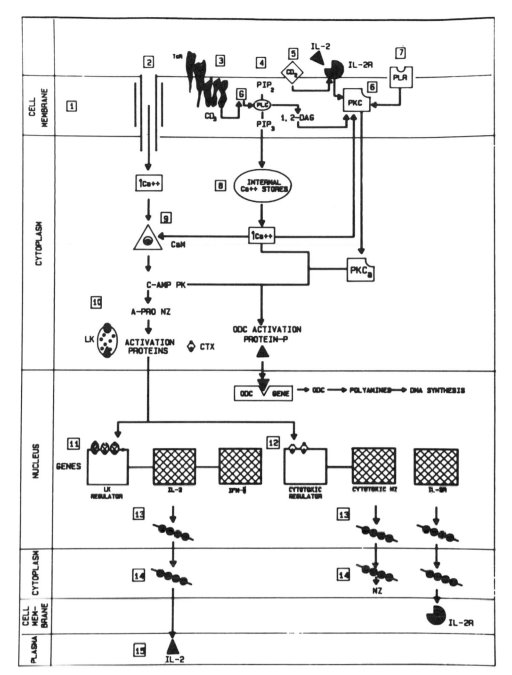

FIGURE 6–14. Cellular site of T lymphocyte inhibition by cyclosporine. Cyclosporine has minimal effects on bulk membrane properties (Site 1), including membrane leaflet order, transmembrane potential, and lysolecithin acyltransferase-mediated incorporation of fatty acids into phospholipids. It has no effect on the calcium channel (Site 2) or on the occupancy of the antigen-specific T cell receptor (TcR), which triggers the phosphorylation of the nonpolymorphic, pentapeptide CD3 complex (Site 3). The consequent coupled reactions of guanosine triphosphate-binding G proteins cause phospholipase C activation (PLC), phosphatidyl-4,5-bisphosphate cleavage to inositol triphosphate and 1,2-diacylglycerol (1,2-DAGH, Site 4), and thereby increase protein kinase C (PKC) activity and intracellular calcium mobilization. The alternate pathways through CD2 (Site 5) or the prolactin receptor (PLR, Site 7) also activate and translocate protein kinase C from the membrane to the cytoplasm (Site 6), thereby stimulating cyclic AMP-dependent protein kinases (C-AMP PK), producing nuclear induction of ornithine decarboxylase (ODC), and generating polyamines necessary for cell division. The figure also shows probable sites of action of cyclosporine. Binding to calmodulin (CaM, Site 9) or, more likely, inhibition of the generation of an activation protein (Site 10), possibly by binding to the prolyl cis-trans isomerase cyclophilin, may prevent the induction of proteins necessary to bind transcriptional enhancers that selectively stimulate genes regulating lymphokines (LK, Site 11) and cytotoxic enzyme (Site 12) expression. Cyclosporine inhibits RNA polymerases (Site 13) only when the drug is present in very high concentrations. Ribosomal translation (Site 14) and post-transcriptional assembly and export (Site 15) remain intact in cyclosporine-exposed cells. IL denotes interleukin; IFN, interferon; NZ, enzyme. (Reprinted from Kahon, B.: N. Engl. J. Med. *321*:1725–1738, 1989.)

103

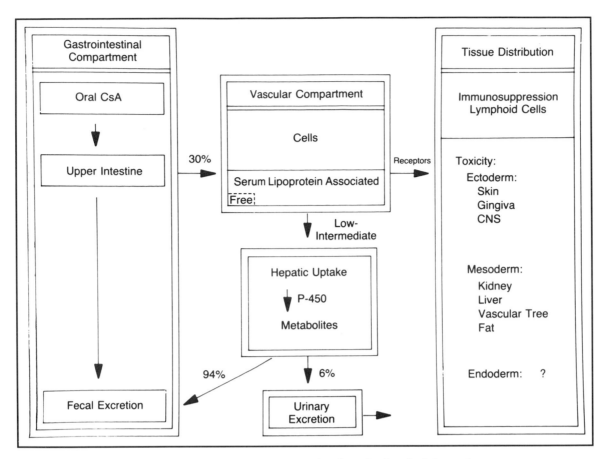

FIGURE 6–15. Disposition of cyclosporine (CsA). The drug is absorbed from the gastrointestinal tract into the vascular compartment, where the major drug fraction becomes cell-associated, and the largest serum fraction binds to lipoproteins, with only a small "free" fraction. The tissue distribution of the drug causes immunosuppression of lymphoid cells on the one hand, and toxicity to ectodermal and mesodermal structures on the other. After the drug is taken up by the liver, it is metabolized by the cytochrome P-450 system, producing metabolites that are primarily excreted in the bile and, to a small extent, in the urine. CNS denotes central nervous system. (Reprinted from Kahan, B.: N. Engl. J. Med. *321*:1725–1738, 1989.)

A. It is composed of hydroxy groups, carbonyl groups, and an amide group (Fig. 6–16) and is virtually insoluble in water. FK506 functions to inhibit IL-2 production, inhibit mouse mixed lymphocyte culture cellular proliferation mediated by helper T cells, inhibit IL-2R expression, and inhibit the generation of murine cytotoxic T cells. Although it inhibits the production of IL-3 and IFN-γ, it does not affect hematolymphopoiesis. In humans, it inhibits the appearance of IL-2 receptors on activated T lymphocytes. Once T cells have been activated, FK506 has no effect. In vivo, it has been demonstrated to prolong the survival of MHC-disparate skin, cardiac, renal, hepatic, and small bowel allografts in laboratory studies. It has been characterized as binding to a cell surface receptor on T lymphocytes and exerting its effect through an intracellular mechanism. It is currently in use in clinical trials as an immunosuppressive agent for liver, bowel, cardiac, pulmonary, and renal allograft recipients. Although FK506 is a potent immunosuppressive agent in allogeneic strain combinations, it is not effective in preventing rejection in xenogeneic (cross-species) combinations.

Two primary drug toxicities have been observed in preliminary clinical trials: (1) anorexia and weight loss, and (2) nephrotoxicity secondary to vascular changes involving fibrinoid necrosis of the small arteries and arterioles.

Rapamycin (RAPA) is another macrolide antibiotic (macrocyclic triene antibiotic) produced by *Streptomyces hygroscopicus*, which was isolated from a soil sample collected from the Vai Atore region of Easter Island. In vitro, RAPA is a potent inhibitor of murine thymocyte proliferation as well as B cell proliferation. In vitro, RAPA is 500 times more potent than cyclosporine in inhibiting mixed lymphocyte reaction (MLR) proliferation. Rapamycin works in a different manner from both cyclosporine and FK506; it

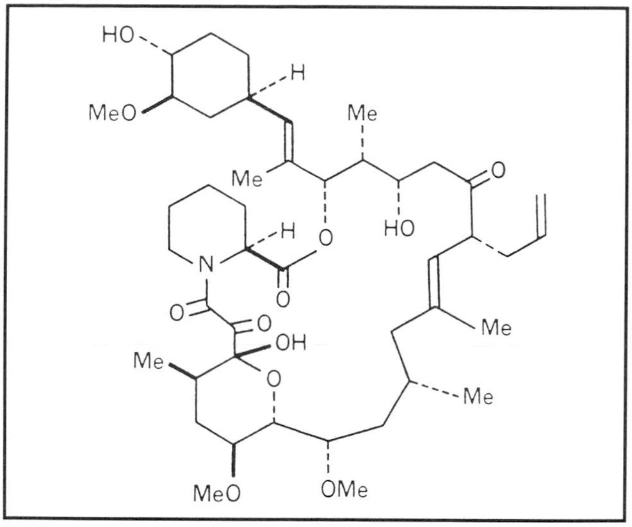

FIGURE 6–16. Chemical structure of FK-506. (Reprinted from Ochiai, T.: A novel immunosuppressive agent: FK-506. Transplant. Immunol. Lett., 7(1), Fig. 1, p. 4, 1990.)

has virtually no effect on IL-2 production. Instead, it strongly inhibits IL-4 and IL-2-driven T cell proliferation. In blocking studies, RAPA did not block the action of cyclosporine, but completely blocked the action of FK506, suggesting that they may compete for a common cellular receptor. In preliminary studies using animal models, rapamycin was potently immunosuppressive in preventing graft rejection. It is currently under evaluation in clinical trials.

Lymphocyte Depletion Measures. A number of clinically important immunosuppressive agents are effective because they function to deplete the host of potentially reactive lymphocytes. The most commonly used agents are antilymphocyte globulin, radiation, and monoclonal antibody therapy. Most act in a relatively nonspecific fashion to produce lymphocyte depletion or inactivation.

Antilymphocyte Globulin. Antilymphocyte globulins (ALG) are polyclonal antibodies produced when lymphocytes are injected into a different species. Antilymphocyte globulin depletes or inactivates T lymphocytes in vivo and as a result interferes with T-cell-mediated reactions, including allograft rejection, delayed-type hypersensitivity (i.e., the tuberculin skin reaction), and the GVH reaction. It has a lesser, but significant, effect on T-cell-dependent antibody production. Lymphocytes coated with ALG are eliminated from the blood by cells in the liver and spleen.

The Role of Monoclonal Antibodies in Transplantation

In 1975, Kohler and Milstein developed the technique for monoclonal antibody production. This simple but elegant technology has revolutionized the

field of immunology, and the application of monoclonal antibodies has had a profound impact upon understanding the biology of transplantation and the immune response, especially rejection. They were awarded the Nobel Prize for their contribution.

The technology for monoclonal antibody production is simple yet elegant. While normal B cells cannot be grown in long-term culture, tumors of the antibody-forming system, called myelomas, can be grown indefinitely. Fusion of a single normal antibody-forming B cell with a self-replicating myeloma cell results in production of a single immortal monoclonal antibody-producing B cell. In effect, a single antibody is immortalized for unlimited production. The resulting hybrid of the two cells is called a hybridoma (Fig. 6–17). Since each individual B cell is able to produce only one antibody, potentially unlimited numbers of monoclonal antibodies can be produced, depending upon which clones of B cells are activated by simulation with a specific antigen. Monoclonal antibodies of great diversity have been generated. In fact, this technology has progressed so rapidly that a national hybridoma repository, the American Tissue Culture Collection, has been organized to facilitate the distribution and availability of hybridomas.

Monoclonal antibodies are used frequently to control rejection in solid-organ transplantation, as well as to monitor changes in lymphocyte subpopulations during immunosuppressive therapy. OKT3 is an anti-CD3 monoclonal antibody which binds to the CD3 present on all mature T cells. When OKT3 binds to the T cell receptor, the receptor is modulated, or changed in conformation, and T cell activity is depressed. OKT3 is frequently used clinically to reverse episodes of acute rejection. It's use is limited by the fact that it too, is immunogenic, and repeated use may result in the formation of anti-idiotypic antibody directed against the OKT3 antibody itself. A number of clinical trials utilizing other monoclonal antibodies directed at various T cell subsets have also been utilized in clinical immunosuppression protocols. Table 6–9 lists some monoclonal antibodies and their targets, only some of which have proven to be useful clinically in transplantation.

Radiation

Radiation was probably the first agent used clinically to produce immunosuppression. Most of the immunosuppressive effects of irradiation are due to changes produced in nucleic acids, especially DNA, which result in inhibition of cellular replication. The effectiveness of radiation is dependent upon the phase of the cell cycle in which the cell is found; cells in the M or G_2 phase are most sensitive to damage. The timing of radiation must be carefully planned to achieve the greatest immunosuppressive effect. As with most immunosuppressive agents, it is most ef-

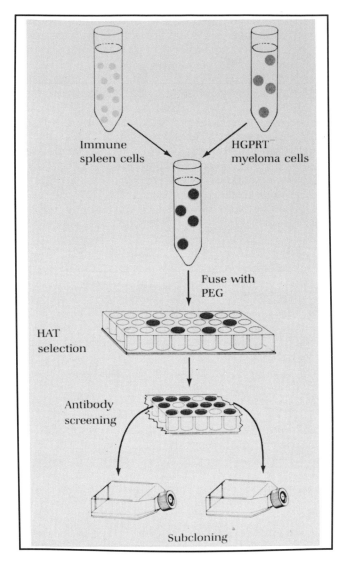

Immune spleen cells

HGPRT⁻ myeloma cells

Fuse with PEG

HAT selection

Antibody screening

Subcloning

FIGURE 6–17. Production of monoclonal antibodies. Immune spleen cells and HGPRT myeloma cells are fused with polyethylene glycol, resulting in hybrid cells. Cells are distributed in microwell plates and grown in HAT medium. Unfused myeloma cells die because they have no HGPRT to use the salvage pathway. Unfused spleen cells are unable to grow in vitro: only fused cells grow (0). Fused cells hybridomas grown in microwells and supernate of each well are tested for specific antibody production. Wells making antibody of interest are subcloned and grown in larger volumes. (Reprinted from Golub, E.: Immunology: A Synthesis. Sunderland, M.A.: Sinauer Associates, Inc., Chapter 6, Fig. 1, p. 95, 1987.)

fective if utilized prior to generation of the rejection response.

Adrenal Corticosteroids

Adrenal cortocosteroids are the immunosuppressive agents most commonly used in clinical practice. The functional effect of steroids is to depress all T cell responses. A decrease in the total blood lymphocyte count occurs within six hours following corticosteroid administration. Glucocorticoids cause emigration of circulating T cells from the intravascular compartments to the lymphoid tissues. Corticosteroids also inhibit the production of T cell lymphokines, which are required to amplify the responses of the activated lymphocytes and macrophages. They exert a lesser effect on the distribution and function of B cells. Corticosteroids block both chemotaxis and phagocytosis by macrophages and neutrophils. The ability of macrophages to respond to lymphocyte-derived signals, such as migration inhibition factor and macrophage activation factor, is blocked, resulting in a decreased number of these cells at the site of inflammatory activity.

Steroids also increase the membrane stability of digestive lysosomal particles in these cells, resulting in a reduction of their inflammatory activity. Inflammation is so intertwined with any substantial immune reaction that the various effects are inseparable. The variety of immunologic activities affected by steroids suggests that their effectiveness against the rejection reaction is probably multifactorial. Steroids alone cannot prevent clinical allograft rejection, but together with other compounds, they are potent in both preventing and reversing rejection reactions.

Hypertension, weight gain, peptic ulcers and gastrointestinal bleeding, personality changes, cataract formation, hyperglycemia, pancreatitis, and osteoporosis are the most frequently encountered toxicities associated with the use of corticosteroids to prevent rejection. A Cushingoid appearance often results form steroid use.

Combination Therapy

The use of a combination of immunosuppressive agents usually allows the surgeon to minimize toxicity yet maximize control of rejection, since lower doses of each individual agent are required. Table 6–10 lists the most frequent agents used clinically.

Other Immunosuppressive Approaches

Blood Transfusion. It was previously shown that blood transfusion prior to renal transplantation may result in improved graft survival. Therefore, transfusion protocols have become part of the preparative regimen at some centers for patients in renal failure who are awaiting transplantation. Sensitization occasionally occurs following the transfusions, but azathioprine administered at the time of transfusion will reduce the rate of sensitization to less than 5 per cent. The mechanism by which these transfusions act is not known, but evidence suggests induction of a possible suppressor cell phenomenon.

TABLE 6–9. REPRESENTATIVE MONOCLONAL ANTIBODIES AVAILABLE TO VARIOUS CLUSTER OF DIFFERENTIATION (CD) ANTIGENS

CD CLASS	MONOCLONAL ANTIBODY	TARGET CELL
CD 3	OKT 3	All T cells
CD 4	OKT 4, Leu3a	Helper and inducer T cells (Class II)
CD 5	Leu1	T cells, B cell subset
CD 8	OKT 8, Leu2	Suppressor and cytotoxic (Class I)
CD 14	Leu M3	Monocytes (granulocytes)
CD 16	Leu 11[a]	NK cells, PMN
CD 19	Leu 12, B4	B cells
CD 20	Leu 16	B cells
CD 34	My10	Hematopoietic stem cells
CD 39	G 28-8	B cells, macrophages

Complications of Immunosuppression

A number of complications are associated with the use of the conventional immunosuppressive agents. Most result from the nonspecific nature of their action (infection and malignancy), while others are end organ toxicities. At times, rejection cannot be controlled and may occur in spite of aggressive combinations and high doses of these agents.

Infection. An increased incidence of infection is observed in transplant recipients who receive immunosuppressive agents. Immunosuppression understandably increases the risk of infection by viral, fungal, and bacterial agents because of the nonspecific mechanism of action. Infection is the most common complication of immunosuppression and is the most common cause of mortality in transplant recipients. Early in the history of kidney transplantation, the majority of deaths occurred as a result of invasive pathogenic bacterial infections. More recently, improved antibiotics and improved immunosuppressive therapy have shifted the spectrum of organisms to opportunistic organisms which are normally weakly pathogenic. Prophylactic antibiotics will erad-icate the more aggressive bacteria, but they leave opportunistic fungal, protozoal, and viral organisms free to colonize the susceptible transplant patient.

Opportunistic fungal and protozoal organisms, normally eliminated by cellular immune mechanisms, become invasive in the face of the T cell depression associated with immunosuppression. *Candida albicans* infections are the most common, and *Aspergillus* species is the second most common cause of fungal infection. *Aspergillus* typically produces upper lobe pulmonary cavities. *Rhizopus oryzae*, *Histoplasma capsulatum*, and *Cryptococcus neoformans* may also invade the lung to produce pulmonary abscesses. *Pneumocystis carinii*, a protozoan, is also a frequent cause of pulmonary infection. It usually produces an alveolar infiltrate with disproportionate dyspnea and cyanosis. Viral infections are very common in kidney transplant recipients. The herpes group of DNA viruses is most frequently encountered. Cytomegalovirus is a frequently encountered offender.

Malignancy. The incidence of malignancy is significantly increased in recipients of transplants, but the rate is not high enough to contraindicate trans-

TABLE 6–10. MECHANISM OF ACTION OF IMMUNOSUPPRESSIVE AGENTS USED IN TRANSPLANTATION

AGENT	CLASSIFICATION	MECHANISM OF ACTION
Azathioprine	Antimetabolite	Purine analog; interference with DNA synthesis
Methotrexate	Antimetabolite	Folic acid antagonists; inhibits DNA and RNA synthesis
Cyclophosphamide synthesis	Alkylating agent	Inhibits DNA and RNA
Cyclosporine	Product of fungus	Inhibits T cell activation and maturation
Antilymphocyte Globulin (ALG)	Lymphocyte depletion compound	Sera directed against T lymphocytes
Steroids	Lymphocyte depletion compound	Produce a decrease in total T lymphocytes
OKT3	Monoclonal antibody	Binds to T cell receptor complex (CD3)
FK506	Product of fungus macrolide antibiotic	Inhibits T cell activation and maturation
Rapamycin	Macrolide antibiotic	Inhibits T cell activation and maturation

plantation. The prevalence of malignancy in patients surviving renal transplantation may be as high as 30 times that of the normal population. Only certain cancers are increased in frequency; the most frequent include lymphomas, sarcomas, and squamous and basal cell carcinomas. Recently, Ebstein-Barr virus-induced lymphomas, which are aggressively invasive, have been reported with cyclosporine therapy. They are referred to as lymphoproliferative disease.

CLINICAL TISSUE AND SOLID ORGAN TRANSPLANTATION

Numerous tissues and organs are now transplanted clinically. The most frequent include kidney, bone marrow, pancreas, liver, heart, and lung. Bone marrow transplantation is still in its inception. It is performed primarily for treatment of hematopoietic and solid tumors and for aplastic anemia from various etiologies. The recipient is conditioned by ionizing irradiation, chemicals, or drugs to "make space" for engraftment. Both autotransplantation (self-self) and allotransplantation are performed. In allotransplantation, a chimera results if engraftment occurs, and in the ideal circumstance, cells of two genetically distinct derivations will coexist and be tolerant of each other. However, untreated bone marrow contains mature T lymphocytes , so that GVH disease may occur when allotransplantation is performed. The more genetically disparate the donor and recipient, the greater the strength of the GVH. T cell depletion of the allogeneic donor bone marrow results in a lower incidence of GVH disease, but recent data indicate that there is a greater rate of failure to engraft if the donor bone marrow is too aggressively T cell depleted.

The major sites of injury due to GVH are those that interact with the outside world: the skin, lymphatic tissues, intestine, and liver. Diarrhea, weight loss, dermatitis, and profound suppression of immune responses result. Control of GVH disease is currently obtained using immunosuppressive agents such as cyclosporine and methotrexate.

Bone marrow transplantation is the only situation in which the transplanted tissue results in the induction of true donor-specific transplantation tolerance and does not require long-term chronic immunosuppressive agents to prolong graft survival.

Because of this unique result, the use of bone marrow to manipulate the immune system for induction of donor-specific transplantation tolerance is being pursued in the laboratory.

FUTURE DIRECTIONS IN PREVENTION OF REJECTION

The current nonspecific immunosuppressive agents have made transplantation possible. However, their nonspecific function in suppressing all aspects of immune function inevitably results in toxicities. Investigative efforts are now being directed to identifying improved, more specific methods of manipulating the immune system to prevent graft rejection. An understanding of the mechanisms involved in the immune response to foreign cells may provide many potential points of vulnerability in activation and deployment of the cells responsible for the rejection reaction which could potentially be manipulated. Potential approaches include (1) immunosuppression by specific antigens, (2) donor-specific transplantation tolerance induced by bone marrow transplantation, and (3) specific, focused immunosuppression by antibodies or suppressor cells. As our understanding of the function of the immune system progresses, other new avenues of experimental immunosuppression will become possible as well. The final goal is to induce a state of donor-specific transplantation tolerance or unresponsiveness to the graft with full preservation of immunocompetence of the recipient to fight infection and eliminate malignant cells which may appear.

Acknowledgment. The authors thank Ms. Michelle Waters for excellent secretarial assistance.

BIBLIOGRAPHY

1. Bach, F.H. and Sachs, D.H.: Transplantation immunology. N. Engl. J. Med. 317-318, 1987.
2. Clark, S.C. and Kamen, R.: The human hematopoietic colony-stimulating factors. Science 236:1229-37, 1987.
3. Cooper, M.D.: Lymphocytes. N. Engl. J. Med. 317:1452-1455, 1987.
4. Dinarello, C.A. and Mier, J.W.: Lymphokines. N. Engl. J. Med. 317: 940-945, 1987.
5. Hood, L.M., Steinmetz, B., and Malissen, C.: Genes of the major histocompatibility complex of the mouse. Annual Review of Immunology.

7

METABOLIC RESPONSE
TO STRESS

PAUL H. KISPERT

All cellular processes require energy. The body is in a constant state of flux, attempting to synthesize new substrates to replace those that are being broken down. The concept of balanced metabolic processes is central to understanding changes that occur in intermediary metabolism. Under normal circumstances in fed, healthy humans, metabolism is tightly controlled to maintain this balance. Injury or infection are stresses that tip this balance in favor of catabolism. The surgical patient is swayed toward catabolism for several reasons. First, such a patient is typically starved for a period before and after the surgery. Second, the imposition of a wound with or without infection dramatically changes the hormonal and metabolic balance in favor of those factors that heal the wound. In general, healing wounds require catabolism of peripheral tissues. While one may look at the array of metabolic changes occurring in response to wounding as being abnormal, these changes are normal for the wounded host and facilitate survival. This chapter describes the normal metabolic fluxes occurring during stress. The most common forms of stress encountered by the surgical patient include starvation, injury, and infection. I will also describe how these metabolic changes help to improve the host's chances for survival after injury.

METABOLIC RESPONSES IN THE BASAL FED STATE

Intermediary metabolism refers to the patterns of use of proteins, carbohydrates, and fats that allow for energy generation and synthetic function. A typical diet reflects the normal patterns of substrate use, approximately a 65·35 mixture of carbohydrate and fats. Ingested carbohydrates are absorbed through the gut and used for energy generation by tissues with obligate glucose needs or stored as glycogen in the liver or muscle. Glucose may be converted to fat and stored for further use. Short-term energy requirements accompanying periods of fasting are met with the breakdown of liver glycogen to glucose. In the presence of insulin, glucose to be used for energy generation is taken up by cells. Similarly, fat stored in adipocytes is released into the circulation as free fatty acids, which are extracted by the peripheral tissues, and further broken down to acetyl-coenzyme A (CoA), which is used to fuel mitochondrial respiration. Protein ordinarily is not used for energy generation but is used for synthesis of other proteins. In times of starvation, however, protein and amino acids are used as a substrate for the generation of glucose. Glucose can be synthesized only from the glycerol component of lipids.

Classically, the metabolic response to injury has been described as an initial ebb phase followed by a flow phase. The ebb phase occurs in the first several hours following injury and is characterized by metabolic changes needed to restore effective circulating volume. The flow phase, lasting from days to weeks, is the catabolic phase characterized by the breakdown of skeletal protein, negative nitrogen balance, and hyperglycemia.

A knowledge of normal carbohydrate, fat, and protein metabolism is necessary to understand the pathophysiology of starvation, injury, and infection. The following sections discuss substrate metabolism and important regulatory steps controlling the flow of these substrates.

CARBOHYDRATE METABOLISM

Carbohydrates, primarily in the form of glucose, provide a rapid energy source for all tissues and are the only source of energy for leukocytes, erythrocytes, the renal medulla, and the nervous system.

The synthesis of glucose, its storage as glycogen, and it's breakdown are tightly controlled by several factors, including the levels of substrates, the energy charge of the cell, and the hormonal environment. After a carbohydrate meal, circulating glucose and insulin levels are high. Glucose is transported across the cell membrane, where it can be used in several ways. It may be stored as glycogen or broken down by glycolysis to form pyruvate, which itself may enter several metabolic pathways.

Glycogen Synthesis and Degradation

Under conditions of high intracellular glucose concentrations and elevated insulin levles, glycogen is synthesized under the action of glycogen synthetase (Fig. 7–1). High levels of insulin signal the fed state, and low levels signal the fasting state. Glycogen, which is a storage form of glucose, can be mobilized readily. The activity of glycogen synthetase is increased by insulin and glucocorticoids. This enzyme is active in its dephosphorylated form. The activities of the enzymes are controlled by reversible phosphorylation, a common mechanism controlling enzyme activation. Phosphorylation of glycogen synthetase, which is stimulated by glucagon and epinephrine, inactivates the enzyme. Glycogen breakdown is facilitated by glycogen phosphorylase,

which is activated by phosphorylation. Phosphorylation is stimulated by epinephrine and glucagon. Muscle glycogen breakdown is more sensitive to epinephrine and hepatic glycogen breakdown is more sensitive to glucagon. Both epinephrine and glucagon act by increasing intracellular levels of cyclic adenosine monophosphate (cAMP). The cAMP activates a protein kinase, stimulating activation and phosphorylation of glycogen phosphorylase and inhibiting glycogen synthetase (Fig. 7–1). It can be appreciated that under conditions of substrate (glucose) abundance, insulin levels are high and favor glycogen synthesis. Under condition of stress in which glucose needs are increased, counterregulatory hormones that activate glycogen phosphorylase (such as glucagon) favor the breakdown of glycogen to glucose. Only the liver can release free glucose. Muscle can synthesize glycogen but cannot release glucose because of a lack of glucose-6-phosphatase, which converts glucose 6-phosphate to glucose.

Glycolysis

The nonreversible breakdown of glucose to pyruvate occurs in the cytosol through a series of steps termed *glycolysis*. Three of these enzymatic steps are irreversible and are outlined in Figure 7–2. The nicotinamide-adenine dinucleotide (reduced)

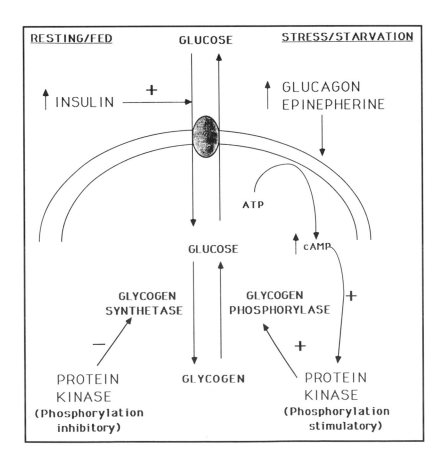

FIGURE 7–1. Glycogen synthesis and breakdown. Glycogen breakdown occurs in the presence of increased glucagon levels. Glucagon results in intracellular cyclic AMP (cAMP) accumulation. cAMP activates protein kinase, resulting in phosphorylation of glycogen phosphorylase and synthetase, favoring glycogenolysis and inhibiting glycogen synthesis. Insulin inhibits phosphorylation and enhances glucose entry into the cell, leading to glycogen synthesis from glucose. (+), activation; (−), inhibition.

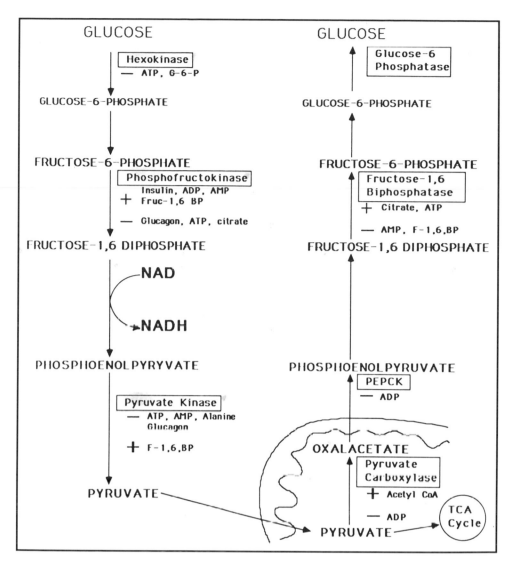

FIGURE 7–2. Glycolysis and gluconeogenesis. Glycoloysis results in the breakdown of glucose to pyruvate, which has many metabolic fates. Three enzyme systems (outlined in squares) are irreversible. Phosphofructokinase (PFK) is the most important in control of glycolysis. Glycolysis is inhibited under conditions of substrate and energy excess (ATP, citrate, insulin) and is activated by substrate and energy depletion (AMP, ADP). Gluconeogenesis is not a simple reversal of glycolysis. Four new enzyme systems are needed. Synthesis of new glucose begins in the mitochondria, but all other steps are cytosolic. Low energy levels (AMP, ADP) inhibit gluconeogenesis while substrate excess (ATP, citrate) enhances glucose synthesis. NADH is produced to be used in the electron transport chain.

(NADH) used in the electron transport chain and pyruvate are generated in this pathway. Depending on the environment, pyruvate may have several metabolic fates, including conversion to lactate or acetyl-CoA for fat synthesis or entry into the tricarboxylic acid (TCA) cycle. Figure 7–2 outlines the inhibitory and stimulatory factors regulating glycolysis. In general, when substrate is abundant and intracellular energy stores (adenosine triphosphate; (ATP) are great, glycolysis is inhibited and glycogen synthesis will be favored. Under conditions in which the cell is energy deprived [decreased ATP, increased AMP and adenosine diphosphate (ADP)], glycolysis will be favored because cellular energy stores are low. Glycolysis may be an aerobic or an anaerobic process. Under aerobic conditions, glucose will rapidly be converted to pyruvate with entry into the TCA cycle for energy generation. Under anaerobic conditions where the TCA cycle is not functional, pyruvate will be converted to lactate with resulting lactic acidosis.

Gluconeogenesis

Certain tissues have obligate glucose needs at a time when glycogen has been depleted and no carbohydrate intake is occurring. Under these circumstances, gluconeogenesis will occur. Gluconeogenesis is more than a simple reversal of glycolysis because three of the glycolytic enzymatic steps are irreversible (Fig. 7–2). Four new enzyme systems must be used under these circumstances (these are outlined in Figure 7–2 and compared with glycolysis). In gluconeogenesis, cytosolic pyruvate must be converted to oxalacetate. This requires entry of pyruvate into the mitochondria for conversion to oxalacetate via a mitochondrial enzyme (pyruvate carboxylase). The mitochondrial membrane is impermeable to oxalacetate so it is shuttled out as malate and converted to oxalacetate in the cytoplasm. Oxalacetate is converted to phosphoenolpyruvate by phosphoenolpyruvate carboxylase (PEPCK). Gluconeogenesis occurs primarily in the liver and secondarily in the kidneys. All of the enzymes of gluconeogenesis are located in the cytoplasms except pyruvate carboxylase, which is located in the mitochondria. Control is reciprocal to that of glycolysis. In general, pyruvate flows to phosphoenolpyruvate and gluconeogenesis is favored when the cell is rich in fuel molecules and ATP (Fig. 7–2).

Aerobic glycolytic tissues, such as leukocytes and erythrocytes, convert glucose to pyruvate and lactate. The lactate and pyruvate released are returned to the liver, where they can enter the gluconeogenesis pathway. This shuttling is termed the *Cori cycle* (Fig. 7–3). The Cori cycle takes on increasing importance under anaerobic conditions in which increased lactate productions occurs, providing substrate to the liver for gluconeogenesis via the Cori cycle.

PROTEIN

No storage form of protein exists. All existing protein has some biologic function. However, under some conditions, amino acids derived from protein may be used to provide carbon precursors to the liver for the synthesis of new glucose. In order for amino acids to be used in the synthesis of glucose, their amino groups must first be removed. This is usually accomplished through transamination with an α-ketoacid to produce the α-keto analogue of the amino acid and a new amino acid (Fig. 7–4). α-Ketoglutarate, glutamate, or pyruvate are the usual amino group receptors for the formation of glutamate, glutamine, or alanine, respectively. Complete oxidation of amino acids occurs mainly in the liver but also in the kidney. The alanine generated through transamination enters the circulation and is transported to the liver, where it is deaminated to pyruvate and can then be used for gluconeogenesis. Similar reactions occur for glutamate and glutamine. However, this generates an amino group that must be eliminated. This is accomplished through the urea cycle (Fig. 7–4), where α-ketoglutamate or pyruvate is regenerated from glutamate or alanine with the production of ammonia by oxidative deamination. The ammonia enters the urea cycle and is subsequently eliminated in the urine. Thus, increased protein catabolism leads to increases in urine urea nitrogen (UUN) loss. Table 7–1 demonstrates how all of the amino acids may be used for energy production through entry as a glycolytic or TCA cycle intermediate or through the formation of ketones. The amino group may also combine with glutamate to form glutamine and be excreted directly by the kidney or in the gut as ammonia.

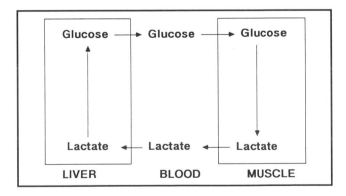

FIGURE 7–3. Cori cycle. The incomplete oxidation of glucose in muscle and leukocytes leads to lactate production. Lactate is returned to the liver, where it is used as a substrate for new glucose formation, ensuring a continuous supply of glucose to these tissues.

TABLE 7–1. PATHWAYS FOR USE OF AMINO ACIDS

Gluconeogenesis	Ketogenesis	Gluconeogenesis and Ketogenesis
Alanine	Leucine*	Isoleucine*
Arginine*		Lysine*
Aspartic acid		Phenylalanine*
Asparagine		Tyrosine*
Cystine		Tryptophan*
Glutamic acid		
Glycine		
Histidine*		
Hydroxyproline		
Methionine*		
Proline		
Serine		
Threonine*		
Valine*		

* Essential amino acids.
Reprinted from Davis, J.H. (ed.): Clinical Surgery. St. Louis, C.V. Mosby Company, 1987, p. 347.

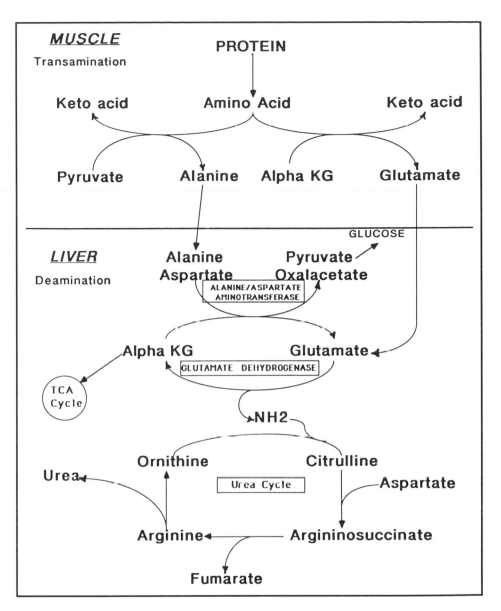

FIGURE 7–4. Transamination, deamination, and the urea cycle. Protein catabolism leads to increases in muscle amino acid levels. The carbon skeletons of these amino acids are transaminated with pyruvate and α-ketoglutarate (KG) to form ketoacids, which can be used by muscle for energy generation. Alanine and glutamate are extracted by the liver, where deamination occurs. The amino group (NH_2) produced is eliminated as urea in the urea cycle.

Through these pathways, all of the carbon skeletons obtained through muscle protein breakdown may be used for energy generation. Under conditions of infection or stress, the amino acids released from muscle are used primarily for the synthesis of new glucose (see later in chapter).

LIPID METABOLISM

Lipids represent the largest energy source in the body and are used by those tissues that are not glucose dependent, including cardiac and skeletal muscle and visceral tissues (liver, pancreas, lung, and fat). The synthesis and catabolism of lipids as well as their regulation will be discussed.

Fatty Acid Catabolism

Many tissues are capable of utilizing fatty acids and glycerol, formed from the breakdown of triglycerides, to generate energy through β oxidation. The glycerol formed can be converted to pyruvate and used in gluconeogenesis. Fatty acids are released into the circulation from adipocytes under the influence of glucagon and epinephrine and are taken up by peripheral tissues (Fig. 7–5). Once in the tissues, β oxidation occurs in the outer mitochondrial membrane. The fatty acid combines with CoA to form fatty acyl-CoA with the subsequent cleavage and formation of acetyl-CoA. Fatty acids with odd numbers of carbon atoms from proprionyl-CoA instead of acetyl-CoA as the final step in fatty acid catabolism. This is converted to succinyl-CoA and

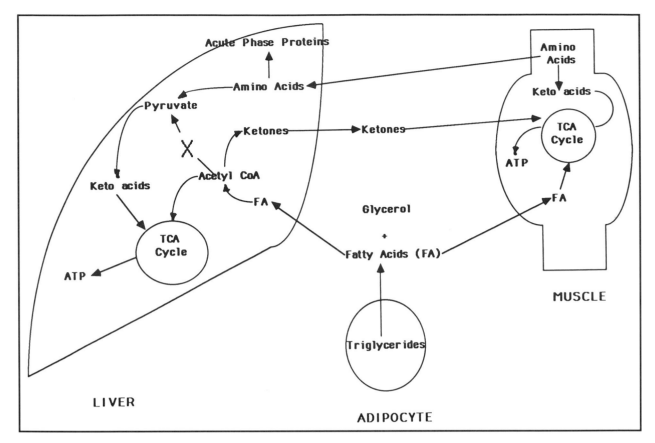

FIGURE 7–5. Fatty acid utilization. Fatty acids (FA) and glycerol are moblizied from adipose tissue. Fatty acids are extracted by the liver for the synthesis of ketones. The acetyl-CoA formed by the oxidation of fatty acids cannot be converted to new glucose (X). Ketones formed in the lever and FA mobilized from adipose tissue can be used by muscle for energy generation, taking the place of glucose during periods in which glucose is unavailable. TCA, tricarboxylic acid.

enters the TCA cycle. Mitochondrial acetyl-CoA can enter several metabolic pathways, including the TCA cycle for the generation of ATP, lipid synthesis, or ketone body synthesis (Fig. 7–6). It is important to note that fatty acids cannot be used in the synthesis of glucose (Fig. 7–5).

Insulin controls fatty acid entry into the mitochondria for oxidation. Insulin favors the synthesis of malonyl-CoA in times of substrate abundance. Malonyl-CoA inhibits the entry of fatty acyl-CoA into the mitochondria by inhibiting the mechanism for mitochondrial entry: carnitine acyltransferase. Inability of fatty acyl-CoA to enter the mitochondria leads to lipogenesis.

Lipid Synthesis

Acetyl-CoA formed during fatty acid catabolism has several fates, including fatty acid synthesis under some conditions. Fatty acid biosynthesis occurs in the cytoplasm, in contrast to lipid oxidation, which occurs in the mitochondria. The rate-limiting and

therefore the most important step in fatty acid synthesis is the conversion of acetyl-CoA to malonyl-CoA (Fig. 7–6). The growing fatty acid chain is elongated by the sequential addition of two carbon units derived from acetyl-CoA. This conversion is controlled by the enzyme acetyl-CoA carboxylase. Fatty acid synthesis occurs under conditions of abundant substrate and energy supplies, which provide clues as to how this enzyme is regulated.

Cytoplasmic citrate (indicating abundant substrate supplies) activates acetyl-CoA carboxylase, favoring fatty acid synthesis. Citrate levels are increased when both acetyl-CoA and ATP are abundant. Acetyl-CoA carboxylase is also inhibited by phosphorylation. Glucagon enhances phosphorylation through increases in intracellular cAMP levels leading to increased activity of protein kinase, which results in enzyme phosphorylation, similar to the mechanism for the contol of glycogen synthesis and degradation. Insulin has the reverse effect and promotes fatty acid synthesis. Palmityl-CoA (a 16-carbon fatty acid), the end product of fatty acid synthesis, inhibits the enzyme. Inhibition of the enzyme will result in the

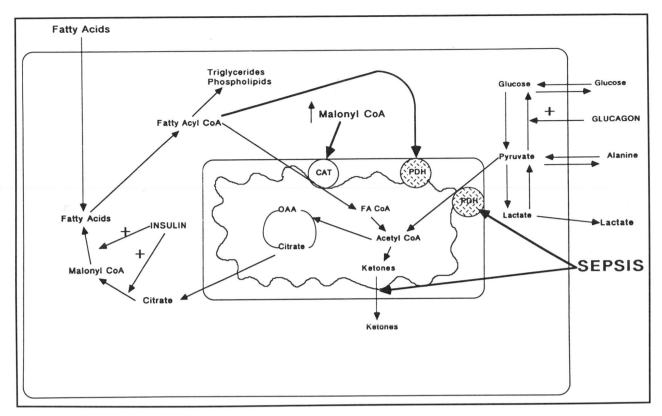

FIGURE 7-6. Fatty acid metabolism. Fatty acids are taken up by cells and converted to fatty acyl-CoA (FA CoA). The fatty acyl-CoA may be used for lipid synthesis or be transported into the mitochondria via carnitine acyltransferase (CAT), where it can be oxidized for energy generation or used for ketone synthesis. Triglyceride synthesis is enhanced by insulin, which stimulates malonyl-CoA formation. Malonyl-CoA inhibits CAT, resulting in increased levels of fatty acyl-CoA in the cytoplasm and increased triglyceride synthesis. Pyruvate dehydrogenase (PDH) is the key enzyme controlling the flow of pyruvate into the mitorchondria or back toward gluconeogenesis. Sepsis inhibits PDH activity through elevated intracellular fatty acyl-CoA levels. This results in the accumulation of pyruvate and lactate facilitating gluconeogenesis. (+), stimulatory; (−), inhibitory, OAA, oxalacetate. (Modified from Vary, T.C., Siegel, J.H., Nakatani, T., et al.: A biochemical basis for depressed ketogenesis in sepsis. J. Trauma 26:20, 1986.)

inhibition of formation of malonyl-CoA from acetyl-CoA and favor the entry of acetyl-CoA into the mitochondria for oxidation. During periods of substrate depletion, hormones such as epinephrine and glucagon favor triglyceride breakdown to free fatty acids (FFAs) in the adipocytes. The FFAs are extracted peripherally and used in oxidation. Fatty acid synthesis is inhibited by low citrate levels, thereby inhibiting acetyl-CoA carboxylase and allowing acetyl-CoA to be oxidized. Fatty acid synthesis is maximal when carbohydrate is abundant and fatty acid levels are low.

Ketone Synthesis and Utilization

Ketones are formed only in the liver and are exported for use to other tissues. The ketone bodies are broken down to acetyl-CoA, which can be used for energy generation by entry into the TCA cycle. In the liver, two molecules of acetyl-CoA are converted to acetoacetyl-CoA and then to acetoacetate or β-hydroxybutyrate. Acetoacetate is formed under the condition of low hepatic glycogen stores, whereas β-hydroxybutyrate is generated when liver glycogen stores are ample. The normal ratio of β-hydroxybutyrate to acetoacetate is 3:1, reflecting the fed state in the liver.

When fatty acids are broken down to acetyl-CoA, why should ketone bodies be formed instead of the acetyl-CoA simply entering into the TCA cycle for energy generation? The reason is that entry of acetyl-CoA into the TCA cycle requires complexing with oxalacetate to form citrate. If glucose availability is low, as occurs in starvation, oxalacetate levels will similarly be depressed because of lower levels of TCA cycle intermediates. In fasting, oxalacetate is used for the formation of glucose (Fig. 7-2) and is unavailable to form citrate by the addition of acetyl-CoA.

Under these conditions, acetyl-CoA is diverted to the synthesis of ketone bodies. It has been found that cardiac muscle and the renal cortex use ketone bodies in preference to glucose. In starvation, 75 per cent of the fuel needs of the brain are met by acetoacetate. Fatty acids are released by adipocytes and converted into acetyl units by the liver, which exports them as acetoacetate. High levels of acetoacetate also inhibit lipolysis by adipose tissues.

Tricarboxylic Acid Cycle and Electron Transport

The ultimate function of substrate oxidation is the generation of energy, primarily in the form of the high-energy phosphate bonds of ATP, to fuel synthetic processes. This process is called oxidative phosphorylation. Electrons in substrate molecules from glycolysis or the TCA cycle are donated to electron carriers with the production of NADH and flavin adenine dinucleotide (reduced) ($FADH_2$). When these molecules donate their electrons through a series of electron carriers to oxygen to form water, a large amount of energy is released that is captured and stored in the phosphate bonds of ATP. Small amounts of ATP are generated through anaerobic glycolysis, but much larger amounts of ATP are generated in an oxygen-rich environment.

The components of the TCA cycle are located in the mitochondrial matrix (Fig. 7–7), whereas the enzymes of the electron transport chain are located on the inner mitochondrial membrane. Substrate enters the TCA cycle as acetyl-CoA or after conversion to one of the intermediates in the TCA cycle. A number of amino acids can be converted to substrates that can directly enter the TCA cycle (Table

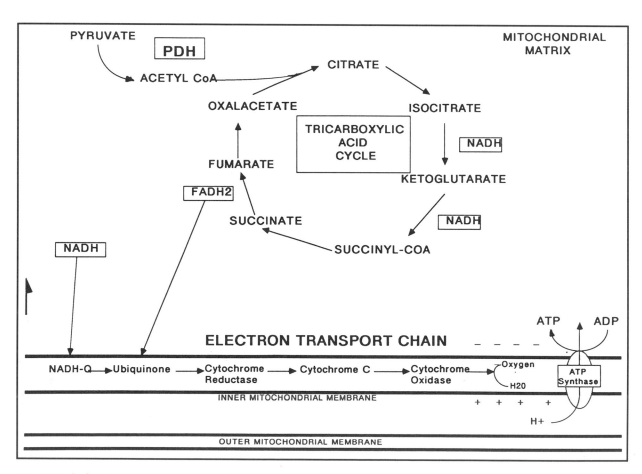

FIGURE 7–7. Tricarboxylic acid cycle and the electron transport chain. Pyruvate, acetyl-CoA, or the carbon skeletons of other amino acids enter the TCA cycle, leading to the production of NADH and $FADH_2$ in the mitochondrial matrix. The electrons transferred to NADH and $FADH_2$ are donated to electon acceptors in the electron transport chain, located on the inner mitochondrial membrane. The transfer of electrons leads to protons (+) being pumped outside the membrane, setting up an electrochemical gradient. The passage of these protons back to the matrix through ATP synthase releases energy for the generation of ATP. (Several intermediate steps in the TCA cycle are omitted.)

7–1). As these substrates are oxidized, electrons are transferred to NAD and FAD to form NADH and $FADH_2$. These electron carriers transfer the electrons to the inner mitochondrial membrane, where they pass down a series of electron carriers with the release of energy. This energy is used to pump protons to the region outside the inner mitochondrial membrane. This creates a potential difference with excess protons (hydrogen ions) outside the membrane. These protons are channeled through ATP synthase. Energy is released as the protons pass down their electrochemical gradient and this energy is used to generate ATP from ADP. Oxygen is the final electron acceptor, with the formation of water. NADH that is generated in the cytosol (from glycolysis) cannot be transported across the mitochondrial membrane. Rather, the NADH transfers its electrons to a carrier that can breach the mitochondrial membrane and the electrons are then transferred back to NAD to reform NADH inside the mitochondria.

OVERVIEW OF INTERMEDIARY METABOLISM IN THE NONSTRESSED STATE

The routes of energy utilization in the normal state and their controlling mechanisms are really quite simple to understand. Substrate use is regulated primarily by the hormonal environment and energy charge of the cell. The energy charge reflects the availability of high-energy bonds in the form of ATP to perform cellular functions. Normal metabolism can be broken down into states of synthesis, where energy and substrate availability is high, and need, where energy and substrate availability is low. In the fed state, synthesis is favored. Glucose and insulin levels are high and favor the synthesis of glycogen from glucose for storage. In addition, much of the glucose that enters the glycolytic pathway goes to form pyruvate. Because energy stores are abundant, pyruvate is converted to acetyl-CoA, which is then used for lipid synthesis. The high existing levels of citrate, ATP, and NADH act as inhibitory influences on the TCA cycle, glycolysis, and the β oxidation pathway of lipids. In this way, synthesis of glycogen and lipids are favored.

In the fasted but nonstressed state, a different set of circumstances exist. Glucose and insulin levels fall and glucagon levels rise. Under these circumstances, the levels of citrate, ATP, and NADH will fall, indicating depressed energy and substrate stores, leading to inhibition of synthesis and favoring the breakdown of glycogen and fatty acids to provide energy. In addition, protein breakdown is favored to provide substrate for the formation of new glucose by gluconeogenesis. Ketone body synthesis is favored because of depletion of oxalacetate, which is used in the synthesis of new glucose, thereby favoring hepatic export of ketone bodies.

Metabolic Changes in Starvation

Starvation is perhaps the most common situation leading to compensatory changes in intermediary metabolism. Surgical patients waiting for operation or diagnostic testing or those with reduced intake secondary to their underlying disease are all starving. An understanding of the adaption to starvation is critical in order to understand the more complex series of changes that occur when injury or infection is superimposed on starvation. The changes in carbohydrate, lipid, and protein metabolism that occur under conditions of starvation are illustrated in Figure 7–8.

All humans have an obligate requirement for carbohydrates, principally glucose. A number of tissues are obligate users of glucose and have variable abilities to adapt to the use of other substrates as starvation progresses. Resting humans have a glucose requirement of approximately 180 gm/day. Most of this (144 gm) is used by the nervous system while a lesser amount (36 gm) is used by other glucose-dependent tissues (erythrocytes, leukocytes, renal medulla). Starvation results in a decrease in serum glucose concentrations as hepatic glycogen stores (which can provide a source of glucose for 18 to 24 hours under resting conditions) are depleted. The depressed glucose levels lead to decreases in insulin secretion and increases in glucagon secretion by the pancreas. In uncomplicated starvation, other counterregulatory hormones such as catecholamines, cortisol, and growth hormone are not elevated, so intermediary metabolism is primarily determined by the opposing effects of glucagon and insulin on intermediary metabolism.

After the depletion of glycogen, what is the source of the glucose necessary to meet the needs of tissues with absolute requirements for glucose? Lipid breakdown is a poor source since only the glycerol portion of the triglyceride molecule can be utilized for new glucose synthesis through gluconeogenesis. Protein is the only other available source of glucose after glycogen is depleted. Breakdown of protein to amino acids with subsequent conversion of the amino acids to their α-keto analogues allows them to be used for gluconeogenesis. Early in starvation, approximately 75 gm of protein per day is catabolized and plasma amino acid levels fall as amino acid extraction increases. This cannot persist forever without oral intake, because humans only have about 6000 gm of protein. After a period of several days, the brain, which has the largest initially obligate requirement for glucose, is able to shift to the use of ketone bodies and thereby minimize its glucose requirement, with a resultant decrease in the need for protein breakdown to supply a source of precursors for glucose synthesis. Protein breakdown drops to 20 gm/day. Ketone body transport across the blood-brain barrier is enhanced, allowing adaptation to occur.

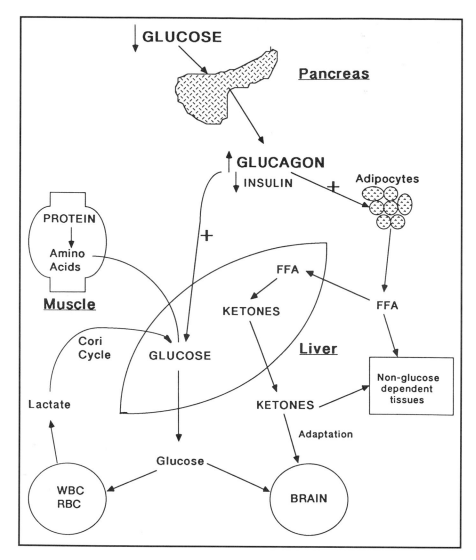

FIGURE 7–8. Starvation. Decreased glucose and insulin levels and increased glucagon levels lead to increased fat mobilization from adipocytes. The free fatty acids (FFA) are transported to the liver for ketone synthesis. Ketones are exported to non-glucose-dependent tissues and the brain after adaptation occurs. Early in starvation, increased muscle proteolysis occurs to provide substrate to the liver for new glucose synthesis needed by tissues with obligate glucose needs. Proteolysis decreases as the brain is able to convert from the use of glucose to the use of ketone bodies for energy generation. Tissues with obligate glucose needs recycle the glucose carbon as lactate, with no net loss of carbon atoms. RBC, red blood cells; WBC, white blood cells.

Gluconeogenesis occurs early in starvation primarily in the liver (90 per cent). As starvation progresses, however, there is a shift of gluconeogenesis to the kidney, where 45 per cent of gluconeogenesis may occur later in starvation.

The decreases in circulating insulin and increases in glucagon also favor the breakdown of lipids. Increases occur in the levels of FFAs, which are used by peripheral tissues for an energy source.

The net result of this adaptation is a shift from the use of glucose to the use of fat and a minimizing of obligate protein breakdown.

Metabolic Changes in Stress and Sepsis

Sepsis and injury are characterized by progressive alterations in the metabolism of substrates used for energy production and synthetic processes. Changes in fat, carbohydrate, protein, and oxygen utilization are well characterized. Energy requirements may increase dramatically, depending on the extent of injury or infection. For example, elective surgery increases energy requirement only about 10 per cent above resting levels, whereas major thermal injury may double resting energy requirements. The hormonal environment changes dramatically in response to these stresses, and this alteration is responsible for many of the changes in patterns of substrate use. The factors responsible for changes in patterns of substrate use are not all defined. Of recent interest, however, is evidence suggesting that macrophage cytokine synthesis, principally interleukin-1 (IL-1), tumor necrosis factor (TNF), and interleukin-6 (IL-6), may affect carbohydrate, protein, and lipid metabolism in septic patients.

Several metabolic changes seen in stress and sepsis are consistently observed:

1. Glucose production by the liver increases and peripheral glucose use is impaired.
2. Skeletal muscle proteolysis and urinary nitro-

gen excretion is enormously increased compared with the fasted state.

3. Lipid is increasingly used as a fuel source to decrease glucose utilization.

The net result of these changes is a hyperglycemic, catabolic immunocompromised patient with marked muscle wasting and organ failure. While the long-term end results of this catabolic state may be injurious, the changes in substrate utilization in the short term are beneficial. It is important to realize that these adaptive changes are important to short-term survival. With the advent of intensive care support, patients are surviving far beyond the evolutionarily anticipated duration of their survival given the severity of their injuries. Because of this, prolonged adaptive responses become maladaptive responses, culminating in organ failure.

Protein Metabolism

Under normal fed conditions, protein degradation is balanced by synthesis. Starvation initially upsets this balance, with an initial increase in protein catabolism to provide substrate for gluconeogenesis. As starvation progresses, protein degradation again falls, sparing muscle and visceral protein stores. Trauma and sepsis upset this pattern of protein sparing. Under these circumstances, protein catabolism proceeds at a rate far exceeding synthesis at a time when nutritional intake is absent and metabolic demands are great. Urinary nitrogen and 3-methylhistidine (a marker of muscle proteolysis) excretion are markedly increased as a result of breakdown of muscle protein leading to muscle wasting.

A logical question to be asked is, why is protein catabolism accelerated in stress and sepsis? The individual should derive some benefit from this "aberration" of protein metabolism (Fig. 7–9). The amino acids released into the plasma from muscle proteolysis are used for new protein synthesis, as oxidative fuels, or as a substrate for gluconeogenesis. Only about 20 per cent of the protein that is broken down is metabolized directly by that organ (muscle, for example) for the generation of energy. The remainder is shuttled to the liver to provide substrate for accelerated gluconeogenesis. Hepatic and muscle glycogen stores are rapidly depleted in the setting of starvation with superimposed catabolism. After depletion of glycogen, in the absence of an exogenous source of glucose, fats must be used or new glucose must be synthesized. The only energy alternatives at this point are protein or lipids (fatty acids or ketone bodies). With the exception of glycerol derived from the breakdown of triglycerides (which accounts for approximately 10 per cent of the carbon skeleton of triglycerides) fatty acids cannot be used for the synthesis of new glucose. Therefore, this leaves protein as the major source of carbon skeletons that can be used in the synthesis of new glucose to satisfy peripheral needs for glucose. Glucose is an absolute requirement of cells infiltrating the wound, which are obligate and voracious users of glucose. If new glucose could not be synthesized from protein, leukocyte function would fail and overwhelming infection would occur. This demonstrates that the short-term effects of muscle proteolysis are beneficial to the host.

A second reason for amino acid release from muscle is the need for new protein synthesis by the liver, the bone marrow, and the wound. Total hepatic protein synthesis is decreased after injury. Specific proteins, the acute-phase proteins, are synthesized at an accelerated rate in injury and infection. These acute-phase proteins include proteins involved in immune functions (third component of complement), coagulation (fibrinogen), opsonization (C-reactive protein), and antiproteases α_2-macroglobulin, α_1-antitrypsin). The benefits of increased synthesis of these proteins after injury should be clear. Significant elevations in C-reactive protein in particular have been noted. C-reactive protein has been demonstrated to play a role in bacterial opsonization, complement activation, and phagocytosis. Antiproteases such as α_1-antitrypsin and α_2-macroglobulin may protect against the systemic effects of proteases released from phagocytic cells at sites of inflammation. Ceruloplasmin and α_2-macroglobulin have been shown to have superoxide scavenging properties. Amino acids derived from skeletal muscle are crucial for the synthesis of acute-phase proteins by the liver. The acute-phase proteins synthesized in the liver are produced at the expense of other proteins such as albumin, which is also produced by the liver. This reprioritization of protein synthesis allows available amino acids to be used for the synthesis of the vital acute-phase proteins and inhibits the synthesis of less essential proteins (albumin and transferin).

Regulation of Proteolysis

It might be expected that, if exogenous glucose were supplied to meet the demands of tissues with obligate glucose needs, proteolysis might be inhibited. This does not appear to be so. In sepsis, administration of excess glucose fails to suppress protein catabolism in a manner similar to that which occurs in starvation-induced proteolysis.

The regulation of proteolysis can be divided into two components, hormonal and nonhormonal. Hormonal regulation involves increases or decreases in counterregulatory hormone production. Nonhormonal regulation relates to the effects that macrophage products have on protein synthesis.

Nonhormonal regulation of protein synthesis by macrophage products, including (IL-1), is postulated as a possible mechanism to induce septic

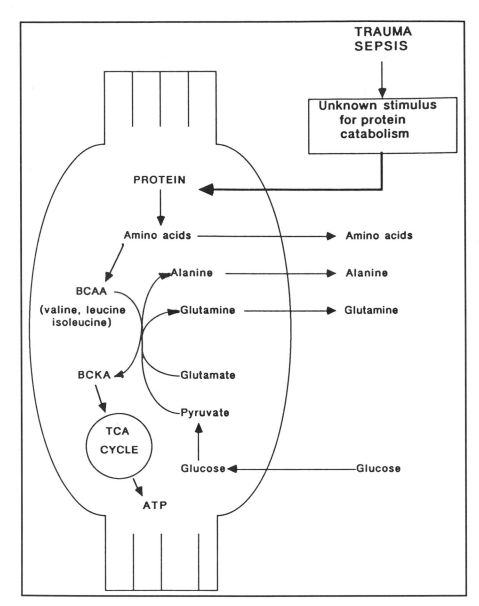

FIGURE 7–9. Skeletal muscle proteolysis. Breakdown of skeletal muscle protein leads to increases in amino acid levels. Amino acids are transaminated with glutamate or pyruvate to form alanine and glutamine, which are formed in quantities much greater than their normal content in muscle. The muscle preferentially uses branched-chain amino acids (BCAA) for energy through transamination with the formation of branched-chain ketoacids (BCKA), which can enter the TCA cycle for energy production.

muscle proteolysis. Proteolysis inducing factor (possibly a breakdown product of IL-1) has been implicated as a mechanism for the initiation of septic proteolysis. Administration of IL-1 in vitro has been demonstrated to increase amino acid release from skeletal muscle. Others have failed to reproduce these findings. Systemic administration of IL-1 and prostaglandin E_2 (PGE$_2$) to dogs has failed to induce proteolysis. Hepatic macrophages (Kupffer cells) have clearly been demonstrated to induce inhibitions of total hepatocyte protein synthesis when the two cells are cultured together in the presence of endotoxin. A combination of cytokines has been demonstrated to reproducibly inhibit total hepatocyte protein synthesis in vitro. Acute-phase protein synthesis has also recently been demonstrated to be under the control of macrophage products. Macrophage-derived IL-6 can reproduce nearly the entire spectrum of augmented acute-phase protein synthesis and depression in albumin synthesis.

Hormonal regulation of protein synthesis has also been noted. Counterregualtory hormones are elevated after injury and sepsis and have been proposed as the cause of accelerated proteolysis. Glucagon promotes gluconeogenesis, amino acid uptake, ureagenesis, and protein catabolism. Cortisol enhances extrahepatic protein catabolism and promotes hepatic utilization of mobilized amino acids for gluconeogenesis, glycogenolysis, and acute-phase protein synthesis. Mixtures of these hormones in concentrations similar to those seen in sepsis have failed to elicit marked elevations in urinary nitrogen excretion. Others have demonstrated modest increases in urinary nitrogen loss when levels of cortisol, epinephrine, and glucagon were administered to normal volunteers in concentration similar to those found in injured patients. Failure to reproduce the septic response of increases in nitrogen loss with hormonal infusion suggests that other factors, perhaps products of activated macrophages, are involved. It would seem logical to propose that the same factors that increase muscle catabolism may be linked to those factors facilitating hepatic acute-phase protein and glucose synthesis, including enhanced hepatic deamination, amino acid oxidation, and urea synthesis.

The implications of this accelerated protein catabolism can be appreciated by the effects that result from it. Marked skeletal muscle wasting occurs, leading to depressed intercostal and diaphragmatic function that culminates in retained secretion, atelectasis, and pneumonia. Protein depletion is associated with immunosuppression and the development of septic complications and nosocomial infection. Altered amino acid metabolism with progressive hepatic failure and decreased clearance of aromatic amino acids

(AAAs) may be associated with the development of encephalopathy and the synthesis of false neurotransmitters that may contribute to the hyperdynamic septic state. In late sepsis, octopamine, an abnormal by-product of tyrosine metabolism, is elevated to concentrations seen in hepatic failure. Elevated octopamine levels may represent diversion of tyrosine away from dopamine and catecholamine synthesis. Octopamine has very little vasoconstrictive effect and may lead to competitive inhibition of the vasoconstrictive effects of catecholamine, resulting in vasodilatation and decreased total peripheral resistance.

A critical concept in understanding alterations in protein metabolism in injury and sepsis is the role of interorgan amino acid cycling. The most significant of these cycles are the skeletal muscle–liver (Fig. 7–10) and muscle-gut (Fig. 7–11) interactions.

The negative nitrogen balance of sepsis is largely due to the breakdown of muscle protein as reflected

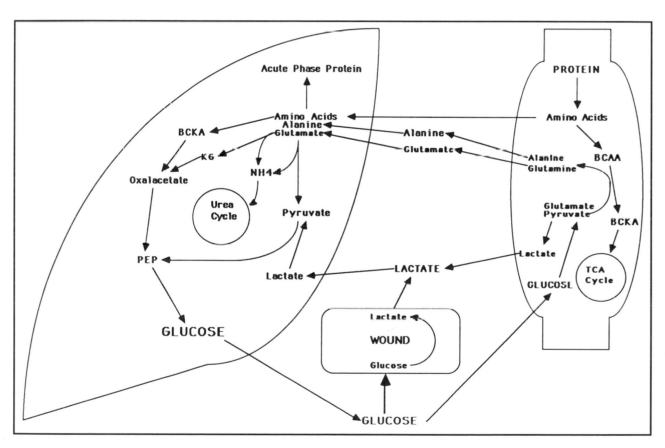

FIGURE 7–10. Substrate cycling between the wound, liver, and skeletal muscle. Skeletal muscle proteolysis leads to increased amino acid release and uptake by the liver. The amino acids taken up by the liver are used for protein synthesis or gluconeogenesis. The new glucose formed by the liver is used by the muscle and wound and lactate is produced. Lactate returns to the liver for new glucose synthesis. Carbon skeletons from the muscle are used for new glucose synthesis by the liver. The continued need for glucose by the wound probably drives gluconeogenesis. BCAA, branched-chain amino acids; BCKA, branched-chain ketoacids, KG, α-ketoglutarate; NH_4, ammonium; PEP, phosphoenolpyruvate.

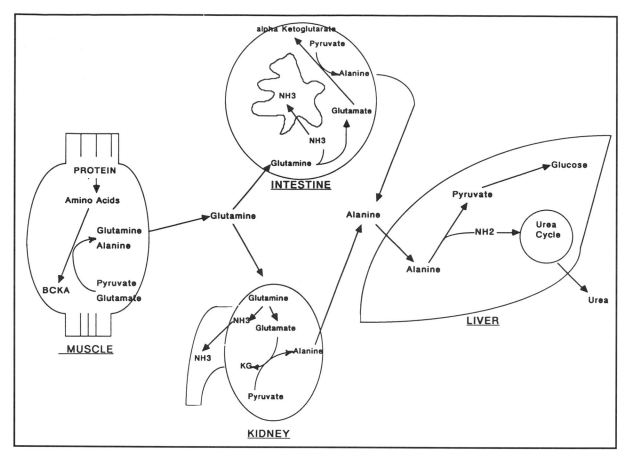

FIGURE 7–11. Glutamine metabolism. Glutamine is generated by skeletal muscle from glutamate by transamination. Glutamine is taken up by the intestine and kidney, where deamination and ammonia elimination occur. The glutamate formed is transaminated with pyruvate to form alanin, which goes to the liver for gluconeogenesis, and α-ketoglutarate (KG), which can be used for energy production by the muscle or kidney. NH_2, amine; NH_3, ammonia.

in increases in 3-methylhistidine excretion in the urine.[6] It appears that larger amounts of urinary nitrogen are lost in septic as opposed to nonseptic trauma. During sepsis, skeletal muscle amino acid release may be three to five times the normal rate (Fig. 7–11). The large UUN loss reflects increased amino acid delivery to the liver with subsequent deamination and increased nitrogen elimination by the urea cycle (Fig. 7–4). Figure 7–10 demonstrates the proposed shuttling of skeletal muscle amino acids to the liver, where they are used for protein synthesis and gluconeogenesis. Muscle amino acids may be released directly into the blood if they cannot be metabolized by muscle. If they are able to be metabolized by muscle, they usually undergo transamination reactions with pyruvate and α-ketoglutarate or glutamate to form alanine, glutamate, or glutamine. These amino acids then enter the circulation and are extracted by the liver, where they undergo deamination with the reformation of pyruvate, α-ketoglutarate or glutamate, and ammonia, then is metabolized as urea. The α-ketoacids

(pyruvate and α-ketoglutarate) can be used by the liver for the synthesis of new glucose, in oxidation by the liver for energy generation to fuel gluconeogenesis, or in ketone synthesis. The new glucose generated re-enters the circulation and travels to wounded or infected tissues where inflammatory cells that are obligate glucose users are present. This facilitates wound repair and clearance of infection by providing the optimal environment for leukocyte function.

The gut is normally thought of as a bystander in the metabolic response. There is evidence, however, that the gut may play an active role in the response to stress through the metabolism of glutamine (Fig. 7–11). Glutamine contains two nitrogen moieties and is an important source or energy for rapidly dividing cells, such as the intestinal mucosa and lymphocytes. Glutamine is an abundant amino acid in the serum and within cells and acts as a major nitrogen carrier from the skeletal muscle to the viscera. It is present in myocytes in concentrations exceeding its normal content in skeletal muscle protein, suggesting net synthesis by the myocyte. In muscle, glutamine is synthesized from glutamate. The branched-chain amino acids (BCAAs) appear to serve as the major nitrogen donor to form glutamine from glutamate. Glutamine is extracted by the liver, kidneys, and intestine (Fig. 7–11). In the kidney, glutamine is deaminated with the formation of glutamate and ammonia, which is excreted in the urine. The carbon skeleton can be used for renal gluconeogenesis or energy production in the Krebs cycle. The glutamate produced from the deamination of glutamine can be transaminated with pyruvate to form alanine, which can be transported to the liver for gluconeogenesis. The gut extracts 20 to 30 per cent of circulaitng glutamine in each pass. In the gut, glutamine is deaminated to form ammonia, which can be excreted in the gut, and glutamate, which can be converted to α-ketoglutarate and enter the TCA cycle. As in the kidney, alanine can be formed and shuttled to the liver. Glutamine may be particularly important for the support of intestinal mucosal integrity. Low concentrations of glutamine have been correlated with intestinal dysfunction and may impair the gut mucosal barrier, facilitating bacterial translocation.

After injury or sepsis, energy production becomes increasingly protein dependent. As sepsis progresses to organ failure, there is a failure to utilize amino acids by the liver and their plasma levels rise, possibly reflecting hepatic failure. The skeletal muscle amino acid release reflects the net effect of muscle proteolysis and synthesis. Amino acids not metabolized by muscle (proline, phenylalanine, tyrosine, and methionine) reach increased levels in the plasma. Alanine and glutamine are released in the plasma in amounts exceeding their normal content in skeletal muscle protein. This reflects muscle transamination to shuttle carbon skeletons to the liver and gut for glucose synthesis, energy production, and protein synthesis as well as to allow oxidation of the amino acid residues. Amino acid transamination has been discussed under normal metabolism. If hepatic insufficiency develops, amino acid clearance is altered and the plasma amino acid profile is changes. Specifically, AAA clearance is impaired and the serum levels of AAAs rise. Branched-chain amino acid clearance is maintained by the liver even in late sepsis. The leucine (BCAA)–tyrosine (AAA) clearance ratio has been used as an index of hepatic function in sepsis, with falling ratios as sepsis and hepatic insufficiency progress.

Lipid Metabolism

The metabolism of lipids and appropriate lipid administration in sepsis and stress is controversial. Authors have advocated both low and high rates of lipid infusion to attempt to minimize protein catabolism and act as an energy substrate.

Fatty acids and ketone bodies can normally act as an energy source for most tissues and as such may substitute for glucose. Fatty acids are mobilized from depots of adipose tissue in response to elevated levels of catecholamines, cortisol, and glucagon in the presence of depressed insulin levels (Fig. 7–8). Elevations in these counterregulatory hormones signal a depressed energy charge in the cells with the need to generate new substrates for energy generation through lypolysis or glycogenolysis. Free fatty acids are transported in the circulation bound to albumin and then enter the cells. In the cytosol, the fatty acids are complexed to CoA to form fatty acyl-CoA. The fatty acyl-CoA is shuttled to the mitochondria via a carnitine-dependent mechanism (Fig. 7–6). Lipid oxidation and ATP formation occur in the mitochondria, and lipogenesis occurs in the cytosol. As more lipid enters the mitochondria for oxidation, TCA cycle intermediates, particularly citrate, increase in concentration. Citrate accumulation results in inhibition of phosphofructokinase, a key enzyme controlling glycolysis. The citrate is ultimately converted to malonyl-CoA. In the cytosol, elevated levels of malonyl-CoA inhibit the carnitine-dependent mechanism responsible for entry of fatty acids into the mitochondria. The inhibition of entry of fatty acids prevents their oxidation and favors the reesterification of fatty acids to triglycerides and storage. In the liver, elevated fatty acid levels also favor the synthesis of ketone bodies for export to other tissues for energy generation. Ketone bodies are utilized by many tissues at times when glucose availablity is diminished.

Starvation results in enhanced fatty acid mobilization and ketone synthesis as insulin levels fall and levels of glucagon rise. In ketotic states, malonyl-CoA levels fall as TCA cycle intermediate levels decrease. As fatty acids are converted to ketones, less fat enters the TCA cycle as acetyl-CoA and less malonyl-CoA is formed, allowing continued mitochondrial entry of fatty acids and thereby allowing fatty acids to be used for ketone synthesis. The depression in TCA cycle intermediates occurs primarily in the liver. In muscle and other tissues, TCA cycle intermediates are not siphoned off for the synthesis of new glucose. Therefore, TCA cycle intermediates fail to fall as drastically, allowing continued entry of acetyl-CoA for energy generation.

Lipid metabolism is altered in stress and sepsis. Endogenous lipids appear to act as a major fuel source in the septic traumatized patient. Marked elevations in triglycerides and increases turnover rates for FFAs have been noted, although FFA levels may be normal. The elevated FFA and glycerol production is thought to result from increased lipolysis due to elevated levels of catecholamine and cortisol and a marked elevation in the glucagon-insulin ratio. The FFAs are used either for oxidation, ketone formation, or resynthesis of triglycerides.

Ketone synthesis by isolated liver preparations

from septic liver cells is depressed compared with that of normal cells. Plasma ketones concentrations in sepsis are lower than expected given the hormonal environment (Fig. 7–6). This may represent an inhibition of carnitine acyltransferase (CAT), which is competitively inhibited by malonyl-CoA. Inhibition of the entry of fatty acids into the mitochondria will result in depressed ketone production. Insulin concentrations are normal or mildly elevated in sepsis and may stimulate malonyl-CoA formation, thereby inhibiting ketogenesis (Fig. 7–6). Impairment in triglyceride clearance may exist because of depression in lipoprotein lipase activity in the muscle and fat of septic animals.

Despite enhanced lipolysis, FFA levels are normal and triglycerides are markedly elevated. Intracellular fatty acyl-CoA levels are elevated with enhanced production of ketone bodies (acetoacetate and β-hydroxybutyrate) but not as high as expected. Plasma ketones do not increase proportionally to muscle needs in sepsis. The high glucagon levels seen in stressed states inhibits acetyl-CoA carboxylase, the enzyme responsible for initiating ketone synthesis, thereby inhibiting ketone synthesis. Therefore, skeletal muscle increasingly relies on other fuel for energy. Elevations in fatty acyl-CoA levels have several important implications in the metabolic response to sepsis. Long-chain fatty acids have been noted to inhibit pyruvate dehydrogenase (PDH), a key regulatory enzyme in intermediary metabolism because it controls the rate at which pyruvate is converted to acetyl-CoA (Fig. 7–12). As fatty acyl-CoA levels rise, acetyl-CoA production from pyruvate falls. Pyruvate is then inhibited from entering the TCA cycle. This results in an accumulation of pyruvate and favors the generation of glucose by gluconeogenesis as well as lactic acid production. Thereby, glucose production by the liver is increased for export to glucose-dependent tissues by the inhibition of PDH. Increased fatty acyl-CoA levels should therefore enhance mitochondrial fat oxidation (fatty acids bypass PDH and directly enter the mitochondria, where they are converted to acetyl-CoA for oxidation), enhance glucose synthesis by increasing substrate (pyruvate) availability for gluconeogenesis, and impair glucose oxidation via the TCA cycle.

With the augmented plasma levels of triglycerides in sepsis, FFAs enter the cells and are converted to fatty acyl-CoA, which enters the mitochondria for oxidation via the carnitine shuttle. If fatty acid entry into the mitochondria is great, TCA cycle intermediates (citrate) increase in concentration. Citrate can leave the mitochondria, where it inhibits phosphofructokinase, thereby inhibiting glycolysis and enhancing gluconeogenesis. In addition, citrate is converted to malonyl-CoA, which inhibits the carnitine-dependent entry of fatty acids into the mitochondria favoring the synthesis of lipids.

Clinically, appropriate administration of lipids in nutritional support of the septic, traumatized pa-

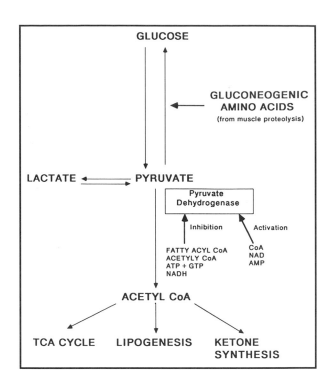

FIGURE 7–12. Pyruvate dehydrogenase (PDH). PDH occupies a key position in intermediary metabolism. Increased activity results in the generation of acetyl-CoA for entry into the TCA cycle, lipogenesis, or ketone synthesis. Inhibition of PDH leads to the accumulation of lactate, pyruvate, and gluconeogenic amino acids, favoring the synthesis of new glucose through gluconeogenesis. Septic inhibition of PDH leads to enhanced hepatic gluconeogenesis and depressed oxidation of substrates by peripheral tissues. GTP, guanosine triphosphate.

tient is still unfolding. At a given level of caloric support, the respiratory quotient (RQ), which is defined as the ratio of carbon dioxide produced to oxygen consumed, is lower in septic than nonseptic patients, suggesting that lipid oxidation may be the favored fuel over carbohydrate. A RQ of 1.0 is consistent with energy production from glucose and a RQ of 0.7 is consistent with fat oxidation. A RQ of 0.85 represents mixed oxidation of fat and carbohydrate. The lower RQ in the septic patient (0.7 to 0.75) is consistent with impaired glucose oxidation and increased gluconeogenesis related to PDH inhibition and with greater reliance on lipid as an energy source.

These findings appear to fit a pattern when considered in the setting of sepsis. Most septic patients initially are starving. They have an absolute requirement for glucose, primarily from their brain and leukocytes in the inflammatory focus, that can only briefly be met by the use of glycogen. This glucose requirement cannot be met by lipids because of the inability of acetyl-CoA resulting from fatty acid breakdown to be converted to pyruvate and subsequently to glucose via the gluconeogenic pathway.

Only about 10 per cent of the carbon in triglycerides in the form of glycerol can be converted to gluconeogenic precursors. Therefore protein, principally from skeletal muscles, is degraded and the amino acids formed are shuttled to the liver, either in the their native form or, after transamination, in the form of alanine or glutamine. Unhindered entry of the amino acid carbon skeletons (after deamination) into the TCA cycles in the liver would decrease the ability of the liver to generate glucose. Basically, if these amino acids entered the TCA cycle they would be unavailable as precursors for gluconeogenesis. Triglyceride mobilization from adipose tissues is dramatically increased. Increased tissue uptake of triglycerides results in increased intracellular levels of fatty acids. These fatty acids perform three functions. First, they can be oxidized by the β oxidation pathway in the mitochondria to generate ATP, some of which is used in gluconeogenesis, which is an energy-requiring process. Second, ketone bodies are formed in the liver for export to peripheral tissues. Third, the long-chain fatty acids may inhibit PDH. This inhibition of PDH will inhibit entry of pyruvate into the TCA cycle, favoring gluconeogenesis from the accumulating pyruvate and preventing the loss of gluconeogenic precursors to the TCA cycle at a time when they are needed for the synthesis of new glucose. Therefore, fatty acids can provide an energy source for the synthesis of glucose (and other cellular synthetic processes) and at the same time inhibit the entry of gluceoneogenic precursors into the TCA cycle. The elevated circulating lipid concentrations may also explain the fatty liver that is often associated with sepsis. At high intracellular fatty acid concentrations, further entry of fatty acids into the mitochondria may be inhibited by elevated malohyl-CoA levels, favoring fat synthesis and accumulation in the liver.

Carbohydrate Metabolism

Hyperglycemia is characteristically observed in the early and late periods after stress. Early hyperglycemia in the ebb phase of injury is related to an inhibition in pancreatic insulin release caused by elevated levels of hormones that diminish insulin release, particularly epinephrine and decreased pancreatic blood flow. This early hyperglycemia increases blood osmolarity and favors restoration of circulating blood volume. Glucose entry into cells (principally skeletal muscle and fat) and its postentry metabolism is facilitated by insulin. Once in the cytosol, glucose enters the glycolytic pathway with the generation of pyruvate and subsequently acetyl-CoA. Glycogen may also be synthesized from glucose under these conditions. The acetyl-CoA may then enter the TCA cycle for energy generation or may be used in fat synthesis after conversion to malonyl-CoA. In the normal postprandial state, plasma insulin levels are elevated and glucose entry into cells is favored, with glucose oxidation and glycogen synthesis. During periods of starvation, insulin levels drop and allow mobilization of fat, glycogen, and ketone bodies for energy production.

Hyperglycemia is commonly encountered in sepsis. This occurs in spite of the fact that glucose uptake by peripheral tissues is increased and glucose utilization and alanine and pyruvate production are increased. The increased glucose uptake by skeletal muscle is not accompanied by glucose oxidation. Failure of complete glucose oxidation leads to increases in the levels of compounds such as pyruvate and alanine, which are shuttled to the liver and used as substrates for gluconeogenesis. Glucose is an essential substrate for a number of tissues, including the central and peripheral nervous systems, leukocytes, erythrocytes, bone marrow, renal medulla, and the healing wound. In general, these tissues are not dependent on insulin for glucose utilization. Approximately 80 per cent of the increased glucose uptake in wounds is secondary to the inflammatory cells. The reticuloendothelial system can provide a major site of glucose utilization during sepsis.

What is the explanation for this hyperglycemia? It is clear that the major reasons for this hyperglycemia are a marked increase in glucose production and an inhibition of its use peripherally. It is thought that glucose oxidation revolves around the activity of PDH (Fig. 7–12). PDH activity seems to decline in sepsis, thereby diminishing the rate at which pyruvate can be converted to acetyl-CoA and enter the TCA cycle. This inhibition results in increased concentrations of pyruvate, alanine, and lactate, which can be shuttled to the liver to form substrate for gluconeogenesis. Because of the rise in these substrates, which is believed to be caused by PDH inhibition, new glucose production in the liver is promoted.

Pyruvate dehydrogenase is an extremely complex enzyme system and the PDH existing in different tissues varies in activity at different times in the course of sepsis. The PDH in skeletal muscle is more sensitive to inhibition in sepsis than is the PDH present in the liver. In fact, skeletal muscle PDH activity declines almost independently of sepsis (maximum inhibition occurs with minimal sepsis). It has been suggested that an early response to sepsis is a decline in skeletal muscle PDH activity. This leads to decreased substrate (glucose) oxidation with release of pyruvate and lactate from muscle. These substrates are shuttled back to the liver for gluconeogenesis. The inhibition of PDH activity is thought likely to be one of the major causes of the hyperglycemia of sepsis (diabetes of sepsis) and trauma and the cause of the relative "insulin resistance." This insulin resistance is a postreceptor phenomenon occurring mainly in skeletal muscle at the level of PDH. Thus, despite the ability of glucose to enter the cell under the influence of insulin (receptor level), glucose oxidation is incomplete and hepatic gluconeogenesis is augmented through increased substrate delivery. The sensitivity of the cellular insulin receptor seems normal in sepsis. The decline in PDH activity may also contribute to the elevated plasma lactate levels and the lactic acidosis in sepsis, which occur in spite of markedly increased blood flow and perfusion.

Other factors contribute to the hyperglycemia of sepsis. Elevated plasma catecholamine levels favor gluconeogenesis. Cortisol antagonizes peripheral glucose use. Plasma glucagon concentrations are markedly increased while insulin levels change little. The glucagon-insulin ratio is high and reversed compared to the postabsorptive state. The elevated glucagon concentration may be resonsible for much of the increased hepatic glucose production seen in sepsis.

Therefore, sepsis seems to be characterized by continued fatty acid oxidation even in the presence of high glucose concentration. The hyperglycemia in some respects correlates with outcome. Septic patients whose glucose tolerance tests were near normal had a 10 per cent mortality rate, whereas an abnormal test carried a 60 per cent mortality rate.

Several important points can be made based on the discussion of substrate metabolism in sepsis:

1. Peripheral glucose demands are great and glucose synthesis is favored more than oxidation.
2. Protein breakdown provides the substrates for hepatic gluconeogenesis as pyruvate, lactate, and amino acids.
3. Enhanced amino acid release from muscle provides substrates for new protein synthesis in the liver, bone marrow, and wound.
4. Fat is increasingly relied upon as the major source of energy production for the cell. Increased fat use provides an energy source that normally would be derived from glucose. Therefore fat substitutes to some degree for glucose and allows glucose to be oxidized by tissues with obligate glucose needs.

ROLE OF CYTOKINES IN INTERMEDIARY METABOLISM

Within the last several years, investigators have proposed that the macrophage and monocyte cell line may be responsible for a number of the sequelae of infection and the development of septic syndromes (Fig. 7–13). Macrophages and their products have also been demonstrated to have effects on carbohydrate, fat, and protein metabolism. Bacterial products, such as endotoxin and other mediators produced in sites of septic or nonseptic inflammation, have been proposed to lead to systemic macrophage activation with synthesis and secretion of

monokines with endocrine, paracrine, and autocrine effects. Endotoxin has been demonstrated to experimentally produce sepsis and death when injected intravenously. The deleterious effects of endotoxin appear to be mediated by macrophage products. Endotoxin is capable of rapidly activating circulating monocytes and tissue macrophages (splenic macrophages, hepatic Kupffer cells, pulmonary alveolar macrophages, and renal mesangial cells) to produce a multitude of monokines, including IL-1, IL-6, TNF, and platelet activating factor (PAF). Infusion of TNF and PAF can reproduce a clinical and metabolic picture of sepsis.

Several mediators synthesized by macrophages are known to alter protein syntheses. Protein synthesis from cultured hepatocytes has been shown to significantly decreased by factors released from Kupffer cells or peritoneal macrophages activated by endotoxin, muramyl dipeptide, gentamicin-killed *Escherichia coli*, and phorbol mystrate. It has been postulated that the failure of protein synthesis by the liver may be a correlate of the hepatic failure of sepsis and organ failure.

While total protein synthesis may decline, the synthesis of specific acute-phase proteins by the hepatocyte may be markedly enhanced in sepsis and trauma. There appears to be a reprioritization of hepatic protein synthesis away from the carrier proteins (albumin and transferin) in favor of the synthesis of acute-phase proteins, including fibrinogen, α_2-macroglobulin, α-antitrypsin, ceruloplasmin, and C-reactive protein. One mechanism regulating the synthesis of these protein appears to involve interactions between Kupffer cells and hepatocytes. Kupffer cells (hepatic macrophages) in the liver are activated in some manner, perhaps involving endotoxin. This may occur through factors reaching the liver by way of the systemic or portal circulation. Translocation of bacteria across an abnormal gut mucosal barrier has been proposed as an activating mechanism for Kupffer cells. This would not seem to be a likely mechanism immediately following injury because the gut's permeability is not changed early enough to account for increases in translocation. This would imply that other mediators, perhaps released from the wound or other inflammatory foci, can be systemically released to activate the Kupffer cell to stimulate hepatocyte acute-phase protein production. The wound might also release factors that directly stimulate hepatocyte protein synthesis.

Activated Kupffer cells and other macrophages and monocytes release IL-6, which is the cytokine that controls the vast majority of hepatocyte acute-phase protein synthesis. Prior suggestions that IL-1 or TNF controls acute-phase protein synthesis are incorrect, although IL-1 and TNF may modulate the effect of IL-6 on the hepatocyte.

The hormonal environment is also important in hepatocyte protein synthesis. Cortisol is required for

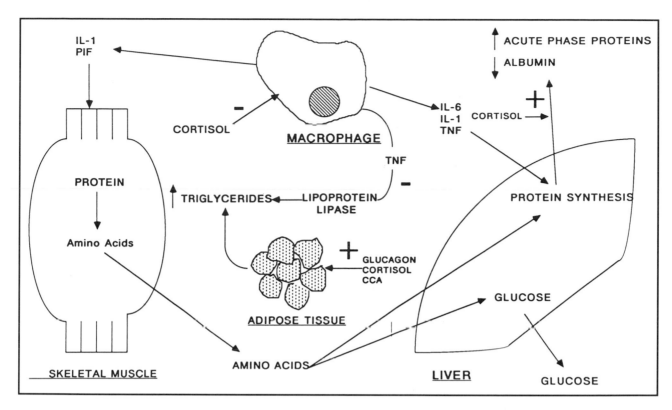

FIGURE 7–13. Role of cytokines in intermediary metabolism. Macrophages synthesize many peptides, termed *monokines,* that can affect protein, fat, and carbohydrate metabolism. Macrophage IL-6 production is primarily responsible for acute-phase protein synthesis. TNF inhibits lipoprotein lipase and leads to hypertriglyceridemia. IL-1 or its breakdown product, proteolysis inducing factor (PIF), may enhance skeletal muscle proteolysis. Increased amino acid release provides new substrate for gluconeogenesis and promotes glucose synthesis and hyperglycemia. CCA, catecholamines.

acute-phase protein synthesis to occur in the presence of IL-6. If corticosteroids are absent, hepatocytes are unresponsive to the effects of IL-6 and no increases in acute-phase protein synthesis occur. Elevations in corticosteroid levels in the postinjury period may thereby facilitate hepatic acute-phase protein synthesis. While TNF and IL-1 are not the major regulators of acute-phase protein synthesis, they may lead to depressions of albumin synthesis and elevations in the synthesis of the third component of complement by the liver. Because albumin synthesis accounts for such a large percentage of hepatic protein synthesis, diminution of albumin synthesis may make amino acids more available for acute-phase protein synthesis. This shunting represents a reprioritization of protein synthesis by the liver.

Lipid metabolism is significantly affected by stress and sepsis. Hypertriglyceridemia is commonly seen. Several mechanisms may account for this. Elevations in catecholamines, cortisol, and glucagon all favor lipolysis from adipose tissues with resulting hypertriglyceridemia. Monokines, particularly TNF, may also play a role.

Endotoxin administered to experimental animals led to marked hypertriglyceridemia. This elevation in triglycerides was not seen in endotoxin-resistant animals. Endotoxin induces TNF release by macrophages, which may partially account for the hypertriglyceridemia. Tumor necrosis factor may have these effects through inhibition of lipoprotein lipase, an enzyme present on the capillary cell membrane responsible for clearing triglycerides. Interestingly, pretreatment of animals with glucocorticoids totally suppressed the effects of endotoxin and TNF release.

Interleukin-1 is a peptide released by macrophages that also has effects on intermediary metabolism. Specifically, IL-1 can accelerate the basal metabolic rate and increase oxygen consumption. In addition, it stimulates the liver to increase amino acid, zinc, and iron uptake from the plasma pool. Interestingly, it also stimulates the pancreatic islets to release insulin and glucagon. Interleukin-1 has also been proposed as a factor responsible for the increases in skeletal muscle proteolysis seen in stressed and septic states.

Tumor necrosis factor, IL-1, and IL-6 seem to be

the cytokines with the most significant effects on intermediary metabolism. One can look at the pattern of hormonal and monokine release and propose a scheme to explain some of the metabolic changes occurring in trauma and sepsis. The macrophage seems to be a cell central to the understanding of this concept. In the traumatized patient, inflammation occurs in wounded tissue. Neutrophils and monocytes accumulate in the wound or inflammatory focus. The wound probably releases monokines that act as hormones. These products could lead to systemic monocyte and macrophage activation and affect parenchymal cells in intimate contact with the macrophages. Liver, lung, and splenic macrophages could be activated by endotoxin in sepsis to produce the effects already described.

Interleukin-1 or an IL-1 breakdown product (proteolysis inducing factor) may augment skeletal muscle proteolysis and amino acid release. These amino acids travel to the liver or gut, where extraction is enhanced by elevated glucagon and cortisol levels. Glucagon release from the pancreatic islets is also enhanced by IL-1. Hepatic macrophages are activated to release IL-6, IL-1, and TNF, which together control and augment hepatocyte acute-phase protein synthesis.

Tumor necrosis factor release leads to hypertriglyceridemia through inhibition of lipoprotein lipase. The triglycerides may be used for energy generation at a time when glucose oxidation is inhibited.

Carbohydrate metabolism may be affected in several ways. Interleukin-1 augments insulin and glucagon release from the pancreas and may stimulate skeletal muscle proteolysis, thereby providing substrate to the liver for gluconeogenesis.

INTEGRATED VIEW OF METABOLISM IN SEPSIS AND TRAUMA

Metabolic pathways and substrate utilization in the normal states are complicated and may become even more so in sepsis and trauma. Certain concepts may be clearer when a clinical case is examined. Consider a multiple trauma patient 10 days after injury who suffered a femur fracture and hepatic trauma requiring laparotomy. This patient has not eaten and has developed fever, tachycardia, and mild hypotension—a picture consistent with sepsis. Given this scenario, how can carbohydrate, lipid, and protein metabolism be integrated into an understandable and sensible picture of metabolic alterations?

At this point, the patient has two problems, starvation and a markedly increased metabolic demand. The metabolic problem in septic patients appears to be mitochondrial in origin and is a progressive inability to fully oxidize substrates for energy generation with a fall in oxygen consumption as sepsis worsens. The glucose requirements of this patient's

fracture, wounds, and inflammatory cells are great at a time when his glycogen stores are depleted. He has normal fat reserves, but fatty acids (except glycerol) cannot be utilized for glucose synthesis. Therefore, protein from skeletal muscle is catabolized with the release of amino acids (particularly alanine), lactate, and pyruvate. The stimulus for muscle proteolysis is not conclusively known, but may be a macrophage cytokine, produced by activated macrophages in injured or infected tissues. Some of these amino acids (primarily BCAAs) are used for muscle energy generation after transamination to form alanine or glutamine. The pyruvate, lactate, and alanine from muscle are also used by the liver for the synthesis of new proteins in the liver (acute-phase proteins), the wound (to promote wound healing), and the bone marrow (for the production of hematopoietic cells) or as substrates for gluconeogenesis by the liver. Thus the muscle protein degradation provides substrate for needed gluconeogenesis and acute-phase protein synthesis. The increased hepatic synthesis of glucose as well as the inhibition of peripheral glucose oxidation accounts for the often-observed hyperglycemia of sepsis.

Fatty acid mobilization from adipose tissue is promoted by elevations in glucagon, catecholamines, cortisol, and TNF and is manifest clinically as hypertriglyceridemia. Fatty acids thus produced are oxidized for ATP production to fuel the syntheses of new glucose and protein, both of which are energy-requiring processes. The elevated fatty acid levels may inhibit PDH, leading to a reduced flow of substrates into the TCA cycle and favoring the accumulation of substrates, such as pyruvate, that are essential for gluconeogenesis. The hormonal response with elevated plasma catecholamine, glucagon, and cortisol concentrations facilitates new glucose formation from amino acids. In addition, epinephrine inhibits insulin release from the pancreatic islets. Cortisol and glucagon both stimulate amino acid mobilization from muscle and hepatic amino acid uptake and new protein and glucose synthesis. The net result is recruitment of muscle amino acids to the liver for hepatic protein synthesis and to the wound and bone marrow for new protein synthesis. In addition, the greatly increased hepatic glucose production provides substrate for tissues with obligate glucose needs, principally the inflammatory cells in wounds or areas of inflammation or infection. The monokine response is not well defined. Macrophages are a cell line that accumulates in injured tissues rapidly after 24 hours, and they are capable of secreting approximately 100 different products. It would seem logical that monokines produced from macrophages in areas of tissue inflammation and injury and infection might escape the confines of the wound and have systemic effects, acting in essence as a hormone. This is the so-called wound factor inducing the systemic changes. The monokines that seem to have the greatest metabolic effects are IL-1, TNF, and IL-6, all of which are mainly macrophage products.

Interleukin-1 or a breakdown product known as proteolysis inducing factor stimulates skeletal muscle proteolysis in vitro with amino acid release as is seen in sepsis. Interleukin-1 also produces increased synthesis of some hepatic proteins. Albumin synthesis is markedly diminished while complement 3 synthesis is augmented. This would allow amino acids that are normally used for albumin synthesis to be used for protein synthesis in other more urgent areas.

Tumor necrosis factor also plays several roles. In the liver, it also inhibits albumin synthesis and augments synthesis of the third component of complement while having little effect on other acute-phase proteins. It also has a significant effect on lipid metabolism through inhibition of lipoprotein lipase and may in part be responsible for the hypertriglyceridemia of infection.

Interleukin-6 has recently been noted to play a significant role in hepatic acute-phase protein synthesis. It is able to elicit the entire spectrum of acute-phase protein synthesis as well as the inhibition of albumin synthesis by the liver. Interleukin-1 has been shown to stimulate release of IL-6 by macrophages and enhance acute-phase protein synthesis in that manner.

As sepsis worsens and organ failure develops, liver function often deteriorates. As liver dysfunction develops, amino acid clearance, particularly of the AAAs, is impaired and the plasma concentration of these amino acids rises. This may have several deleterious effects. The AAAs may be metabolized to false neurotransmitters, which may compete with catecholamines for binding sites on sympathetic nerve terminals. This may lead to vasodilatation and hypotension. The rapidity with which septic vasodilatation develops suggests that some other rapidly acting mechanism must be involved. Recent evidence suggests that nitric oxide, formed from the metabolism of L-arginine, may play a role in sepsis. Nitric oxide is an extremely potent vasodilator produced by many cell lines. Local production of nitric oxide by endothelial cells in sepsis leads to vascular smooth muscle relaxation and vasodilatation. The full role of nitric oxide in septic vasodilatation remains to be investigated.

The elevated plasma AAA concentration probably also predisposes to the development of septic encephalopathy. Aromatic amino acids compete with other neutral amino acids (mainly BCAAs) for transport across the blood-brain barrier through a common neutral amino acid carrier. Once in the brain, the AAAs are postulated to be converted to an abnormal neurotransmitter and an encephalopathic picture may be produced. As hepatic function worsens, acute-phase protein synthesis and the synthesis of coagulation proteins is depressed. Glucose metabolism is maintained until very late in the course of hepatic failure, when hypoglycemia replaces hyperglycemia as the abnormality of glucose metabolism. The development of fatty liver is a common finding. The etiology may relate to abnormalities of hepatic lipid metabolism and oxidation. As fat is used for energy generation, intramitochondrial citrate and then cytosolic malonyl-CoA levels are elevated. The elevated malonyl-CoA levels inhibit the carnitine shuttle mechanism, preventing fatty acids from entering the mitochondria for oxidation. This results in the accumulation of fatty acyl-CoA in the cytosol and favors lipogenesis and the development of a fatty liver. Depressions in intracellular carnitine concentrations in sepsis may also play a role in the failure of fat to enter the mitochondria.

Much of the above synopsis of the changes in metabolism that occurs in sepsis and trauma is controversial and much more investigation is needed to confirm some of the hypotheses presented here. This overview may provide a useful framework within which to think about the metabolic changes in sepsis and trauma as seen in the surgical patient. There is no doubt that as our understanding of septic metabolism improves, the scheme presented will be modified.

BIBLIOGRAPHY

1. Howard, R.J., and Simmons, R.L.: Surgical Infectious Disease. Norwalk, CT, Appleton and Lange, 1988.
2. Deitch, E.A.: Multiple Organ Failure: Pathophysiology and Basic Concepts of Therapy. New York, Thieme Medical Publishers, 1990.
3. Davis, J.M., and Shires, G.T.: Principles and Management of Surgical Infections. Philadelphia, J.B. Lippincott, 1991.
4. Davis, J.H., Drucker, W.R., Foster, R.J., Gamelli, R.L., Gann, D.S., Pruitt, B.A., and Sheldon, G.F.: Clinical Surgery. St. Louis, C.V. Mosby Co., 1987.
5. Siegel, J.H.: Trauma: Emergency Surgery and Critical Care. New York, Churchill Livingstone, 1987.
6. Stryer, L.: Biochemistry. New York, W.H. Freeman and Company, 1988.
7. Cahill, G.F. Jr.: Starvation in man. N. Engl. J. Med. 282:668, 1970.

8

SHOCK

ANDREW B. PEITZMAN

Shock is a clinical syndrome which results from tissue perfusion inadequate to maintain normal metabolic and nutritional activities. Although direct histotoxic factors probably play a role in the development of the syndrome, the common denominator in all forms of shock is low blood flow to vital organs. Even though inadequate oxygen delivery is a common feature of all shock, *primary* failure in substrate availability (hypoxia) or extraction (cyanide poisoning) is not included in the definition. In the clinical setting, one is confronted with a patient in shock, the origin of which may not be apparent. Since shock may progress rapidly to death, treatment is initiated empirically while the specific cause is sought.

The term "shock," therefore, essentially describes a generalized dysfunction of the normal cardiovascular homeostatic mechanisms. It is important to understand these circulatory mechanisms prior to discussing the treatment of shock. The major components of cardiovascular regulation fall into two categories: factors which are related primarily to cardiac pump functioning, circulating the blood volume, and vasomotor tone; and microcirculatory factors such as blood viscosity and aggregation of cellular components. The clinical syndrome of shock results from derangement of any one or a combination of these factors.

Shock can be classified into four types according to etiology: cardiogenic shock, vasogenic shock, neurogenic shock, and hypovolemic shock. Cardiogenic shock is circulatory failure caused by failure of the heart to serve as an adequate pump (e.g., acute myocardial infarction, arrhythmias, or myocardial depression). Vasogenic shock is circulating failure associated with a decrease in peripheral arterial resistance and increase in central venous capacitance: septic shock and shock associated with multiple organ failure are prototypes. Neurogenic shock is a central failure of the autonomic nervous system to maintain peripheral vascular resistance, as in spinal anesthesia or a high spinal cord section. Hypovolemic shock is circulatory failure due to a loss of intravascular volume—whole blood, plasma, extracellular fluid, or a combination of these. These categories of shock differ in certain of their pathophysiologic features and in many components of their treatment. Each will be reviewed, with the goal of this chapter being to define common principles.

NORMAL RESPONSE TO HYPOVOLEMIA

The circulatory system has an effective homeostatic mechanism to control blood flow to various tissues. These interrelated controls include autonomic control of cardiac contractility and peripheral vascular tone; hormonal adrenergic and nonadrenergic response to stress and volume depletion, which supplement this autonomic control; and local mechanisms that are organ specific and regulate local blood flow. Loss of circulating blood volume is the primary disturbance in hypovolemic shock from which low cardiac output and hypotension result. The body's response to acute hypovolemia (e.g., hemorrhage) involves both neural and humoral components. The nervous system is the first to respond to either pain or acute loss of circulating volume. Sympathetically mediated vasoconstrictor responses occur almost immediately after hypovolemia or pain. Thus the capacitance of the circulation is reduced.

The receptor for this control system resides primarily in the baroreceptors that are located in the aortic arch and carotid sinus. These sensors respond within seconds to changes in blood pressure caused by adjusting sympathetic tone to maintain blood pressure. Changes in blood pressure slow the rate of normal afferent impulses from arterial baroreceptors. These impulses are integrated primarily in the medulla and normally inhibit vasoconstriction. Thus, slowing incoming impulses increases sympathetic discharge. Concurrently, the vagal center is inhibited and parasympathetic tone is reduced.

The brain and heart are favored organs in hypovolemic shock, and flow to these organs will be maintained until all compensation fails. Hypoperfusion of the brain will induce additional and even more potent activation of the vasomotor center of the medulla, increasing sympathetic output even further. This intense outpouring of sympathetic signals becomes active when arterial blood pressure falls to 50 torr, and is maximal when arterial pressure is less than 15 torr.

This sympathetic response to acute hypovolemia has several major cardiovascular effects: arterioles constrict in most areas and thus increase total peripheral resistance; capacitance veins increase their mural tone, decreasing their capitance so that venous return is augmented. Cardiac performance—both rate and strength of contraction—increase. The arterial vasoconstriction is not homogeneous, so that a marked redistribution of blood flow occurs. Although sympathetic stimulation causes constriction of cardiac and cerebral vessels, metabolic vasoregulation in these organs prevents excessive local vasoconstriction, so that perfusion is maintained. Blood flow to other (so called nonvital) tissues thus decreases significantly. Renal blood flow may be re-

duced to as little as 5 to 10 per cent of normal, and flow to the splanchnic circulation, skin, and skeletal muscle decrease greatly.

The venous circulation normally holds two thirds of the circulating blood volume. The venous system is thus the capacitance side of the circulation. In response to hypovolemia, these capacitance vessels contract, thus preserving cardiac filling pressure by returning more blood to the heart as total circulating blood volume decreases. The constrictor responses which are seen in early hypovolemic shock are mediated by norepinephrine and epinephrine, which are released into the circulation from the adrenal medulla, as well as being mediated by direct effects of local sympathetic activity on vascular walls.

HORMONAL RESPONSES TO ACUTE HYPOVOLEMIA

Hypovolemia also initiates complex endocrine responses. The plasma levels of adrenocorticotro-

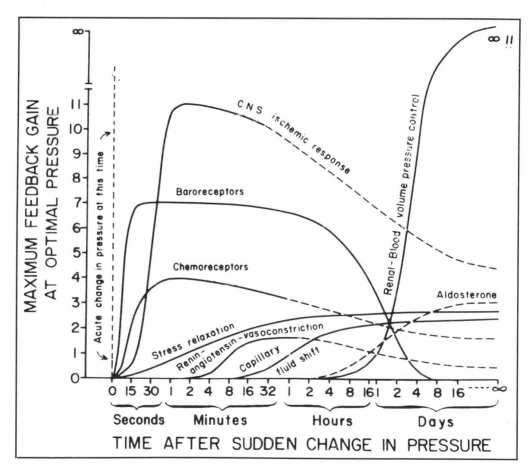

FIGURE 8–1. Potency of various arterial pressure control mechanisms at different time intervals after the onset of a disturbance to the arterial pressure. Note especially the infinite gain of the renal-body fluid pressure control mechanism that occurs after a few days' time. (Reprinted from Guyton, A.C.: Textbook of Medical Physiology. Philadelphia, W.B. Saunders Co., Fig. 21–3, p. 248, 1981.)

pin (ACTH), glucagon, growth hormone, and cortisol increase (Fig. 8–1). The renin-angiotensin-aldosterone axis is stimulated in hypovolemia via hypoperfusion of the juxtaglomerular apparatus. A release of antidiuretic hormone (ADH) also results from hypovolemia. The ADH increases resorption of water in the distal tubule of the kidney and also causes splanchnic vasoconstriction. Growth hormone promotes gluconeogenesis and lipolysis. Glucagon similarly opposes the effects of insulin by promoting gluconeogenesis, lipolysis, and glycogenolysis. In addition, glucagon has a direct inotropic effect on the heart. Hyperglycemia results from the gluconeogenesis, glycogenolysis, and inhibition of insulin release by epinephrine and norepinephrine. There also may be tissue resistance to insulin in shock states. Glucagon, growth hormone, catacholamines, and tissue insulin resistance combine to increase blood sugar and osmolarity. This tends to shift fluid from the cells and interstitium to the vascular bed and thus to help maintain circulating volume.

The sympathetic cardiovascular mechanisms in response to hypovolemic shock are augmented by ADH, glucagon, and angiotensin. Hormonal effects also limit further loss of fluid or salt via the kidneys. The end result of these hormonal responses is to maximize cardiovascular function, conserve salt and water for circulating volume, and provide nutrients and oxygen to the heart and brain.

MICROCIRCULATORY CHANGES

An equally important, but less often discussed mechanism in the maintenance of central blood volume is autoregulation of local blood flow. Autoregulation may be defined as regulation of microvascular tone by local tissue mediators in response to pressure change or tissue metabolic needs. Such microcirculatory changes are a major component of the homeostatic response to shock. When microcirculatory autoregulation fails, shock may become irreversible.

In hemorrhagic shock, sympathetic response causes vasoconstriction of the larger arterioles (90 to 150 microns). There is also early dilation of 20- to 50-micron arterioles. This constriction of larger arterioles and the dilation of smaller arterioles will lower hydrostatic pressure within the capillary. This causes a flux of fluid from the extracellular space into the capillary. This represents a prime mechanism of capillary refilling and hemodilution which is observed three to four hours after hemorrhage. Furthermore, hyperglycemia increases the osmotic gradient, which promotes the influx of fluid from the interstitium into the capillary by altering the forces in the Starling equation. The end result of these mechanisms is partial restoration of intervascular

volume by a relative diminution in interstitial volume.

These compensatory mechanisms allow a patient to sustain a substantial blood loss and recover without treatment. In this compensated state of hypovolemia, tissue perfusion may be lower than normal, and anaerobic metabolism may be apparent as lactic acidosis. However, the microcirculation is not blocked irreversibly and is not so impaired that progressive tissue dysfunction occurs. Dysfunction at this time in hemorrhagic shock can be reversed by adequate intravascular volume replacement. If the volume loss continues or is inadequately treated, a vicious cycle may develop. Further depression of cardiac output will cause further tissue and microcirculatory changes; this will create negative feedback to the heart and cause further cardiac decompensation. This transition from simple hypovolemia to irreversible dysfunction (progressive shock to irreversible shock) is often subtle (Fig. 8–2). In fact, many authors do not believe in the entity of irreversible shock and redefine it as simply inadequate resuscitation.

PROGRESSIVE SHOCK

Several studies have suggested that progressive cardiac deterioration occurs with hemorrhagic shock. Certainly as venous return diminishes, cardiac output falls. Current studies suggest that myocardial dysfunction may be a late component of progressive hemorrhagic shock. It probably does not occur early during hypovolemia. This late myocardial dysfunction may be due to sympathetic exhaustion or possibly to a myocardial depressant factor which is released from ischemic tissue.

FLUID SHIFTS AND CELLULAR CHANGES

As previously discussed, a decrease in capillary perfusion pressure promotes movement of interstitial fluid into the capillary, increasing intravascular volume at the expense of extracellular (ECF) volume. Studies using a triple isotope technique demonstrated that this ECF volume deficit persisted when shed blood or shed blood plus plasma was used as volume resuscitation of these animals. Furthermore, returning shed blood alone to the animals resulted in an 80 per cent mortality in 24 hours, returning shed blood plus plasma resulted in a 70 per cent mortality in 24 hours. These studies demonstrated that infusion of shed blood plus lactated Ringer's solution, an ECF mimic, returned the mea-

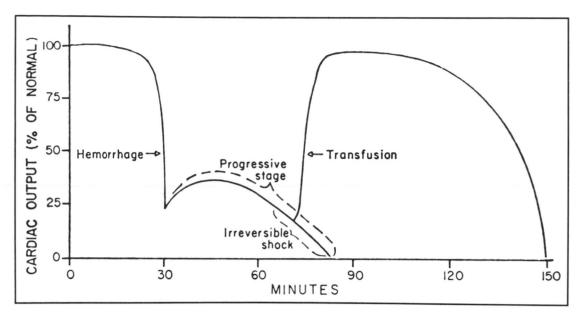

FIGURE 8–2. Failure of transfusion to prevent death in irreversible shock. (Reprinted from Guyton, A.C.: Textbook of Medical Physiology. Philadelphia, W. B. Saunders Co, Fig. 28–6, p. 338, 1981.)

sured ECF volume to near control levels, and more importantly, decreased the mortality to 30 per cent in 24 hours.

The marked reduction in ECF volume seen in prolonged hemorrhagic shock is greater than could be accounted for by vascular refilling from the interstitial space. Further studies by these investigators demonstrated that cellular dysfunction also occurred in prolonged hemorrhagic shock with loss of cell membrane integrity, cell membrane dysfunction, and uptake of interstitial fluid by the injured cells.

These early studies were performed primarily on skeletal muscle. Skeletal muscle transmembrane potential difference decreased in prolonged hemorrhage shock. This depolarization of the cell membrane was proportional to both the degree and duration of the shock states. Intracellular chloride, sodium, and water content increased in prolonged shock, associated with this membrane depolarization. With this cellular swelling, there was marked decrease in the extracellular water volume in hemorrhagic shock. Since skeletal muscle mass makes up 50 per cent of body mass, skeletal muscle cells may be a principle site of cellular fluid and electrolyte sequestration after prolonged hemorrhagic shock.

Electron microscopic studies have further corroborated these findings. Ultrastructural changes in the skeletal muscle of animals subjected to hemorrhagic shock have demonstrated intracellular edema, spreading of the myofibrils, and distortion of the mitochondria. Several studies have demonstrated dysfunction of the mitochondria in prolonged shock. This is important because the mitochondria are the primary source of adenosine triphosphate (ATP) production. The impairment of the mitochondria results in profound loss of cellular and membrane functions.

In shock states, there is also lysosomal disruption with resultant release of the lysosomal enzymes, and intracellular autodigestion occurs. With adequate resuscitation, these cellular and cell membrane changes can be reversed. After volume resuscitation using shed blood and lactated Ringer's solution in baboons, not only was the hypotension reversed and muscle PD returned to baseline, but the abnormalities in electrolyte and water shifts also returned to normal.

These studies suggest that a defect in sodium potassium active transport mechanism across the cell membrane occurs in hemorrhagic shock. Because this active transport is dependent upon ATP, intracellular energy depletion has been suggested as a cause of this persistent cellular dysfunction. However, several studies have shown that cell membrane dysfunction can occur despite normal ATP stores in both the skeletal muscle and red blood cells.

Widespread membrane dysfunction occurs in hemorrhagic shock resulting in fluid shifts and tissue dysfunction. However, the specific mechanism responsible for this dysfunction remains unclear. To date, the only treatment that has been documented to consistently reverse these changes is adequate volume resuscitation, including nonsanguinous solutions. Appropriate volume resuscitation is mandatory to abort microcirculatory damage that may result in severe tissue dysfunction and irreversible shock.

IRREVERSIBLE SHOCK

If hypotension if profound enough and of significant duration, what was previously adequate volume resuscitation may fail to reverse the process. This condition has been referred to as irreversible shock. As stated, some authors believe this represents inadequate resuscitation. The clinical distinction between progressive and irreversible shock is often difficult to make, except in retrospect. This irreversible state of hemorrhagic shock can be created in a dog model by the spontaneous uptake of a set volume, usually 30 to 50 per cent, of previously shed blood after an interval of shock. Despite the return of all shed blood at this point and further fluid resuscitation, survival is usually not possible after this "uptake phase." The precise mechanisms responsible for this irreversibility are ill defined. It is likely that activation of mediators create a vicious cycle which cannot be broken with simple volume resuscitation.

Loss of autoregulation of the microcirculation may be a major factor in the irreversibility of the shock state. Even brief experimental hemorrhage may be followed by a nearly complete cessation of blood flow in the skeletal muscle for 5 to 20 minutes. The major site of this constriction is in the larger arterioles. This maldistribution of blood flow occurs in the muscle bed during the resuscitation phase, which may contribute to the progression of the shock state, despite restoration of the blood pressure. Sludging of red blood cells, white blood cells, or platelets and increasing microvascular viscosity also may play a major role in the progression of hemorrhagic shock. Flow may stop in some microvessels and continue in adjacent bypass capillaries. Thus, measurable resistance to tissue flow may not change even when local tissue perfusion has been severely decreased. This problem complicates any gross analysis of pressure or flow during shock.

This reuptake of blood that marks the onset of irreversibility probably occurs as a loss of vasomotor tone. This loss of vasomotor tone is due to either local mediator release or to vasomotor paralysis. Flint et al. found that in prolonged shock, arteriolar dilation occurred despite continued hypovolemia and high circulatory levels of norepinephrine. Large arterioles showed a persistent constriction response and a lower sensitivity to norepinephrine. Smaller arterioles and venules dilated in irreversible shock. Worsening tissue acidosis further exacerbates these mechanisms. This vasomotor failure or loss of autoregulation may be due to resistance to catacholamines and is probably a major determinant in irreversible shock.

THE TREATMENT OF HEMORRHAGIC SHOCK

Resuscitation of the patient in shock consists of simultaneous evaluation and treatment. A delay in appropriate volume resuscitation may result in irreversible organ injury. Resuscitation that is initiated prior to a definitive diagnosis must be directed toward those elements which are common to most forms of shock. During this initial treatment, the patient is evaluated primarily for signs of adequate tissue perfusion, which is best judged by assessing organ system function.

First (as with any critically ill patient) a patent airway and adequate ventilation must be assured. Therapy is then directed toward rapid restoration of the blood volume. The primary treatment of hemorrhagic shock is replacement of the blood and cessation of the hemorrhage.

In the treatment of hypotension, the patient is often placed in Trendelenburg position to increase central blood volume and arterial pressure. However, in a recent study, the Trendelenburg position was found to have no consistent effect on venous return or systemic vascular resistance in normal or hypotensive patients. Furthermore, cerebral perfusion and pulmonary function may be compromised in patients who are placed in the Trendelenburg position.

Military antishock trousers (MAST) are widely used in the emergency treatment of hemorrhagic shock. Until recently, it was thought that MAST suits had their effect by causing an autotransfusion of blood from the periphery to the central circulation by squeezing blood out of the capacitance vessels in the legs and abdomen. However, recent data demonstrates that the autotransfusion is a minimal effect, maximally 4 ml/kg. The primary mechanism for the maintenance of blood pressure with use of the MAST suit is by increasing total peripheral resistance and by decreasing the size of the perfused vascular bed. Utilization of the MAST suit may also have utility in the early treatment of patients with a neurogenic shock, septic shock, or hypotension secondary to vasodilators. Pulmonary edema is an absolute contraindication to use of the MAST suit. Proper application and removal of the garment are critical for its safe utilization. A recent prospective study has demonstrated no difference in outcome in trauma patients where MAST suits have been used.

If the patient presents in hemorrhagic shock, volume may be replaced with packed red blood cells or whole blood. How much blood or crystalloid solution is necessary for adequate volume replacement in the bleeding patient? Restoring normal tissue perfusion rather than simply having evidence of normal blood pressure must be the goal. Due to the previously described homeostatic mechanisms, the systemic arterial blood pressure may be maintained within the normal range until the patient has lost 20 to 30 per cent of his blood volume. Thus, if only blood pressure is used as an index of volume resuscitation, inadequate amounts of fluid would be given. More appropriate indicators of adequate fluid resuscitation include adequate urine output, 0.5 to 1 ml/kg/hr, normal heart rate, adequate capillary refill, and normal sensorium, in addition to restoration of blood pressure. Restoration and maintenance of normal organ system function must be the goal and endpoint in volume resuscitation of these patients. Central filling pressures are often used as endpoints in volume resuscitation. Several studies suggest that central filling pressures, specifically the central venous pressure, and the pulmonary artery wedge pressure (PAWP) may not reliably predict cardiac preload in critically ill patients. In addition, a recent study also demonstrated that direct measurements of left atrial pressure may not reliably indicate optimal fluid resuscitation in hemorrhagic shock. When sufficient volume was given to baboons in resuscitation of hemorrhagic shock so that left atrial pressure returned to baseline, large volumes of crystalloid solution were required and resulted in an equally large urinary output. In the group which was resuscitated to maintain a normal blood pressure, outcome was the same, and fluid requirements were significantly less. Furthermore, fluid resuscitation to either a normal blood pressure or normal central filling pressure did not result in normal blood volume, even 18 hours after hemorrhagic shock. Thus, the compensatory mechanisms that protect the organisms during shock are still in effect 18 hours after seemingly appropriate resuscitation.

Certain metabolic functional parameters have also been monitored as possible endpoints of volume resuscitation. These include oxygen consumption, tissue pH, transmembrane potential difference, or transcutaneous oxygen content. Our most reliable indices in the resuscitation of the patient remain adequate urine output, adequate capillary filling, normal sensorium, and restoration of the heart rate.

The hematocrit does not indicate volume status of the patient. It merely indicates the balance between the red blood cells and nonsanguinous fluid in the vascular space. If the hematocrit is too high, there will be a resultant increase in viscosity, and resistance to flow increase appears. A hematocrit lower than approximately 30 per cent decreased oxygen delivery substantially and may increase patient mortality. An optimal hematocrit is probably between 30 to 45 per cent. As previously discussed, infusion of asanguinous fluid in addition to packed red blood cells is necessary for maximal survival after hemorrhagic shock. The basic choice of nonsanguinous fluid is between a crystalloid solution or a colloidal solution. Considerable controversy has resulted from this debate.

The premise for giving albumin-containing solutions, or crystalloids, is based on the Starling equation. This presumes that with the increase in plasma colloid osmotic pressure (PCOP) caused by the albumin infusion, fluid will be drawn from the interstitium, and in particular, from the lung. In theory, this would make resuscitation more effective, with fewer pulmonary complications. Two assumptions are applied here. First, that the alveolar capillary membrane is impermeable to albumin. Second, that there is no mechanism for rapid removal of albumin from the lung interstitium. However, the albumin content in lung interstitium may be 70 per cent of that in plasma. Thus, changes in PCOP cause minimal change in the osmotic gradient between the lung interstitium and the capillaries. Furthermore, under normal conditions, the pulmonary lymphatics very effectively clear albumin and fluid from the lung interstitium. Interstitial fluid accumulation must increase approximately tenfold before this lymphatic system is overwhelmed with resultant pulmonary edema. Hypoproteinemia alone does not lead to pulmonary edema. Although it is likely that low PCOP may contribute to an increase in lung water when hydrostatic pressures are high, the use of colloid for acute volume replacement or resuscitation has never been shown in a prospective study to be beneficial. The substantial increase in the cost of colloid solutions as opposed to crystalloid solutions argues against their routine use.

Both the volume of fluid infused and the rate of fluid administration are important in the restoration of normal circulation. An excess of either fluid will be detrimental. Furthermore, several studies have demonstrated that successful resuscitation can be achieved with red blood cells plus salt solution, or red blood cells plus colloid solution.

SEPTIC SHOCK

Septic shock is usually due to gram-negative or gram-positive bacteria, but may be caused by viruses, fungi, parasites, or rickettsiae. Patients are often presumed to have sepsis on the basis of their clinical presentation, when no organisms have actually been cultured from the bloodstream. Despite major advances in hemodynamic monitoring and antibiotic therapy, the mortality from septic shock remains as high as 50 to 70 per cent. When patients die from sepsis, this rarely occurs during the clinical episode of septic shock. The majority of the patients die later after a lingering course, after they have progressed to the syndrome of multiple system organ failure. Similarly, sepsis is the most frequent cause of adult respiratory distress syndrome.

Patients in septic shock usually present with hypotension, high cardiac output, warm skin, mental status changes, and respiratory alkalosis. It is a hyperdynamic state that is the usual presentation for patients with septic shock. However, approximately 25 per cent of septic patients will present with hypodynamic sepsis with low cardiac output and signs of vasoconstriction. These patients may be indistinguishable from patients in hypovolemic shock. These two presentations probably represent a continuum of the same disease, with the major variables being peripheral vascular tone, myocardial function, and intravascular volume. This hypodynamic state is often seen late in the course, when therapy has failed and vascular tone is lost.

Predisposing Factors to Sepsis

Many variables predispose to the development of sepsis. The incidence of sepsis is increased by the use of broad spectrum antibiotics, better early care of multiple-trauma patients, the extremes of age, and the wider use of immunosuppression. Patients receiving chemotherapy and those with acquired immunodeficiency syndrome are also at increased risk of developing sepsis. In addition to the increased susceptibility of infection in these patients, diagnosis and successful treatment are also much more difficult in the immunosuppressed population.

The Reticuloendothelial System

A common theme in the development of sepsis is decreased effectiveness of the immune system in these patients. The reticuloendothelial system (RES) is a major component of the immune system. The RES functions to clear the blood of platelet aggregates, bacteria, and other particulate matter. There is impairment of these functions after burns, trauma, or sepsis. Furthermore, the RES can be overwhelmed in previously healthy patients by physiological stress. In patients with uremia, liver disease, diabetes mellitus, starvation, or malignancies, there is also impairment of RES function. Patients with diabetes mellitus have abnormal neutrophil chemotaxis and impaired lymphocyte function. The microvascular disease in patients with diabetes may also impede the response of components of the immune system. Cirrhosis has been documented to be a very poor prognostic factor if associated with infection. In patients suffering multiple trauma or burns, abnormal neutrophil chemotaxis has been demonstrated, as well as depressed lymphocyte responsiveness.

Early studies suggested that anergy or failure of delayed hypersensitivity reaction, was a marker for host resistance in surgical patients. However, more recent studies have demonstrated that the anergy usually follows—rather than precedes—the onset of major complications. Current data suggest that responsiveness to skin antigens after injury is not useful in a quantitative or predictive sense.

The spleen functions as a filter within the reticuloendothelial system. It clears bacteria and debris from the circulation. Previous splenectomy increases the risk of overwhelming septicemia. This risk varies, dependent upon the initial indication for splenectomy. The risk of overwhelming postsplenectomy infection is highest in those patients who have had splenectomy performed for hematologic disease, as opposed to those patients who have a splenectomy following trauma.

Nutritional factors may be important in the development of sepsis, in particular by their interaction with the immune system. As stated, there does seem to be an association between malnutrition and anergy. There may be an abnormality of neutrophil chemotaxis in malnourished patients. Abnormal immune function has been documented to occur with deficiencies of copper, iron, phosphate, zinc, vitamin A, vitamin B_{12} or pyridoxine.

Pathophysiology of Septic Shock

The initiating event in hemorrhagic shock is decreased blood volume, which results in diminished cardiac output and decreased organ perfusion. In hemorrhagic shock, a loss of vasoregulation is a late phenomenon, following prolonged inadequate tissue perfusion. By contrast, in septic shock this loss of autoregulation and tissue dysfunction occur early and persist, despite supranormal cardiac output. Possible mechanisms for this observed impairment in vasoregulation include arteriovenous shunting, direct histotoxicity, or vasoderegulation. Unlike a hypovolemic shock state, histotoxicity implies that septic shock may represent as primary cellular disease from which circulatory dysfunction results. Vasoderegulation implies that the high cardiac output and organ dysfunction may be due to dysfunction of vasoregulatory mechanisms such that blood flow is not preferentially directed to metabolically active tissues.

The pathophysiology of progression from hyperdynamic to hypodynamic sepsis is not well defined. The factors which probably play a role in this transition include relative hypovolemia, right ventricular dysfunction secondary to an early increase in pulmonary vascular resistance, impaired left ventricular function, or resistance of the cardiovascular system to catacholamines. In all forms of shock, the heart will eventually fail. In primate models of bacterial sepsis, ventricular dysfunction is significant within three to six hours. Furthermore, there are some data for the existence of a humoral myocardial depressant factor causing a fall in cardiac output late in sepsis.

An abnormally low arteriovenous oxygen difference is the hallmark of hyperdynamic sepsis. Early studies indicated that this may be due to arteriovenous shunting. However, current data does not support this as being the mechanism for the low arteriovenous oxygen difference. These studies suggest that the microcirculatory dysfunction in septic shock appears to be due to either hypoperfusion of some capillary beds with a high output maintained by excessive perfusion of those capillaries that remain open, or to a generalized inability of the peripheral tissues to metabolize oxygen.

Adequate volume loading seems to be important in the development of hyperdynamic septic shock. Furthermore, prognosis for survival is higher in patients with hyperdynamic septic shock as opposed to those with hypodynamic septic shock. In addition, a study demonstrated that septic dogs quickly decompensated when minimal blood loss was superimposed on the sepsis. These data suggest that adequate venous return with adequate volume loading is mandatory in the development of the hyperdynamic state.

The primary circulatory derangement in sepsis seems to be loss of vasoregulation. As a result of this, areas of hypoperfusion and hyperperfusion may exist simultaneously within the same microvascular beds. The establishment of the hypoperfusion of the microvascular beds seems to be a fundamental component of septic shock. The survival of the patient or development of multiple-system organ failure will depend upon persistence of the microcirculatory failure, local toxic factors, enhanced aggregation of the cellular components within the microvascular tree, cell toxicity, and inadequate resuscitation. Prompt reversal of this microcirculatory process is critical in the mangement of sepsis.

Organ Failure and Sepsis

As stated, patients rarely die during the acute hypotensive episode of sepsis. Rather, these patients will progress to develop multiple-system organ failure. This is discussed further in a later chapter. Late mortality from septic shock can be predicted based on the number of organ systems involved in multiple-system organ failure. The organs which are most commonly involved include the lung, kidney, liver, gut, coagulation system, and the heart.

Treatment

Mortality from septic shock remains 50 to 70 per cent. Early drainage of the septic focus is important. For patients with infections that are amenable to surgical drainage, the mortality is approximately 50 per cent. On the other hand, only 23 per cent of patients with infections which are not amenable to surgical drainage will survive the sepsis. This in part represents different patient populations. Thus, when we initially assess a patient in septic shock, an aggressive search for the source is important in treatment and outcome.

Fluid Resuscitation

The patient should be aggressively volume resuscitated during an apparent episode of septic shock. Endpoints in this should be restoration of normal sensorium, blood pressure, and urine output. Urine output is not as reliable a monitor of fluid therapy as during the treatment of hemorrhagic shock, since renal tubular impairment may increase urine volume with impaired concentrating function. The pulmonary wedge pressure is often used to assess the adequacy of intravascular volume in critically ill patients. However, in septic patients, multiple studies have demonstrated that the PAWP is actually a poor indicator of left ventricular preload. Proposed mechanisms for this are changes in left ventricular diastolic compliance or an altered relationship between PAWP and left atrial pressure in septic patients.

Whether the patient presents in hyperdynamic or hypodynamic sepsis, prompt volume resuscitation is central to the management of these patients. Several authors have proposed that oxygen consumption (VO_2) may be the critical endpoint in volume resuscitation of critically ill patients. An abnormally low oxygen consumption is a poor prognostic sign; however, it is usually preceded by hemodynamic deterioration. The progression from low to increasing values for oxygen consumption may indicate appropriate resuscitation in the treatment of septic shock. However, the single measurement of a supernormal oxygen consumption at one point during sepsis does not correlate with survival.

Drug Therapy

Volume expansion alone improves the hemodynamic status of most septic patients. In those patients that do not respond to aggressive volume resuscitation, it may be necessary to add an inotropic agent. Either dopamine or dobutamine is effective in supporting the circulatory system in septic shock. Administration of vasoconstrictive agents, in an attempt to enhance perfusion of the heart and brain, may be necessary in acute hypotension, but it compromises overall systemic perfusion. Thus, the use of inotropes should not be necessary unless the patient remains resistant to volume infusion.

A source for the bacteremia is often documented when a patient develops an episode of clinical sepsis. Organism-specific antibiotic treatment is associated with better outcome than inappropriate antibiotic therapy for the septic patient. Blood cultures should be a routine part of the work-up of the septic patient. Urine and sputum should also be obtained for culture. Careful clinical examination, looking for localizing signs of infections, is imperative. Draining a septic focus increases a patient's chance of surviving a septic episode. Since antibiotic therapy must be initiated prior to return of the bacterial culture, this therapy should be based on the probable source of the sepsis. Mortality has been shown to double when inappropriate antibiotics are used in the treatment of septic patients.

Adjuvant Therapy in Sepsis

Minimal improvement in mortality from sepsis is a testimony to our inadequate understanding of the processes that lead to sepsis and multisystem organ failure. Even with appropriate antibiotics, drainage of an abscess, and appropriate fluid resuscitation, the mortality rate is still substantial for septic shock.

Several studies have addressed the use of steroids in the treatment of septic shock. This was first supported by Schumer's study in 1976. However, several recent studies have demonstrated that steroids have no long-term benefit in the treatment of septic shock and may actually increase mortality. Thus, at the present time, steroids are not recommended as routine treatment of septic shock.

Experimentally, blockage of prostaglandin synthesis for treatment of septic shock with the opiate antagonist naloxone, held promise. However, the clinical studies have produced conflicting results.

Depression of the RES by fibronectin deficiency has been documented during sepsis. Several studies have suggested that treatment with fibronectin infusion will not only reverse the fibronectin deficiency, but also will improve metabolic and pulmonary function in these patients. Similar to the other adjunctive measures that we have mentioned, the clinical data is still controversial in this regard. Recent evidence suggests there may be benefit from a monoclonal antibody to endotoxin. However, at the present time there are no proven adjuvant therapies in the treatment of septic shock, beyond the administration of fluids, antibiotics, and early drainage of the infection.

CARDIOGENIC SHOCK

Cardiogenic shock may be defined as any condition in which the heart cannot pump sufficiently to maintain the body's needs. This may represent inadequate cardiac output due to acute myocardial infarction, chronic myocardial dysfunction, arrhythmia, or from an obstructive cause. The obstructive causes of cardiogenic shock include acute pulmonary embolism or cardiac tamponade. These differ from the other causes in that the myocardium is normal. We will discuss cardiogenic shock due to acute myocardial dysfunction.

Cardiogenic shock may be defined as shock secondary to acute myocardial dysfunction with a systolic blood pressure less than 90 torr, or 30 torr less than baseline in a hypertensive patient; cold, clammy, cyanotic skin; urine flow less than 20 ml/hour; and altered mental status. The criteria for cardiogenic shock are not as well defined for chronic heart failure.

The mortality from cardiogenic shock due to acute myocardial infarction remains quite high, ranging from 80 to 100 per cent. Typical pharmacologic interventions may increase hemodynamics but have not modified the mortality. The intraaortic balloon pump or the left ventricular assist device may be used to stabilize the acutely unstable patient with cardiogenic shock.

In order to develop cardiogenic shock secondary to acute myocardial infarction, 35 to 40 per cent of the left ventricular myocardium must be infarcted. Cardiac compensatory mechanisms in the setting of decreased pump function include increased heart rate, increased sympathetic stimulation, increased preload, cardiac chamber dilatation, hypertrophy of the left ventricle, and increased compliance of the left ventricle. Ventricular hypertrophy and increased compliance generally require time to develop and are not really applicable in the setting of acute myocardial dysfunction. In the chronic state, they are important. This is represented by the typical Frank-Starling curve with the relationship between left ventricular volume for changes in pressure.

As in other forms of shock, a vicious cycle develops in cardiogenic shock. Due to impaired pump function and decreased cardiac output, compensatory mechanisms to increase peripheral vasoconstriction are activated in an attempt to maintain blood pressure. This stimulation of the sympathetic nervous system causes catecholamine release. This induces arterial vasoconstriction, increased heart rate, increased venous tone and venous return, and increased cardiac inotropy.

These mechanisms to maintain peripheral blood pressure will increase afterload and further impede cardiac performance. These vasoconstrictor mechanisms are then further stimulated, and the cycle continues. It should be noted that in treating a patient with an acute myocardial infarction, other diagnostic possibilities exist. These include ventricular septal rupture, acute mitral regurgitation secondary to papillary muscle rupture, right ventricular infarction, free ventricular wall rupture, left ventricular aneurysm, or hypovolemia.

As stated earlier, the mortality from acute cardiogenic shock still approximates 80 per cent. Clinical estimates of hemodynamic status in the setting of acute myocardial failure are often incorrect, and invasive monitoring is frequently indicated. The goal in the treatment of acute myocardial failure should be maintaining organ perfusion and cardiac viability by maximizing myocardial oxygen supply while minimizing myocardial oxygen demand. The major reason for doing this is the fact that the peri-infarction zone is a potentially salvageable area of the myocardium. With inappropriate treatment and increasing myocardial oxygen demand, the infarct may extend—and thus deleteriously effect the patient's outcome. Furthermore, optimal filling pressures are important in maximizing outcome in acute cardiogenic failure. Available data suggest that the optimal pulmonary wedge pressure should be from 15 to 20 torr.

NEUROGENIC SHOCK

The clinical presentation of neurogenic shock is different from that classically seen in hypovolemic shock. The blood pressure may be low, however the patient is often bradycardic, and has warm, dry, and even flushed skin. Hemodynamic measurements made during neurogenic shock reveal that the patient has a decreased cardiac output, but this is secondary to a decrease in resistance of the arteriolar vessels, as well as a decrease in venous tone. Thus, the patient is normovolemic, with tremendously increased reservoir capacity in both the arterial and venous side, thus decreasing venous return to the heart and acutely decreasing cardiac output.

The typical setting for neurogenic shock is after a spinal anesthetic or a spinal cord injury. As with other forms of shock, if the hypotension is not corrected, a reduction of blood flow to the viscera will result in organ failure. Shock due to a high spinal anesthesia can be treated effectively with a vasopressor such as ephedrine. Treatment of spinal shock may be more difficult when it is due to a spinal cord injury. These patients require extensive volume resuscitation and may require a vasopressor as well. In the management of these patients, our goal is to balance the volume expansion with the risk of vasopressor administration. Slight volume overexpansion is much less of a risk than excessive vasopressor use. At least temporarily, the MAST suit may support the peripheral vascular resistance with neurogenic shock.

This chapter has reviewed the basic pathophysiology of shock. The common denominator in all forms of shock is inadequate tissue perfusion to maintain normal organ function. The outcome after the onset of shock depends upon the severity of the shock, the duration of the shock, the underlying cause of the shock, preexisting diseases, and the reversibility of the shock. Prompt and effective treatment is essential to achieve maximal outcome.

BIBLIOGRAPHY

1. Calvin, J.E., Driedgen, A.A., Sibbald, W.J., et al.: Does the pulmonary capillary wedge pressure predict left ventricular preload in critically ill patients? *Crit. Care Med. 9:*437, 1981.
2. Carroll, G.C. and Synder, J.V.: Hyperdynamic severe intravascular sepsis depends on fluid administration in cynomolgus monkey. *Am. J. Physiol. 243:*R313, 1982.
3. Civetta, J.M.: A new look at the Starling equation. *Crit. Care Med. 7:*84, 1979.
4. Cunningham, J.N., Jr., Shires, G.T., and Wagner, Y.: Cellular transport defects in hemorrhagic shock. *Surgery 70:*215, 1971.
5. Drucker, W.R., Chadwick, C.D.J., and Gann, D.S.: Transcapillary refill in hemorrhage and shock. *Arch. Surg. 116:*1344, 1981.
6. Flint, L.M., Cryer, H.M., Simpson, C.J., et al: Microcirculatory norepinephrine constrictor response in hemorrhagic shock. *Surgery 96:*240, 1984.
7. Gann, D.S., and Amaral, J.F.: Endocrine and metabolic responses to injury. *In* Schwartz, S.I. (ed.): Principles of Surgery. New York, McGraw-Hill Book Co., 1989, pp. 1–69.
8. Guyton, A.C.: Textbook of Medical Physiology. Philadelphia, W.B. Saunders Co., 1981.
9. Kaufman, B.S., Rackow, E.C., and Falk, J.L.: The relationship between oxygen delivery and consumption during fluid resuscitation of hypovolemic and septic shock. *Chest 85:*336, 1984.
10. McNamara, J.J., Suehiro, G.T., Syehiro, A., et al: Resuscitation from hemorrhagic shock. *J. Trauma 23:*552, 1983.
11. Peitzman, A.B.: Principles of circulatory support and treatment of hemorrhagic shock. *In* Snyder, J.V. (ed.): Oxygen Transport in the Critically Ill. Chicago, Year Book Medical Publishers, 1987, pp. 407–418.
12. Peitzman, A.B., Corbett, W.A., Shires, G.T., III, et al.: Cellular function in liver and muscle during hemorrhagic shock in primates. *Surg. Gynecol. Obstet. 161:*419, 1985.
13. Shires, G.T., Cunningham, J.N., Baker, C.R.F., et al.: Alterations in cellular membrane function during hemorrhagic shock in primates. *Ann. Surg. 176:*288, 1972.
14. Shires, G.T., III, Peitzman, A.B., Albert, S.A., et al.: Response of extravascular lung water to intraoperative fluids. *Ann. Surg. 197:*515, 1983.
15. Shoemaker, W.C., and Hauser, C.J.: Critique of crystalloid versus colloid therapy in shock and shock lung. *Crit. Care Med. 7:*117, 1979.
16. Sibbald, W.J., Paterson, N.A.M., Holliday, R.L., et al.: The Trendelburg position: Hemodynamic effects in hypotensive and normotensive patients. *Crit. Care Med. 7:*218, 1979.
17. Thal, A.B., Robinson, R.G., Nagamire, T., et al: The critical relationship of intravascular blood volume and vascular capacitance in sepsis. *Surg. Gynecol. Obstet. 143:*17, 1976.

9

TUMOR BIOLOGY

MITCHELL C. POSNER

Normally the body's cellular ecosystem is in balance. Each cell type emerges from the germ cell and maintains its life cycle, its territory, and its population within limits. In cancer, these rules are broken as a cell type evolves that is capable of relentless proliferation, local invasion, and distant dissemination. The mechanisms underlying initiation, regulation, and progression of tumor growth and the host defenses against it are just beginning to be elucidated. Although surgery has been and remains today the principal method for the treatment of solid tumors, it often fails to control the disease; for this reason, adjuvants to surgical extirpation, including radiation, chemotherapy, and immunotherapy, are increasingly being evaluated in controlled clinical trials. This multimodality approach to the treatment of malignancy requires recognition by surgeons of the biologic nature of malignancy. Active laboratory investigation and technical progress in the fields of molecular and cellular biology, genetics, and immunotherapy have markedly advanced the current state of our knowledge concerning the origin and progression of cancer. It is therefore essential that all students of surgery understand the biologic principles of oncology.

CHARACTERISTICS OF THE MALIGNANT CELL

Cancers are classified by the cell type from which they arise (Table 9–1). About 90 per cent of cancers arise from epithelial cells, and most maintain some of the functions of the original differentiated cell type, e.g., melanomas make melanin; basal cell tumors make keratin. In fact, their close resemblance to non-transformed cells is a property that sometimes permits one to tailor the therapy to the tumor cell itself, as in the hormonal control of tumors arising from hormonally dependent tissues. In contrast, the cells of a tumor are most often heterogeneous, and this lack of uniformity sometimes accounts for the failure to control tumor progression and metastases. Understanding tumor origin and evolution may well determine future therapeutic directions.

The Origin of Tumors

Normal tissue development is a result of an ongoing process whereby descendants of a small population of rapidly proliferating cells undergo differentiation to a mature state. The cell of origin, or stem cell, not only has the capacity for rapid proliferation but also is able to renew itself. The stem cells appear to be regulated by one or several specific growth

TABLE 9–1. CANCER INCIDENCE AND CANCER DEATH IN THE UNITED STATES, 1989

CANCER TYPE	NEW CASES	DEATHS
Epithelial cancers (carcinoma)	851,900	402,650
Digestive organs	227,800	123,000
Reproductive organs	181,800	52,200
Respiratory system	171,600	147,100
Breast	142,900	43,300
Urinary organs	70,200	20,200
Oral cavity/pharynx	30,600	8650
Skin (melanoma)	27,000	8200
Hemopoietic/immune cancers		
Leukemias/lymphomas	79,100	65,500
Central nervous system/ eye cancers	16,900	11,300
Gliomas, neuroblastomas, etc.		
Bone, connective tissue cancers	7700	4300
Sarcomas		
All Other	54,400	38,250
TOTAL	1,010,000	522,000

Modified from Silverberg, B.S., and Lubera, S.A.: Cancer statistics, 1989. Cancer, *39:*3–20, 1989.

factors for which they have receptors. Neoplasia occurs when control of the processes of cell division and differentiation is altered or lost.

Evidence exists that cancers are unicellular (clonal) in origin, even though most tumors contain vessels, fibroblasts, and other normal supporting structures. For example, identical immunoglobulin markers have been shown to be present in all cells of each given B cell tumor, even though different B lymphocyte tumors bear a different immunoglobulin marker. Studies examining the X-linked enzyme, glucose 6 phosphate dehydrogenase (G6PD), demonstrate loss of heterozygous expression in tumor-bearing patients. The clonal origin of tumor cells means that neoplasms are generated from a single altered cell followed by expansion of that clone. The alternative hypothesis—that tumors have a multicellular origin and that a subpopulation of cells has a selection bias that confers a growth advantage over other cells—is much less likely.

Therefore, on a genetic level, most cancers are probably initiated by a change in the cellular DNA sequence of a single cell. The alternative hypothesis involves a modification in the pattern of gene expression, an epigenetic change, as the initiating event in the malignant process. Although epigenetic alteration frequently occurs during normal cellular differentiation and is a heritable process, it is unlikely to initiate carcinogenesis. For most tumors, carcinogenesis equals mutagenesis: chemical carcinogens tend to cause local changes in the nucleotide sequence, ionizing radiation causes chromosome breaks and translocation, and viruses insert foreign DNA into the genome.

There are five lines of evidence that genetic mutations cause cancer.

1. Agents that damage DNA are frequently carcinogenic, and most carcinogenic agents are mutagens.
2. There is increased incidence of cancer in patients with genetically determined deficiency in the enzymes necessary to repair DNA damage.
3. Inherited disorders associated with increased chromosomal aberrations predispose to some cancers.
4. Heritable human cancers have been identified.
5. The clonal origin of cancer indicates that tumors arise from a single altered cell.

Several models have been proposed to explain on a genetic level the transformation of a normal cell to a malignant cell. Studies suggest that the number of mutations required for malignant transformation of a normal cell is between five and seven. This multihit model would require a mutation frequency that is unrealistic for any carcinogen at a dose that is nonlethal. An alternative model is based on the stem or progenitor cell and its capacity for either self-renewal or differentiation to a mature cellular form. After a single mutation, stem cells are "sensitized," but still retain their ability to either differentiate or proliferate. If cell differentiation occurs before a second "hit" (mutagenic event), that cell is no longer a target for transformation and the mutation is lost. If, however, a second, third, fourth, etc. mutation occurs, self-renewal is enhanced, and differentiation is either aborted or abnormal. A third model does not involve mutation, but hypothesizes the differential expression of particular genes.

Regardless of the proposed mechanism, it is evident that any change in the genome (point mutations, deletions, insertions, translocation, or amplification) may predispose to the development of cancer. Although almost all cancers are initiated by mutations, defects in DNA repair can accelerate it. This is seen in several heritable genetic disorders. Xeroderma pigmentosum, Bloom's syndrome, Fanconi's anemia, and ataxia telangiectasia have well-described defects in DNA repair. Other evidence suggests that some mutant cells develop similar defects.

Cancer cells in general have a very unstable karyotype. As seen in the abnormal nuclear morphology that characterizes them. This instability is further manifested by a propensity for duplicated or translocated chromosomes in culture and gene amplification or deletion. This propensity suggests a defect in one or several genes governing cell division. The vulnerability of the cell division process and augmented mutability can be exploited in designing therapeutic regimens in cancer.

Alternatively, genetic changes can result in the cell acquiring a selective advantage. Gene amplifications in response to chemotherapy may induce the emergence of a multidrug resistance gene (mdrl). This gene codes for a cell membrane ATPase that serves as a lipophilic drug pump, excluding all such drugs from the cell. Other types of genes are also amplified in some cancers, providing the cell with a defense against therapeutic attack.

Mechanisms of Carcinogenesis. The relationship between chemicals and cancer has been recognized for over two centuries since John Hill described a correlation between nasal cancer and snuff in 1761 and Percival Pott (1775) recognized the high incidence of scrotal cancer in chimney sweeps. Chemical carcinogenesis appears to be a multistep process. The first step, *initiation,* involves exposure to the chemical that, in its reactive form, interacts with DNA and irreversibly alters the molecular target. Initiators are all mutagenic. The second step in chemical carcinogenesis is termed *promotion.* It is a slow, reversible process whereby initiated cells are stimulated by promoting agents to develop into tumor cells. The promoters may be the carcinogen itself or another stimulus, which need not be a mutagen. Among the best tumor promoters are the phorbol esters, which can directly activate protein kinase C that is part of the phosphatidyl inositol intracellular signaling pathway.

The final step, *progression,* involves the stepwise maturation of relatively few tumor cells into a fully malignant neoplasm. Progression involves the natural selection of altered cells by an environment relatively favorable to the mutant's growth, as well as the intrinsic potency of the altered cell.

Radiation carcinogenesis causes multiple defects in DNA, such as base damage or single- or double-strand breaks. Either error-prone repair or no repair may lead to mutations or chromosomal derangements. Ionizing and ultraviolet radiation frequently act as both initiators and promoters in the carcinogenic process. Other environmental or host factors surely have an impact on whether full malignant potential is realized; that is, such factors are determinants of progression.

Evidence exists in experimental animal systems for a viral etiology in various tumors. Early work by Ellerman and Bang in 1908 and Rous in 1911 demonstrated that filtered cell-free extracts of animal tumors could induce tumor formation in normal animals, suggesting a viral cause. Subsequent work has led to the identification of DNA- or RNA-containing tumor viruses responsible for malignant transformation. Both RNA- and DNA-containing tumor viruses ultimately act by insertion of the genetic code into the host genome. The "infected" cells acquire immortality by expression of specific viral genes that code for uninterrupted growth (Table 9–2).

Oncogenes and the Molecular Genetics of Carcinogenesis. Although phenotypic heterogeneity is common in cancers so that no two tumors likely involve exactly the same genes, all cancers exhibit accelerated cell proliferation. Changes in a relatively small number of genes responsible for regulating cell proliferation can induce uncontrolled cell division. There are two general types of genes in this realm—those that stimulate and those that inhibit cell proliferation. Thus, two mechanisms exist for the deregulation of cell division. The stimulatory gene can be made hyperactive and is then referred to as an oncogene. The normal allele governing stimulation is called a proto-oncogene. The oncogene is expressed as the dominant gene. The second mechanism involves inactivation of the inhibitory gene. For this to influence cell division, homozygosity is required (a recessive gene), in which case the lost gene is called a tumor-suppressor gene.

The system has been best studied in viral tumorigenesis. Both DNA and RNA viruses (especially retroviruses) can cause cancer by inducing mutations, even though most viruses probably operate as promoters, especially in humans. The viruses can initiate cancer by either inserting viral DNA into the host genome (most DNA tumor viruses and some RNA viruses) or in the form of an extrachromosomal plasmid (RNA retroviruses and some DNA tumor viruses). Some DNA tumor viruses insert a viral gene directly into the host genome, thereby forcing the cell into uncontrolled division. In this instance, the viral gene acts as an oncogene causing malignant transformation. Other DNA viruses, via protein products of the viral gene, alter the host's DNA in such a way that the host control of division is subverted to replicate the viral genome. By contrast, some RNA retroviruses (so called because they reverse the normal process of DNA transformation to RNA) act by incorporating a host proto-oncogene into itself, so that the gene product promoting division is produced in excess and acts as an oncogene causing cancerous transformation. Other retroviruses utilize cellular reverse transcriptase, so that DNA copies of the viral RNA are inserted at sites close to the proto-oncogene in the host genome. This mechanism for genetic alteration is termed insertional mutagenesis, and the resulting oncogene is inherited by daughter cells of the host cell. Many of the protein products of oncogenes code for growth factors, growth factor receptors, or for gene-regulating proteins (Table 9–3). Inappropriate expression of these genes leads to events conducive to carcinogenesis. In addition to the hyperactivation of proto-oncogenes, loss of tumor-suppressor genes may be responsible for malignant transformation.

Oncogenes and Proto-oncogenes in Human Malignancy. Expanding on the discovery of viral oncogenes in RNA tumor viruses, investigators pro-

TABLE 9–2.   VIRUSES AND HUMAN CANCER

VIRUS GROUPS	HUMAN EXAMPLE	ASSOCIATED TUMOR
DNA Viruses		
Hepadna	Hepatitis B	Hepatocellular carcinoma
Papova A	Papilloma	Benign warts, cancer of uterine cervex
Herpes	Epstein-Barr	Burkitt's lymphoma, nasopharyngeal cancer
RNA Viruses		
Retrovirus	Human T-cell leukemia (HTLV-1) Human immunodeficiency (HIV-1)	Adult T-cell leukemia/ lymphoma, Kaposi's sarcoma

Modified from Alberts, B., Bray, D., Lewis, J., Raff, M., Roberts, K., and Watson, J.D. (eds.): The Molecular Biology of the Cell, 2nd ed. New York, Garland Publishing, Inc., 1989. Table 21–3, p. 1204.)

TABLE 9–3.   ONCOGENES ORIGINALLY IDENTIFIED THROUGH THEIR PRESENCE IN TRANSFORMING RETROVIRUSES

ONCOGENE	PROTO-ONCOGENE FUNCTION (where known)	SOURCE OF VIRUS	VIRUS-INDUCED TUMOR
abl	Protein kinase (tyrosine	Mouse, cat	Pre-B-cell leukemia sarcoma
erb-A	Thyroid hormone receptor	Chicken	(Supplements action of v-erb-B)
erb-B	Protein kinase (tyrosine): epidermal growth factor (EGF) receptor	Chicken	Erythroleukemia, fibrosarcoma
ets	Nuclear protein	Chicken	(Supplements action of v-myb)
fms	Protein kinase (tyrosine): macrophage colony-stimulating factor (M-CSF) receptor	Cat	Sarcoma
fos	Nuclear transcription factor	Mouse	Osteosarcoma
mil/raf	Protein kinase (serine/threonine)	Chicken/mouse	Sarcoma
myb	Nuclear protein	Chicken	Myeloblastosis
myc	Nuclear protein	Chicken	Sarcoma, carcinoma
H-ras	G-protein	Rat	Sarcoma, erythroleukemia
K-ras	G-protein	Rat	Sarcoma, erythroleukemia
el	Nuclear protein	Turkey	Reticuloendotheliosis
ros	Protein kinase (tyrosine)	Chicken	Sarcoma
sis	Platelet-derived growth factor, B chain	Monkey	Sarcoma
src	Protein kinase (tyrosine)	Chicken	Sarcoma

Modified from Alberts, B., Bray, D., Lewis, J., Raff, M., Roberts, K., and Watson, J.D. (eds.): Molecular Biology of the Cell, 2nd ed. New York, Garland Publishing, Inc., 1989, p. 1207.)

posed a model for the development of cancer in humans. It is based on the finding that DNA sequences homologous to the region that codes for malignant transformation in viruses are present in human cells. These proto-oncogenes and their protein products, when expressed in normal cells, appear to be responsible for vital functions in growth and development of the cells and normal tissue. Activation of these proto-oncogenes by either point mutation, amplification, or translocation may result in loss of regulation and differentiation, as well as increased proliferative activity associated with malignant transformation. These oncogenes have been detected in human malignancy (Table 9–3) by direct transfer of specific DNA (transfection) into normal cells with subsequent transformation to a malignant cell. What role these oncogenes actually play in the development of human cancers is not known at present. In fact, a viral cause for most human cancers has not been demonstrated. However, it is hoped that advances in genetic technology and improved understanding of oncogenes and their function in the malignant process will lead to methods for control of tumor growth.

The Stem Cell Hypothesis.   Whatever the mutagen, stem cells would appear to be the ideal progenitor cell of a neoplastic clone. Alterations of stem cell function result in changes in differentiation and self-renewal properties that are consistent with neoplasia. The presence of stem cells in tumors has been suggested by the finding that cells with an accelerated growth capacity have a tendency to form colonies. Colony-forming assays of human tumors have detected a subpopulation of cells with a high growth potential. The microenvironment necessary for successful colony formation suggests that stem cells may have receptors that respond to factors (growth factors, hormones, mitogens, etc.) that turn on the malignant machinery (Table 9–4). The milieu bathing the stem cells may well determine whether normal or neoplastic tissue will be the final product.

The stem cell model has far-reaching implications with regard to treatment. Those cells with the capacity for regeneration would seem to be the proper target for prospective treatment, even though this subpopulation represents only a small percentage of the detectable tumor volume. A random partial reduction in tumor mass may not translate into potential cure since those cells responsible for sustaining growth are not "killed." The effects of therapy aimed at stem cells can sometimes be evaluated in vitro by utilizing the colony-forming assay.

Tumor Cell Heterogeneity

Regardless of the origin of the tumor cell, a mature malignant neoplasm comprises multiple populations of cells that exhibit different biologic characteristics. The heterogeneity within a solitary neoplasm involves many different cell properties, including morphology, proliferative capacity, karyotype, cell surface markers, hormone receptors, biochemical products, antigenicity, immunogenicity, drug resistance, invasive potential, and metastatic behavior. The mechanism for tumor cell heterogeneity is not known, but may entail some or all of the following: (1) development of subclones with different biologic properties and distinct genetic subtypes during expansion from a single cell to a measurable

TABLE 9–4. GROWTH FACTORS INVOLVED WITH MALIGNANT TRANSFORMATION

GROWTH FACTOR	ASSOCIATION WITH MALIGNANCY
Epidermal growth factor (EGF)	EGF receptor is homologous to product of erb-B oncogene (erythroleukemia). Human tumors (breast carcinoma, glioblastoma) have EGF receptor abnormalities.
Platelet-derived growth factor (PDGF)	PDGF is homologous to protein product sis-oncogene (sarcoma). Products of some tumors (sarcoma, breast cancer) are PDGF-like peptides that may act as autostimulators.
Transforming growth factor (TGF)	TGF competes with EGF for EGF receptor. TGF-EGFR complex results in autostimulation (breast cancer).
Macrophage colony-stimulating factor (CSF-1)	CSF-1 is homologous to protein product of fms oncogene (sarcoma).
Bombesin	Bombesin is autocrine growth factor in human small-cell lung cancer.
Fibroblast growth factor	Basic form stimulates angiogenesis.

Modified from Buick, R.N., and Tannock, I.F.: Properties of malignant cells. *In* Tannock, I.F., and Hill, R.P. (eds.): The Basic Science of Oncology. New York, Pergamon Press, 1987, pp. 127–139.

tumor; (2) variable vascular supply to different regions of a developing tumor with resultant nonuniform distribution of nutrients leading to cell loss, cell death, or cellular dysfunction; and (3) relative levels of differentiation among cells so that, at each differentiation tier, distinct cellular properties are dominant. The mechanism of clonal evolution is the most widely accepted explanation for cellular heterogeneity within a neoplasm. Intratumoral heterogeneity is considered to be a major causative factor in tumor progression as it permits the natural selection process to operate to its greatest advantage.

Tumor Progression

With time, tumors tend to become more aggressive and evolve toward a more malignant phenotype.

Foulds described tumor progression as a series of steps along a spectrum with orderly progression from a benign tumor to premalignant stage (e.g., carcinoma in situ) and eventually to a fully malignant neoplasm. Nowell hypothesized that this biologic and clinical progression was a function of acquired genetic variability within developing subclones. As tumors develop from a single transformed cell, genetic alterations occur and, coupled with selective pressures of the host environment, result in subpopulations of cells with a greater tendency toward malignant behavior (Fig. 9–1). As the process evolves, increased genetic instability increases the probability of further genetic alterations. Many mutations are lethal or result in alterations incompatible with growth. However, some mutations confer a selective growth advantage, and that subpopulation becomes dominant within the tumor and is responsible for properties associated with tumor progression. Multiple subpopulations within the tumor not only define tumor heterogeneity but interactions between different cell lines may also enhance genetic instability. Any number of host factors, such as immunologic pressures, hormones, growth factors, and microenvironmental influences including therapeutic manipulations, may provide selective advantage to a specific subclone.

Although tumor initiation is normally a mutagenic event, tumor progression is not inevitable for every event. It has been estimated that in a lifetime, every gene will have undergone mutation on 10^{10} separate occasions. Thus, tumor progression must involve natural selection. The selective advantage of a mutant depends on the nature of the mutant and on certain environmental conditions, which are sure to promote the cancer once the mutation has occurred. Certain substances are tumor promoters; for example, phorbol esters, a plant product that directly activates protein kinase C. Similarly, surgical wounds, chronic inflammation, and infection are probably tumor promoters—effective after the mutation, but ineffective at initiating mutations themselves.

Tumor progression is associated with recognizable clinical and biologic properties. The most obvious and clinically relevant is that of invasion and metastasis. Tumor progression appears to involve an increase in the subpopulation of cells with accelerated growth potential, which may also explain the tendency toward a less differentiated state. The production and release of specific tumor-associated proteins may predispose toward invasion and metastases. Likewise, diminished antigenicity and acquired drug resistance confer on the tumor an improved ability to avoid both internal and external mechanisms of cell death and promote progression. These aspects of tumor progression and heterogeneity in part explain the past and present difficulty in controlling tumor growth and suggest avenues of investigation in the future.

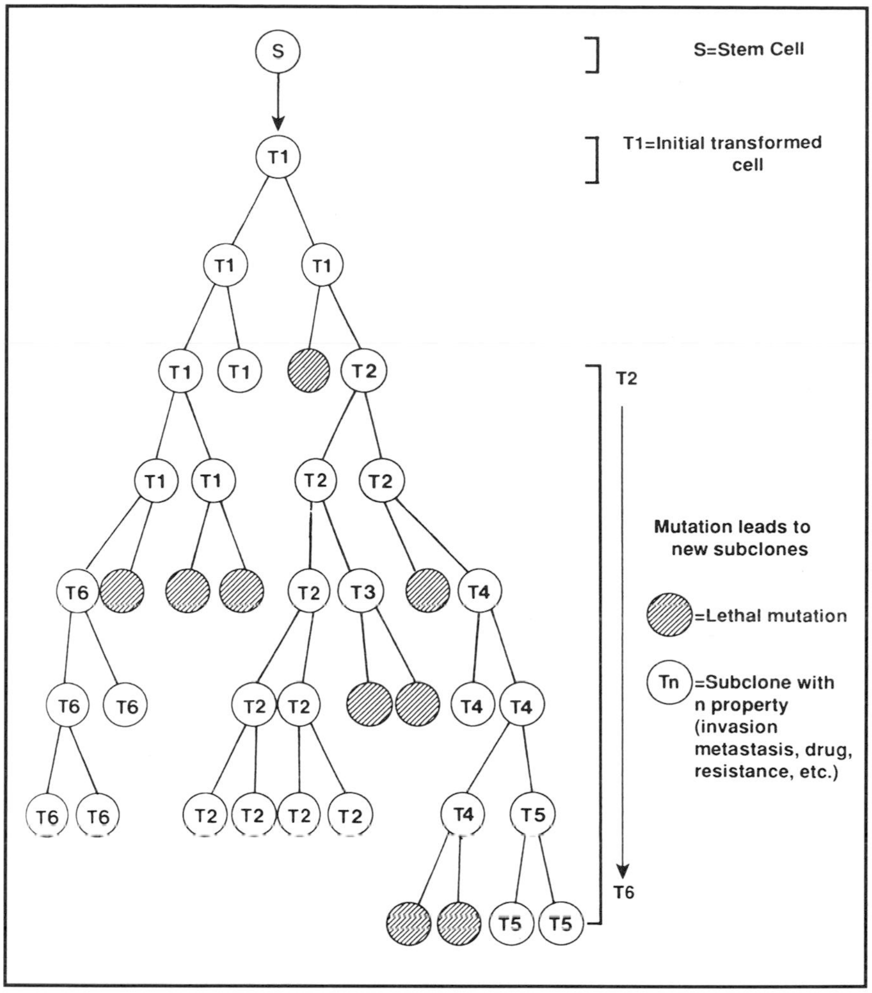

FIGURE 9–1. The clonal evolution of tumors. Subpopulations of cells (subclones) arise from a single transformed cell by mutation, resulting in a heterogenous population. Some mutations are lethal, whereas others result in properties (invasion, metastasis, etc.) that are associated with tumor progression. (Adapted from Nowell, P.C.: The clonal evolution of tumor cell populations. Science, *194:* 24, 1976, Figure 1, p. 24. Copyright 1976 by the AAAS.)

Properties of Transformed Cells

Normal cells, as well as malignant cells, can be cultured outside of their normal environment, allowing comparison between the transformed cell and the normal cell. The characteristic properties that distinguish the malignant cell include (1) loss of density-dependent or contact inhibition, allowing malignant cells to form colonies; (2) anchorage independence, i.e., the ability of malignant cells to grow in suspension or semisolid medium; (3) the lesser need of malignant cells for serum to sustain growth, a reflection of a presumed greater autonomy from growth factors; (4) increased refractility and random orientation, i.e., disorganization in malignant growth; (5) secretion of specific proteins, such as plasminogen activator, laminin, etc., by malignant cells, which may herald the development of invasive properties, and (6) cell cycle differences. None or all of these properties may be responsible for tumor growth in vivo.

TUMOR GROWTH AND CELL CYCLE KINETICS

Tumor growth is marked by cell division in excess of cell loss/death and decreased sensitivity of the tumor to normal control mechanisms. The study of tumor growth is hindered in that the clinically detectable growth is only a small fraction of the total growth period. Furthermore, the heterogeneity exhibited by tumors ensures the presence of widely variant growth rates among different tumors and among subpopulations of cells within a tumor. In fact, the cells responsible for proliferation comprise only a small percentage of the total cells present. Newer methods for the study of cell proliferation have provided insight into cell cycle dependent growth and kinetics during tumor progression. Although the logistics of such studies in human tumors are complicated by the availability of tissue and the timing of its removal, the differences in cell cycle kinetics between normal and malignant tissue, as well as between proliferating and nonproliferating cells within the neoplasm, present an opportunity for future treatment innovation.

Tumor Growth

The inability to control tumor growth eventually results in the host's demise. Tumor growth is estimated by measuring volume expansion over a period of time. One might expect to produce a curve during tumor expansion that indicates exponential growth, i.e., continued increase in volume over the period of observation. This concept of exponential growth is probably valid during an undefined time interval in almost all tumors. However, human tumor growth is not as straightforward as an exponential growth curve implies and is described more accurately by Gompertzian growth, at least after the tumor is large enough to be detected clinically and is subject to observation. Gompertzian growth is characterized by progressive slowing of tumor growth with time as depicted in Figure 9–2.

An explanation for the reduction in growth rate as tumor size increases can be found in the heterogeneous nature of malignant neoplasms. Studies utilizing advanced techniques in studying cellular proliferation reveal nonuniform growth rates among regions of a tumor. One mechanism for the intratumoral heterogeneity is variable tumor vascularity; as proliferation occurs, cells are progressively distanced from their feeding blood vessel. When the

parallel distance between tumor blood vessel and the advancing edge of tumor growth reaches 150 to 200 μm, necrosis occurs. A diffusion gradient for essential nutrients develops, and when nutrient concentration falls to a critically low level, cells can no longer sustain themselves. Deoxyribonucleic acid (DNA) labeling experiments have shown that the percentage of cells synthesizing DNA decreases at increasing distance from the nutrient vessel. These nondividing cells add to tumor volume, yet do not contribute to the tumor growth rate; hence, the leveling off of the growth curve. Tumor angiogenesis factor(s) is a protein(s) released by tumor cells that mediates endothelial cell production and blood vessel ingrowth into the tumor. Yet, DNA labeling methods reveal that DNA synthesis in the endothelial cells of tumor vessels is usually diminished relative to DNA synthesis in surrounding tumor cells. This discrepancy in DNA synthesis could also explain the retarded growth rate with increasing tumor volume.

Before it is clinical detectable, the actual growth rate of a tumor can only be estimated. A tumor will not be detected until it weighs at least 1 gram (30 doublings = 10^9 cells). A lethal tumor burden of 10^{12} cells only requires ten more doublings. Thus, the vast majority of tumor growth takes place before its clinical recognition. Observations of human tumors treated and studied to recurrence suggest exponential growth during the major portion of a tumor's preclinical expansion. The need to establish a nutrient blood supply and avoid host factors deleterious to the malignant process may cause a lag phase early in tumor development as depicted in Figure 9–3.

Tumor Cell Kinetics

An understanding of the normal cell cycle is essential to the study of tumor cell kinetics and its influences on tumor growth and treatment (Fig. 9–4). Not all cells are actually proliferating nor do cells simultaneously divide or have equivalent cell cycle phase durations. After mitosis (M), a new cycle is initiated and cells enter the G1 phase. During this phase, ribonucleic acid (RNA) and protein synthesis occurs. Normal cells may mature and through their protein products carry out cellular functions associated with normal tissue differentiation during G1. Once this occurs, the capacity for regeneration is lost. In tumors this process of maturation and differentiation is less operative, and cells either enter a nonproliferative resting phase (G0) or continue on in the cycle. The next phase is the S phase or phase of active DNA synthesis. The number of tumor cells that enter the S phase is probably a small proportion of the total cells. These cells are responsible for maintaining the proliferative pool, i.e., the stem cells. Before mitosis occurs, cells enter the G2 phase

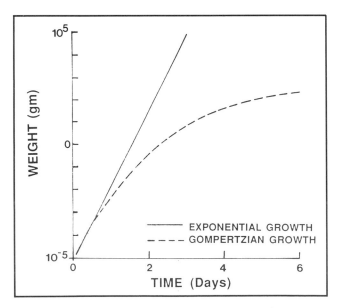

FIGURE 9–2. Curves depicting tumor growth. Human tumor growth more closely parallels the Gompertzian curve, i.e., a reduction in growth rate as tumor size increases. Gompertzian growth is a result of intratumoral heterogeneity. (Adapted from Sugarbaker, E.V.: Interdisciplinary cancer therapy: Adjuvant therapy. Curr. Prob. Surg., 6:1–69, 1977. Figure 2, p. 10.)

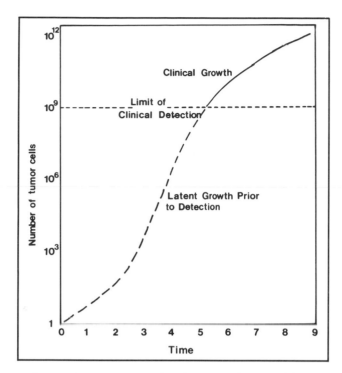

FIGURE 9–3. Curve estimating growth rate of human tumor before clinical detection. The early lag phase may be due to inadequate vascular and metabolic supply during initial tumor growth. Exponential growth predominates before the tumor becomes apparent clinically. (Adapted with permission from Tannock, I.F.: Tumor growth and cell kinetics. *In* Tannock, I.F., and Hill, R.P. (eds.): The Basic Science of Oncology. New York, Pergamon Press, 1987. Figure 9–3, p. 143.)

phase, they retain the capacity to do so. Local environmental stimuli, such as growth factors, hormones, or even changes brought about by such cancer treatment as radiation or chemotherapy, can stimulate these cells to enter the proliferative state and divide. Tumors contain other nonproliferating cells, which include nonmalignant supportive cells and cells that have differentiated to a greater or lesser extent and are unable to divide.

Newer techniques have explained in greater detail the cell cycle as it relates to malignancy. Radioisotopic labeling with tritiated thymidine (^3H) provides an estimate of the number of cells undergoing DNA synthesis and the duration of the cell cycle phases. From this, one can calculate the proportion of cells that is actually proliferating (growth fraction). This subpopulation, in human tumors, is relatively small yet vitally important to tumor growth and therapy. Cycle-specific chemotherapy is geared toward this group of cells. Yet, the large number of nonproliferating cells and high cell loss make tailoring therapy toward this subpopulation difficult. In addition, the ability to study this clonogenic population adequately as a separate entity is limited.

The application of flow cytometry techniques has also fueled cell kinetic studies. Flow cytometry utilizes fluorescence to measure the number of cells containing different quantities of DNA. Based on known DNA content during specific cell phases (2N or diploid=G1, 4N or tetraploid=G2, aneuploid=S), the proportion of cells within each cell cycle phase can be measured. This technique and innovations in its applicability hold some promise for determining response to therapy and prognosis.

in which further protein synthesis occurs. Cells in the G2 phase possess the tetraploid or 4N DNA content as opposed to the diploid (2N) number of chromosomes in the G1 phase. After mitosis, cells enter the G1 phase in which the cell either recycles, differentiates, or enters the nonproliferative pool (G0). Although cells are not actively proliferating in the G0

METASTASES

The dissemination of cancer cells from a primary tumor to distant sites is the single most germane aspect of cancer biology confronting oncologists.

FIGURE 9–4. The normal cell cycle. Cells in the nonproliferative (Go) phase retain their capacity to divide, although they may be dormant for a period of time. Go phase cells can re-enter the cell cycle if provoked by external stimuli or they may go on to die. (Adapted from Tannock, I.F.: Cell kinetics and chemotherapy: A critical review. Cancer Treat. Rep., *62*: 1117–1133, 1988, Figure 1, p. 1118.)

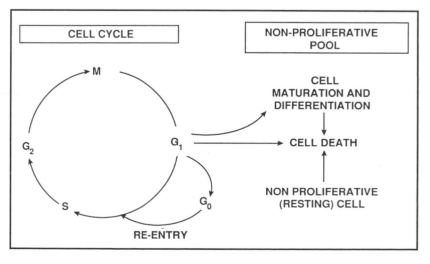

Metastasis is characteristic of the malignant process. Controversy surrounds not only how metastases occur but also when they occur, how we can prevent them, and how we should treat them. So, although traditional resectional therapy of a primary tumor is designed to prevent its spread, our failures far outweigh our success in achieving this goal because clinically covert metastasis has already occurred.

Mechanisms of Metastases

The spread of tumor cells can occur by a number of nonmutually exclusive routes. Direct invasion along tissue planes and into various body cavities is a way in which tumor cells might travel from their site of origin, although this is not the primary mode of dissemination. In most tumors, hematogenous and lymphatic spread is clearly the predominant route. Invasion of surrounding normal tissue may result in blood vessel or lymphatic invasion and eventual embolization to distant sites. Properties of malignant neoplasms that promote infiltration of host tissues are thus an important component of successful dissemination. Sometimes the presence of proteolytic enzymes within tumors (Fig. 9–5) has been detected in vitro and, along with hydrolytic enzymes and collagenases, can result in breakdown of basement membranes. Subsequent endothelial damage promotes adherence of tumor cells to blood vessels, as well as penetration of the vessel wall.

Hematogenous spread of tumor cells results in widespread distant metastases. Not only do the properties of malignant cells determine whether tumor cells enter the bloodstream but also host factors mediate the metastatic process. The release of tumor cells into the bloodstream does not ensure the eventual establishment of a metastatic colony. Circulating tumor cells have been identified in patients during and after operation, but do not necessarily result in metastases. Further proof of this phenomenon is provided by data from patients who have peritoneovenous shunts in place for malignant ascites, which does not necessarily result in increased rates of metastases. This phenomenon has been confirmed in experimental animal models. It appears that the release of tumor cells into the circulation is a necessary but insufficient factor in predicting metastases; most circulating cells die. There is, however, a correlation between the number of malignant cells released by the primary tumor and the number of cells that survive to become metastases. There is also evidence to suggest that the number of tumor cells in the bloodstream correlates with size of the primary tumor and the length of time it is clinically detectable. This correlation, of course, has therapeutic implica-

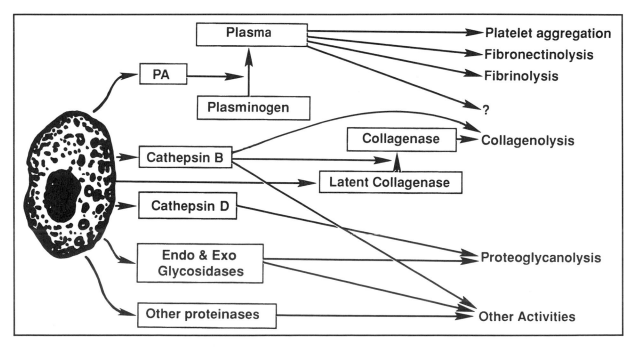

FIGURE 9–5. Malignant cells may produce proteolytic enzymes, collagenases, and hydrolytic enzymes that promote the malignant process. (Adapted from Nicholson, G.L., et al.: Metastatic cell attachment to and invasion of vascular endothelium and its underlying basal lamina using endothelial cell monolayers. *In* Nicholson, G.L., and Milas, L. (eds.): Cancer Invasion and Metastasis: Biologic and Therapeutic Aspects. New York, Raven Press, 1984. Figure 4, p. 157.)

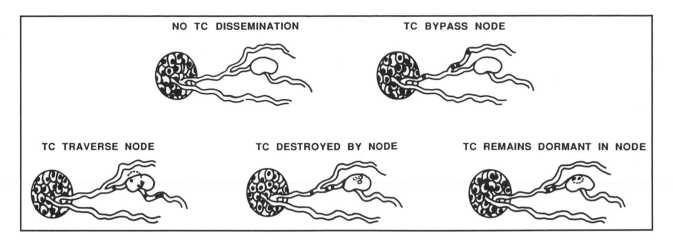

FIGURE 9–6. Illustration of the multiple pathways available to a tumor cell and its relation to the regional lymph node. (Adapted from Fisher, B.: The surgical dilemma in the primary therapy of invasive breast cancer: A critical appraisal. Curr. Prob. Surg., *10:*1–53, 1970. Figure 2, p. 40.)

tions for the timing and necessity for surgical extirpation of the primary neoplasm.

The other major route for dissemination of tumor cells is via the lumphatic system. As with hematogenous spread, tumor cells can enter the lymphatics by invasion. Once tumor emboli gain access to the lymphatic network, there are multiple pathways available (Fig. 9–6). Tumor cells may be carried to the first lymph node they encounter where they become lodged and establish growth. Alternatively, they may traverse collateral pathways to stop in more distal lymph nodes whether the more proximal lymph node is involved or not, producing a "skip" metastasis. It was and to some degree still is surgical teaching that lymph nodes function as barriers to tumor cell dissemination. If resection encompassed the primary neoplasm and surrounding lymph nodes before tumor cells escape from this anatomic barrier, surgical cure would be obtained. Although in select tumor types this may be true, in many instances even in the absence of involved lymph nodes, tumors recur at distant sites despite "curative" en bloc resection. This has been shown clinically both in melanoma and breast cancer through prospective randomized trials. In the laboratory, tumor cells labeled with radioactive isotopes rapidly enter efferent lymphatics once they have encountered a lymph node and are not trapped. Both properties of the tumor cells themselves and host factors dictate whether tumor emboli become trapped by lymph nodes or escape the "filter." Experimental evidence suggests that tumor cells are not confined to either the lymphatic system or bloodstream. These two networks are interconnected, and tumor emboli in the lymphatic system may pass into the blood vascular system or vice versa.

The Metastatic Process— Tumor-Host Interactions

It is important to keep in mind that many factors influence whether metastases occur and how they travel from the primary tumor to a distant host site. The complex metastatic process involves many steps and requires that tumor cells pass through each stage unscathed. The necessary steps for the formation of metastases include (1) release of tumor cells from the primary neoplasm, (2) invasion of the vascular system, (3) embolization in the circulation to a distant site, (4) arrest at a new location with adherence to the endothelial surface and formation of cell aggregates, (5) extravasation and infiltration of surrounding parenchyma, and (6) establishment of a new microenvironment capable of supporting tumor cell proliferation. Tumor cell survival will not occur if the cell is adept at only one stage and fails at others. Release of tumor cells into either the blood or lymphatic channels is necessary before they can invade and embolize. This release is dependent on the rate of tumor growth, extent of necrosis, mechanical stress, increase in cellular activity of certain enzymes, and decreased levels of proteins involved in cell adhesion.

Once released and throughout the metastatic process, host factors play a major role in determining cell survival. A minority of cells will actually avoid the rigors of host defense mechanisms, which include mechanical stress, lack of nutrient supply, and immune surveillance. The immune system most probably plays a critical role in prevention of metastases. Experimental models have shown that the greater the immunogenicity expressed by a tumor cell, the less capable it will be at forming metastases. Arrest of tumor cells may involve both thrombus formation and endothelial damage that is conducive to adherence. As mentioned earlier, the production of tissue destructive enzymes facilitates extravasation into the surrounding parenchyma. Once a cell has invaded new territory, new tumor growth is critically dependent on environmental conditions that are properly suited to nurture cell proliferation. The presence of growth factors or inhibiting factors influences the establishment of metastases. Likewise, proper nutritional conditions are necessary to support tumor growth, which requires an adequate blood supply for delivery of essential metabolites.

The complementary interaction between tumor cell and host emphasized in this review is not a new concept. One hundred years ago, Paget theorized that specific cellular properties, matched with specific organ miroenvironments appropriate for a particular cell to grow, were required for metastatic growth. The "seed and soil" hypothesis is yet another example of the biologic heterogeneity of malignant neoplasms, specifically metastases. The path through the metastatic cascade as described above is arduous, with only a minute percentage of cells capable of navigating its course. Is this a random event, or are specific cells selected by the properties they possess to survive and form metastases? There is considerable evidence that the latter is true and

that the "seeds" are cells within the heterogeneous tumor aggregate with specific metastatic capability. These cells vary in their proficiency for metastatic growth.

Two models have been used to test for metastatic heterogeneity within the primary neoplasm. In vivo selection entails implantation of parent tumor cells at a primary site followed by harvesting of metastatic tumor cells. These cells are then serially passed, with selection at each passage for cells that constitute a metastatic lesion. This technique described by Fidler results in the capture of cells with increased metastatic proficiency (Fig. 9–7A). The in vitro procedure takes advantage of one cell property known to contribute to the metastatic phenotype and selects for cells with that attribute. It is then determined whether the selected variant has increased metastatic potential when compared with the heterogeneous parent tumor (Fig. 9–7B). Organ specificity demonstrated for some cell populations may reflect either specific cellular attributes conducive to organ-specific growth or host factors that influence cellular proliferation. It appears that the development of metastases is not a random event, but a selective process based on a unique relationship between tumor cells with heterogeneous metastatic capability and host factors.

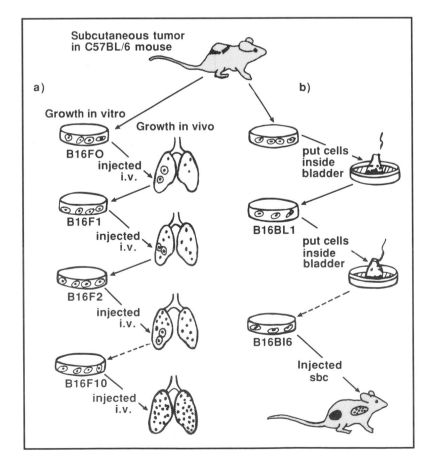

FIGURE 9–7. Metastatic heterogeneity within tumors as exemplified by selection of cell populations with variable and highly specific metastatic properties. *a*, B16F10 cells are selected by serial passage of cells that form lung metastases. *b*, B16BL6 cells are selected by their ability to invade the mouse bladder wall. (Adapted from Hill, R.P.: Metastasis. *In* Tannock, I.F., and Hill, R.P. (eds.): The Basic Science of Oncology. New York, Pergamon Press, 1987. Figure 10.9, p. 167.)

Heterogeneity in Metastases

As with the primary neoplasm, heterogeneity exists among multiple metastases in the same organism and within individual metastases. Tumors tend to progress to a more malignant, unstable form with time. The more malignant the tumor, the greater the tendency toward genetic instability and genetic alteration. It therefore follows that metastatic neoplasms comprise cells with a greater probability for genetic alterations, resulting in increased heterogeneity. This has therapeutic implications as chemotherapy or radiotherapy affects certain cells yet leave others unharmed. Since evidence exists that cells within a tumor stabilize and regulate neighboring cells, selecting out certain subpopulations by therapeutic manipulations can result in greater instability. The interlesional and intralesional heterogeneity present in metastases may well be the most important factor with regard to developing "curative" treatment. Unless 100 per cent cell kill is achieved, the remaining cells will be a fertile ground for variants resistant to conventional therapy. If 99.9 per cent of a one cubic centimeter tumor containing 10^9 cells is destroyed, that still leaves 10^6 cells. Thus, what would seem to be a highly effective treatment might unleash a more virulent subtype lacking the regulatory control imposed by surrounding cells. This is an argument for a multimodality approach in an attempt to kill all cells at the earliest possible time. Waiting for recurrence might allow selective processes to act and complicate curative attempts.

Heterogeneity in metastatic neoplasms also involves such factors as antigenicity and immunogenicity. These properties may well affect the cells' capability to metastasize and avoid immune mechanisms primed to prevent cell proliferation. Host factors are equally important in determining the formation of metastases. The finding that certain tumors have a predilection for forming metastases in specific organs is as much a consequence of a suitable microenvironment as it is a function of cellular properties. Organ specificity does not appear to be dependent on hemodynamic parameters or a first-pass phenomenon. The "soil" must be appropriate for growth to occur.

IMMUNOLOGY AND CANCER

The role of the immune system in tumor development and progression and manipulation of the immune system as a therapeutic alternative for the treatment of cancer are being studied actively. A basic understanding of tumor immunology is therefore warranted for any surgeon involved with the care of cancer patients.

The immune system's major function is to recognize and eliminate foreign agents. It accomplishes this task by determining what is "self" and what is "non-self" and mounting a response to whatever is perceived as non-self. If a substance is recognized as non-self, it is said to be antigenic. If the immune system is able to respond against the foreign agent, it is termed immunogenic. Tumor cells can be thought of as foreign, and therefore, one function of the immune system would be to recognize tumor as non-self and destroy it before tumor progression. Tumor-specific antigens may be expressed by some tumor cells in the process of transformation from a normal cell to the malignant phenotype. However, although some tumors are antigenic, others do not have specific antigens recognized by the host as foreign and therefore will not invoke an active response against it. As with other cellular properties, primary neoplasms and metastases are made up of a heterogeneous population of cells that express varying degrees of antigenicity or immunogenicity. Another type of immunity, termed natural immunity, may be specific for tumor cells and is mediated through cellular mechanisms.

Alterations in the tumor cell would appear to be likely as cells progress from benign to malignant and as they become more virulent, eventually resulting in metastases. Changes caused by genetic mutations or expression of genes not normally "turned on" may result in the production of new proteins that are antigenic. Whether these new antigens are immunogenic or not will determine whether a response will be elicited. It would seem that if the alteration causes a moderate phenotypic change away from normal self, it would invoke a response from the immune system. From a practical standpoint, these tumor-associated antigen determinants may prove to be invaluable as a means of tumor detection and possible tumor-directed therapy. Tumor markers, such as carcinoembryonic antigen (CEA), human chorionic gonadotropin (HCG), alpha-fetoprotein (αFP) etc., are antigens expressed on cancer cells (Table 9–5). These antigens are also expressed on normal cells in utero to a lesser degree than tumor cells and in other disease states not associated with malignancy. Because of their ubiquitous expression on both normal and abnormal cells, the immune system does not eliminate these cells, i.e., the antigen is not immunogenic. These antigens are of use in monitoring recurrent disease in patients after tumor reduction. In the future, tumor-specific antigens may be of use in the early detection of malignancy. The same may be true for monoclonal antibodies, which are antibodies exquisitely specific for single antigens detected on tumor cells; they are currently being used for diagnosis and imaging of many different histologic types of malignancy. Their use is limited by cross-reactivity with normal cells, as well as by the fact that small tumors, the key to early detection, express less antigen and are poor targets for the antibody. In addition, the possibility of linking monoclonal antibodies with cytotoxic drugs, radioisotopes, or other tumor cell toxic agents exists.

TABLE 9–5. USEFUL AND POTENTIALLY USEFUL TUMOR MARKERS

Tumor Marker	Associated Cancer
Carcinoembryonic antigen (CEA)	Colon, rectum, lung, breast, ovary, pancreas, hepatocellular carcinoma
Alpha-fetoprotein (AFP)	Hepatocellular carcinoma, nonseminomatous testicular tumors
Human chorionic gonadotrophin (HCG)	Gestational trophoblastic disease, germ cell testicular tumors, lung, ovary
Prostate-specific antigen (PSA)	Prostate
Prostatic acid phosphatase (PAP)	Prostate
CA-125	Ovary, endometrial, pancreas
CA 19-19	Pancreas, colorectal
DU-PAN 2	Pancreas
CA 15-3	Breast
Calcitonin	Medullary carcinoma thyroid

Once the immune system recognizes a tumor as non-self, how does it eliminate it from the host? There are a number of effector mechanisms by which the immune system can mediate tumor cell destruction. Antibody can bind directly to specific antigens on a tumor cell and by activation of the complement system kill the tumor cell directly. Another method involving antibody is termed antibody-dependent cellular cytotoxicity (ADCC). Killer cells of the monocyte/macrophage lineage with a receptor for a portion of the antibody bind to the antibody and mediate the death of the tumor cell to which the antibody is already bound (Fig. 9–8). T cells can also mediate tumor cell destruction. Cytotoxic T- lymphocytes specific for tumor-associated antigens have been isolated and in association with major histocompatibility (MHC) molecules can bind to the cell surface antigen by a receptor mechanism, thereby resulting in lysis of the targeted tumor cell. Attempts to improve the efficacy and increase the yield of these effector cells are actively being pursued in the laboratory. Another type of cell, the natural killer (NK) cell, has the capability to spontaneously eliminate cultured tumor cells without previous exposure to specific antigens. The NK cell is derived from a subpopulation of lymphocytes termed null cells. These cells appear to be morphologically distinct from T and B cells and are not limited by MHC antigens as are the other cells. NK cells may be involved in immune surveillance. Studies have shown an inverse relationship between NK cell activity and spontaneous tumor occurrence. NK cells are unable or minimally able to lyse fresh tumor cells.

Unlike NK cells, another type of killer cell also derived from the null lymphoid subpopulation can, in the presence of the lymphokine interleukin-2 (IL-2), lyse fresh tumor cell targets. These cells, referred to as lymphokine-activated killer (LAK) cells, are non-MHC restricted in their cytotoxicity and are capable of lysing, in addition to fresh tumor preparations, cultured normal and malignant cells.

Recently a lymphoid population that resides within growing tumor has been identified with specific MHC-restricted tumor cell lytic activity. These tumor-infiltrating lymphocytes (TIL) can be generated from single cell suspensions of harvested tumor in the presence of IL-2. TILs have been isolated from a wide variety of murine and human tumors and possess markedly enhanced tumor cell kill activity when compared with LAK cells.

BIOLOGIC PRINCIPLES OF CANCER THERAPY

The principles of cancer treatment are to some extent based on biologic properties of the cell and tumor growth and therapy attempts by altering or manipulating these properties, to selectively abort tumor cell proliferation while sparing normal tissue growth. The ability to achieve this goal determines the efficacy of any one therapeutic modality. The different types of cancer treatment take advantage of various biologic mechanisms and exert their own biologic effects in order to achieve this goal.

Radiation Therapy

Radiation therapy damages cells by transferring energy and causing ionization (complete displacement of an electron) or excitation (partial displacement) of atoms or molecules. It does so by one of the following three methods: (1) photons (x-rays and gamma rays) collide with charged particles (electrons) and transfer their energy, (2) charged particles (electrons and protons) are themselves delivered to the target and their energy is directly absorbed, or (3) uncharged particles (neutrons) collide with nuclei and create charged particles. All three methods produce a particle that transfers energy in its path of motion. The amount of linear energy transferred (LET) determines the biologic effect of any radiation dose. Cellular damage may occur indirectly through the production of free radicals when energy is absorbed by the aqueous portion of the cell. Alternatively and most important is the direct damage to DNA by ionizing radiation. On a molecular level, this damage results in single- or double-strand DNA breaks, base changes, or aberrant cross-links. The relative ability or inability of DNA to repair itself may well determine cell viability. On a cellular level, it is the reproductive capacity of the cell that is biologi-

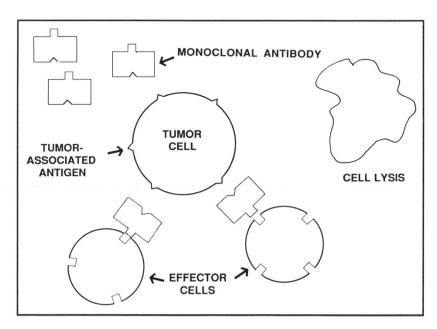

FIGURE 9–8. Antibody-dependent cellular cytotoxicity. Monoclonal antibody binds to specific antigen on tumor targets. In addition, the same antibody has a receptor for killer cells and, when coupling occurs, mediates lysis of the cell. (Adapted from Tannock, I.F.: Immunotherapy and the potential application of monoclonal antibodies. *In* Tannock, I.F., and Hill, R.P. (eds.). The Basic Science of Oncology. New York, Pergamon Press, 1987. Figure 20.7, p. 333.)

cally critical. Even low doses of radiation inhibit reproductive capacity, although the cell may divide once or even more times before the cell progeny eventually becomes sterile. In addition, radiation may cause a delay in mitosis—the cell pauses in the cell cycle resulting in synchronization of cell cycle events, which may effect cell killing.

Survival curves have been generated for both malignant and normal cells that have been exposed to ionizing radiation (Fig. 9–9). There are no definable differences between benign and malignant cells in the slope (D_0) of the exponential portion of the survival curve. However, the initial shoulder region of the curve can vary considerably among different cell lines and is a function of the cells' ability to repair radiation damage. At low doses of radiation, a large portion of the sublethal damage incurred is repaired. If a single dose of radiation is split into two doses separated by an interval of time, repair occurs, and a larger total dose is required to achieve the same biologic effect. This action is the basis for fractionation of radiation treatments in the clinical setting. In addition, different cell populations have differing capacities for sublethal damage repair. Multiple small fractions of radiation can therefore selectively preserve tissues (lung, gastrointestinal mucosa, etc.) with a greater capacity for repair of damage. Cell survival is also dependent on the cells' position in the cell cycle. Experimental evidence suggests that cells in the G2 or M phase are most sensitive to radiation, whereas S phase cells have a high probability for survival (Fig. 9–10). As alluded to earlier, radiation tends to eventually synchronize the surviving cells in a more sensitive phase. However, this synchrony is short lived and is probably not clinically significant. Probably the most important factor in determing the biologic effect of radiation is oxygen. Significantly higher doses of radiation are nec-

essary under hypoxic conditions to produce the same cell killing achieved in the presence of oxygen. Therefore, methods for improving oxygen delivery to the tumor cell target are actively being investigated.

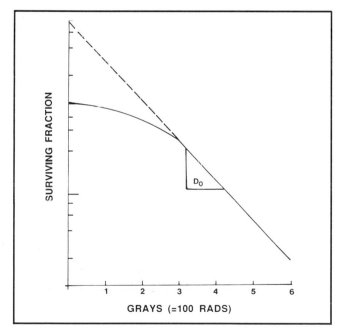

FIGURE 9–9. Survival curve for cells exposed to ionizing radiation. The initial shoulder represents repair of sublethal damage, resulting in inefficient cell killing. Do represents the proportion of cells killed by a given radiation dose. (Adapted from Hellman, S.: Principles of radiation therapy. *In* Devita, V.T., Hellman, S., and Rosenberg, S.A. (eds.): Cancer: Principles and Practices of Oncology, 3rd ed. Philadelphia, J.B. Lippincott Co., 1989. Figure 15–8, p. 258.)

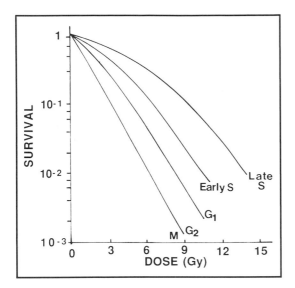

FIGURE 9–10. Survival curves for cells exposed to radiation during different phases of the cell cycle. (Adapted with permission from Sinclair, W.K.: Cyclic x-ray responses in mammalian cells in vitro. Radiation Res., *33:* 620–625, 1968. Figure 7, p. 632.)

The ability to control tumor growth with radiotherapy is a complex process that is dependent on numerous factors. Tumor response to radiation therapy is illustrated by the sigmoid-shaped dose-tumor control curve (Fig. 9–11). The dose of radiation required to control the tumor is dependent on the number of stem cells (cells with a large proliferative capacity) and their radiosensitivity. Due to the heterogeneous nature of tumors, all tumors vary with respect to these critical factors, a characteristic that tends to decrease the slope of the dose-tumor control curve. The larger the pool of proliferative cells in a given tumor, the earlier the expression of radiation damage and tumor regression. Similar results are seen in normal tissues in which acute injury occurs in tissues with rapid cell renewal (bone marrow, gastrointestinal tract mucosa, skin, etc.), whereas lesser responses are seen in tissues with decreased turnover capacity (liver, lung, kidney, or CNS). It is the relative sensitivity of the tumor versus the tolerance of normal tissue that determines the dose of radiation therapy and its efficacy. This principle is termed the therapeutic ratio and is illustrated in Figure 9–12.

Separation of the two sigmoid curves (tumor control and complications) is a favorable event and is achieved through fractionation of radiation treatment. The biologic events underlying this advantage involve four identifiable cellular processes: repair, regeneration, redistribution, and reoxygenation. Repair of damage induce by radiation will tend to reduce the tissue response to any given radiation dose. Regeneration will increase the number of targets at risk during radiation, resulting in a decreased

response. An increased total dose of radiation is required to achieve the same biologic effect in the presence of repair and cellular regeneration. Redistribution refers to the subsequent progression of cells, initially in more resistant phases of the cell cycle, to more sensitive phases during the course of fractionated therapy. Reoxygenation of hypoxic cells will increase the sensitivity of tumor during fractionated radiation. Redistribution and reoxygenation should result in a reduction in total dose needed to produce an equivalent biologic damage. Reoxygenation is mainly applicable to tumors, whereas the other three processes affect all tissues. Clinically, during fractionated radiotherapy, repair and repopulation appear to be predominant factors in the response of normal tissue and are critically dependent on fraction size, number of fractions, and the length of treatment. Manipulation of these factors and the creation of new fractionation schedules in order to derive a selective advantage—greater tumor response with minimal normal tissue damage—are important components of experimental radiotherapy. Hyperfractionation and accelerated fractionation in which smaller fraction sizes given more than once a day over a shorter total time period take advantage of relatively greater repair of late damage than early damage and may achieve a therapeutic gain. Other approaches, such as the use of hypoxic cell radiosensitizers, increasing oxygen delivery, and radioprotectors of normal tissues, are being evaluated to improve the therapeutic ratio.

Chemotherapy

Although chemotherapeutic agents differ with respect to the biologic mechanisms underlying there mode of cellular damage, all of these drugs are simi-

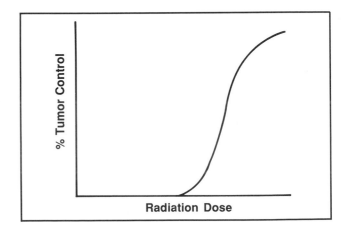

FIGURE 9–11. Sigmoid dose-response curve for tumors. (Adapted from Hellman, S.: Principles of radiation therapy. *In* Devita, V.T., Hellman, S., and Rosenberg, S.A. (eds.): Principles and Practice of Oncology, 3rd ed. Philadelphia, J.B. Lippincott Co., 1989. Figure 15–19, p. 264.)

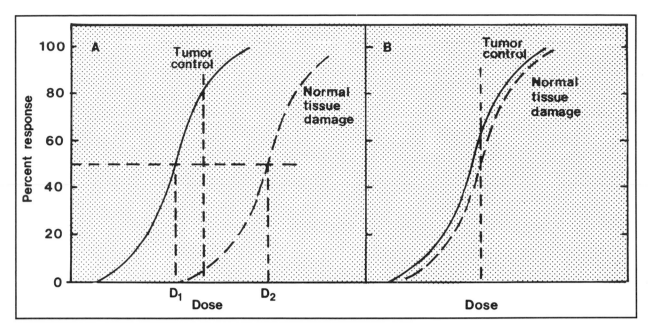

FIGURE 9–12. Dose-response curves illustrating the concept of therapeutic ratio. *A*, Shifting the tumor control curve to the left allows greater tumor control at a dose that incurs minimal normal tissue damage. *B*, When the two curves approximate each other, the risks of treatment outweigh the benefits of tumor control. (Adapted with permission from Hill, R.P.: Experimental radiotherapy. *In* Tannock, I.F., and Hill, R.P. (eds.): The Basic Science of Oncology. New York, Pergamon Press, 1987. Figure 16.7, p. 262.)

lar in that their ultimate goal is the destruction of stem cells. The classes of drugs available are listed in Table 9–6. As with radiation therapy, cell survival curves can be generated, and the number of cells surviving treatment is dependent on the concentration of the drug being administered. The amount of drug reaching a tumor and the cells within a tumor is highly variable and dependent on properties of the cell, drug, and environment. In addition, since tumors are composed of a heterogeneous cell population, tumor cells differ with respect to a number of factors that influence cell survival.

One factor that determines the efficacy of drug-dependent cell kill is the cells' capacity for division. The majority of chemotherapeutic agents have greater activity against rapidly proliferating cells. For some agents (alkylating agents, 5-FU), the relationship between cell survival and dose is exponential throughout the spectrum of drug doses. For other agents (antimetabolites, cytosine arabinoside, and vinca alkaloids), cell survival decreases exponentially at low doses and then plateaus at higher doses. This response may be explained by the drug being most effective during one specific phase of the cell cycle. Cell cycle specificity is another factor that determines drug activity. Alkylating agents exert their effects in two phases, G2-M and at the G1-S boundary. Antimetabolites are specific for cells in the S phase, as are tubulin-binding agents (vincristine, vinblastine, cytosine arabinoside etc.) that disrupt the formation of the mitotic spindle, a process that be-

gins during DNA synthesis. Other drugs exert their maximal effect during one phase, but affect all other phases to a lesser degree. Repair of damage caused by anticancer drugs probably affects cell survival, but is less well documented than repair of radiation-induced damage.

Probably the most important factor determining the clinical effectiveness of chemotherapy is drug resistance. Some cells exhibit resistance to drugs during their initial exposure to the agent (intrinsic resistance), whereas other cells acquire resistance during therapy. A great deal of evidence supports a genetic role in drug resistance. Point mutation or gene amplification is probably the initiating genetic event in drug resistance. The excess production of the target enzyme for methotrexate, dihydrofolate reductase, reduces the relative effectiveness of methotrexate and is a well-established example of gene amplification resulting in drug resistance. Some cells possess resistance to a variety of drugs with different mechanisms of action. Multiple drug resistance is caused by defective intracellular transport of drug across the cell membrane associated with the expression of a specific glycoprotein. Regardless of the exact cause of drug resistance, its presence may well determine the optimal scheduling of drug therapy. The Goldie-Coldman hypothesis suggests that as tumor size increases so does the likelihood of drug-resistant cells being present. Therefore, the earlier that drug treatment is instituted, the greater the chance of cure.

TABLE 9-6. MAJOR CLASSES OF ANTICANCER DRUGS

Alkylating Agents

Nitrogen mustard
Cyclophosphamide
Ifosfamide
Melphalan
Chlorambucil
Busulfan
Nitrosoureas
    BIS-cloroethylnitrosourea (BCNU)
    Cyclohexylnitrosourea (CCNU)
    Methylyclohexylnitrosourea (Methyl-CCNU)

Antimetabolites

Methotrexate
5-Fluorouracil
Cytosine arabinoside
Purine analogues
    6-mercaptopurine
    6-thioguanine

Antitumor Antibiotics

Bleomycin
Doxorubicin
Daunorubicin
Mitomycin C
Actinomycin D
Mithramycin

Plant Alkaloids

Vinblastine
Vincristine
Etoposide (VP-16)

Miscellaneous Synthetic Agents

Cisplatin
Carboplatin
Dacarbazine (DTIC)
Procarbazine
Mitoxantrone

The mechanism for producing lethal cell toxicity differs among the different classes of chemotherapeutic drugs. Alkylating agents possess electron-deficient side groups that can form covalent bonds with electron-rich groups on biologic molecules. The interaction of these agents with DNA bases results in cross-linking of DNA strands and single-strand breaks. Antimetabolites are synthetic compounds that resemble normal metabolites and act as competitive substrates for enzymes critical to DNA and RNA synthesis. Methotrexate resembles folic acid, which in its reduced form is necessary to complete the biosynthetic pathway to DNA synthesis. Methotrexate inhibits DNA synthesis by acting as a competitive inhibitor of dihydrofolate reductase, the enzyme necessary to form reduced folate. 5-Fluorouracil re-sembles the pyrimidine bases, uracil and thymine, and competitively inhibits thymidylate synthesis, thereby resulting in reduced DNA synthesis. Doxorubicin and bleomycin act by inserting themselves between base pairs, resulting in unwinding of the DNA double helix. The vinca alkaloids, vincristine and vinblastine, by binding to the protein tubulin, prevent the formation of a normal mitotic spindle and therefore disrupt DNA synthesis. Cisplatin acts in a similar fashion to the alkylating drugs and causes cross-linking of DNA strands.

As with radiotherapy, the efficacy of anticancer drugs is determined by the therapeutic index: the ability to deliver a drug dosage sufficient to cause lethal tumor cell damage yet minimize damage to normal cells. Normal cell toxicity is most apparent in tissues with a high rate of cellular division (bone marrow, intestinal mucosa, etc.), as would be predicted by the drugs' affinity for proliferating cells. Treatment regimens are designed to optimize tumor cell kill, yet the dosage and frequency of administration of drug are severely limited by normal tissue tolerance. Tumor cure requires 100 per cent tumor cell kill, or relapse is likely to occur. Cure is rarely achieved with solid tumors even though "complete remission" is obtained, since at the lowest limits of clinical detection the likelihood of viable tumor cells still being present is high. In addition, due to the need to limit toxicity, lower doses in multiple courses are necessary. This lengthens treatment time and increases the probability of developing drug-resistance clones.

Different approaches in treatment have been utilized in order to improve the therapeutic index. Combining chemotherapy with surgery or radiation therapy may improve response rates by presenting a smaller tumor burden to the administered agent. Smaller tumors contain less cells and may have a higher percentage of rapidly proliferating cells, thereby increasing the sensitivity to chemotherapy. Delivery of chemotherapy before surgery or radiation (neo-adjuvant chemotherapy) may be advantageous. Small, virgin tumors have an intact blood supply, which may allow more drugs to reach the target. The Goldie-Coldman hypotheses would suggest there is also less opportunity for drug-resistant clones to develop the earlier that drug therapy is instituted. Finally, presence of the primary tumor has been shown in animal studies to suppress the growth of metastases, and its removal results in an early burst of metastatic activity. Treatment with chemotherapy only and before tumor excision may prevent the accelerated growth of metastases. Other approaches include (1) using substances, such as dimethylsulfoxide (DMS0), that have been shown to induce differentiation and halt the proliferative process; (2) administering drugs that may block one of the steps in the metastatic cascade, (i.e., anticoagulants or platelet inhibitors—dipyridamole, PG-I$_2$, etc.) to prevent the thrombotic arrest of circulating tumor cells, (3) regional delivery of drugs directly to the tumor, i.e., intra-arterial infusion for hepatic metastases and intrathecal administration for CNS tumors; and (4) linking anticancer drugs to antibodies directed against tumor-specific antigens (bifunctional antibody).

The most common means of attempting to improve the therapeutic ratio is through combination chemotherapy. By administering multiple drugs at one time, one hopes to improve tumor response while taking advantage of the differential normal tissue toxicity associated with each drug. This potentially allows higher drug doses to be administered. The use of combination chemotherapy also reduces the chance of a cell population arising that is cross-resistant to all the drugs administered in that combination. Whether drugs given in combination are synergistic or additive is difficult to discern. Investigators are constantly searching for more effective means of delivering cytotoxic agents to the tumor cell target.

Hyperthermia

For centuries it has been recognized that cells exposed to elevated temperatures may be destroyed. Recently, the use of hyperthermia as a form of cancer therapy has attracted considerable interest. Cell survival curves, similar to those after radiation exposure, show decreasing cell survival with increasing temperatures above 41° C (Fig. 9–13). Cell killing is exponential at higher temperatures after an initial shoulder region. The initial shoulder is due to the cells' ability to repair sublethal damage. At temperatures below 42.5° C the curve plateaus with longer exposure time because of the development of thermotolerance. Thermotolerance decays with time, increasing cell sensitivity, suggesting that fractionated heat exposure may optimize therapy. The amount of cell kill is critically dependent on both exposure time and temperature, with minor changes of either variable resulting in major biologic effects.

A number of factors have been shown to modify the cellular effects of hyperthermia. Cell cycle position influences thermal sensitivity. Cells in either the S or M phase appear to be most sensitive. Both acidic pH and an environment depleted of nutrients improve cell killing during heat exposure. These two factors, and not intrinsic cell sensitivity, probably explain the relative sensitivity of malignant cells to hyperthermia when compared to normal cells. Tumor cells are generally poorly perfused, resulting in reduced nutrient levels and drops in pH secondary to anaerobic glycolysis. Since blood flow is the primary route for dissipation of heat, tumors with inadequate perfusion would tend to retain heat as opposed to normal tissues with an adequate blood supply. All of the above provide a rationale for hyperthermia treatment since tumors can theoretically

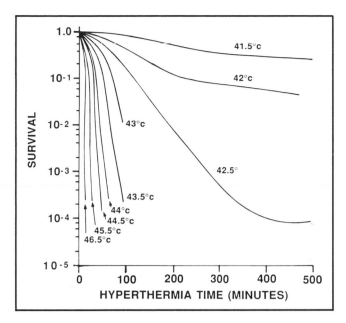

FIGURE 9–13. The effects of varying temperatures on cell survival. The flattening of the survival curve after prolonged exposure of tumor at lower temperatures is due to thermotolerance. (Adapted from Dewey, W., Hopwood, L., Sapareto, S., and Gerweck, L.E.: Cellular responses to combinations of hyperthermia and radiation. Radiology, *123:* 463–474, 1977. Figure 1, p. 464.)

be heated to higher temperatures than normal cells. The mechanism of thermal cell killing is not clearly understood, but appears to involve cell membrane damage, protein denaturation, or nuclear damage.

Hyperthermia both sensitizes cells to radiation and targets cells not sensitive to radiation damage, i.e., hypoxic cells. Therefore, combining the two modalities has theoretical advantages. Heat also appears to enhance the effect of cytotoxic agents and may be used to improve the efficacy of chemotherapy. Mechanisms explaining the enhancing effect of hyperthermia include (1) increased DNA damage and inhibition of DNA repair, (2) increased drug activation, and (3) cell membrane damage resulting in increased drug permeability. The effectiveness of hyperthermia is limited by our current technology and inability to provide uniform, well-controlled heating of targeted tissue. Most reports of the effects of hyperthermia are anecdotal, and its role as an effective cancer treatment can only be assessed in controlled clinical trials.

Hormones

Hormones exert their effects by binding to specific receptors on a cell. They then interact directly or via a second messenger, such as cyclic adenosine monophosphate, with the cell's genome to alter gene expression. This interaction may result in malignant transformation or altered protein products that fuel the proliferative process. Three routes are used for transfer of an intercellular message to its target receptor. The first involves an endocrine effect whereby the secreted hormone travels in the blood to a cell in a different location. Paracrine cells produce growth factors that act on phenotypically different neighboring cells. Autocrine cells secrete growth factors that act upon the cell from which the growth factor originated. Hormones have been documented to significantly influence cellular differentiation and have been implicated as etiologic agents in certain cancers, i.e., endometrial and breast cancer are associated with estrogen, and prostate cancer is associated with androgens. Although the mechanism of malignant transformation is not completely understood, this hormone-tumor cell relationship can be manipulated to obtain a therapeutic advantage by blocking either the hormone itself or a growth factor that directly stimulates tumor growth.

The hormonal treatment of breast cancer has evolved over the last three decades from surgical obliteration of the ovaries, adrenals, or pituitary gland to administration of estrogens, progestins, or androgens to the current use of antiestrogens (Tamoxifen). Tamoxifen apparently competes with estradiol for the estrogen receptor and effectively reduces estrogen stimulation of the cell. Whether tumor growth is inhibited by direct reduction of estrogen concentration at the cell or is a result of decreased production and release of growth factor necessary for tumor progression is unclear. However, the presence of hormone receptors does correlate with therapeutic response and prognosis.

Hormonal manipulation is also successful in the treatment of advanced prostate cancer. Marked tumor regression and long-term remissions have been produced with orchiectomy, estrogen (DES) and antiestrogen (Flutemide) administration, or the use of a gonadotropin-releasing hormone agonist (Leuprolide). The luteinizing hormone-releasing hormone agonists, work via feedback inhibition of the pituitary axis to subsequently decrease the release of testosterone. Other tumors not considered to be hormone sensitive may be responsive to hormonal therapy if hormones or growth factors responsible for tumor growth are eventually identified.

Immunotherapy

Manipulation of the immune system to actively recognize antigens specifically associated with tumors and that are not present on normal cells continues to evolve as a form of cancer therapy. Although tumor-specific antigens have been demonstrated in human tumors, the expression of these antigens in a tumor composed of a heterogeneous group of cells is variable and may be weakly immunogenic or nonimmunogenic. These antigens can also be expressed to a lesser degree on some normal cells. Hence, targeting effective immunotherapy to the tumor is a difficult clinical problem.

Early attempts at immunotherapy focused on active nonspecific stimulation of the immune system by such agents as *Bacillus Calmette-Guerin, Corynebacterium parvum,* and levamisole. In theory, generalized immunomodulation would result in enhanced immune reactivity toward tumor. However in practice, this generalized stimulation of the immune system has had limited success. Active specific immunization with killed primary tumor cells has also been attempted. Its broad application and effectiveness have been hindered by (1) failure to augment an immune reaction in a host previously exposed to the antigen throughout tumor growth; (2) lack of specificity of tumor-specific antigens that are present and expressed variably by normal cells, thereby effectively limiting tumor cell targeting; (3) heterogeneity between the primary tumor and metastases; (4) "downregulation" of MHC antigen expression by tumors, thereby camouflaging the malignant cell from recognition by lymphocytes; and (5) release of substances by tumors that act as suppressors of the immune mechanisms. Other approaches to immunotherapy involve attempts at more specific stimulation of the immune system through passive immunotherapy. Monoclonal antibodies, as mentioned earlier, are antibodies bred against specific tumor antigens, providing a large pool of activated immunoglobulins directed toward malignant cells. At present, their use has been limited to attempts at early detection and imaging of many types of human malignancy. Linking these biologic agents with other forms of cytotoxic therapy (anticancer drugs or radioisotopes) has potential as a form of cancer therapy. Another alternative is adoptive immunotherapy whereby effector cells with known and improved capability for tumor lysis are systemically or locally transferred to the tumor-bearing host. These effector cells may take the form of cytotoxic T lymphocytes, natural killer (NK) cells, or activated macrophages. Animal studies have shown that lymphocytes cultured in the presence of high concentrations of the biologic response modifier interleukin-2 acquire cytotoxic activity against tumor cells, but not normal cell targets. These lymphokine-activated killer (LAK) cells have subsequently been demonstrated to cause tumor regression of established murine hepatic and pulmonary metastases in animals. Clinical studies have also shown a limited response in human malignancy, mainly melanoma and renal cell carcinoma. Augmentation of NK cell lineage, where the cytotoxic effector property appears to reside, with biologic response modifiers, such as the interferons, is also under investigation.

Finally, isolation of lymphocytes that reside within tumors should theoretically be highly specific to the tumor cells with which they were once associated during tumor growth. In the presence of IL-2 these TILs can be expanded and in murine models have exhibited potent cytolytic activity. Initial clinical trials in human melanoma are encouraging, and TILs appear to be the most effective immunotherapeutic effectors identified to date. Obviously, further investigation is warranted as manipulating the highly specific antitumor activity of TILs may lead to very effective immunotherapy for human solid tumors.

BIBLIOGRAPHY

1. Tannock, I.F., and Hill, R.O. (eds.): The Basic Science of Oncology. New York, Pergamon Press, 1987.
2. Devita, V.T., Hellman, S., and Rosenberg, S.A. (eds.): Cancer: Principles and Practice of Oncology, 3rd ed. Philadelphia, J.B. Lippincott Co., 1989.
3. Ruddon, R.W. (ed.): Cancer Biology. New York, Oxford University Press, 1981.
4. Alberts, B., Bray, D., Lewis, J., Raff, M., Roberts, K., and Watson, J.D. (eds.): Molecular Biology of the Cell, 2nd ed. New York, Garland Publishing, Inc., 1989.
5. Nicholson, G.L., and Milas, L. (eds.): Cancer Invasion and Metastasis: Biologic and Therapeutic Aspects. New York, Raven Press, 1984.
6. Tannock, I.: Cell kinetics and chemotherapy: A critical review. Cancer Treat. Rep., 62:1117–1133, 1978.
7. Sugarbaker, E.V., Ketcham, A.S., and Zubrod, G.F.: Interdisciplinary cancer therapy: Adjuvant therapy. Curr. Prob. Surg., 6:1–69, 1977.
8. Fisher, B.: The surgical dilemma in the primary therapy of invasive breast cancer: A critical appraisal. Curr. Prob. Surg., 10:1–53, 1970.
9. Sutherland, R.M., Rasey, J.S., and Hill, R.P.: Tumor biology. Am. J. Clin. Oncol., 11:253–274, 1988.
10. Nowell, P.C.: Mechanisms of tumor progression. Cancer Res., 46:2203–2207, 1986.
11. Weinstein, I.B.: The origins of human cancer: Molecular mechanisms of carcinogenesis and their implications for cancer prevention and treatment. Cancer Res., 48:4135–4143, 1988.

Part III

PHYSIOLOGY AT THE ORGAN LEVEL

10

RESPIRATORY PHYSIOLOGY

MORRIS I. BIERMAN

STRUCTURE AND FUNCTION

Normal ventilation begins with the passage of air through the upper airway, which consists of the mouth, nose, pharynx, larynx, and trachea. This anatomic region is involved in both respiratory and nonrespiratory functions, such as speech, cough, and smell. There are two basic respiratory functions. First, these passages serve as a conduit for the movement of air both into and out of the lung, and second, they serve to protect the lower airway from a variety of insults. Air is warmed and humidified during its passage into the lung, and particulate matter is filtered out. A variety of reflexes involving the upper airway serve to protect the lower respiratory tract from foreign material. These reflexes depend on a extensive network of neural innervation, as well as on fine muscle control. Insults interfering with these reflexes may result in compromise of the airway.

There are 23 generations of the airways ranging from a mean diameter of 18 mm at the trachea to 0.3 mm at the alveolar ducts (Table 10–1). With each generation of airways the number of passages approximately doubles. These airways can be classified into three groups. First are the proximal cartilaginous airways consisting of the trachea and mainstem lobar, segmental, and small bronchi. Second are the membranous bronchi that lack cartilaginous support in their walls and include the bronchioles and terminal bronchioles. The final group comprises the distal gas exchange ducts that consist of the respiratory bronchioles, alveolar ducts, and alveolar sacs. The average therapeutic bronchoscope with an outer diameter of 5 mm is not capable of visualizing below the level of the fourth generation (segmental) bronchi. The vast majority of the lung thus cannot be visualized directly.

This pattern of branching airways that increase in number at each level has several functional implications. First, the more proximal cartilaginous airways and membranous bronchi lack alveoli and thus do not participate in gas exchange. These comprise the anatomic dead space and have been defined as the conducting zone. The respiratory zone comprises the more distal airways that do contain alveoli. Second, at approximately the level of the terminal bronchioles there is a tremendous increase in the cross-sectional area of the airways. Inspired air moves by bulk flow down to this level whereupon its forward velocity slows drastically and diffusion becomes the major mode of gas transport. The majority of the airway resistance therefore occurs in the region of bulk flow, i.e., the upper airways and cartilaginous bronchi. Finally, from a single airway (the trachea) one ends up with approximately 300 million terminal units (the alveoli). This creates a tremendous surface area for gas exchange to occur.

The primary lobule or acinus is defined as that portion of the lung distal to a terminal bronchiole. It represents the basic functional respiratory unit in the lung. The respiratory bronchioles contain alveolar outpouchings that gradually increase in number distally. They culminate in the formation of the alveolar sacs, which are the last generation of the air passages and contain about 17 alveoli each. The primary lobule (acinus) therefore typically contains 3 orders of respiratory bronchiole, 3 orders of alveolar ducts, and 17 alveolar sacs for a total of approximately 2300 alveoli. Note that the distance from the terminal bronchiole to the furthest alveolus is only approximately 5 mm. There are felt to be 130,000 primary lobules in the lung.

The alveoli are the smallest units of gas exchange, with a mean diameter of only 0.2 mm at functional residual capacity. They are larger in the nondependent regions of the lung (i.e., the apex in the upright patient) because the pleural pressure is more negative in these regions than at the base of the lung. Their walls are composed of a squamous epithelium; however, the intimately intertwined capillary network and its contents form a large portion of their walls. The alveolar walls also contain connective tissue fibrils, nerve endings, and possibly small numbers of macrophage and polymorphonuclear leukocytes.

163

TABLE 10–1. STRUCTURAL CHARACTERISTICS OF THE AIR PASSAGES

	GENERATION (MEAN)	NUMBER	MEAN DIAMETER (mm)	AREA SUPPLIED	CARTILAGE	MUSCLE	NUTRITION	EMPLACEMENT	EPITHELIUM
Trachea	0	1	18	Both lungs	U-shaped	Links open end of cartilage			
Main bronchi	1	2	13	Individual lungs	U-shaped				
Lobar bronchi	2 → 3	4 → 8	7 → 5	Lobes	Irregular shaped and helical plates	Helical bands	From the bronchial circulation	Within connective tissue sheath alongside arterial vessels	Columnar ciliated
Segmental bronchi	4	16	4	Segments					
Small bronchi	5 → 11	32 → 2 000	3 → 1	Secondary lobules					
Bronchioles Terminal bronchioles	12 → 16	4 000 → 65 000	1 → 0·5		Absent	Strong helical muscle bands		Embedded directly in the lung parenchyma	Cuboidal
Respiratory bronchioles	17 → 19	130 000 → 500 000	0·5	Primary lobules		Muscle bands between alveoli	From the pulmonary circulation		Cuboidal to flat between the alveoli
Alveolar ducts	20 → 22	1 000 000 → 4 000 000	0·3			Thin bands in alveolar septa		Forms the lung parenchyma	Alveolar epithelium
Alveolar sacs	23	8 000 000	0·3						

Reprinted from Nunn, J.F.: Applied Respiratory Physiology, 3rd ed. London, Butterworths, 1987. Table 1.1, p.7.

The airways are lined with a specialized epithelium that serves a number of functions at different levels. The bronchi possess a ciliated pseudostratified columnar epithelium that gives way to a cuboidal epithelium at the end of the conducting zone. Several types of cells can be found within this epithelium. The ciliated cells are derived from a multipotential stem cell found at the base of the epithelium. The coordinated beating of these cilia is crucial to the removal of mucus and particulate matter from the lower airways. Goblet cells are present down to the level of the terminal bronchioles and are responsible for the secretion of mucins. The larger cartilaginous bronchi also contain submucosal glands that secrete water, electrolytes, and mucins into the lumen. Smooth muscle, connective tissue, lymphoid tissue, and nerve endings are also found in the bronchial walls. A wide variety of drugs, neuronal reflexes, inhalational agents, and immunologic factors all can have a profound influence on the functions of the bronchial epithelium. It should also be noted that this epithelium is easily damaged by direct contact (i.e., suctioning) and a variety of noxious agents.

The alveolar epithelium is composed of a number of specialized cells. The main component is the type I pneumatocyte, which is a squamous cell that participates in gas exchange. This cell has no capability to reproduce itself. The type II pneumatocyte serves two major functions. First, it functions as a stem cell with the capability of producing new alveolar epithelial cells. Also, this cell is responsible for the production of surfactant, which lowers the surface tension in the alveolus, thereby stabilizing the alveoli. The type II pneumatocyte does not participate in gas exchange.

Other cells found within the respiratory mucosa include the nonciliated epithelial cells known as Clara cells, which are found in the terminal bronchioles. The function of these cells has not yet been determined. Alveolar macrophages play a crucial role in the removal of debris from the air spaces. These cells are derived from mononuclear cells in the circulation and pass freely through the interstitial space into the alveoli. They are the predominant cell type recovered from the normal lung when bronchoalveolar lavage is performed. Mast cells are also found throughout the airways. These cells participate in immunologic processes involving the lung. Neutrophils are not generally found within the normal alveolus, but may appear in disease states.

PULMONARY MECHANICS

The mechanical properties of the respiratory system are those that define the movements of the lung, chest wall, and respiratory gases. In order to discuss these issues it is first necessary to define the divisions of lung volume (Fig. 10–1). The total lung capacity (TLC) is the volume of gas contained within the lung at maximal inspiration. The vital capacity (VC) is the greatest volume that can be exhaled during a maximal expiratory effort. It is not possible to empty the lung completely during exhalation due to the collapse of small airways at low lung volumes. That quantity of gas remaining in the lung after maximal exhalation is known as the residual volume (RV). The tidal volume is defined as the quantity of air moved during a normal respiratory excursion. The functional residual capacity (FRC) is the quantity of air remaining in the lungs after a normal exhalation. It includes the sum of the residual volume and that volume of air that can be exhaled to RV from the tidal breath (the expiratory reserve volume). The

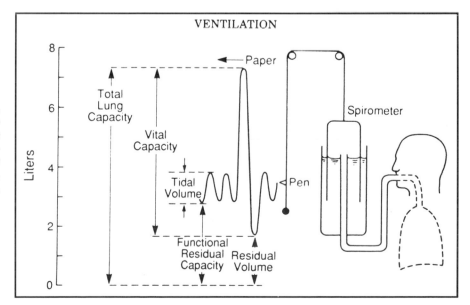

FIGURE 10–1. Lung volumes. Note that the functional residual capacity and residual volume cannot be measured with the spirometer. (Reprinted from West, J.B.: Respiratory Physiology—The Essentials, 4th ed. Baltimore: Williams & Wilkins Co., 1990. Figure 2.2, p. 13.)

inspiratory capacity is that quantity of air that can be inhaled from FRC. It includes the tidal volume plus the amount of air that can be inhaled subsequently up to TLC (the inspiratory reserve volume). The closing volume is a measure of the lung volume at which small airways begin to close with decreasing lung volumes. Aging or some disease processes (i.e., emphysema) can cause the lung to lose some of its elastic recoil, resulting in airway closure at larger lung volumes than normal. In some cases, airway closure may begin to occur at lung volumes greater than FRC. Areas of the lung distal to the closure may be perfused but are not ventilated, which may result in a deterioration of gas exchange.

The spirometer can be used to measure the volumes of air that can be moved into and out of the lung with respiratory effort. Because it is not possible to empty the lungs completely with maximal exhalation, specialized techniques are needed to measure any lung volume that includes the residual volume, i.e., the TLC, FRC, and RV itself. These typically involve the use of a helium dilution technique, a nitrogen washout method, or the body plethysmograph. The closing volume also requires special techniques for measurement, and it is usually expressed as a percentage of the vital capacity or total lung capacity. The details of these methods are beyond the scope of this chapter, but can be found in the references listed.

The lung is an elastic structure with an inherent tendency to recoil any time that it is stretched beyond its resting volume. This recoil is due to the network of collagenous and elastic fibers that are within the interstitial compartments of the lung and to the surface tension forces within the alveoli.

These surface tension forces are created by the air interface with the liquid film lining the alveoli. If one fills the lung with saline, the air-liquid interface is eliminated, thus negating these surface tension forces, and lower pressures are needed to inflate the lung to any given volume, i.e., improved compliance. Surface tension forces also affect the individual alveoli through the law of Laplace. This principle states that the pressure within a spherical alveolus is directly proportional to its surface tension and indirectly proportional to its radius. Therefore, two alveoli of different sizes but with the same surface tension would have different internal pressures. Smaller alveoli would have higher internal pressures than larger ones, thus causing the smaller alveoli to empty into the larger ones. Obviously the lung would be a very unstable structure if these surface tension forces were not decreased.

Surfactant, a phospholipid secreted by the type II pneumatocyte of the alveolus, lowers these surface tension forces. The reduction in surface tension is greater at smaller alveolar volumes. Surfactant, through its action on surface tension, thus has several important roles. First, it improves the compliance of the lung, thereby making it easier to in-flate. Second, it stabilizes the lung by preventing smaller alveoli from emptying into larger ones. Lastly, these surface tension forces tend to pull fluid from the vascular space as the alveoli collapse. By reducing this tendency, surfactant helps prevent fluid accumulation in the alveoli.

The chest wall is also an elastic structure that has a tendency to return to its resting position when displaced from it. The resting position of the chest wall occurs at approximately 75 per cent of the vital capacity. At lower volumes there is a tendency for the chest wall to recoil outward, whereas at greater volumes there is a tendency for the chest wall to recoil inward toward its resting volume.

The interplay of these two elastic structures, lung and chest wall, defines the elastic properties of the total respiratory system. The functional residual capacity is achieved when the inward tendency of the lung to recoil is exactly balanced by the outward tendency of the chest to expand. It is not until over 75 per cent of the vital capacity is obtained that both the lung and chest wall recoil in the same direction. These elastic properties of the lung and chest wall thus interplay to determine the subdivisions of the lung volume. Deformities of the chest wall, such as obesity and kyphoscoliosis, can have important effects on these lung volumes. Likewise, abnormalities within the lung parenchyma that affect these elastic properties also have similar effects. For example, such disorders as pulmonary fibrosis increase the elastic recoil of the lungs and thus decrease the FRC. Conversely, emphysema decreases the elastic recoil of the lung, resulting in an increase of the FRC.

Inspiration is initiated with contraction of the inspiratory muscles, which results in expansion of the chest cavity and a drop in the pleural pressure. As the lung expands, the alveolar pressure falls in relation to the mouth pressure, thus creating a pressure gradient down which fresh air flows into the lung. To initiate this flow three forces must be overcome: (1) tissue resistance, which is largely created by the elastic forces of the lung and chest wall as described above; (2) flow resistance within the airways; and (3) the inertial forces in the lung, thorax, and air. These inertial forces are felt to be minimal.

Resistance to air flow occurs mainly in the upper airway and in the larger parenchymal airways. Nasal breathing accounts for up to two thirds of the total airway resistance during quiet breathing. The oropharynx, larynx, and trachea contribute approximately 25 per cent of the airway resistance during quiet breathing, but up to 50 per cent if the minute ventilation is elevated. The peripheral airways (less than 2 mm in diameter) contribute less than 20 per cent of the total airway resistance. This is because, although they are small in size, the tremendous increase in the total cross-sectional airway at this level slows the forward velocity of the entrained air, and diffusion, rather than bulk flow, becomes the chief mode of gas transport. These small airways have been described as a "silent zone," as considerable narrowing of them must occur before the effects can be detected in the standard pulmonary function tests.

The resistance to gas flow in the airways is dependent on a number of factors, including the dimensions of the airways (length and especially radius) and the characteristics of the inhaled gas (viscosity and density). Expiratory flow resistance is also affected by the dynamic compression of the airways with forced expiratory efforts, especially at low lung volumes.

Gas flow in the airways can be characterized as being either turbulent, laminar, or transitional between the two. Laminar airflow is characterized as streamlined flow that is parallel to the sides of the tube. Resistance to such flow is proportional to the length of the airway and viscosity of the gas. Also, it is inversely proportional to the fourth power of the radius of the airway. Very small changes in the airway diameter thus can have a marked effect on resistance to this type of flow.

Turbulent flow represents a deterioration of the orderly progression of laminar flow. It occurs in the setting of high flow rates, areas of changing diameter, sharp bends, and at branch points in the airways. The driving pressure is related to the gas flow rate and the density of the gas (not viscosity in contrast to laminar flow).

The distribution of laminar and turbulent flow in the airways is thus dependent on the velocity of the air flow, airway diameter, and the ratio of the density of the gas to its viscosity. In the majority of the airways the flow is transitional between the two types, with fully developed turbulent flow probably only occurring in the trachea at high minute volumes (increased flow rates) and pure laminar flow most likely only occurring in the very small peripheral airways. Administration of a gas of low density, such as helium, reduces the resistance to turbulent flow and makes turbulent flow less likely to occur. Lung volume also has an effect on airway resistance. At increased lung volumes the airways are larger in diameter, thus reducing resistance to flow through them. At small lung volumes airway resistance increases. The level of bronchial muscle tone also has an important effect on the airway luminal diameter and therefore the resistance to air flow. Parasympathetic stimulation via the vagus nerve results in bronchial muscle constriction. Beta 2 adrenergic receptors on the bronchial smooth muscle cause bronchodilation, whereas alpha sympathetic stimulation has a bronchoconstrictor effect.

Reflex constriction of the bronchial smooth muscle is mediated via vagal afferents. A number of different stimuli can cause reflex constriction, including physical manipulation (i.e., laryngoscopy), foreign bodies, cold air, and chemical stimuli, i.e., nitrogen dioxide, sulphur dioxide, gastric acid. Other mediators of bronchoconstriction include histamine and certain arachidonic acid mediators, i.e., some prostaglandins and leukotrienes.

During exhalation an additional source of flow resistance comes from the dynamic compression of the airways. It has been demonstrated that the peak expiratory flow is dependent on patient effort, but after that flow is reached, increasing effort no longer causes the flow rate to increase. In fact at any given lung volume below 70 per cent of TLC there is a maximal attainable flow rate that cannot be increased with extra effort. This limitation is due to dynamic compression of the airway with forced efforts and the pressure drop that occurs along the airways with expiration.

With forced expiration alveolar pressure increases, forming a gradient for gas to flow from the alveoli to the airway opening. The air passages are also subjected to this increased pressure, which tends to narrow them (Fig. 10–2). At some point the pressure within the airway equals the applied expiratory pressure. Beyond this point (closer to the airway

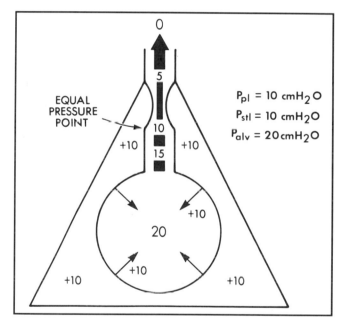

FIGURE 10–2. Schematic diagram of the equal pressure point concept. At a particular lung volume during forced expiration, pleural pressure (Ppl) = 10 cm H_2O, and static recoil pressure (Pst1) = 10 cm H_2O. The sum of these pressures, alveolar pressure (Palv) = 20 cm H_2O, is the driving pressure that must be dissipated as air flows along the airway to the mouth, where the pressure is zero. Accordingly, there must be a point along the airway at which the pressures inside and outside the wall are the same: the equal pressure point. Downstream (toward the mouth) from the equal pressure point, the airway is compressed because the pressure surrounding it is greater than the pressure in the lumen. (Adapted from Murray, J.F.: Respiration. *In* Smith, L.H., and Thier, S. (eds.): Pathophysiology. Philadelphia, W.B. Saunders Co., 1985, pp. 753–854.)

opening) the external pressure exceeds that in the airway, causing compression of the airway and thus limiting gas flow. Increasing effort will only cause compression more proximally in the airway so that the flow limitation remains. This situation should be contrasted with inspiration in which expansion of the lung tends to widen the airways so flow is not limited by effort. Expiratory flow is thus related to many factors, including effort (at high lung volumes), lung volume, elastic recoil of the lung, airway resistance, and the cross-sectional area of the airways.

The practical application of this principle occurs with pulmonary function testing. The forced expiratory volume in 1 second (FEV1) is related to effort only in the initial part of the measurement, i.e., at high lung volumes when flows are effort dependent. As the patient continues to exhale, flow then becomes independent of effort. Flow measured between 25 and 75 per cent of the VC is also relatively independent of patient effort (FEF 25-75). These measurements are very reproducible as they are not completely dependent on patient effort and thus are useful for diagnostic purposes.

Each inspired breath is not uniformly distributed throughout the lung. In the upright position there is a gradient of pleural pressure from the apex of the thorax to the base, which is created by gravity due to the weight of the lung. Pleural pressure thus increases from nondependent to dependent portions of the thorax. Alveoli in the nondependent areas are subjected to a greater distending pressure than those at the base and are therefore larger in size at FRC. This larger size also places them on a flatter portion of their compliance curve so that there is less increase in volume for a given change in pressure than for the smaller alveoli in the nondependent parts of the lung. As a result, with inspiration the basilar alveoli increase in size more than at the apex so that the total ventilation to the base is greater than that to the apex. One important physiologic consequence is that, because blood flow is also favored in dependent (basilar) parts of the lung, the ventilation/perfusion ratio is maintained so that gas exchange is optimal.

This gradient in pleural pressure has a somewhat different effect at low lung volumes. In this situation, the intrapleural pressure at the base may actually exceed the airway pressure, resulting in airway compression. Furthermore, the alveoli in the upper portions of the lung will be on a more favorable portion of their compliance curve. With inspiration the upper alveoli will expand, whereas no expansion of the basilar alveoli will occur until the local pleural pressure dips below the airway pressure. The end result is that at low lung volumes the nondependent portions of the lung ventilate better than those at the base. This compression of the airways occurs even in normal subjects at low lung volumes. With aging and the loss of some elastic recoil in the lung, the intrapleural pressure is lessened. This exaggerates this

effect so that airway closure may occur at higher lung volumes and possibly even at FRC,. This is one explanation for the decreased pulmonary efficiency found in older patients.

It should also be noted that the tidal breath may not be evenly distributed to all alveoli, even within a single region of the lung. This is due to local factors that may influence air flow into different areas of the lung. For example, regional decreases in compliance or increases in resistance cause those areas to fill slower than other alveoli. Again depending on the relationship to the pulmonary blood flow, there can be profound influences on ventilation/perfusion ratios, resulting in important effects on gas exchange.

THE PULMONARY CIRCULATION

The lung has a dual circulation, each of which serves a unique function. The bronchial circulation is derived from the systemic circulation (aorta or the upper intercostal vessels), comprises 0.5 to 2 per cent of the cardiac output, and provides nutrients to all the airways proximal to the terminal bronchioles. Most venous drainage from these vessels goes through bronchial veins into the azygous, hemizygous, or intercostal veins. Because a small portion of the bronchial venous drainage empties directly into the main pulmonary circulation, it comprises part of the shunt that can be found in the normal lung. It should be noted that, unlike the main pulmonary vasculature, these vessels have the capability to proliferate and may form the major vascular innervation to scar tissue and tumors within the lung.

The distal branches of the pulmonary artery follow the airways to the terminal respiratory units where the arterioles branch extensively such that the extensive capillary network formed maximizes the surface area available for gas exchange. The pulmonary venules and veins travel in the loose connective tissue in the lung, but not as intimately associated with the airways as is the arterial circulation.

The pulmonary circuit is a high-flow, low-pressure system, with the pressures being about one sixth that of the systemic arteries. The pulmonary capillary and venous pressures are, however, similar to the systemic circulation.

The pulmonary circulation contains 10 to 20 per cent of the total blood volume depending on posture, sympathetic tone, administered drugs, and cardiac function. The pulmonary circuit accepts the entire cardiac output at very low driving pressures, thus reflecting the low resistance of this circuit. Although low, the pulmonary vascular resistance is dependent on a number of factors.

The pulmonary vascular resistance is unique in its ability to decline with increasing vascular pressures. Two factors are responsible. First, as pulmonary arterial pressure rises, additional vessels are recruited,

[handwritten in left margin: ? all depends on flow rate]

thereby expanding the vascular bed and limiting the pressure increase. Second, the existing open vessels undergo further distension. This second effect is the predominant one, limiting the increase in pulmonary vascular resistance as pressures rise.

Pulmonary vascular resistance is also dependent on lung volume. At larger lung volumes the pulmonary vessels are stretched open so that the resistance they offer is lessened. At even higher lung volumes, however, the pulmonary capillaries are stretched thinner, which, as expected, will increase resistance. The overall effect is that, with inflation of the lung from a low lung volume, the pulmonary vascular resistance first falls as the extra-alveolar vessels are opened. As the lung is progressively inflated, resistance then starts to rise as the capillary bed is stretched thinner and thus creates greater resistance.

Other factors play a role in determining the pulmonary vascular resistance. The smooth muscle of the vessels are subject to both sympathetic and parasympathetic influences. Parasympathetic activation via acetylcholine has a weak vasodilatory action. Norepinephrine and epinephrine have a vasoconstrictor action and isoproterenol a vasodilator action based on their interactions with alpha and beta receptors, respectively. Other mediators with constrictor activity include histamine, serotonin, thromboxane A_2, and prostaglandins PGF and PGE. Vasodilators also include bradykinin, PGE1, and prostacyclin.

Disease processes that decrease the size of the pulmonary vascular bed may have a profound effect on pulmonary vasculature resistance. Due to the distensibility of this circuit, as well as the ability to recruit additional vessels, a large portion of the pulmonary vasculature must be obstructed or destroyed before substantial increases in pulmonary vascular resistance and pressure are noted. A wide variety of processes, ranging from emphysema to surgical resection, may result in destruction of the pulmonary vascular bed. Emboli may be thrombotic in nature or nonthrombotic (air, fat, amniotic fluid). Embolic events may create pulmonary hypertension not only because of their direct blockage of the pulmonary vascular bed but also due to a variety of mediators that may be released at the time of their impaction.

One of the crucial regulators of pulmonary vascular tone is the alveolar pO_2. Unlike the systemic circulation, the pulmonary vessels have little smooth muscle within their walls; thus, the degree of active control over them is weak. Redistribution of the blood flow by manipulation of the arteriolar tone as in the systemic circulation does not generally occur. Hypoxic vasoconstriction, however, is an important means of regulating the distribution of pulmonary flow and maintaining the optimal ventilation-perfusion relationships. In regions of alveolar hypoxia, the arteries constrict, resulting in a redistribution of the pulmonary blood flow away from the hypoxic region. This is largely the effect of the alveolar pO_2, rather than the arterial pO_2. The mechanism of this response is unknown. It does not seem to be dependent on neural connections nor has any particular mediator of this effect been isolated. It appears to be a direct effect of the alveolar hypoxemia on the local arterial vasculature. A number of vasodilators, such as nitroprusside, may "release" this phenomenon, which results in the perfusion of poorly ventilated hypoxic areas and therefore worsening arterial hypoxemia.

Given the low pressure nature of the pulmonary circuit, it should not be surprising that gravitational forces play an important role in the distribution of the pulmonary blood flow. There is a gradient of increasing hydrostatic pressure from the apex of the lung to its base in the upright patient. This creates several regions or zones that can be described based on the interplay of the alveolar distending pressure, pulmonary arterial pressure, and the pulmonary venous pressure (Fig. 10–3).

Zone I occurs at the apex of the lung and is a region where the alveolar pressure can sometimes be greater than the pulmonary artery or venous pressure so that no blood flow can occur. This does not occur in the normal lung as pulmonary arterial pressure is generally sufficient to overcome the alveolar pressure. If, however, arterial pressure is reduced (i.e., hypovolemia) or alveolar pressure is raised (i.e., mechanical ventilation), then zone I conditions can occur. Note that this ventilated but not perfused lung then functions as dead space and may have a significant effect on gas exchange.

Below zone I the pulmonary arterial pressure increases due to the hydrostatic gradient and is greater than the alveolar pressure. Venous pressure remains below both the pulmonary arterial and distending alveolar pressures. This lower venous pressure defines zone 2 where blood flow is determined by the difference between the pulmonary arterial and alveolar pressure. Venous pressure only has an effect on the blood flow when it exceeds the alveolar pressure.

In zone 3, the pulmonary arterial and venous pressures are greater than the alveolar pressure so that the alveolar pressure has no role in determining the blood flow. Here the pulmonary arterial pressure is the greatest so that the vessels are more distended, and more of them are recruited so that vascular resistance is minimized.

A fourth zone has been described in the most dependent part of the lung at low lung volumes (residual volume). In zone 4 there is a reduction in pulmonary perfusion, even though the relationship of the pulmonary arterial, venous, and alveolar pressures is unchanged as in zone 3. This occurs because vascular resistance is increased as the extra-alveolar vessels become compressed. In addition, should airway closure occur, local hypoxia may increase the resistance further because of hypoxic vasoconstriction. This will reduce the perfusion through this zone even more.

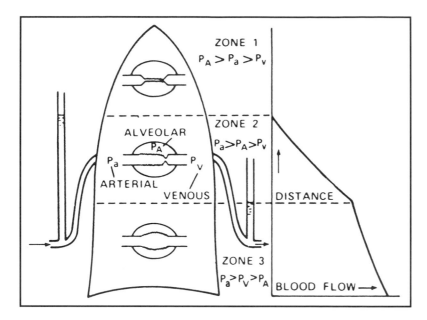

FIGURE 10–3. Model to explain the uneven distribution of blood flow in the lung based on the pressures affecting the capillaries. (Reprinted from West, J.B.: Respiratory Physiology—The Essentials, 4th ed. Baltimore, Williams & Wilkins Co., 1990. Figure 4.9, p. 41.)

GAS EXCHANGE

It is the intimate apposition of the alveolar air with the microcirculation that allows the lung to accomplish the exchange of oxygen and carbon dioxide. If the lung was a perfect gas exchanger, the alveolar pO_2 and pCO_2 would exactly equal the arterial pO_2 and pCO_2 as the blood leaves the lung, so that there would be no alveolar-arterial difference for either gas. In reality the lung is not perfect so that a small alveolar-arterial gradient exists for oxygen and carbon dioxide.

Diffusion is the process by which the molecules of a gas move from an area of high partial pressure through random motion to a region of lower partial pressure until an equilibrium is established. In the case of the lung a dynamic equilibrium is obtained due to the phasic nature of respiration, with the net movement of oxygen into the blood and carbon dioxide into the exhaled gas.

In a purely physical sense the degree and rate of gas diffusion across permeable membranes are directly related to the difference in partial pressures and the area of the membrane. Diffusion is *inversely* proportional to the thickness of the membrane. In addition, diffusion is dependent on the solubility and molecular weight of the gases involved. For example, carbon dioxide diffuses 20 times faster than oxygen because of its higher solubility. The large surface area of the lung at the blood-gas interface (50 to 100 square meters), as well as its thin surface (less than 0.5 μm), makes it uniquely constructed for rapid diffusion.

At sea level the alveolar pO_2 breathing room air is approximately 105 mm Hg. Given the pO_2 in the mixed venous blood entering the pulmonary capillaries of 40 mm Hg there is a large diffusion gradient down which oxygen will cross through the alveolar-capillary membrane and into the blood. The administration of supplemental oxygen greatly increases the alveolar pO_2, thereby enhancing the gradient for diffusion. Conversely, at high altitudes the pO_2 of the inspired air is much lower so that the gradient for diffusion is decreased. Similarly, a decrease in the inspired concentration of oxygen also diminishes the diffusion gradient. Carbon dioxide enters the pulmonary capillary with a partial pressure of 46 mm Hg and diffuses down its partial pressure gradient into the alveolus after which it equilibrates so that the end capillary pCO_2 is approximately 40 mm Hg.

It has been estimated that the average erythrocyte traverses the pulmonary capillary in approximately 0.75 seconds. Diffusion equilibrium for oxygen occurs within only 0.25 seconds, and CO_2 reaches equilibrium even faster. The lung therefore has a large reserve before diffusion becomes limited. In fact, diffusion limitation can only be demonstrated in normal subjects under conditions of decreased transit time (i.e., exercise) with a lowered diffusion gradient, (i.e., low alveolar pO_2) as at high altitudes. Most other processes that limit the diffusion process involve loss of functional membrane area. These include the destruction of pulmonary capillaries due to disease or surgical resection, poor alveolar ventilation, or impaired perfusion. Pathologic thickening of the diffusing membrane is rarely the cause of hypoxemia without the actual obliteration of alveolar spaces.

Thus, any process that interferes with diffusion will exaggerate the difference between the alveolar and arterial pO_2 and pCO_2 because of the inability of the pulmonary capillary blood to equilibrate with the alveolar gas. Yet, changes in ventilation or in the inspired concentration of gases will not change the alveolar-arterial difference. For example, hypoxemia will occur while breathing at high altitudes because alveolar-arterial equilibration occurs at the lower pO_2. Similarly, when alveolar ventilation is reduced, the alveolar pO_2 is also reduced so that equilibration across the alveolar capillary membrane takes place at a depressed pO_2. Alveolar hypoventilation results in elevation of the pCO_2 within the alveolus so that the arterial pCO_2 equilibrates at a higher level.

Pure hypoventilation is an uncommon cause of hypoxemia clinically. It can be seen in disorders that depress the central nervous system, such as with the administration of sedatives or anesthetic agents. It may also be seen in neuromuscular diseases that interfere with respiratory muscle function, such as myasthenia gravis or Guillian-Barre syndrome.

In clinical medicine the major cause of abnormal gas exchange is not abnormalities of diffusion or ventilation, but the mismatching of ventilation and perfusion. In the perfect lung the level of perfusion exactly matches that of ventilation so that maximal transfer of oxygen and carbon dioxide can occur. Equilibration takes place such that there is no difference between the alveolar and arterial pO_2 or pCO_2. The perfect lung would have no areas where ventilation would exceed perfusion resulting in "wasted" ventilation. Likewise, the perfect lung would have no areas where perfusion would be "wasted" by flowing through areas that are ventilated inadequately. Yet, all lungs have some mismatching of ventilation and perfusion that results in some inefficiency of gas exchange. Such inefficiencies are the major cause of the normal alveolar-arterial difference for oxygen and carbon dioxide. The degree to which this mismatch occurs significantly affects the gas exchange that is seen in disease states.

As has been described in an earlier section, there is a hydrostatic gradient in blood flow through the normal lung such that it is greater at the base and then decreases toward the apex. Similarly, ventilation also is increased at the base of the lung and decreases toward the apex due to differences in regional compliance. The rate at which ventilation and perfusion change as one moves from base to apex is not the same in that the blood flow falls off more rapidly. This results in an increasing ratio of ventilation to perfusion (V/Q) from the base of the lung to the apex. This inhomogeneity of V/Q ratios is one factor that accounts for the alveolar-arterial gradient found in even the normal lung.

It is important to note that the abnormalities of oxygenation or carbon dioxide excretion created by relative overventilation of some lung units (high V/Q) will not compensate for the underventilation of others (low V/Q). This occurs because of the nature of the oxyhemoglobin and CO_2 dissociation curves. For example at high pO_2s the hemoglobin becomes fully saturated, and further elevation of the pO_2 thus adds little to the total oxygen content (dissolved oxygen + hemoglobin bound) of the blood and cannot compensate (i.e. increase total oxygen content) for the inadequate oxygenation contributed by areas of low V/Q ratio.

In regions of the lung that are overventilated (high V/Q) relative to their perfusion, a portion of the total ventilation is essentially "wasted." In the extreme case the alveoli are ventilated but completely unperfused (V/Q = infinity), and thus they become part of the "dead space." Dead space is defined as regions of the lung that are ventilated but not perfused and can be divided into two parts. The anatomic dead space is composed of those airways without alveoli that obviously cannot participate in gas exchange. The size of the anatomic dead space in milliliters is roughly equal to the body weight in pounds. The second component of the dead space is the alveolar dead space that is composed of alveoli that are ventilated but not perfused. The physiologic dead space is defined as the sum of the alveolar and anatomic dead space.

Ventilation of the dead space decreases the amount of ventilation available to better perfused areas of the lung. The total minute ventilation is defined as the exhaled tidal volume multiplied by the respiratory rate. It can be divided into the alveolar ventilation and the dead space ventilation. The effect of increasing the dead space ventilation is to lower the alveolar ventilation unless total minute ventilation increases to compensate for it. The physiologic dead space is usually quantified as the ratio of dead space to the tidal volume (Vd/Vt). This can be calculated from the measurement of the mixed expired pCO_2 and the arterial pCO_2. The normal ratio is 0.2 to 0.35. Many factors can influence the size of the dead space, including age, posture, lung volume, artificial devices (i.e., endotracheal tubes, face masks etc.), hypoperfusion, embolism, and diseases that destroy the pulmonary vasculature.

In regions where perfusion greatly exceeds ventilation a portion of the perfusion is "wasted" as it is not adequately exposed to the alveolar gas for full equilibration to occur. In the extreme case, an area of the lung may be completely unventilated yet still be perfused (V/Q = 0), resulting in a shunt. Shunts can be described as being anatomic or physiologic. Anatomic shunts are those where desaturated blood is directly mixed with oxygenated blood (a right-to-left shunt) through direct vascular connections, i.e., a patent foramen ovale or a pulmonary AV malformation. Physiologic shunt (also known as venous admixture) refers to the contribution to the arterial blood from areas of relative hypoventilation to perfusion, i.e., low V/Q regions. The effect of venous admixture is to hinder the efficiency of gas exchange by returning to the arterial circulation blood that has not fully equilibrated with the alveolar gas, thus resulting in a gradient between the alveolar and arterial pO_2 and pCO_2.

In the normal lung there is a range of ventilation-perfusion ratios from the apex to the base. This partially accounts for the normal alveolar-arterial oxygen gradient that is present. In addition to this inherent V/Q mismatch, there is a certain amount of normal shunting that arises from two sources. First, connections between the bronchial circulation and the postalveolar pulmonary capillaries form a pathway by which desaturated blood is added to the circulation. In addition a small amount of desaturated blood empties directly into the left ventricle from the thesbian veins of the heart. In general the normal shunt comprises only about 5 per cent of the cardiac output.

In disease states a wide range of ventilation-perfusion ratios can be found. Regional differences in airway mechanics and compliance may exaggerate the normal regional differences in ventilation through the lung. Similar differences in perfusion result in a wide range of V/Q ratios that increase the alveolar-arterial gradient and thus lead to increased inefficiency of gas exchange. Some areas of high V/Q ratio act as dead space, whereas other areas of low V/Q ratio act effectively as a shunt. The net effect is that the arterial oxygenation declines. Note that V/Q mismatch also interferes with carbon dioxide excretion. The body senses this tendency for the carbon dioxide to rise and responds by increasing the total minute ventilation, which thus restores the pCO_2 to normal. If the body is unable to raise its minute ventilation as, for example, in respiratory muscle fatigue, then the pCO_2 will rise and the pH will fall.

The degree of pure shunt can be differentiated from other causes of V/Q mismatch by the response to the administration of 100 per cent oxygen. Shunted blood is never exposed to alveolar gas so that in a patient with a significant shunt the administration of pure oxygen will have little impact on the shunted blood or blood coming from alveoli with very low V/Q ratios. This is in contrast to regions of the lung with V/Q mismatch in which, given enough time for equilibration, the arterial pO_2 will eventually rise. If one measures the alveolar-arterial difference on 100 per cent oxygen, one finds that the effect of the shunted blood is to augment this discrepancy. The arterial pO_2 will rise because of the effects on nonshunted blood, but the alveolar-arterial oxygen gradient will be magnified due to the effects of the shunt.

OXYGEN/CARBON DIOXIDE TRANSPORT

Oxygen is transported in the blood in two forms: the dissolved form that is carried in physical solution and that which is carried by hemoglobin in the red blood cells. The oxygen content of the blood is defined as the sum of the dissolved and hemoglobin-bound oxygen. Oxygen delivery is the amount of oxygen transported to the tissues per minute and is the product of the cardiac output and the oxygen content.

The amount of dissolved oxygen in the blood is a function of the partial pressure of oxygen, representing 0.003 mL O_2/100 mL blood for each mm Hg of pO_2. Note that at the normal pO_2 of 100 mm Hg this represents only 0.3 mL O_2/100 mL of blood. Hemoglobin is capable of carrying 1.34 mL of oxygen per gram of hemoglobin. The total amount of hemoglobin-bound oxygen is determined by the saturation of the hemoglobin and the absolute amount of hemoglobin in the blood. Under normal conditions the amount carried by the hemoglobin measures 19.58 mL O_2/100 mL blood. Thus, the dissolved oxygen represents only approximately 1 per cent of the total oxygen content. In terms of oxygen transport the mildly hypoxic and anemic patient therefore benefits far more from a transfusion than from an elevation of pO_2.

The hemoglobin molecule consists of four protein chains, each of which carries a heme moiety. The amino acid sequence of the protein chains determines the type of hemoglobin. The heme moiety that actually binds the oxygen contains iron in the ferrous state (+2). Each molecule of hemoglobin thus can carry four molecules of oxygen.

A variety of hemoglobin forms have been found normally and in pathologic conditions. Normal adult hemoglobin consists of two alpha and two beta chains. Fetal hemoglobin (HbF), which has a higher affinity for oxygen than adult hemoglobin, has two alpha and two gamma chains. Hemoglobin A2 forms 2 per cent of the adult hemoglobin and contains two alpha and two delta chains. A large number of abnormal hemoglobins have been identified by abnormal sequences of amino acids in the protein chains. Sickle hemoglobin (HbS), for example, has a valine substitution for glutamic acid in the beta chains. This results in a decreased solubility in the deoxygenated form, which causes a change in the shape of the hemoglobin to a sickle configuration under hypoxic conditions. The iron in the heme moiety can be oxidized to the ferric (+3) form by a variety of agents, such as nitrites and sulfonamides, resulting in the formation of methemoglobin. Methemoglobin is incapable of combining with oxygen and can be reduced back to the ferrous form with ascorbic acid or methylene blue.

The hemoglobin saturation can be related to the oxygen tension (pO_2) though the oxygen dissociation curve (Fig. 10–4). The curve has a characteristic shape that defines a number of important properties. First, at high levels of pO_2 the curve becomes quite flat, meaning that there is progressively less increase in hemoglobin saturation and therefore blood oxygen content as the pO_2 is increased. In this range, minor fluctuations in the pO_2 have little effect on total oxygen content. Furthermore, oxygen loading in the lung is enhanced as a large partial pressure gradient for oxygen diffusion is maintained even

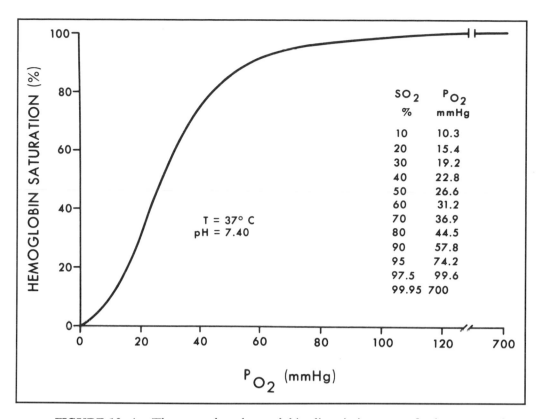

FIGURE 10–4. The normal oxyhemoglobin dissociation curve for humans. Values for hemoglobin saturation (S_{O2}) at different P_{O2} values, under standard conditions of temperature and pH, are indicated. (Data from Severinghaus JW.: Blood oxygen dissociation line charts: Man. *In* Altman, P.C., and Dittmer, D.S. (eds.): Respiration and Circulation. Bethesda, Federation of Experimental Biology, 1971, pp. 204–206. Reprinted from Murray, J.F.: The Normal Lung, 2nd ed. Philadelphia, W.B. Saunders Co., 1986. Figure 7.7, p. 174.)

though the hemoglobin becomes fully saturated. Conversely, on the initial portion of the curve the shape of the pO_2 and saturation curve is steeper so that small changes in partial pressure have a large effect on saturation. This is advantageous at the tissue level as it means that only a small partial pressure gradient is needed between the capillaries and the oxygen in order to unload the hemoglobin. In the hypoxemic patient the consequence of this linear relationship is that the patient's oxygen content and therefore oxygen delivery can be seriously compromised by any small decline in arterial pO_2. Conversely, significant improvement can occur through the administration of supplemental oxygen that increases the pO_2 of the arterial blood.

This oxygen dissociation curve can be shifted to the right or left by a number of conditions. The P50 is a measure of the partial pressure of oxygen needed to saturate 50 per cent of the hemoglobin and thus serves as a marker of the position of the dissociation curve. The normal P50 corresponds to a pO_2 of 26.6 mm Hg. A shift of the curve to the left (a lower P50) implies that less partial pressure is needed to saturate the hemoglobin; thus, it is a marker of increased affinity of the hemoglobin for oxygen. A shift to the right (higher P50) indicates that additional partial pressure is needed to saturate the hemoglobin; thus, its affinity for oxygen is decreased.

The dissociation curve may be shifted to the right (increased P50) under several conditions. An elevated temperature, increased pCO_2, or a decreased pH cause a shift to the right. 2,3-Diphosphoglycerate (2,3-DPG) is manufactured in red blood cells and serves to lower the affinity of hemoglobin for oxygen in the erythrocyte, thereby favoring the unloading of oxygen to the tissues. Carbon dioxide affects the affinity of hemoglobin for oxygen mainly through its effect on pH, which is known as the Bohr effect. At the tissue level these changes enhance the unloading of the hemoglobin.

The oxygen dissociation curve is shifted to the left (lower P50 or increased oxygen affinity) under conditions opposite to the above. An increased pH, lower pCO_2, or lower temperature all cause a left shift of the oxygen dissociation curve. Note that such conditions occur in the lungs relative to the tissues, thus enhancing the oxygenation of the blood in the lung. A deficiency of 2,3-DPG as may occur when red blood cells are stored in the blood bank under certain conditions can also cause a shift to the right, thereby interfering with oxygen unloading at the tissue level.

Carbon monoxide can have a profound effect on the transport of oxygen in the blood. Carbon monoxide binds to hemoglobin with an affinity 240 times that of oxygen. Therefore, at very low partial pressures of carbon monoxide the hemoglobin will become fully saturated with it so that little is available for oxygen transport. Furthermore, carbon monoxide causes a left shift of the oxygen dissociation curve, thus interfering with the unloading of oxygen at the tissue level. It is crucial to note that carbon monoxide does not interfere with the amount of oxygen carried in the blood in the dissolved form, i.e., pO_2. A patient who has been exposed to a large dose of carbon monoxide may therefore have a relatively normal pO_2, yet have a serious deficiency of oxygen-carrying capacity.

Oxygen saturation can be assessed noninvasively to varying degrees. Cyanosis refers to the bluish discoloration of the skin and mucous membranes caused by sufficient quantities of desaturated hemoglobin (felt to be at least 5 grams reduced hemoglobin per 100 mL of capillary blood) in the circulation. It can be difficult to detect in anemic patients and under varying conditions of ambient light and skin pigmentation. Pulse oximetry utilizes the absorption of specific wavelengths of light by oxygenated and deoxygenated hemoglobin through the tissues to give a more precise noninvasive measure of arterial saturation.

Carbon dioxide is carried in the blood in three forms. The dissolved carbon dioxide is that portion carried in physical solution in the blood. Carbon dioxide is 20 times more soluble than oxygen in blood. However, dissolved carbon dioxide accounts for only 5 per cent of the total CO_2 in the arterial blood.

Most of the carbon dioxide is carried as bicarbonate, which is formed from the dissociation of carbonic acid. This process occurs when CO_2 diffuses into erythrocytes where it combines with water in the presence of the enzyme carbonic anhydrase to form carbonic acid. The carbonic acid then disassociates without the need for a special enzyme into bicarbonate and hydrogen ions. The bicarbonate diffuses out into the plasma in exchange for chloride ions. The intracellular hydrogen ions may then react with hemoglobin, especially in the reduced form, so that the presence of deoxygenated hemoglobin actually enhances carbon dioxide transport.

The third form in which carbon dioxide is carried in the blood is in the form of carbamino compounds. These are formed from the combination of carbon dioxide with the terminal amine group in some blood proteins. Hemoglobin is the most important of these proteins. Deoxygenated hemoglobin has approximately 3.5 times the ability to combine with

carbon dioxide as does oxygenated hemoglobin. In terms of the total CO_2 content of the blood, the carbamino compounds account for only a small proportion of the total carbon dioxide content.

The presence of reduced (deoxygenated) hemoglobin enhances the carrying of carbon dioxide in the blood for the two reasons noted above. Clearly, this is of benefit at the tissue level where oxygen is unloaded and then carbon dioxide must be carried away. This property by which deoxygenated hemoglobin enhances carbon dioxide transport is known as the Haldane effect. The ability of the hemoglobin to forms carbamino compounds accounts for most of the Haldane effect.

A carbon dioxide dissociation curve can be constructed much like the oxygen dissociation curve (Fig. 10–5). It differs from the oxygen dissociation curve in that it is much more linear and steeper. A different curve can be constructed for each level of hemoglobin saturation because of the Haldane effect.

CONTROL OF RESPIRATION

The control of the respiratory system is complex because not only is it concerned with the exchange of oxygen and carbon dioxide but it also plays a role in a number of nonrespiratory functions. These other functions are voluntary, such as speech; partially voluntary, such as eating; and also completely involun-

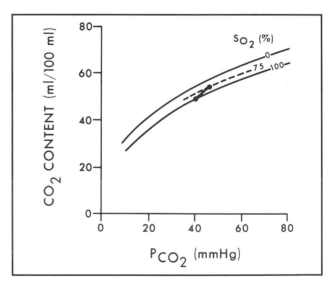

FIGURE 10–5. Normal CO_2 equilibration (dissociation) curves for whole blood at 0, 75, and 100 per cent oxyhemoglobin saturation (S_{O2}). The heavy line connecting the two points shows the usual extent of the Haldane effect in arterial and venous blood. (Reprinted from Murray, J.F.: The Normal Lung, 2nd ed. Philadelphia, W.B. Saunders Co., 1986. Figure 7.10, p. 180.)

tary, such as acid-base homeostasis. The system undergoes controls at many different levels, including the brain, spinal cord, and peripheral organs (lungs, airways, respiratory muscles, and the like). A number of reflexes involve several of these levels; however, it is possible to override some of these reflexes and control the system on an entirely voluntary basis.

The respiratory system is regulated by controllers within the central nervous system (CNS), sensors in both the periphery and CNS, and effector mechanisms involving the upper airway, lungs, and muscles of respiration. The degree of regulation is enormous, ranging from unconscious rhythmic respiration to the precise respiratory control of the professional singer. These control mechanisms integrate the respiratory function of the lungs with a wide variety of nonrespiratory functions, such as speech, eating, singing, sneezing, and coughing.

The medulla is the location of the main controllers of automatic respiration. There are two bilateral groups of respiratory neurons that most likely interact to form the basic respiratory rhythm, although the precise mechanism for this occurrence is unclear. The dorsal respiratory group (DRG) consists mainly of inspiratory neurons, whereas the ventral respiratory group (VRG) has neurons with both inspiratory and expiratory activity. It is felt that the DRG most likely receives information from visceral afferents from the ninth and tenth cranial nerves. After processing them, the DRG transmits its modifications both through inspiratory neurons in the VRG and through inspiratory neurons (mainly phrenic) in the spinal cord. The VRG receives inputs from the DRG and projects its axons onto other spinal motor neurons, especially the intercostal, abdominal, and accessory muscles of respiration. The VRG does not appear to be a site for the integration of afferent sensory information in contrast to the DRG, nor does it transmit any impulses to the DRG.

Other centers of respiratory control have also been identified. Two areas have been localized in the pons and most likely act on the other medullary centers to modify respiratory activity. These include the apneustic center, which appears to play a role in terminating inspiration, and the pneumotaxic center, which is felt to play a role in controlling the pattern of breathing in response to afferent stimuli, such as hypoxia or hypercarbia. The voluntary control of breathing originates from the cerebral cortex. These neuronal pathways are separate from those that govern automatic respiration.

At the spinal cord level, local reflexes are integrated with efferent information from the supraspinal centers. The peripheral respiratory efferents are modified by a large variety of receptors located within the respiratory muscles, airways, and lung. These include stretch receptors within the smooth muscle of the airways and irritant receptors in the nasal mucosa, upper airways, and tracheobronchial tree. Juxtapulmonary-capillary (type J) receptors are located in the walls of the pulmonary capillaries or the interstitium and respond to a variety of influences. Afferent signals travel within the vagus (tenth) nerve or other cranial nerves in the case of the upper airway. Receptors located in muscles, tendons, and joints can also affect ventilation and play an important role in modifying the respiratory response to increased workloads.

The chemical control of breathing is regulated both peripherally and centrally. Peripheral chemoreceptors are found in the carotid and aortic bodies, although in the human the influence of the aortic bodies is felt to be minimal. The carotid body is a complex network of axons, blood vessels, and specialized cells that lies at the bifurcation of the common carotid arteries. Afferent signals travel through the carotid sinus nerve to the CNS via the ninth cranial nerve. Some efferent input to the carotid bodies appears to come from sympathetic fibers originating from the superior cervical ganglion. The actual chemosensitive cell in this complex collection of neurons and specialized cells is unknown.

The carotid body chemoreceptors increase their activity in response to a decreased arterial pO_2 (not arterial oxygen content), increased arterial pCO_2, or low arterial pH. Two simultaneous stimuli have a synergistic effect on the carotid body output. The carotid bodies also respond to decreased blood flow, as may occur with hypotension or in vasoconstricted states. It is felt that the carotid bodies are solely responsible for the hypoxic ventilatory response. They contribute approximately 20 to 30 per cent of the response to breathing increased carbon dioxide mixtures, with the central chemoreceptors having a more important influence. They also play an important role in the ventilatory response to the acute metabolic acidosis of exercise.

Central chemoreceptors have also been isolated. Three bilateral areas in the medulla, independent of the central respiratory control areas (VRG, DRG), have been identified. These chemoreceptors react in response to the pCO_2 and pH in the cerebrospinal fluid (CSF). Unlike the peripheral chemoreceptors, they do not respond to hypoxemia. They are isolated from the systemic circulation by the blood-brain barrier. It should be noted that carbon dioxide readily diffuses into the CSF across the blood-brain barrier as contrasted to hydrogen ions and bicarbonate. This accounts for the observation that the ventilatory response to a respiratory acidosis is greater than that to a metabolic acidosis for the same change in pH.

Hypoxic drive is mediated by the response of the carotid bodies to a decreased arterial pO_2. A reduction in the oxygen content (i.e., anemia) does not stimulate respiration as long as the pO_2 is maintained. The ventilation-pO_2 response curve (Fig. 10–6) is hyperbolic such that a significant rise in ventilation does not occur until the pO_2 drops below 60 mm Hg. The response to hypoxemia varies widely and may

do not respond to ↓O_2 [handwritten margin note]

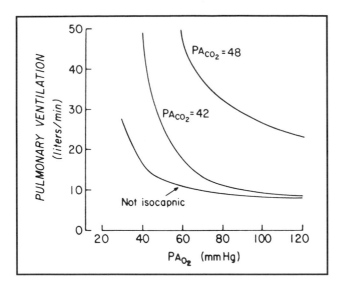

FIGURE 10–6. Ventilatory responses to alterations in alveolar O_2 (P_{AO2}) under both nonisocapnic and two levels of isocapnic conditions. (Data from the study of Loeschcke, H.H., and Gertz, K.H.: Einfluss des O_2-Druckes in der Einatmungsluft auf die Atemtätigkeit des Menschen, geprüft unter Konstanthaltung des alveolaren CO_2-Druckes. Pflügers Arch. Ges. Physiol., *267*:460–477, 1958. Reprinted from Burger, A.J.: The control of breathing. *In* Murray, J.F., and Nadal, J.A. (eds.): Textbook of Respiratory Medicine. Philadelphia, W.B. Saunders Co., 1988. Figure 7–6, p. 161.)

be absent in some otherwise normal people. Hypoxic sensitivity deceases with increasing age, acclimatization to high altitudes, and the administration of sedatives. Decreased hypoxic sensitivity contributes to disease states in some patients with chronic lung disease and morbid obesity. Exercise and hypercapnia enhance the response to hypoxemia.

The hypercapnic drive is largely mediated by the central chemoreceptors, with the carotid bodies accounting for only 20 to 30 per cent of the response to an increased pCO_2. In contrast to the hypoxic response, the hypercapnic response is linear within the clinical range and quite sensitive (Fig. 10–7). Hypoxemia potentiates the response to hypercarbia. Again, there is a wide variation among individuals. At very high levels, carbon dioxide acts as a respiratory depressant (pCO_2 over 70 mm Hg). The CO_2 response curve decreases with age, endurance training, sedation, anesthetics, and in some disease states.

RESPIRATORY MUSCLE PHYSIOLOGY

The diaphragm is the most important muscle of inspiration. It consists of a central tendinous portion from which its muscular fibers originate. The muscular portion of the diaphragm can be divided into its crural and costal portions. The crural portion

attaches to the first three lumbar vertebrae, as well as to the medial and lateral arcuate ligaments. The costal portion attaches to the xiphoid process and the lower six ribs. The motor innervation of the diaphragm is from the phrenic nerve (cervical roots 3, 4, and 5), whereas sensory innervation originates from intercostal nerves.

Functionally the diaphragm should be thought of as a piston, with the muscular portion forming its sides and the dome of the diaphragm forming the top of the piston. Contraction of the muscular fibers results in a piston-like downward displacement of the dome of the diaphragm so that the thoracic cavity is expanded while the abdominal compartment is compressed. This same action also serves to elevate the lower ribs.

Other muscles may also play a role in inspiration. These include the scalenes, external intercostals, parasternal internal intercostals, and the sternocleidomastoids. Traditionally these have been considered to be "accessory" muscles of inspiration because they were felt to be active only during times of increased respiratory efforts. However, more recent evidence suggests that the scalene muscles and the parasternal intercostal muscles may be active even during quiet respiration. The parasternal internal intercostal muscles, which have interchondral attachments as opposed to the more lateral internal intercostals that have interosseous attachments be-

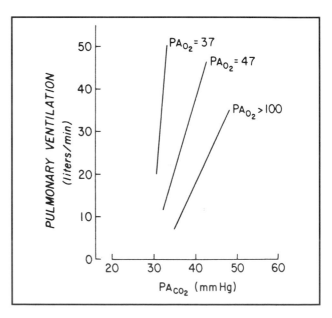

FIGURE 10–7. Ventilatory responses to alterations in alveolar CO_2 (P_{AOC2}) at three different levels of alveolar O_2 (P_{AO2}). (Data from Nielsen, M., and Smith, H.: Studies on the regulation of respiration in acute hypoxia. Acta Physiol. Scand., *24:*293–313, 1952. Reprinted from Burger, A.J.: The control of breathing. *In* Murray, J.F., and Nadal, J.A. (eds.): Textbook of Respiratory Medicine. Philadelphia, W.B. Saunders Co., 1988. Figure 7–5, p. 161.)

tween the ribs, have an inspiratory function by elevating the ribs and depressing the sternum. The scalene muscles (medial, posterior, and anterior) arise from the transverse processes of the lower cervical vertebrae and insert on the upper two ribs. They also serve to elevate the rib cage. The sternocleidomastoids, which raise the sternum and expand the upper rib cage, and the external intercostals, which also elevate the ribs, are most likely true "accessory" muscles that are active only during times of increased inspiratory efforts.

At rest, expiration is a passive event as the lung and chest wall recoil from their expanded position back to their resting position at FRC. With increased respiratory effort, expiration becomes an active phenomenon, with the abdominal muscles playing the most important role. They lower the rib cage and increase the intra-abdominal pressure, which forces the diaphragm back to its resting position. The interosseous portion of the internal intercostal muscles also has an expiratory function by lowering the ribs.

Recently, much attention has been given to the role of the respiratory muscles in ventilatory failure. Failure of the respiratory muscle pump can be a primary cause of ventilatory failure (i.e., Guillian-Barre syndrome) or an important contributing cause when the respiratory muscles become fatigued. Respiratory muscle fatigue can arise from factors that increase the demands on the respiratory muscles such as increased airway resistance or poor lung compliance, or from factors that compromise the energy stores of the respiratory muscle pump, such as low cardiac output states or malnutrition.

NONRESPIRATORY FUNCTIONS OF THE LUNG

The lungs have a number of important functions that are not directly related to gas exchange. Because the lung receives virtually the entire venous return, it is well situated to filter out particulate matter that would otherwise affect the arterial circulation. Thrombotic emboli originating from the deep venous system are probably the most common such matter. However, a wide variety of nonthrombotic emboli have been documented. These include air,

fat, amniotic fluid, and septic emboli. Paradoxical embolization is said to occur when embolic material bypasses the lungs and gains access directly to the systemic circulation, generally via intracardiac shunts.

The lung also plays a major role in the metabolism of certain vasoactive substances. The most well known is the conversion of angiotensin I into the powerful vasoconstrictor angiotensin II within the lung utilizing angiotensin-converting enzyme (ACE). The lung is a major site of this conversion (although not the only site) due to the large amount of ACE associated with the extensive pulmonary endothelium. Other substances that are extensively removed or inactivated by the lung include bradykinin, serotonin, norepinephrine, ATP, AMP, certain prostaglandins, and leukotrienes.

SUMMARY

Virtually all surgical procedures have some impact on lung function either directly as with a pneumonectomy or indirectly as through the effects of anesthesia or analgesics. This impact is evident in the large number of respiratory complications that can occur in the postoperative period. Such complications can be trivial, or they can contribute significantly to the patient's perioperative morbidity and mortality. A thorough knowledge of basic pulmonary physiology is mandatory not only to understand the potential impact of surgical procedures on the respiratory system but also to effectively treat and prevent these potential complications.

BIBLIOGRAPHY

1. Murray, J.F.: The Normal Lung, 2nd ed. Philadelphia, W.B. Saunders Co., 1986.
2. Nunn, J.F.: Applied Respiratory Physiology, 3rd ed. London, Butterworths, 1987.
3. West, J.B.: Respiratory Physiology—The Essentials, 4th ed. Baltimore, Williams & Wilkins Co., 1990.
4. Murray, J.F., and Nadel, J.A. (eds.): Textbook of Respiratory Medicine. Philadelphia, W.B. Saunders Co., 1988.

11

CARDIAC FUNCTION

ROBERT D. DOWLING *and* BARTLEY P. GRIFFITH

CARDIAC FUNCTION

The heart is a muscular blood pump that, in the average man, weighs 320 gm and, in the average woman, 280 gm. The heart consists of four chambers: two atria and two ventricles.

The atria are low-pressure, thin wall chambers, whereas the ventricles are high-pressure chambers. The muscle cell layer of the ventricle consists of a complex spiral of cells, the fiber orientation of which provides for a maximum decrease in left ventricular size with a minimal increase in tension development. The heart and the root of the great vessels are surrounded by the pericardium, which is a fibrous sac consisting of a fibrous and serous layer. The fibrous layer of the pericardium serves to limit the motion of the heart. The serous layer of the pericardium is divided into a parietal layer that lines the fibrous pericardium and a visceral layer that is applied to the surface of the heart. The visceral layer of pericardium is also called the epicardium. The space between the visceral and parietal layers contains a few milliliters of serous fluid, which serves to lubricate the heart within the confines of its sac. The one-way flow of blood through the heart is achieved by the presence of valves between the atria and ventricles and at the openings of the aorta and pulmonary artery. The atrioventricular valves are supported by chordae tendineae—fibrous strands connecting the ventricular papillary muscle to the edge of the valve leaflets. The chordae tendineae function to bring the valve leaflets together and prevent their eversion into the atria during ventricular systole.

Innervation

The heart is innervated by both components of the autonomic nervous system. Cardiac parasympathetic fibers originate in the medulla oblongata and travel to the heart via tha vagus nerve. Although there is considerable overlap, the main supply to the sinoatrial node (SAN) is from the right vagus nerve,

whereas the main supply to the atrioventricular node (AVN) is via the left vagus nerve. The ventricles are poorly innervated with parasympathetic nerve fibers. The postganglionic sympathetic nerve fibers travel to the heart via the great blood vessels from the paravertebral chain of ganglia (C2 to T2). The entire heart is richly innervated with postganglionic sympathetic fibers that form an extensive epicardial plexus. Some of the postganglionic sympathetic fibers join the vagus nerve and are distributed to the SAN and AVN. Sensory endings for afferent impulses are located in the walls of the coronary arteries, the myocardium, and the pericardium. The sensory nerves travel with both sympathetic fibers and the vagus nerve.

Blood Supply

The blood supply to the heart is of major importance, as the leading cause of death in the United States is coronary artery disease. The right and left coronary arteries are the first two branches of the aorta; they originate at the base of the sinuses of Valsalva behind the aortic valve cusps (Fig. 11–1). The right coronary artery (RCA) arises from the anterior (right) aortic sinus and runs to the right in the atrioventricular groove. Early in its course, the right coronary artery gives off branches to the right ventricle, as well as to the sinoatrial node artery that supplies the right atrium and the SAN. The right coronary artery then passes to the inferior border of the heart where it gives off small branches that supply the right atrium and the right ventricle and a constant marginal branch that descends along the right ventricle to the apex of the heart. The right coronary artery then continues around to the posterior heart where it gives off an AVN artery and its largest branch, the posterior interventricular artery. The RCA continues on to anastomose with the circumflex branch of the left coronary artery (LCA), while the posterior interventricular artery courses in the interventricular groove to the apex of the heart,

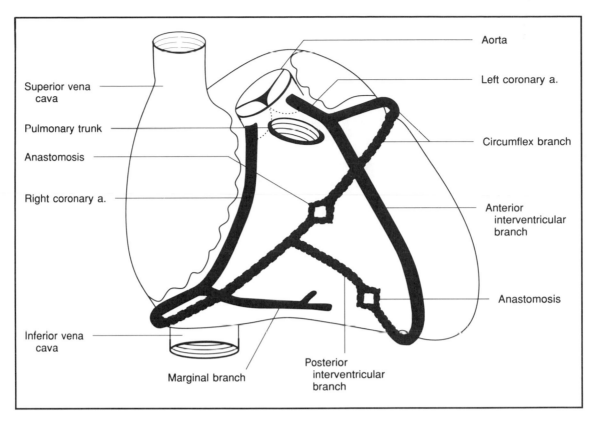

FIGURE 11–1. The major coronary arteries. Usually, the right and left coronary arteries share equally in the blood supply, but the posterior interventricular branch comes off the circumflex in about 15 per cent of hearts. (Reprinted from Moore, K.L.: Clinically Oriented Anatomy, 2nd ed. Baltimore, Williams & Wilkins, 1985. Figure 1–57.)

supplying both ventricles and part of the interventricular septum.

The left coronary artery (left main coronary artery) arises from the left aortic sinus and passes between the main pulmonary artery and the left atrium (Fig. 11–1). After emerging from behind the pulmonary artery, the LCA divides into two main branches, the left anterior interventricular branch (left anterior descending artery) and the left circumflex artery. The left anterior descending coronary artery continues in the interventricular groove to the apex of the heart, supplying both ventricles and the interventricular septum. The circumflex artery follows the coronary groove around the left border of the heart to the posterior surface of the heart, giving off a marginal branch along the way. The circumflex artery terminates by anastomosing with the right coronary artery.

The coronary sinus is the main vein of the heart, and its major tributaries are the great cardiac vein, the middle cardiac vein, and the small cardiac vein (Fig. 11–2). The great cardiac vein drains the area supplied by the left coronary artery. The middle cardiac and small cardiac veins drain the area of the heart supplied by the right coronary artery. The anterior cardiac veins begin on the anterior surface of the right atrium and travel across the coronary groove to empty directly into the right atrium. The oblique vein of the left atrium empties into the coronary sinus. The thesbian veins (venae cordis minimi) begin in the myocardium and empty directly into the atria.

A plexus of lymphatics is formed in both the endocardium and epicardium. The efferent lymphatics travel with the coronary arteries, eventually emptying into pretracheal lymph nodes.

Embryology

The cardiovascular system is the first system to develop in utero. After conception the early embryo obtains nutrients by diffusion from surrounding tissue. However, the embryo grows so rapidly that by the end of the third week simple diffusion of nutrients is no longer able to sustain life. Thus, early development of the cardiovascular system is essential, and circulation of blood occurs by the beginning of the fourth week postconception.

The cardiovascular system is derived from mesenchymal tissue that is referred to as angioblastic tissue. This angioblastic tissue forms angiogenic clusters

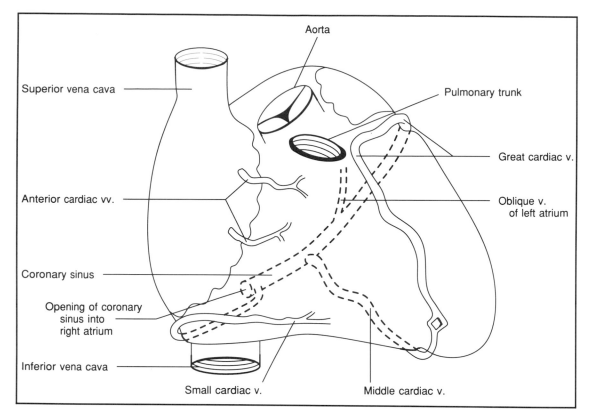

FIGURE 11–2. Anterior view of the cardiac veins. The coronary sinus runs in the posterior coronary sulcus and enters the right atrium. Although most veins empty into the coronary sinus, some small veins empty directly into the chambers. (Reprinted from Moore, K.L.: Clinically Oriented Anatomy, 2nd ed. Baltimore, Williams & Wilkins, 1985. Figure 1–66.)

that coalesce to form a plexus of blood vessels. The central portion of this plexus is known as the cardiogenic area, and it is here that the paired cardiogenic cords appear. The cardiogenic cords fuse in the midline to form a single heart tube (Fig. 11–3) that continues to differentiate to form a primitive atrium and common ventricle. Differentiation continues with formation of septa that divide the heart into four chambers (Fig. 11–4).

Formation of the cardiac septa occurs between the 27th and 37th days postconception. Partition of the primitive atria occurs by formation and subsequent modification of two distinct septa (septum primum and septum secundum) and fusion of the septa with the endocardial cushions (Fig. 11–4). The septum primum, so named because it is the first septum to develop, grows downward from the roof of the primitive atrium toward the endocardial cushions. The opening between the free edge of the septum primum and the endocardial cushions is called the foramen primum. The foramen primum eventually disappears as the septum primum continues to grow downward toward the endocardial cushions, with which it will eventually fuse. Before the foramen primum disappears, perforations occur in the upper portion of the septum primum. These perforations

coalesce to form the foramen secundum. This is followed by the formation of the septum secundum from the roof of the primitive atrium to the right of the septum primum. The septum secundum grows downward and eventually overlaps the foramen secundum. The portion of the septum primum that is attached to the roof of the atrium gradually disappears. The foramen that exists in the septum primum is now overlapped by the septum secundum and is referred to as the foramen ovale.

Simultaneous with the formation of the atrial septa, outgrowths of mesenchymal tissue form in the AV canal, which is the area between the primitive atrium and ventricles. These outgrowths eventually fuse, allowing for complete division of the atria and ventricle chambers.

Formation of the ventricular septum also occurs during the fourth to sixth week postconception. The ventricular septum has a muscular and a membranous portion. Formation of the muscular portion of the septum occurs by outgrowth and fusion of the medial walls of the primitive ventricle. The membranous portion of the ventricular septum is formed by the inferior aspect of the endocardial cushions that normally fuses with the muscular septum.

Abnormalities in septum formation are the most

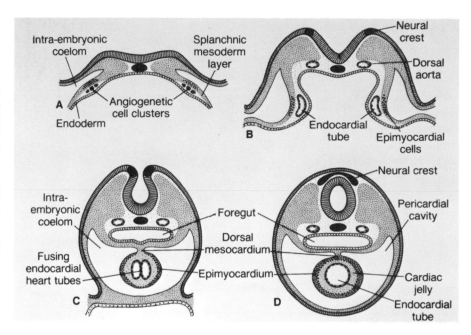

FIGURE 11–3. Schematic transverse sections through embryos during early development, showing the formation of a single heart tube from paired primordia. *A*, Early presomite embryo (approximately 17 days); *B*, late presomite embryo (approximately 18 days); *C*, at four somites (approximately 21 days); *D*, at eight somites (approximately 22 days). (Reprinted from Sadler, T.W.: Langman's Medical Embryology, 5th ed. Baltimore, Williams & Wilkins, 1985. Figure 12–3, P. 171.)

common cause of congenital heart defects. Abnormalities in formation of the atrial septum account for 10 to 15 per cent of all patients with congenital heart disease. The most common type of atrial septal defect, ostium secundum defect, is caused by either inadequate development of the septum secundum or excessive resorption of the septum primum (Fig. 11–5). A less frequent type of atrial septal defect is the ostium primum defect, which results from incomplete fusion of the septum primum with the endocardial cushions. An ostium primum defect is also referred to as an incomplete endocardial cushion defect. A complete endocardial cushion defect is a more severe anomaly that is characterized by an atrial septal defect and incomplete formation of the mitral and tricuspid valves and the ventricular septum. Ostium primum defects are found in 20 to 30 per cent of children with Down's syndrome.

An atrial septal defect results in shunting of blood from the left atrium to the right atrium. The left ventricle is much thicker than the right ventricle and as a result is less distensible (less compliant). This results in a normal left atrial pressure of 7 to 10 mm Hg. The thin-walled right ventricle is more distensible (more compliant), and therefore, normal right atrial pressures are only 4 to 5 mm Hg. The pressure difference that results from the difference in ventricular compliance results in a left-to-right shunt. During the first years of life, the compliance of the right ventricle progressively decreases as the workload of the right ventricle is much less after birth. For this reason, the flow across an atrial septal defect will increase during the first years of life.

Calculation of shunt flow is possible and is often combined with findings on physical examination to determine the need for operation. The ratio of pulmonary blood flow (Q_p) to systemic blood flow (Q_s) is

the number *most* must frequently used when describing the magnitude of shunt flow. Pulmonary blood flow is given by the equation:

$$Q_p = O_2 \text{ consumption } / \text{ SA } O_2 - \text{Pa } O_2$$

(Eq. 1)

where SA O_2 is the oxygen content of arterial blood in mL/L and PA O_2 is the oxygen content of pulmonary artery blood in mL/L.

Oxygen content is determined by the level of hemoglobin and the saturation of the blood. When fully saturated, 1 gm of hemoglobin is able to combine with 1.34 mL O_2. The O_2 content is expressed mathematically by the equation:

$$O_2 \text{ content (mL/min)} = 1.34 \times \text{hemoglobin concentration} \times \% \text{ saturation}$$

(Eq. 2)

Systemic blood flow is given by the following equation:

$$Q_s = O_2 \text{ consumption/SA } O_2 - \text{MV } O_2$$

(Eq. 3)

where SA O_2 is the oxygen content of arterial blood and MV O_2 is the oxygen content of mixed venous blood.

When the ratio Q_p/Q_s is used, oxygen consumption is cancelled from the equation, and the ratio can be obtained by determination of O_2 saturation.

$$Q_p/Q_s = \text{SA } O_2 2 - \text{MV } O_2 / \text{SA } O_2 - \text{PA } O_2$$

(Eq. 4)

With a pure left-to-right shunt the ratio Q_p/Q_s will be greater than 1, whereas with a pure right-to-left shunt the ratio will be less than 1.

Most atrial septal defects result in a pulmonary flow that is two to four times the flow in the systemic circulation. The decreased systemic flow results in retarded growth, which is referred to as the gracile

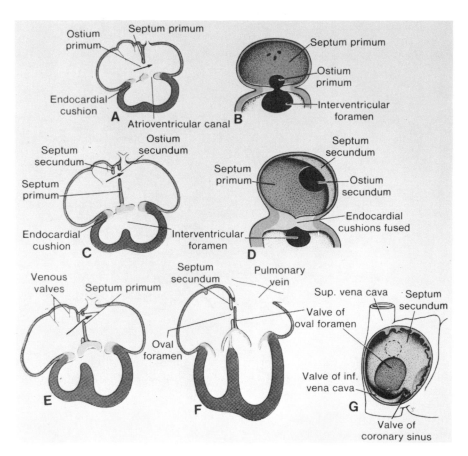

FIGURE 11–4. The cardiac septa are formed between the 27th and 37th days postconception. Partitioning of the primitive atrium occurs by the formation and subsequent modification of two distinct septa (septum primum and septum secundum) and fusion of the septa with the endocardial cushions. The septum primum (*A*), so named because it is the first septum to develop, grows downward from the roof of the primitive atrium toward the endocardial cushions. The opening between the free edge of the septum primum and the endocardial cushion is referred to as the ostium or foramen primum (*B*). The ostium primum disappears as the septum primum continues to grow downward and eventually fuses with the endocardial cushions (*C*). Before the foramen primum disappears, perforations occur in the upper portion of the septum primum. These perforations coalesce to form the foramen secundum (*D*). This is followed by formation of the septum secundum from the roof of the primitive atrium and to the right of the septum primum (*D,E*). The septum secundum grows downward and eventually overlaps the foramen secundum (*F*). The portion of the septum primum that is attached to the roof of the atrium gradually disappears. The foramen that exists in the septum primum and is now overlapped by the septum secundum is referred to as the foramen ovale (*G*). (Reprinted from Sadler, T.W.: Langman's Medical Embryology, 5th ed. Baltimore, Williams & Wilkins, 1985. Figure 12–13, p. 178.)

habitus, whereas the increased pulmonary flow results in an increased susceptibility to pneumonia and decreased exercise tolerance. Long-term effects of an atrial septal defect with its attendant left-to-right shunt are atrial arrhthmias caused by right atrial hypertrophy and an increase in pulmonary vascular resistance. The increase in pulmonary vascular resistance is due to progressive sclerosis of the vascular bed, which may eventually become irreversible. These changes in the pulmonary vascular bed result in right ventricle hypertrophy. In patients who

develop these irreversible changes, the increase in pulmonary vascular resistance eventually produces pulmonary pressures that are equal to systemic pressures. At that point, the compliance of the two ventricles is equal, and the result is a balanced shunt. Further increases in pulmonary vascular resistance result in continued right ventricle hypertrophy. The compliance of the left ventricle eventually exceeds the compliance of the right ventricle, and flow across the septal defect is reversed, resulting in a right-to-left shunt. This is termed the Eisenmenger syn-

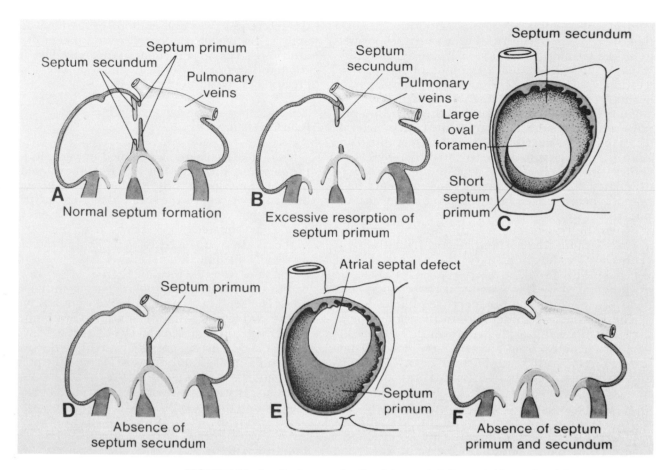

FIGURE 11–5. Pathogenesis of atrial septal defects. *A*, Normal atrial septum formation. *B* and *C*, Ostium secundum defect caused by excessive resorption of the septum primum. *D* and *E*, Similar defect caused by failure of development of the septum secundum. *F*, Common atrium or cor trilocular biventriculare—complete failure of the septum primum and septum secundum to form. (Reprinted from Sadler, T.W.: Langman's Medical Embryology, 5th ed. Baltimore, Williams & Wilkins, 1985. Figure 12–18, p. 183.)

drome and is characterized by typical manifestations of a right-to-left shunt, such as clubbing, cyanosis, and polycythemia.

Ventricular septal defects also result in a left-to-right shunt of blood. The amount of flow across a ventricular septal defect is a function of the size of the defect and the pulmonary vascular resistance. Manifestations of a ventricular septal defect are cardiac failure and pulmonary hypertension. Patients with ventricular septal defects have also been shown to be at an increased risk of bacterial endocarditis and are more likely than patients with atrial septal defect to develop Eisenmenger syndrome.

Simultaneous with the development of the septa, development of the proximal heart into the ventricular outflow tract and the great vessels takes place. The proximal heart is referred to as the bulbis cordis. The proximal one third of the bulbis cordis develops into the trabeculate portion of the right ventricle. The middle third of the bulbis cordis, referred to as the conus cordis, develops into the out-flow tracts of both ventricles. The distal one third of the bulbis cordis is referred to as the truncus arteriosus and develops into the proximal aorta and the proximal pulmonary artery. Septum formation is also crucial in allowing normal development of the truncus arteriosus into the proximal aorta and pulmonary artery. Two ridges arise from the opposing sides of the truncus arteriosus, spiral around each other, and eventually fuse to form the aorticopulmonary septum, which divides the truncus into an aortic and pulmonary channel. Similar ridges develop in the cordis conus, dividing the outflow tracts of the two ventricles and fusing with the aorticopulmonary septum.

Congenital defects related to abnormal development of the truncus arteriosus and the conus cordis are relatively common. The most common abnormality in this group is the tetralogy of Fallot, which is caused by anterior displacement of the truncoconal septum. The result is a narrowed right ventricular outflow tract (infundibular pulmonic stenosis), a ventricular septal defect, and a malpositioned aorta that overrides both ventricles. The fourth abnormality in the tetralogy is right ventricular hypertrophy, which occurs as a result of the pulmonary stenosis. Tetralogy of Fallot is the most common cause of cyanotic congenital heart disease.

Failure of descent and fusion of the aorticopulmonary septum results in a persistent truncus arteriosus. This is characterized by a single artery (the truncus) originating from the heart and the presence of a ventricular septal defect. The pulmonary artery originates from the truncus. These patients have cyanotic heart disease, and the prognosis is usually poor.

When the truncoconal septum fails to spiral in a normal fashion, the aorta originates from the right ventricle and the pulmonary artery from the left ventricle. This anomaly, referred to as transposition of the great vessels, is a frequent cause of cyanotic heart disease and requires operative repair.

The arterial system develops at the same time as the heart. Paired dorsal aorta form that eventually fuse. Branchial arches with their corresponding aortic arch vessels originate in the truncus arteriosus and terminate in the dorsal aorta. There are a total of six aortic arch vessels. All are obliterated in whole or in part except the third, fourth, and sixth. The third forms the common carotid and the internal carotid arteries, the fourth aortic arch on the right forms the proximal portion of the right subclavian artery, and the left fourth forms part of the arch of the aorta. The sixth aortic arch on the right becomes the proximal right pulmonary artery, whereas the left sixth arch becomes the ductus arteriosus.

Abnormal development of the arterial system is relatively uncommon. Double aortic arch is caused by persistence of the right dorsal aorta and results in formation of a vascular ring that encircles both the trachea and the esophagus. Right aortic arch is caused by obliteration of the left fourth aortic arch and persistence of the right. Interruption of the aortic arch results from obliteration of the fourth aortic arch and is usually associated with a patent ductus arteriosus, i.e., a persistent sixth arch. The most common abnormality of arterial development is coarctation of the aorta (Fig. 11–6).

Fetal Circulation

The fetal circulation is designed not only to meet the needs of the fetus but also to allow immediate modifications in response to changes occurring at birth. The placenta is the site of gas exchange for the fetus so that pulmonary blood flow is irrelevant (Fig. 11–7). Oxygenated blood returns from the placenta to the fetus via the umbilical vein. Half of the blood carried by the umbilical vein flows to the liver via the portal sinus, whereas the other half bypasses the liver by flowing through the ductus venosus to the vena cava. The septum secundum in the right atrium directs most blood through the foramen ovale into the left atrium and ventricle. The blood that reaches the right ventricle mostly passes through the ductus arteriosus to the descending aorta because the pulmonary vascular resistance is higher than the systemic vascular resistance in utero. Approximately half of the blood in the aorta returns to the placenta via the paired umbilical arteries (Fig. 11–7).

The result of fetal circulation is that the head is supplied with well-saturated blood directly from the placenta via the left ventricle while less well-saturated blood from the superior vena cava flows to the rest of the body.

Changes at Birth

Soon after birth, the three shunts (ductus venosis, foramen ovale, and ductus arteriosus) close, and the pulmonary and systemic circulation are separated. Constriction of the muscular umbilical arteries that

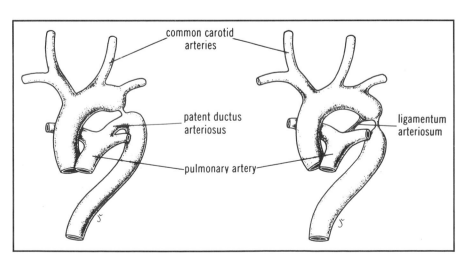

FIGURE 11–6. Coarctation of the aorta. *A*, Preductal type; *B*, postductal type. The caudal part of the body is supplied by large, hypertrophied intercostal and internal thoracic arteries. (Reprinted from Sadler, T.W.: Langman's Medical Embryology, 5th ed. Baltimore, Williams & Wilkins, 1985. Figure 12–36, p. 201.)

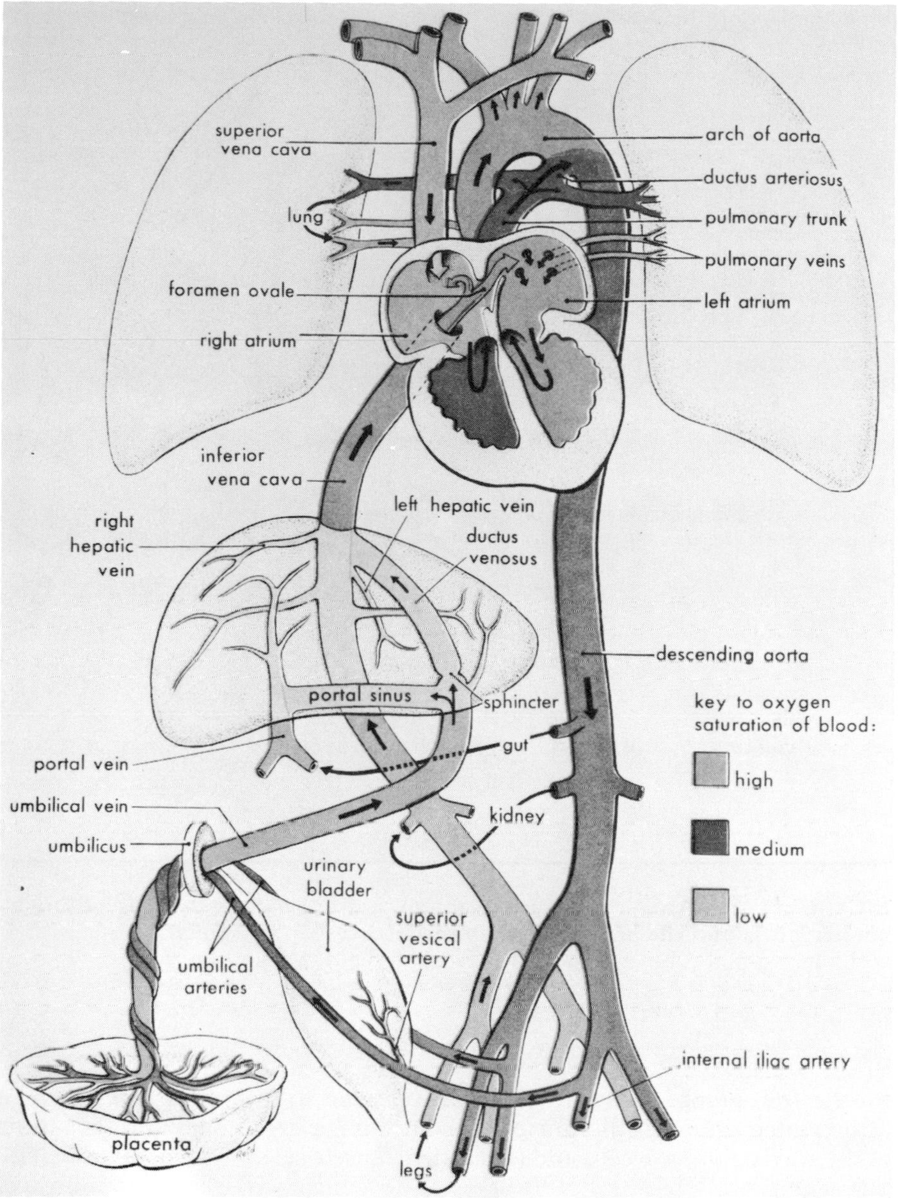

FIGURE 11–7. Scheme of the fetal circulation. Three shunts permit most blood to bypass the liver and the lungs: (1) The ductus venosus, (2) the foramen ovale, and (3) the ductus arteriosus. (Reprinted from Moore, K.L.: The Developing Human, 3rd ed. Philadelphia, W.B. Saunders Co., 1982. Figure 14.38, p. 334.)

occurs at birth initiates the process, causing a marked increase in systemic vascular resistance and systemic blood pressure. The hypoxia that results from loss of placental gas exchange stimulates the respiratory center, and the newborn starts to breath. The hypoxic ductus venosus is stimulated to constrict and close. Ventilation of the lungs drops the pulmonary vascular resistance, which in turn allows for a corresponding increase in pulmonary blood flow and drop in pulmonary vas pressure. The increase in pulmonary blood flow produces an increase in left atrial volume and pressure. Simultaneously, right atrial pressure falls as a result of decreased placental blood flow and constriction of the ductus venosus. Left atrial pressure quickly exceeds right atrial pressure, and the flap over the foramen ovale is forced to close and fuse. The pressure changes in the systemic

and pulmonary systems cause a reversal of flow in the ductus arteriosus. The high oxygen content of the aortic blood causes constriction of the ductus and functional closure by 12 hours after birth. The mediators of shunt closure are unknown, but the degree of muscular hypertrophy of the vessels and their sensitivity to sympathomimetic amines, bradykinin, angiotensin, and prostaglandins are probably involved.

Functional Anatomy of the Cardiac Muscle

The heart is made up of striated muscle, which differs from skeletal muscle in the following ways (Fig. 11–8): (1) cardiac muscle cells are connected longitudinally in a series through specialized areas

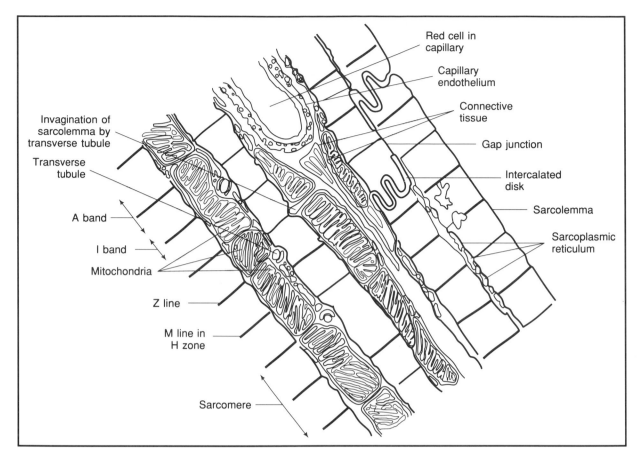

FIGURE 11–8. An electron micrograph of cardiac muscle showing large numbers of mitochondria and the intercalated discs with nexi (gap junctions), transverse tubules, and longitudinal tubules. (Reprinted from Berne, R.M., and Levy, M.N.: The cardiac pump. *In* Berne, R.M., and Levy, M.N. (eds.): Physiology, 2nd ed. St. Louis, C.V. Mosby Co., 1988. Figure 28–2, p. 432.)

on the cell membranes (sarcolemma) referred to as intercalated discs, (2) the nucleus is centrally located in the cardiac muscle cell, and (3) cardiac muscle cells bifurcate.

Intercalated Discs. The intercalated disc is a specialized area of adjacent myocardial cell membranes. Its function is twofold. First, it serves as a path of low resistance that allows for rapid conduction of electrical impulses from muscle cell to muscle cell. The electrical resistance through the intercalated disc is one four hundredth the resistance through the other areas of the cell membrane. Although the heart is not a true syncytium, these pathways of low resistance allow the cardiac muscle to contract as one. Since the atria and ventricles are separated by a ring of fibrous tissue, the heart is considered to be composed of two functional syncytia, atrial and ventricular, with the action potential of the atrial syncytium being conducted through the fibrous ring to the ventricular syncytium through the AVN. If the AVN is not functioning and accessory pathways are not available, the atrial syncytium does not spread to the ventricular syncytium, and heart

block results. The second function of the intercalated disc is to maintain a firm union between adjacent myocardial cells to permit transmission of tension from one cell to the next, allowing the atria and ventricles to function as single contractile units.

Contractile Apparatus. The contractile cells of the heart contain groups of myofibrils densely packed in a linear arrangement that extends the length of the cell (Fig. 11–8). Each myofibril is divided at regular intervals by transverse bands referred to as Z lines. The area between two Z lines is referred to as a sarcomere and is the functional unit of the myocardium. The contractile proteins of cardiac muscle and their three-dimensional configuration are identical to that of skeletal muscle. Thick filaments composed of myosin are present in the A band, and thin filaments composed primarily of actin are found in the I band. The thin filaments extend into the A band where interaction between actin and myosin takes place (see Chapter 21).

Cardiac muscle cells also differ from skeletal muscle cells in two ways in terms of the morphology of the transverse tubular system. The transverse tubular system (T system) is made up of a series of transverse invaginations of the cell membrane that release calcium when the muscle cell is depolarized and thus play a major role in excitation-contraction coupling. Not only is the T system larger in cardiac muscle than skeletal muscle but the cardiac T system also is found at the level of the Z line, rather than at the A-I junction as in skeletal muscle. This arrangement allows for more rapid and prolonged excitation-coupling, which is crucial in allowing effective ventricular contraction.

One major difference between skeletal muscle, which can operate anaerobically for short periods of time, and cardiac muscle, which must operate repetitively, is the relative scarcity of mitochondria in skeletal muscle. Cardiac muscle, by contrast, is rich in mitochondria necessary for ATP synthesis for continuous energy. For similar functional reasons, the myocardium has a rich capillary network for O_2, nutrient, and water exchange. Thus, the interstitial fluid of the heart is continuous and well supplied by capillaries. The T tubular system brings the interstitium close to the myofibrils, and an intercellular network of tubules (sarco tubules) that surrounds the myofibrils is in intimate proximity with the interstitium at T tubular sites. Thus, there is minimal interference to the transfer of extracellular fluid to the inside of the cell or to the capillary.

The Pacemaker and the Conduction System

The heart beats automatically and rhythmically because it initiates its own beat, and the conduction system allows for orderly propagation of the action potential to all areas of the myocardium. The conduction system is made up of the sinoatrial node (SAN), the internodal atrial pathways, the atrioventricular node (AVN), the bundle of HIS, the bundle branches, and the Purkinje system. Table 11–1 lists the unique functions of these separate components.

Sinoatrial Node. The SAN acts as the normal cardiac pacemaker. It occupies a small area, 3 × 10 mm, and is located under the epicardium on the posterior wall of the right atrium at the junction of the right atrium with the superior vena cava. The sulcus terminalis marks this junction on the epicardial surface, and the crista terminale marks the junction on the endocardial surface. The SAN is made up of two cell types, P (pacemaker) cells and T (transition) cells. The P cells are small and round and stain poorly (pale). The T cells are thin, elongated cells. P cells act as pacemaker cells, and the T cells interconnect P cells with the interatrial and internodal pathways. Three pathways connecting the SAN to the AVN have been described.

Atrioventricular Node. The three interatrial pathways converge on the atrioventricular nodal complex, which is located beneath the right atrial endocardium at the base of the interatrial septum. The AVN complex has three components: junctional fibers, the atrioventricular node proper, and the bundle of His. Although the normal time for transmission from the SAN to the AVN is .04 seconds, a delay in conduction occurs at the AVN to allow the atria time to empty their contents into the ventricles. This delay in conduction is attributed to a decreased conduction velocity in the junctional fibers and AVN, as well as a slow rate of development of the action potential in the AVN proper. In addition, the refractory period is prolonged in the node so that a rapid atrial rate is incompletely transmitted to the ventricle. A decrease in the action potential occurs secondary to decremental conduction so that the magnitude of the voltage diminishes from one end of the impulse path to the other.

The impulse passes from the AVN to the bundle of His, which is continuous with the anterior part of the AVN proper. The bundle of His then enters the interventricular septum where it divides into right and left bundle branches to supply the right and left ventricles, respectively. The terminal bundle branches penetrate into the ventricular wall and terminate on ventricular myocardial cells with which they are continuous. As the bundle of His exits from the AVN, the cell morphology changes; the cells

TABLE 11–1.   FUNCTIONS OF COMPONENTS OF THE CONDUCTION SYSTEM

COMPONENT	FUNCTION	VELOCITY OF TRANSMISSION (m/sec)	TIME OF TRANSMISSION (msec)
SA node P cells T cells	Initiation of electrical activity	0.05	
Atrial pathways	Conduction of action potential to AV node	0.5 to 1.0	40
AV node	Delay	0.5 to 1.0	80–120
Bundle of His	Rapid transmission of impulse to ventral myocardium to allow coordinated, forceful ejection	3 to 4	30
Myocardium	Contraction with ejection blood	0.4 to 1.0	10–30

become larger and are referred to as Purkinje cells. Purkinje cells are specialized to allow rapid transmission of action potentials. This rapid transmission is most likely a result of the increased number of nexi between adjacent Purkinje cells. The conduction velocity in Purkinje fibers is 1.5 to 4.0 m/sec, which is four to six times as fast as cardiac muscle. The combination of rapid transmission of the action potential through the Purkinje system and the intimate relationship of the Purkinje cells to myocardial cells allows for almost simultaneous contraction of the ventricular muscle mass (Table 11–1). The total time from the entry of the impulse into the bundle of His until it reaches the terminal Purkinje fibers is 0.03 seconds. The total time for spread of the action potential through the ventricular muscle is also only 0.03 seconds.

The Cardiac Action Potential

Cardiac action potentials are more complex than those of skeletal muscle and nerve. The cardiac action potential is prolonged (more than 300 msec) compared to a few milliseconds for the action potential for a muscle or nerve. Although the action potential of muscle or nerve is biphasic, the cardiac action potential consists of five different phases.

Action Potential Phases.   The resting transmembrane potential in nonpacemaker myocardial cells is 80 to 90 mV, with the inside negative with respect to the outside. Figure 11–9 shows a typical action potential of a cardiac muscle cell, and Figure 11–10

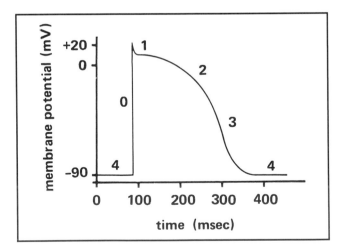

FIGURE 11–9.   The cardiac action potential (shown here for a Purkinje fiber) lasts over 300 msec and consists of five phases. Phase 0 (upstroke) corresponds to depolarization in skeletal muscle, and phase 3 (repolarization) corresponds to repolarization in that tissue. Phases 1 (early repolarization) and 2 (plateau) have no clear counterpart in skeletal muscle, whereas phase 4 (diastole) corresponds to the resting potential. (Reprinted from Katz, A.M. Physiology of the Heart. New York, Raven Press, 1977. Figure 14.2, p. 230.)

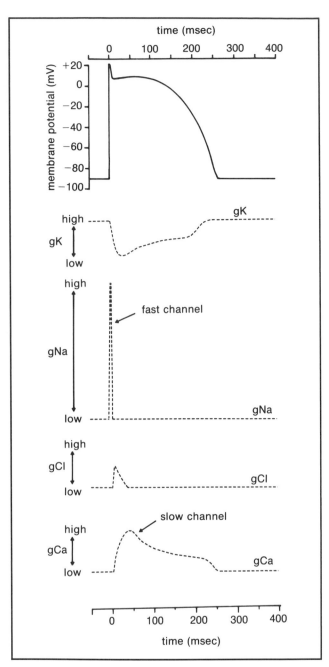

FIGURE 11–10.   The action potential in a Purkinje fiber. The typical action potential (*top*) accompanies changes in conductance for potassium (gK), sodium (gNa), chloride (gCl), and calcium (gCa). An increase in gNA or gCa augments inward current flow, whereas increasing gK or gCl augments outward current flow. (Reprinted from Katz, A.M.: Physiology of the Heart. New York, Raven Press, 1977. Figure 14.7, p. 237.)

shows the ionic mechanisms responsible for the changes in action potential. After stimulation, there is an extremely rapid phase of depolarization (Phase 0) lasting 1 to 2 msec. The transmembrane potential becomes momentarily positive by 15 to 30 mV. This reversal of polarity is referred to as overshooting and lasts 6 to 15 msec. As in skeletal muscle and nerves, the rapid depolarization is due to a rapid increase in sodium permeability. The depolarization is followed by a brief period of rapid repolarization—phase 1—that is caused by an increased chloride permeability and a decrease in the sodium permeability. The plateau phase 2, which lasts about 100 msec, is caused by (1) a rapid rise in calcium permeability with a prolonged fall to baseline, (2) a fall in the potassium permeability with a slow return to baseline, and (3) a stable, low chloride permeability that prevents short-circuiting of the potential during the plateau. The net effect of the permeability changes and ion fluxes that occur during the plateau phase is a gain in intracellular sodium and calcium and a small loss of potassium. Calcium is available for binding to the actin-myosin complex. Sodium and potassium levels are maintained by the sodium-potassium ATPase pump.

The plateau phase of the action potential is followed by repolarization-phase 3. Repolarization is caused by a return of the calcium permeability to normal and an increase in K permeability. Phase 4 of the action potential is the resting membrane potential, which in nonpacemaker cells is stable at -80 to -90 mV.

Action Potential in Pacemaker Cells. Cells in the SAN, AVN and Purkinje fibers do not have a stable resting potential, i.e., they are capable of progressive diastolic depolarization in phase 4 of the action potential. Figure 11–11 compares the action potential of a pacemaker cell to a cell without pacemaker function. Progressive diastolic depolarization allows the transmembrane potential to increase until the threshold is reached and an action potential is initiated and propagated. Because P cells in the SAN normally undergo this spontaneous depolarization at a faster rate than other cells, they control the rate of the heart. The maximum negative membrane potential of SAN cells is less negative than nonpacemaker cells because P cells are more permeable to Na than are nonpacemaker cells. The action potential in the SAN is illustrated in Figure 11–11. The maximum negative membrane potential, which is typically between -55 to -60 mV, is achieved immediately after the previous action potential. Diastolic depolarization then occurs due to a progressive decline in K permeability. When the threshold potential is reached, a slow phase 0 occurs. Cells of the SAN lack a distinct phase 1 and 2 and have a prolonged phase 3.

Control of Heart Rate. Although local factors, such as temperature, blood pH, and tissue stretch, can affect the pacemaker, the principal extranodal control of heart rate is the autonomic nervous system. There are three mechanisms by which neurotransmitters of the autonomic nervous system modify the discharge frequency of pacemakers cells and thus alter the heart rate: a change in the slope of diastolic depolarization, a change in the threshold

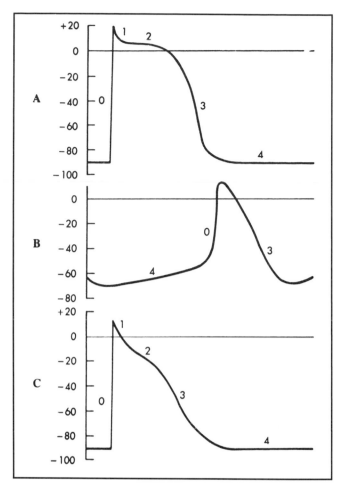

FIGURE 11–11. Action potentials in a ventricular cardiac muscle fiber (A), a pacemaker cell (B), and an atrial myocyte (C). (Reprinted from Berne, R.M., and Levy, M.N.: Cardiovascular Physiology, 5th ed. St. Louis, C.V. Mosby Co., 1986. Figure 2–17, p. 23.)

potential, and a change in the maximum negative membrane potential. Figure 11–12 shows how these three mechanisms may be employed to slow the rate of pacemaker discharge.

Effect of Parasympathetic Innervation

Although the heart is under the tonic influence of both divisions of the autonomic nervous system, the parasympathetic tone is predominant at rest. It is for this reason that complete denervation of the heart, as occurs with cardiac transplantation, results in an increase in resting heart rate. The vagal parasympathetics release acetylcholine (ACh) as the neurotransmitter. The right branch of the vagus nerve is the predominant supply to the SAN, and the left branch of the vagus is the dominant supply to the AVN. The main effect of parasympathetic stimulation is on the SAN, with a lesser effect on the AVN and an even lesser effect on atrial muscle. The ven-

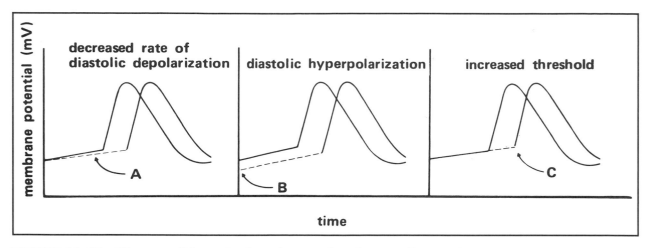

FIGURE 11–12. Three possible mechanisms that can slow the rate of pacemaker discharge (*solid line*, control; *dashed line*, slowed): decreased rate of diastolic depolarization (*arrow A*), diastolic hyperpolarization (*arrow B*), and increased threshold (*arrow C*). The first two of these changes result from vagal stimulation. Accelerated pacemaker discharge can occur through sympathetic stimulation, which increases the rate of diastolic depolarization (but also the degree of hyperpolarization.) (Reprinted from Katz, A.M.: Physiology of the Heart. New York, Raven Press, 1977. Figure 14.14, p. 253.)

tricles are poorly supplied by the parasympathetic division.

Vagal stimulation slows heart rate by causing both a hyperpolarization (more negative maximum membrane potential) and a decrease in the slope of diastolic depolarization (Fig. 11–12). It does so by increasing K^+ permeability, which is responsible for polarization. Thus, vagal stimulation serves to shorten the duration of the atrial action potential (Fig. 11–13). The major effect of ACh in the AVN is to slow conduction. Parasympathetic stimulation of atrial myocytes has a negative inotropic effect, causing a shortened refractory period. The mechanism is the same for atrial muscle—a slower inward current and faster repolarization. At physiologic doses ACh has little or no effect on the bundle of His, bundle branches, or Purkinje fibers.

The effect of parasympathetic stimulation is short-lived because acetylcholine is rapidly degraded by the rich cholinesterase supply at the SAN and AVN.

Effect of Sympathetic Innervation

The sympathetic nervous supply to the heart originates in the lower two cervical and upper six thoracic segments of the spinal cord. The postganglionic fibers are transmitted to the heart along the great blood vessels and richly innervate the SAN, the AVN, and both the atrial and ventricular myocardium.

Catecholamines are the neurotransmitters of the sympathetic supply of the heart. They cause both a hyperpolarization and an increase in the rate of diastolic depolarization. Hyperpolarization, which would tend to decrease the heart rate, is more than offset by the increase in slope of phase 4 (diastolic depolarization), and the net result is an increase in heart rate. Figure 11–14 shows the effect of sympathetic stimulation of the SA node. Similar effects are seen on the Purkinje fibers. The slope of phase 4 is determined by the K permeability. In the presence of catecholamines, K permeability is decreased,

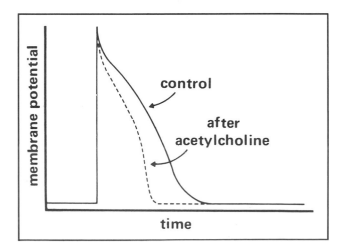

FIGURE 11–13. Atrial action potential after vagal stimulation. The duration of the action potential is shortened because the slow inward current is reduced and the outward potassium currents that cause repolarization are increased. (Reprinted from Katz, A.M.: Physiology of the Heart. New York, Raven Press, 1977. Figure 19.10, p. 363.)

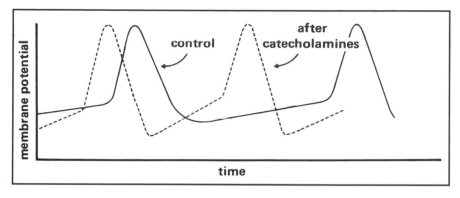

FIGURE 11-14. Effects of catecholamines, or sympathetic stimulation, on the SA node. (Reprinted from Katz, A.M.: Physiology of the Heart. New York, Raven Press, 1977. Figure 19.13, p. 367.)

and the slope of phase 4 is increased. The effect of sympathetic stimulation is longer-lived than that of parasympathetic stimulation because enzymatic breakdown of the neurotransmitter does not occur in the sympathetic system. Instead, the catecholamines released by the fibers of the sympathetic nerves are taken back up by the nerve endings and are washed away in the blood.

The Baroreceptor Reflex (Marey's Law of the Heart)

A number of physiologic reflexes play a role in controlling heart rate. Marey in 1859 noted that there was an inverse relationship between systemic arterial blood pressure and heart rate. This reflex is referred to as Marey's law of the heart or the baroreceptor reflex. The mechanoreceptors for arterial tension in the wall of the aortic arch and the carotid sinus at its bifurcation transmit afferent impulses along the vagus (aorta) and the ninth (glossopharyngeal) cranial nerve (carotid) to the vasomotor center of the medulla oblongata. Increased tension depresses sympathetic tone and increases parasympathetic activity. Both of these factors act to decrease the heart rate; a decrease in tension causes the reverse. The baroreceptor reflex plays a major role in the regulation of heart rate and blood pressure in response to changes in position.

Atrial Receptors. In 1915, Bainbridge reported that, at a constant arterial blood pressure, the heart rate could be increased by volume infusion. This Bainbridge reflex is mediated via pressure-sensitive receptors in both atria. Atrial distension results in a decrease in efferent vagal activity and an increased heart rate. The sympathetics are not involved.

There is a second mechanism by which right atrial pressure results in an increase in heart rate. Right atrial distension stretches the fibers of the SAN. Cells of the SAN respond to an increased stretch by increasing their rate. This response is an inherent property of the SAN cells.

Ventricular Receptors. Sensory receptors are located near the endocardial surface of both ventricles. Afferent impulses are transmitted to the vasomotor center via vagal fibers. An increase in pressure results in increased vagal efferent activity and a reflex decrease in heart rate, as well as a decrease in systemic peripheral resistance.

THE CARDIAC CYCLE

The period from the end of one heart contraction to the next is called the cardiac cycle. In the normal heart, the electrical and mechanical events occurring in each cycle are initiated by an action potential that is spontaneously generated by the SAN. Each cardiac cycle consists of a period of relaxation called diastole followed by a period of contraction called systole. The events of the cardiac cycle are best understood by simultaneous measurements of aortic pressure, atrial pressure, and ventricular volumes and by EKG tracing (Fig. 11–15).

Function of the Atria

In diastole the atria serve both as a conduit and a reservoir of blood from the venous system to the ventricles. In systole, the atria act as a primer pump of the ventricles, filling them just before ventricular systole. This permits the ventricles to maintain low pressure for most of diastole, which serves to minimize oxygen consumption. Atrial systole, which plays a greater role at higher heart rates, increases the volume of blood in the ventricles by approximately 30 per cent. At rest, the heart is able to maintain cardiac output in the absence of atrial systole. In a diseased heart or at high heart rates, the compensatory mechanisms may not be adequate, and cardiac failure will supervene. In this situation, sequential atrial-ventricular pacemakers are occasionally employed to restore the benefit obtained to cardiac output from atrial systole.

Atrial Pressure Tracings. The normal atrial pressure is 4 to 8 mm Hg. The three pressure waves that are seen in the atria during the cardiac cycle are the a, c, and v waves (Fig. 11–15). The a wave is a result of atrial systole. Figure 11–15 shows the increase in left ventricular volume during the a wave. The c wave reflects the beginning of ventricular sys-

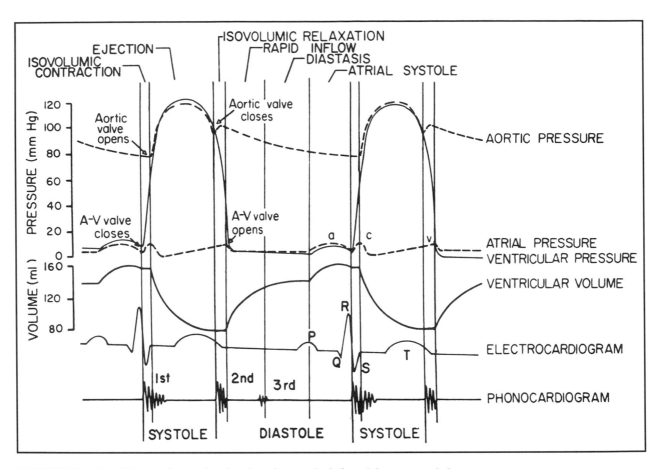

FIGURE 11–15. The cardiac cycle, showing changes in left atrial pressure, left ventricular pressure, aortic pressure, ventricular volume, the electrocardiogram, and the phonocardiogram. (Reprinted from Guyton, A.C.: Human Physiology and Mechanisms of Disease, 4th ed. Philadelphia, W.B. Saunders Co., 1987. Figure 8.4, p. 83.)

tole, during which the AV valves are forced backward toward the atria and the contracting ventricle pulls on the atria. The v wave reflects the accumulation of blood in atria with closed AV valves. The v wave disappears when the AV valve opens.

Ventricular Mechanical Events

Diastolic filling of the ventricles is divided into three phases. The first phase, the period of rapid filling, occurs after the AV valves open. During the middle third of systole, the atria simply act as a passive conduit of blood from the venous sytems to the ventricles. This period of diastole is referred to as diastasis to emphasize the low rate of blood flow. By the end of the middle third of diastole, 70 per cent of ventricular filling has occurred. The last one third of diastole is the period of atrial contraction.

Ventricular Systole. The period of ventricular systole is divided into two phases: the period of isometric or isovolumic contraction and the period of ejection. The ventricular pressure rapidly rises as systole begins. The AV valves are quickly closed as

the ventricular pressure rapidly exceeds that of the atria. The closing of the AV valves results in the first heart sound and marks the beginning of the period of isometric contraction. The ventricles continue to contract with the AV valves and the semilunar valves closed for 20 to 30 msec until the ventricular pressure exceeds the diastolic pressure in the aorta or pulmonary artery. The semilunar valves are forced open, marking the end of the period of isometric contraction and the beginning of the period of ejection. Blood is then rapidly ejected from the ventricle, with the majority of emptying occurring in the first quarter of systole. Ventricular emptying is completed in the first three quarters of systole (Fig. 11–15). Protodiastole, despite its name, occurs in the last quarter of systole. It is the brief period when ventricular pressure is less than aortic pressure, but blood continues to leave the ventricle as it has built up momentum.

The end of protodiastole marks the end of ventricular systole. The aortic valve is forced closed as the ventricular pressure falls below that of the aorta. The closing of the semilunar valves results in the second heart sound and marks the beginning of the period of isometric relaxation. While the ventricular pressure is rapidly falling, there is a period of 30 to 60 msec when the ventricular pressure remains greater than atrial pressure and the ventricle is relaxing with the AV and semilunar valves closed. Once the ventricle pressure falls below the atrial pressure, the AV valve is forced open, ending the period of isometric relaxation and beginning the period of rapid ventricular filling.

Volume Measurements

During systole, the ventricles do not empty completely. The difference between the volume at the end of diastole (the end-diastolic volume; EDV) and the end-systolic volume is the stroke volume (the amount of ejected blood). Under resting conditions the normal stroke volume approximates 60 to 70 mL. The normal EDV in the resting state is approximately 130 cc. The ratio of the stroke volume to the EDV is referred to as the ejection fraction, and normal values are 55 to 65 per cent. Cardiac output is defined as the total output of either the left or right ventricle per minute. Normal cardiac output in the resting state is approx 5L/min. When averaged over a period of time, the outputs of the left and right ventricle are identical.

Cardiac output is determined by the amount of blood ejected with each contraction (the stroke volume) and the number of contractions occurring per minute (the heart rate).

$$CO = (HR) \times (SV). \qquad \text{(Eq. 5)}$$

Control mechanisms that determine the heart rate have been previously discussed. Control of stroke volume is the next topic.

REGULATION OF CARDIAC FUNCTION

Cardiac output in the resting state is 4 to 6 L/min. Increases up to six or seven times the resting cardiac output can occur during strenuous exercise. The myocardium can adjust to changes in hemodynamics by two major mechanisms: intrinsic and extrinsic regulation. Intrinsic regulation relies on properties intrinsic to cardiac muscle and therefore can occur in the absence of any nervous or hormonal control. Extrinsic regulation, on the other hand, refers to changes in myocardial performance that occur as a result of chemical and neural influences.

Intrinsic Regulation of Cardiac Function

Preload: The Frank-Starling Law of the Heart. Preload is defined as the force acting on a muscle just before contraction. The relationship be-

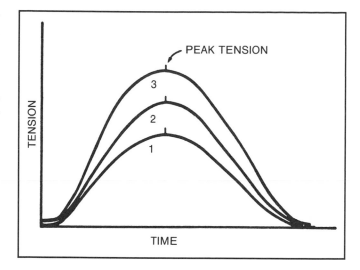

FIGURE 11–16. Diagram of isometric twitches from isolated cardiac muscle produced by progressively increasing preloads. Twitches obtained at different times are superimposed. Notice the increase in resting muscle tension and peak tension development in beats 1 to 3 and that, as peak tension rises, the time to peak tension remains constant. (Reprinted from Wist, J.B. (ed.): Best and Taylor's Physiologic Basis of Medical Practice, 11th ed. Baltimore, Williams & Wilkins, 1985. Figure 2.93, p. 198.)

tween preload and tension developed during the contraction of skeletal muscle has been discussed. Figure 11–16 shows the tension developed as a function of initial muscle length in an isolated whole muscle preparation. A similar curve would be obtained if a single muscle fiber was studied. As the preload is increased, the length of the muscle is increased, and the tension developed during contraction increases to a maximum and then declines as stretching continues. This response is explained by the sliding filament hypothesis of muscle contraction, which states that there is a certain muscle length at which interaction between contractile proteins is at a maximum and contraction is greatest. For cardiac and skeletal muscle, the maximum tension is developed at a sarcomere length of 2.2 μM. Thin actin filaments extending from the Z line are 1 μM in length; therefore, thin filaments occupy 2.0 μM of the sarcomere. The central 0.2 μm is felt to be free of reactive sites. At shorter muscle lengths, overlap of actin filaments decreases the actin-myosin interaction, and at longer lengths some sites on the actin molecules are no longer available for interaction. The result in both instances is a decrease in developed tension. This relationship between muscle length, as determined by preload, and developed tension applies to the heart and is referred to as the Frank-Starling law of the heart. To quote Starling, "The energy of contraction is proportional to the initial length of cardiac muscle fiber." Although increases in preload will result in increases in developed tension, the time-to-peak tension is not changed by changes in preload (Fig. 11–16). In the intact heart, the initial length of the muscle fiber before contraction is a function of the end-diastolic volume.

The Starling law of the heart is best illustrated in Figure 11–17. The end-diastolic volume is plotted on the x-axis, and the stroke volume is plotted on the y-axis. As the EDV increases as a result of increased venous return, muscle fiber length is increased and thereby stroke volume increases up to point A. This is the point at which there is maximum interaction of the contractile proteins. When EDV is less or more than this value, interaction of actin and myosin is less and contraction is not as strong. Therefore, by the Frank-Starling mechanism the heart is able to adjust to changes in diastolic filling by appropriate changes in cardiac output. In other words, the heart is able to "pump what it gets."

In clinical practice no method exists with which to rapidly determine ventricular EDV and stroke volume. However, there is a linear relationship between left atrial pressure and left ventricular EDV (LVEDV). Placement of a pulmonary artery catheter allows for serial measurements of pulmonary capillary wedge pressure, which in turn is a direct reflection of left atrial pressure. Furthermore, measurements of cardiac output are possible with a pulmonary artery catheter. Therefore, a modified Starling curve can be made by substituting pulmonary capillary wedge pressure for LVEDV on the x-axis and substituting cardiac output for stroke volume on the y-axis (Fig. 11–18). This approach is often used clinically to determine optimal filling pressures in patients with poor cardiac function before operative intervention.

Afterload. Afterload is defined as the tension that a muscle must develop before it can begin to

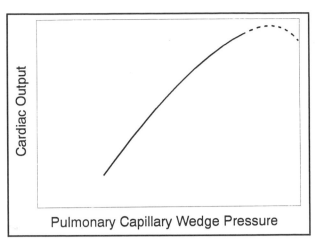

FIGURE 11–18. The Starling curve, illustrating the relationship of EDV to stroke work occurring at a given level of contractility.

shorten. The afterload of the left ventricle is a function of the aortic pressure, the peripheral vascular resistance, the distensibility and capacitance of the vascular system, the the viscoelastic properties of blood. The major determinant of afterload, and the factor that is most easily measured, is the aortic pressure. An increase in the afterload will increase the amount of energy required for contraction. Because more work goes into raising intraventricular pressure to the point where it is above the aortic pressure, less work will be available for ejection of blood. The result of an increase in afterload therefore is a decrease in stroke volume. A decrease in afterload has the opposite result: less energy is required to raise the intraventricular pressure, more energy is available for ejection, and stroke volume is increased. This is the mechanism by which afterload reduction is used to increase the output of a failing heart.

Myocardial Contractility. We have seen that the work of the heart can be varied by changes in the fiber length as measured by end-diastolic volume. The work of the heart can also be varied independent of changes in fiber length. Changes in the ability of the heart to do work at a constant fiber length are referred to as changes in contractility. Thus, the Starling curve shown in Figure 11–18 represents the relationship of EDV to stroke work at a given level of contractility. Since different contractile states exist, there are a number of Starling curves, one for each contractile state. Figure 11–19 shows a family of Starling curves. Starling curves further to the left represent an increased state of contractility, whereas curves further to the right are progressively decreasing contractile states. Positive inotropic agents, such as beta agonists, glucagon, and cardiac glycosides, induce an increased contractility. Negative inotropic agents—atropine or some of the calcium channel blockers—decrease the contractile state of the heart.

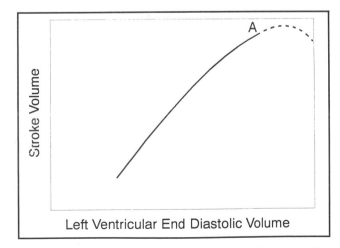

FIGURE 11–17. The Starling law of the heart. As the EDV increases as a result of increased venous return muscle fiber, length is increased and thereby stroke volume increases up to point A. This is the point at which there is maximum interaction of the contractile proteins.

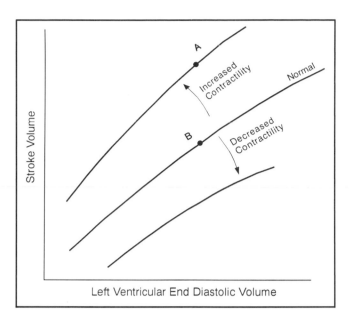

FIGURE 11–19. Points A and B occur at the same fiber length, but the stroke volume of A is greater than that of B. Point A therefore represents an increase in myocardial contractility.

Current evidence suggests that two molecular mechanism are responsible for changes in cardiac contractility. One is a change in the myosin molecule, which would result in improvement in actin-myosin kinetics. This is felt to be a long-term mechanism. The second mechanism is alteration in the amount of intracellular calcium during the action potential, which is felt to be responsible for rapid changes in cardiac contractility.

The Force-Frequency Relationship. The force of contraction is also a function of the contraction frequency. This rate-dependent variation in the intensity of contraction is referred to as the Bowditch staircase, the treppe phenomemon, or the force-frequency relationship. Bowditch studied this relationship by measuring the tension developed at different heart rates. He found that an increase in heart rate resulted in a progressive increase in tension until a new plateau of tension was reached. A decrease in heart rate resulted in a progressive decrease in the tension developed until a plateau was reached at a lower tension. In isolated papillary muscle, tension generated can be increased to up to five times the original value by increases in contraction frequency. In summary, each stimulation frequency is associated with a characteristic tension, and changes in the stimulation frequency cause directly proportional changes in tension.

This progressive increase in generated tension due to an increased heart rate is felt to be caused by progressive increases in intracellular calcium. Calcium enters the cell during systole and exits during diastole. At higher heart rates a larger percentage of the cardiac cycle is spent in systole, and calcium in-

flux is greater than calcium egress. As the intracellular calcium level is increased, a new steady state is eventually reached in which calcium influx is once again equal to calcium egress. An increase in intracellular calcium is also responsible for the increase in force of contraction seen after a premature systole. This phenomena is referred to as post extrasystolic potentiation and is due to an increased influx of calcium that occurs as the result of the extra systole.

Thus, there are at least four ways to influence the stroke volume: (1) altering the preload; changing the fiber length by changing end-diastolic volume, which means that one moves along a single Starling curve; (2) altering the myocardial contractility, i.e., moving to a Starling curve to the left of normal; (3) producing a change in afterload; and (4) changing the heart rate to alter the contractile state of the heart.

Alterations in preload and in the contractile state of the heart are the major physiologic mechanisms employed in regulating stroke volume. The Frank-Starling law is more important in adjusting to a minor variation in venous return as occurs with respiration or changes in position. Larger increases in cardiac output, such as occur during exercise, are affected by an increased contractile state.

Excitation-Contraction Coupling

Excitation-contraction coupling refers to the mechanism by which an action potential leads to contraction of the myocytes. As in skeletal muscle, the proper concentrations of Na^+, K^+, and Ca^{++} are necessary for optimal contraction. Calcium is the major ion involved in contraction. Under resting circumstances, the intracytoplasmic concentration of calcium is low. To achieve contraction this concentration must be increased. The major questions to be answered are how does an action potential result in an increase in intracytoplasmic calcium and how does this increased calcium level lead to contraction of the cell. When an action potential reaches the cell, the wave of depolarization also spreads down the T-tubules, which are invaginations of the cell membrane located in close proximity to the sarcoplasmic reticulum where calcium ions are concentrated and stored. Depolarization in the T-tubules results in the opening of calcium channels in the sarcoplasmic reticulum and the sarcolemma, causing the release of calcium in the vicinity of the contractile proteins. Thus, in this straightforward manner an action potential results in an increase in intracytoplasmic calcium.

The next issue to be addressed is how this increased calcium concentration leads to contraction of the cell. We have previously stated that the functional unit of the myocyte is the sarcomere and the major contractile proteins are actin and myosin. When actin and myosin are allowed to interact, contraction occurs as described by the sliding filament hypothesis. In the resting state (low intracytoplasmic calcium), actin and myosin are prevented from interacting by the presence of troponin, which is the major regulatory protein involved in contraction. Troponin is bound to the thin filaments. In the presence of high intracytoplasmic calcium, binding of up to four calcium ions to troponin occurs, resulting in a conformational change of the thin filaments. This change in structure of the thin filaments allows for interaction of actin and myosin, which results in formation of cross-bridges and contraction. The amount of calcium that is available to the contractile proteins during the action potential is one of the factors determining the strength of contraction. As noted above, the regulation of this calcium flux is one of the mechanisms by which alterations are made in the contractile state of the heart.

Excitation-contraction coupling is the mechanism by which the action potential results in the actual contraction of the cell. As in skeletal muscle, the proper concentrations of Na^+, K^+, and Ca^{++} are necessary for optimal contraction. Na^+ is necessary for propagation of the action potential. The influx of Ca^{++} to the generally low Ca^{++} myoplasm triggers contraction. A low concentration of K^+ is necessary to maintain polarization. Thus, high K^+ concentrations lead to loss of polarization and cardiac arrest in diastole. In contrast, high Ca^{++} interstitial fluid concentrations lead to contraction and arrest in contraction. T-tubules are present in both cardiac and skeletal muscle. When the action potential reaches the cell, the wave of depolarization also spreads down the T-tubules. The T-tubules are intimately associated with sarcoplasmic reticulum where calcium ions are concentrated and stored. Depolarization in the T-tubules results in the opening of calcium channels in the sarcoplasmic reticulum and the sarcolemma causing the release of calcium in the vicinity of the contractile proteins. The calcium ions bind to troponin, causing a change in the three-dimensional configuration of troponin. This change, in turn, allows for the interaction of actin and myosin associated with shortening of the filaments. Unlike skeletal muscle, in cardiac muscle there then occurs a significant flux of calcium across the T-tubule membrane. This calcium flux is important for two reasons. First, the terminal cisternae of the sarcoplasmic reticulum are not as well developed as in skeletal muscle and consequently release less calcium in response to depolarization, and second, the prolonged influx of calcium allows for the prolonged duration of action of the myocardial cells. Morphologically, the T-tubules of cardiac muscle are well suited for this purpose, being five times the size of those found in skeletal muscle. Moreover, the extracellular fluid surrounding the T-tubule is rich in negatively charged glycoproteins, which allow for accumulation of calcium ions. After phase two of the action potential, calcium is actively transported into the sarcoplasmic reticulum and across the sarcolemma into the extracellular fluid in exchange for Na^+. The amount of calcium available to the contractile proteins during the action potential is one of the factors that determines the strength of contraction. As noted above, the regulation of this calcium flux is one of the mechanisms by which alterations are made in the contractile state of the heart.

Inotropic Agents

Digitalis. Knowing the molecular basis for excitation-contraction coupling and alterations in contractility, it is possible to understand the mechanisms of action of commonly used inotropic agents. The first inotrope introduced in the clinical arena, digitalis, was derived from the foxglove plant. Intensive study of the mechanism by which digitalis improves contractility has shown that the site of action of this drug is the Na-K ATPase dependent pump. Digitalis acts as a poison to decrease the efficiency of the pump, with the result being an increase in intracellular sodium. Sodium is better able to compete with calcium at a second pump, the normal function of which is to exchange Ca^{++} for Na^+. The net result is an increase in intracellular calcium, which as noted above results in increased contractility.

Catecholamines. Catecholamines act through a mechanism completely different from that of digitalis. They mediate changes in the adenylate cyclase system and increase the level of intracellular cyclic AMP, which acts in turn to control the calcium channels in the cell membrane. The result is an increse in the amount of calcium that moves across the membrane during phase two of the action potential. Increases in intracellular calcium cause an increase in the contractile state of the heart.

There are three different types of adrenergic receptors—alpha, beta, and dopaminergic—and catecholamines differ in their ability to stimulate these receptors. Alpha adrenergic receptors consist of alpha-1 and alpha-2 receptors. Alpha-1 receptors are postsynaptic receptors found predominantly on vascular smooth muscle with a lesser concentration on the heart. Stimulation of the alpha-1 receptors of the heart results in a positive inotropic effect and a negative chronotropic effect. Phenylephrine, norepinephrine, and epinephrine, in that order, are the clinically available agonists with the most alpha-1 activity. Alpha-2 receptors are presynaptic receptors that mediate inhibition of neurotransmitter release. Stimulation of alpha-2 receptors results in a decrease in the release of catecholamines.

Beta receptors are also divided into two classes. Beta-1 receptors are found predominantly in the heart, whereas beta-2 receptors are found primarily in smooth muscle and glandular tissue. Stimulation of beta-1 receptors causes a positive chronotropic effect and inotropic effect; stimulation of beta-2 receptors results in vasodilation and relaxation of bronchial, uterine, and gastrointestinal smooth muscle. Beta receptors are also involved in carbohydrate metabolism and cause renin release.

Norepinephrine, epinephrine, and dopamine are naturally occuring catecholamines that differ in their selectivity for alpha and beta receptors. The relative potency of these compounds for the different receptors is shown in Figure 11–20.

Norepinephrine. Norepinephrine is the immediate precursor to epinephrine. Chemically, norepinephrine differs from epinephrine by the absence of a methyl group on the terminal amine of norepinephrine. Norepinephrine and epinephrine are equally potent in their ability to stimulate beta-1 receptors. Norepinephrine is a much more potent alpha-1 agonist and has minimal beta-2 activity, whereas epinephrine is a poor alpha-1 agonist and a strong beta-2 agonist.

Administration of a low or moderate dose of norepinephrine causes widespread vasoconstriction (alpha effect) and a positive inotropic effect. The result is an increase in systolic blood pressure, diastolic blood pressure, and mean arterial blood pressure (Fig. 11–20). The increased blood pressure causes a reflex decrease in heart rate. The increase in the vascular resistance usually counteracts the positive inotropic effect, with the result being a decrease in cardiac output. Norepinephrine also causes an increase in myocardial oxygen consumption and may, by stimulation of the alpha receptors of the coronary arteries, cause a decrease in oxygen delivery. It is for this reason that norepinephrine should be avoided when treating patients with ischemic heart disease. The main indication for norepinephrine, if any, is hypotension associated with a low systemic vascular resistance, as occurs with sepsis.

Epinephrine. Epinephrine is formed by the addition of a methyl group to the terminal amine of norepinephrine. As noted above, epinephrine and norepinephrine are equipotent in their effect on beta-1 receptors. However, unlike norepinephrine, epinephrine has little alpha activity and is a strong beta-2 agonist.

Epinephrine administration at low to moderate doses has a positive inotropic effect (beta-1 effect) and causes a decrease in systemic vascular resistance

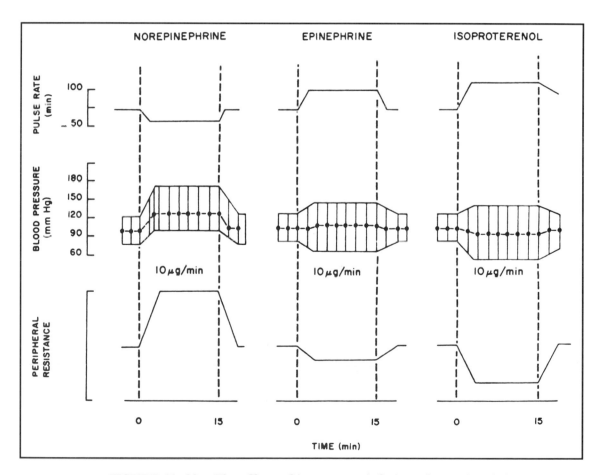

FIGURE 11–20. The effects of intravenous infusion of norepinephrine, epinephrine, and isoproterenol in humans. (Reprinted from Gilman, A.G., Rall, T.W., Nies, A.S., and Taylor, P. (eds.): Goodman and Gilman's The Pharmacological Basis of Therapeutics, 8th ed. New York, Pergamon Press Inc., 1990. Figure 10–1, p. 193.)

(beta-2 effect). This results in an increase in systolic blood pressure, a decrease in diastolic blood pressure, and no change in mean blood pressure (Fig. 11–20). Beta-1 stimulation also has a positive chronotropic effect. Cardiac output is increased due to increased myocardial contractility in the face of decreased vascular resistance.

At high doses of epinephrine, alpha-1 activity predominates over beta-2 activity because of the larger number of alpha-1 receptors. The effect of high-dose epinephrine is therefore similar to the effect of norepinephrine administration.

Dopamine. Dopamine is the immediate precursor to norepinephrine. Dopamine stimulates dopaminergic, beta, and alpha receptors. It also causes the release of norepinephrine from nerve terminals. At low doses, 1 to 3 mcg/kg/min, stimulation of dopaminergic receptors occurs. Dopaminergic receptors are found in the renal and mesenteric vascular bed, and stimulation of these receptors by low-dose dopamine causes vasodilation of the renal and mesenteric vasculature. This results in an increase in renal blood flow, glomerular filtration rate, and sodium excretion. At higher doses of dopamine, 3 to 10 mcg/kg/min, stimulation of beta receptors occurs, with the result being a positive inotropic and chronotropic effect. Systolic and mean blood pressure are increased, whereas diastolic blood pressure is usually unchanged (Fig. 11-20). At higher doses (10 to 20 mcg/kg/min), the stimulation of alpha receptors predominates. Diastolic blood pressure and mean blood pressure are further increased, and the salutary effect on renal blood flow is lost. Cardiac output may be decreased by the increase in systemic vascular resistance. At doses above 20 mcg/kg/min, an almost pure alpha effect is seen, with the result being similar to the infusion of norepinephrine.

Isoproterenol. Isoproterenol is a synthetic amine with almost exclusive beta activity. Infusion of isoproterenol results in a significant increase in heart rate and cardiac output. Diastolic blood pressure is decreased, and mean blood pressure and systolic blood pressure are decreased or unchanged. Isoproterenol is not frequently used because it causes a marked increase in heart rate and myocardial oxygen demand.

Dobutamine. Dobutamine is a synthetic sympathomimetic amine with predominantly beta-1 and beta-2 activity. Administration of dobutamine results in an increased contractile state of the heart, a decrease in systemic vascular resistance, and an increase in cardiac output and coronary blood flow. Dobutamine also results in an increased heart rate, but with conventional doses the increase is less than seen with dopamine or isoproterenol. Dobutamine usually does not cause an imbalance between myocardial oxygen consumption and oxygen delivery because the increased demand, due primarily to a modest increase in heart rate, is offset by increased cardiac output and coronary vasodilation (beta-2 effect), which results in increased coronary blood flow.

Coronary Blood Flow

The first branches of the aorta are the right and left coronary arteries. These two vessels, which communicate poorly, supply the heart with an average blood flow at rest of approximately 250 mL/min.

The blood flow through the coronary vessels varies with the phase of the cardiac cycle. During systole the pressure in the wall of the left ventricle is similar to the pressure in the aorta, and as a result little flow of blood occurs. During diastole, the pressure gradient between the aorta and left ventricular wall rapidly rises as the ventricle relaxes. Blood flow to the left ventricle peaks at the beginning of diastole and actually reaches zero flow in early systole. Flow to the right ventricle is more constant, as the pressure developed in the right ventricle wall during systole remains significantly lower than aortic pressure. The blood flow to the right ventricle has two peaks: one occurring at the peak aortic pressure and the second at the beginning of diastole.

Oxygen extraction from coronary blood is higher than in any other tissue. Since oxygen extraction is nearly maximized in the resting state, significant increases in oxygen delivery can only occur by increasing blood flow. The regulation of blood flow to the myocardium is mainly determined by local metabolic factors. Patients with significant coronary artery disease have fixed lesions that do not allow for an increase in flow in response to metabolic demands. The result is an imbalance between myocardial oxygen consumption and oxygen delivery that may result in either reversible ischemia (angina) or cell death (myocardial infarction).

Mechanical Circulatory Support

Mechanical devices that provide support to a failing heart have been in clinical use since the introduction of the Roller pump by DeBakey in 1934. Refinements in bioengineering have allowed for the successful clinical use of total artificial hearts (TAH) with external power sources, and further advances are likely to provide a completely implantable TAH.

Attention here is focused on the intra-aortic balloon pump (IABP), which remains the most frequently used method of providing mechanical support. Circulatory assist with an intra-aotic balloon pump requires placement of the catheter tip in the descending thoracic aorta. The intra-aortic balloon pump catheters vary in size from 9 1/2 to 12 French. Balloon volumes vary from 10 to 40 mL. In addition to the balloon, catheters in use today include a central lumen through which central aortic pressure can be monitored.

Insertion of the intra-aortic balloon catheter is almost always accomplished through a percutaneous approach to the femoral artery. Correct position after placement must be verified by a chest roentgenogram or with fluoroscopy.

The mechanical action of the balloon is to inflate immediately after closure of the aortic valve and to deflate just before the opening of the aortic valve. Inflation during diastole results in an increased diastolic blood pressure and thereby an increase in coronary blood flow. Deflation during systole allows for decreased aortic impedance, which results in a decreased afterload. Afterload reduction results in a decreased left ventricular end-diastolic volume and, in turn, a decreased preload. Therefore, when timed appropriately, inflation and deflation of the intra-aortic balloon result in an increased coronary blood flow, a decrease in afterload, and a decrease in preload.

Appropriate timing of balloon inflation and deflation is essential in achieving these physiologic effects. The balloon should inflate with every other beat, with half of the normal volume being delivered to the balloon. Ideally, inflation occurs immediately after closure of the AV valve. When a radial arterial line is used to time inflation, inflation should coincide with the occurrence of the dicrotic notch. Deflation is adjusted to provide a decrease of 10 to 15 mm Hg in the diastolic pressure of an augmented beat and to maximize reduction of the next ventricular systole.

One of the most frequent indications for the intra-aortic balloon pump is postoperative left ventricular power failure. LV power failure is frequently a result of an intraoperative ischemic event and, in that instance, is often reversible. However, pump failure is associated with preoperative LV dysfunction (ejector fraction of less than 30 per cent), is associated with a poor prognosis, regardless of the nature of circulatory support. Overall, 85 per cent of patients placed on the intra-aortic balloon pump after open heart surgery are discharged from the hospital.

Circulatory assist with the intra-aortic balloon pump has been shown to be an effective treatment for patients with angina that is refractory to medical management. When support with the intra-aortic balloon pump is required for angina, it should be closely followed by a cardiac arteriogram and revascularization. Circulatory assist with the intra-aortic balloon pump is also effective therapy for complications of acute myocardial infarction, including pump failure, ventricular septal defect, acute mitral regurgitation, and ventricle arrhythmias. In a setting of postinfarction and ventricular septal defects, assist with the intra-aortic balloon pump may decrease the left-to-right shunt by up to 30 per cent.

Circulatory assist with the intra-aortic balloon pump is often used before open heart surgery. Most clinicians feel that it is clearly indicated in patients with angina refractory to medical therapy and in patients with complications of acute myocardial infarction. Other indications, which are shown in Table 11–2, are frequently employed, but remain somewhat controversial.

Complications as a result of placement of an intra-aortic balloon pump occur in 10 to 30 per cent of patients. The most frequent complication is vascular insufficiency distal to the femoral insertion site. It is usually treated with removal of the catheter, but on occasion requires thrombectomy or repair of the femoral artery or both. In instances when the intra-aortic ballon pump is felt to be absolutely essential, a femoral-femoral bypass graft can be performed, which enables the intra-aortic balloon pump to remain in place. Other complications of intra-aortic balloon counterpulsation include would infection, local hemorrhage, embolism, aortic dissection, and thrombocytopenia.

PERICARDIUM

The pericardium is a fibrous sac that surrounds the heart. A serosal layer is present on the inner surface of the pericardium. This layer is reflected onto the heart at the visceral pericardium. The pericardium is attached to the sternum, the diaphragm, and the root of the great vessels. Normally, there is 15 to 50 cc of pericardial fluid, and intrapericardial pressure is equal to intrapleural pressure.

The pericardium functions to maintain the heart in a relatively fixed position and serves as a barrier to infection. However, no significant adverse effects occur as a result of the absence of the pericardium.

Inflammation of the pericardium is caused by a number of conditions, including viral, fungal, and bacterial infections; trauma; tuberculosis; radiation therapy; amyloidosis; tumors; drug reactions; and acute myocardial infarction. Acute pericarditis is associated with chest pain and typical EKG changes in the presence of a friction rub. These typical EKG changes are ST segment elevation in the precordial leads, ST segment depression in lead AVR, and depression of the PR segment. Late changes in the EKG consist of symmetric T wave inversion and eventual return of the EKG to normal.

Pericardial effusion, although frequently hemodynamically insignificant, can progress to cardiac tamponade. The compliance of the pericardium is nonlinear. Once the upsloping portion of the pressure volume curve is reached, small increases in fluid volume produce large increases in intrapericardial pressure. Eventually, the intrapericardial pressure will equal the diastolic pressures in the right and left heart, and tamponade will occur when the right atrial, left artrial, left ventricular diastolic, and right ventricular diastolic pressures are equal. Restriction of diastolic filling occurs as a result of the increased intrapericardial pressures. Preload is thereby decreased, and cardiac output falls. Compensatory tachycardia ensues, and a pulsus paradoxis (a decrease in 10 mm Hg in systolic blood pressure on inspiration) is present. Findings of systemic hypotension with increased venous pressures and a small flat heart are referred to as Beck's triad and are typical of cardiac tamponade. Treatment of cardiac tamponade is by pericardiocentesis and, on occasion, resection of a portion of the pericardia.

CORONARY ARTERY DISEASE

The incidence of coronary artery disease (CAD) has been declining for more than 25 years, yet CAD remains the major cause of death in the United States. Ninety-nine per cent of lesions of the coronary arteries are atherosclerotic with rare lesions occurring secondary to syphilis, connective tissue disease, arteritis, or embolus. Risk factors for coronary artery disease have been identified and include increased serum cholesterol, increased serum low density lipoprotein, hypertension, smoking tobacco, diabetes mellitus, decreased high density lipoprotein, increased serum triglyceride levels, obesity, and a family history of coronary artery disease.

Coronary artery disease may present with angina, acute myocardial infarction, heart failure, arrhythmias, or sudden death. Angina is caused by the imbalance between oxygen delivery and oxygen demand, such that oxygen demand exceeds oxygen delivery. A decrease in oxygen delivery occurs as a result of fixed coronary artery lesions or, on occasion, spasm of the coronary arteries. Any activity that increases oxygen demand above the level of oxygen supply will result in angina. The diagnosis of angina is usually readily made by obtaining a history of exertionally- induced chest discomfort that is relieved by rest and laboratory evidence of reversible ischemia. The electrocardiogram, performed either during symptomatic episodes or during an exercise stress test, is often able to document myocardial ischemia by the appearance of ST segment depression. In patients with a negative EKG stress test, a history suggestive of angina, or an equivocal stress test, radionuclide angiography is indicated. A localized defect in perfusion that occurs during exercise and disppears at rest identifies an ischemic area of myocardium.

Treatment of angina is directed at improving the balance between oxygen supply and demand by either decreasing demand or increasing supply. Attempts to halt progress of the responsible lesions should be made. Reduction of serum cholesterol by dietary and pharmacologic interventions, cessation of smoking, control of hypertension, and weight loss should be attempted.

Medical therapy of angina involves the use of explosives (nitrates) and blockers (beta and calcium channel). Nitrates favorably alter the oxygen balance in a number of ways. They cause smooth muscle relaxation that results in venodilation and decreased venous return to the heart. This decrease in preload causes a decrease in wall tension and therefore a decrease in myocardial oxygen consumption. The decrease in wall tension, as well as the direct effect of nitrates in the coronary arteries, results in an increase in the blood flow to the subendocardium. Nitrates have also been shown to decrease flow through collaterals and to dilate pericardial collaterals. Animal studies have shown that nitroglycerin increases blood supply to ischemic areas of myocardium. By the above methods, nitrates both decrease oxygen demand and increase oxygen supply.

The major effect of beta blockers in the treatment of angina is to decrease oxygen demand. This effect occurs by decreasing the heart rate, blood pressure, and contractile state of the heart. Beta blockers have been shown to reduce the frequency of anginal episodes and increase the anginal threshold. Calcium channel blockers decrease myocardial oxygen demand by reducing afterload and contractility. Oxygen supply is increased by the direct dilatory effect on coronary arteries of calcium channel blockers.

Unstable angina is generally defined as an increase in anginal episodes in a patient with previously stable angina or as angina that is refractory to medical therapy. The presence of angina refractory to all medical therapy is an indication for placement of an intra-aortic balloon pump and coronary arteriography to determine the suitability of the coronary vessels for a bypass operation. Acute myocardial infarction occurs as a result of a localized area of myocardial ischemic necrosis.

Myocardial infarction is believed to be a result of acute thrombosis of the coronary artery occurring in a patient with underlying coronary artery atherosclerosis. Coronary spasm of an interplaque hemorrhage may also result in irreversible cell loss. The territory supplied by the left anterior descending artery is most frequently involved in infarction, followed by the areas supplied by the right coronary artery and, less frequently, the areas supplied by the left circumflex artery. Diagnosis of acute myocardial infarction is made by history and physical examination, evaluation of serial EKGs, and serial determinations of the myocardial band isoenzymes of creatine phosphokinase. The volume of tissue involved in an infarction is proportional to the peak level of the MB band of creatine phosphokinase.

Management of patients with acute myocardial infarction has consisted of EKG monitoring to allow rapid diagnosis and treatment of arrhythmias, nitrates and beta blockers to improve the oxygen balance, analgesic sedation, and oxygen. Invasive monitoring with heart lines, pulmonary catheters, and urinary catheters is frequently required in patients with hemodynamic instability. Profound cardiogenic shock after acute infarction often occurs in the face of an intra-aortic balloon pump.

Recent data have accumulated to suggest that fibrinolytic therapy is of benefit to patients who present within 4 to 6 hours of the onset of symptoms or in patients with evolving infarction. Tissue plasminogen activators are presently the drug of choice as they are felt to have less of a systemic effect than urokinase or streptokinase. If fibrinolytic therapy appears to have resulted in myocardial salvage, cardiac catheterization should be performed, but angioplasty may be done if an amenable lesion in the affected artery is found. Operative revascularization may be required in some of these patients.

Catecholamines

The synthesis of catecholamines begins with the hydroxylation of tyrosine to DOPA and is outlined in Figure 11–21. Dopamine is the main neurotransmitter of the extrapyramidal system, norepinephrine is the transmitter of most sympathetic postganglionic fibers, and epinephrine is the major hormone of the adrenal medulla.

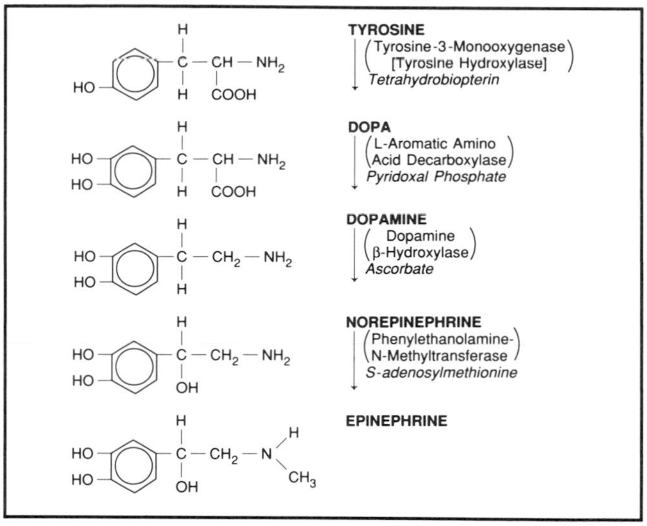

FIGURE 11–21. Steps in the enzymatic synthesis of dopamine, norepinephrine, and epinephrine. (Reprinted from Gilman, A.G., Rall, T.W., Nies, A.S., and Taylor, P. (eds.): Goodman and Gilman's The Pharmacological Basis of Therapeutics, 8th ed. New York, Pergamon Press, Inc., 1990. Figure 5–3, p. 102.)

TABLE 11–2. CHARACTERISTICS OF SUBTYPES OF ADRENERGIC RECEPTORS*

RECEPTOR	AGONISTS	ANTAGONISTS	TISSUE	RESPONSES
α_1†	Epi ≥ NE >> Iso Phenylephrine	Prazosin	Vascular smooth muscle	Contraction
			Genitourinary smooth muscle	Contraction
			Liver†	Glycotenolysis, gluconeogenesis
			Intestinal smooth muscle	Hyperpolarization and relaxation
			Heart	Increased contractile force, arrhythmias
α_2‡	Epi ≥ NE >> Iso Clonidine	Yohimbine	Pancreatic islets (β cells)	Decreased insulin secretion
			Platelets	Aggregation
			Nerve terminals	Decreased release of NE
			Vascular smooth muscle	Contraction
β_1	Iso > Epi = NE Terbutaline	ICI 118551	Smooth muscle (vascular, bronchial, gastrointestinal, and genitourinary)	Relaxation
			Skeletal muscle	Glycogenolysis, uptake of K$^+$
			Liver†	Glycogenolysis, gluconeogenesis
β_3§	Iso = NE > Epi BRL 37344	ICI 118551 CGP 20712A	Adipose tissue	Lypolysis

* This table provides examples of drugs that act on adrenergic receptors and of the location of subtypes of adrenergic receptors. Abbreviations are epinephrine (Epi); norepinephrine (NE); isoproterenol (Iso); phospholipase C (PLC); inositol-1,4,5-triphosphate (IP$_3$); diacylglycerol (DAG).

† In some species (e.g., rat), metabolic responses in the liver are mediated by α_1 receptors, whereas in others (e.g., dog), β_2 receptors are predominantly involved. Both types of receptors appear to contribute to responses in humans.

‡ At least two subtypes of α_1- and α_2-adrenergic receptors are known, but distinctions in their mechanism of action and tissue location have not been defined.

§ Metabolic responses in adipocytes and certain other tissues with atypical pharmacologic characteristics may be mediated by this subtype of receptor. Most β-adrenergic antagonists (including propranolol) do not block these responses.

Reprinted from Gilman, A.G., Rall, T.W., Nies, A.S., and Taylor, P. (eds.): Goodman and Gilman's The Pharmacological Basis of Therapeutics, 8th ed. New York, Pergamon Press, Inc., 1990. Table 5–3, p. 108.

Adrenergic Receptors

A description of the classification and characteristics of adrenergic receptors is essential to understanding the effects of sympathomimetic aminas.

Three types of beta receptors have been described. Beta-1 receptors are found in the heart and in the juxtaglomerular cells. Stimulation of the beta-1 receptors in the heart results in an increased contractile state, an increased chronotropic effect (increased heart rate), and an increased conduction velocity. The stongest beta-1 agonist is isoproteronol, followed by epinephrine and then norepinephrine. Dopamine is a strong beta-1 agonist with little beta-2 activity. Stimulation of beta-1 receptors in the juxtaglomerular cells results in an increased production of renin.

Beta-2 receptors are found in smooth muscle, skeletal muscle, and in the liver. Stimulation of smooth muscle beta-2 receptors results in relaxation of the muscle fibers. Stimulation of beta-2 receptors in skeletal muscle leads to glycogenocysis, whereas beta-2 stimulation of the liver leads to glycogenolysis and glyconeogenesis. Terbutrine has strong beta-2 activity with minimal beta-1 agonist effect.

Beta-3 receptors, which have only recently been isolated, are believed to be involved with regulation of lypolysis from adipose tissue.

Two types of alpha receptors have been described. Previously an anatomic concept of alpha-1 receptors as postsynaptic and alpha-2 receptors as presynaptic was standard teaching. Recently, postsynaptic alpha-2 receptors have been described, and the anatomic concept has been replaced by a structural and physiologic classification (Table 11–2). From a cardiovascular point of view, the most important alpha receptors (both alpha-1 and alpha-2) are located on vascular smooth muscle, and stimulation of these receptors results in contraction. Distribution of alpha receptors and the physiologic effects of alpha receptor stimulation on other organ systems are outlined in Table 11–2.

BIBLIOGRAPHY

1. Berne, R.M., and Levy, M.N.: The cardiac pump. *In* Berne, R.M., and Levy, M.N. (eds.). Physiology, 2nd ed. St. Louis, C.V. Mosby Co. 1988, pp. 431–450.
2. Guyton, A.C.: Human Physiology and Mechanisms of Disease, 4th ed. Philadelphia, W.B. Saunders Co. 1987.
3. Berne R.M, and Levy, M.N.: Cardiovascular Physiology, 5th ed. St. Louis, C.V. Mosby Co. 1986.
4. Gilman, A.G., Rall, T.W., Nies, A.S., and Taylor, P. (eds.): Goodman and Gilman's The Pharmcological Basis of Therapeutics, 8th ed. New York, Pergamon Press, Inc., 1990.
5. Moore, K.L.: The Developing Human, 3rd ed. Philadelphia, W.B. Saunders Co. 1982.
6. Moore, K.L.: The thorax. *In* Clinically Oriented Anatomy, 2nd ed. Baltimore, Williams & Wilkins, 1985, pp. 49–148.
7. Katz, A.M.: Physiology of the Heart. New York, Raven Press, 1988.
8. Sadler, T.W.: Langman's Medical Embryology, 5th ed. Baltimore, Williams & Wilkins, 1985.

12

VASCULAR PHYSIOLOGY

MARSHALL W. WEBSTER *and* FUAD RAMADAN

In *De Motu Cordis,* published in 1628, William Harvey (1578-1657) first described the closed circulation of blood. That book is considered by many to be the most important and most valuable book in the history of medicine. Systemic blood pressure was first measured in a horse in 1733 by Stephen Hales (1677-1761). In 1828 the mercury hemodynameter was invented by Jean Leonard-Marie Poiseuille (1799-1869), who first described the factors controlling the flow of fluids through cylindrical tubes. Notable contributions by Ernest Henry Starling (1866-1927) and others gave vascular physiology a firm foundation in anatomy, physics, biochemistry, and now molecular biology.

GENERAL STRUCTURE AND FUNCTION

The systemic circulation is made up of all the blood vessels between the aortic root and the right atrium. It consists of conduits spanning a broad spectrum of sizes, structural characteristics, and functions. Each segment of the circulation has an ideal and distinctive combination of size, wall thickness, wall composition, cross-sectional area, and blood flow velocity that best fulfills its function. Figure 12–1 summarizes the different sizes and structural compositions of the various vessels in the systemic circulation. The aorta and large arteries have thick walls with high collagen and elastin contents and function primarily to deliver and distribute blood under high pressure to the various tissue beds. Smaller arteries and arterioles, with larger proportions of smooth muscle, act as variable resistors, dynamically directing blood flow to individual organs and tissue beds according to changing local needs. The microcirculation, consisting of capillaries and venules with walls that are one cell layer thick, delivers oxygen, nutrients, and biologically active substances to individual cells and collects carbon dioxide, metabolic byproducts, and locally synthesized agents for transport to other locations. The cutaneous microcirculation has the auxiliary role of contributing to the control of body temperature. The venous system is a collection network that also has a capacitance function that moderates the volume of blood returned to the right heart as part of the control of cardiac output. The lymphatic system primarily collects surplus interstitial fluid and protein from the interstitial spaces and returns it to the venous system.

The circulation is a continuous closed system, and although brief pooling may occur, cardiac output must equal the sum of the regional flows. Further, the pulmonary and systemic flows must remain equal over time.

The proportion of the blood volume contained in each segment of the systemic circulation is shown in Table 12–1. At any time the major portion of the blood volume is in the venous circulation, which acts as a reservoir. Although only 5 per cent of the blood volume is in the capillary bed, the total surface area of the capillary bed is enormous. The capillary beds and sinusoids of the spleen, liver, splanchnic veins, and subcutaneous plexi may also act as specific blood reservoirs.

ARTERIAL STRUCTURE AND FUNCTION

All arteries are formed by an intima, a media, and an adventitia. The intima consists of a thin monolayer of endothelial cells, usually oriented along the long axis of the artery. A thin layer of glycoprotein, the glycocalyx, covers the luminal surface. Beneath the endothelium is a fibrillar layer, the basal lamina, which bonds the endothelial cells to the subendothelial connective tissue. The internal elastic lamina separates the intima from the media. The media comprises smooth muscle cells in an elastin and collagen matrix, which may be up to 500 μm thick. The smooth muscle cells tend to be oriented circumferentially or helically. The elastin permits distension of the artery while the collagen bundles provide tensile strength, limit distension, and prevent disruption.

203

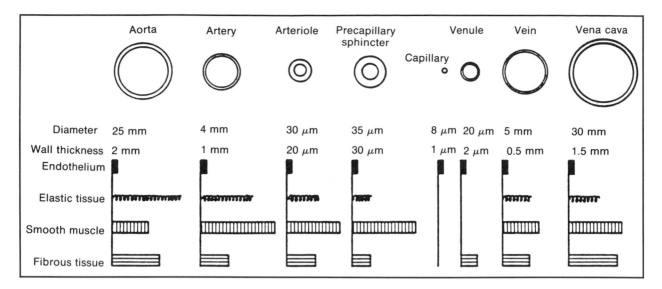

FIGURE 12–1. Dimensions and structural constitutients of the various vessels of the systemic circulation. (Modified from Burton, A.C.: Physiol. Rev., *619*–642, 1954. Reprinted from Selkurt, E.E. (ed.): Physiology, 4th ed. Boston, Little, Brown and Co., 1976.)

The thickness of the media is closely related to the radius of the artery. The adventitia is separated from the media, in some arteries, by an external elastic lamina. The adventitia consists of sparse fibroblasts with layers of elastin and collagen fibers, adding further strength to the wall. It merges with the loose connective tissue that surrounds all vessels.

There is a gradual diminution in the size of the arteries as they progress from the aorta to the precapillary arterioles. This is accompanied by a progressive increase in total cross-sectional area and a proportional reduction in blood flow velocity (Table 12–2). The elastic or conducting arteries (aorta, innominate, subclavian, common carotid, and common iliac arteries) have a large elastin component in the media that allows distension, blood pooling, and storing of potential energy during cardiac systole and then recoil during diastole after aortic valve closure (Windkessel effect). This capacitance function serves to modulate a more uniform flow and pressure into the distributive and muscular arteries, also known as resistance arteries. The muscular arteries

that comprise most of the arterial tree are characterized by dense smooth muscle in the media that is capable of changing luminal size. Blood flow can be directed into individual regional beds according to varying needs. The smooth muscle in the media not only has the ability to contract and maintain arterial tone but also can synthesize connective tissue proteins. The thickness of the media in arteries varies depending on the internal pressure and external forces to which they are exposed, e.g., the media is thicker in arteries of the lower extremity than the upper extremity. Where arteries are subject to bending or stretching (e.g., the popliteal), the intima may contain smooth muscle fibers. The large arteries and veins are also characterized by vasa vasora that nourish the adventitia and outer media, since the vessel wall is too thick to be nourished by diffusion from the lumen alone. The wall of a typical muscular artery is shown in Figure 12–2.

The left heart output is distributed to the regional beds in basal conditions as shown in Table 12–3.

TABLE 12–1.   VASCULAR DIMENSIONS

Vessel Type	Fraction of blood Volume (%)
Arteries	10
Capillaries	5
Venules and small veins	54
Large veins	21
Heart	10

TABLE 12–2.   RELATIONSHIP BETWEEN ARTERIAL SIZE, CROSS-SECTIONAL AREA, AND BLOOD FLOW VELOCITY

Vessel	Diameter (cm)	Cross-sectional Area (cm^2)	Flow Velocity (cm/sec)
Aorta	2	3	30
Arteriole	3×10^{-3}	800	0.1
Capillary	8×10^{-4}	3500	0.026
Vena cava	3	7	14

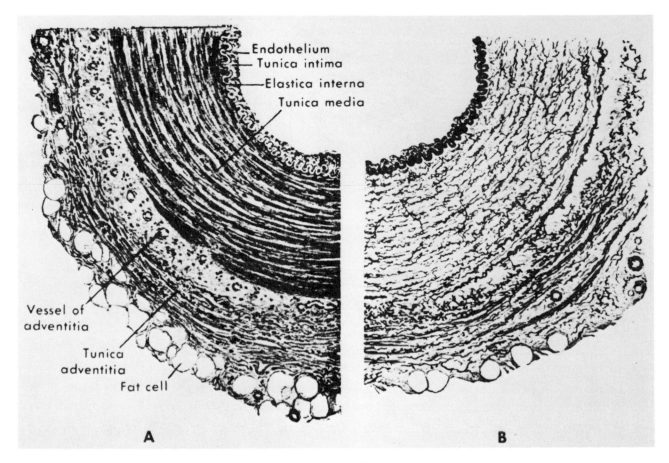

FIGURE 12-2. Wall of a small artery in cross-section, showing the concentric arrangement of tunica intima, media, and adventitia. *A,* Stained with hematoxylin and eosin; *B,* stained with orcein to reveal the elastic tissue component. (Reprinted from Fawcett, D.W.: Blood and lymph vascular systems. *In* A Textbook of Histology, 11th ed. Philadelphia, W.B. Saunders Co., 1986. Figure 12–1, p. 368.)

TABLE 12–3. PERCENT OF CARDIAC OUTPUT DISTRIBUTED TO INDIVIDUAL REGIONAL BEDS UNDER BASAL CONDITIONS

	DISTRIBUTION OF NORMAL LEFT HEART OUTPUT		
	(%)	(mL/min)	(mL/min/100 gm)
Brain	14	700	50
Heart	4	200	70
Bronchi	2	100	25
Kidneys	22	1100	360
Liver			
Portal	(21)	(1050)	
Arterial	(6)	(300)	
Muscle (inactive state)	15	750	4
Bone	5	250	3
Skin (cool weather)	6	300	3
Thyroid gland	1	50	160
Adrenal glands	0.5	25	300
Other tissues	3.5	175	1.3
Total	100.0	5000	– – –

Reprinted from Guyton, A.C.: Textbook of Physiology, 7th ed. Philadelphia, W.B. Saunders Co., 1986. Table 20–1, p. 230.

Considerable variation can occur normally or in pathologic states. In general, metabolically active tissues, such as the endocrine glands and liver, require higher flows. The kidneys require high flow to permit plasma filtration. Muscle under basal conditions needs little perfusion, but flow may increase 20 to 25 times the basal levels with strenuous exercise. Changes in regional distribution are based either on local need or systemic circumstances. Regional flows may be determined by local control or may be mediated by nervous or humoral pathways.

MICROCIRCULATION STRUCTURE

The microcirculation comprises arterioles, metarterioles (or terminal arterioles), precapillary sphincters, capillaries, venules, and arteriolarvenular anastomoses (or thoroughfare channels). Although the exact configuration of these structures varies in different organs, a general scheme is shown in Figure 12–3. Each arteriole feeds a microcircula-

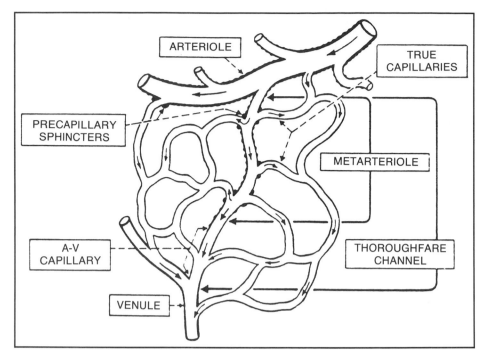

FIGURE 12–3. A microcirculatory unit. (Reprinted from Zwiefach, B.W.: Factors Regulating Blood Pressure. New York, Josiah Macy Jr. Foundation, 1949.)

tory unit consisting of 10 to 100 capillaries, which results in a dramatic increase in cross-sectional area and reduction in blood flow velocity (Table 12–2), thereby allowing prolonged contact times for metabolic exchanges to take place. These exchanges between the circulation and the extravascular compartment occur mainly across capillaries and venules, with the venous end being more permeable to water and solutes than the arterial end.

In addition to these differences within the same circuit, significant permeability differences exist between the capillary beds of different tissues. The smooth-muscle-rich precapillary sphincters function to control flow into regional beds by varying resistance according to the specific metabolic needs. This smooth muscle constrictor function is under both neural and humoral control. The capillary network is most dense in tissues with the highest metabolic activity. The total surface area of the capillary bed is estimated at 250 to 700 square meters, but of course, only a small proportion (approximately 25 per cent) of capillary beds are open at any one time. Venules are formed by converging capillaries and merge to give rise to the collecting venules that drain the microcirculatory unit. Muscular venules, along with small veins, act as postcapillary resistance vessels, which, together with the precapillary sphincters, determine capillary hydrostatic pressure and therefore greatly influence transcapillary exchange. Venules and small veins also are the major capacitance vessels of the vascular system and hold the major portion of the blood volume. Direct arteriovenous anastomoses, usually side branches from terminal arterioles, may shunt blood directly into the venous bed, bypassing the capillary bed. Both adrenergic and cholinergic nerve endings are found in the arteriovenous anastomoses. In the skin, these arteriovenous anastomoses play an important role in regulating heat loss and controlling body temperature. Their functional significance in other tissues is unclear.

The flow through the capillary bed can also be controlled by autoregulation. Increased local flow or reactive hyperemia occurs as a response to the accumulation of metabolic byproducts, such as lactic acid, and is independent of innervation.

The capillaries are 5 to 12 μm in size, with an average length of 0.5 to 1.0 mm (Fig. 12–4). Most permit passage of only a single red cell, and some capillaries may be so small as to allow only plasma flow. Red blood cells are normally deformable, which allows them to squeeze through the smaller capillaries. The degree of deformability can be measured by a number of techniques, including filtration through micropore filters and laser diffraction methods. Such measurements have demonstrated a tendency for red cells to become more rigid in certain disease states, such as atherosclerosis and diabetes. This increase in rigidity is an adverse rheologic factor, and pharmacologic agents, such as pentoxifylline, have been employed in an attempt to restore greater deformability. White blood cells are normally less deformable than red cells and have a greater tendency to obstruct the microcirculation, one white cell being equivalent to 700 to 1000 red cells. Their presence can have a tremendous impact on the pathophysiology of certain clinical situations, such as shock or reperfusion, in which white cells cause significant microcirculatory obstruction.

Several anatomic varieties of capillaries have been

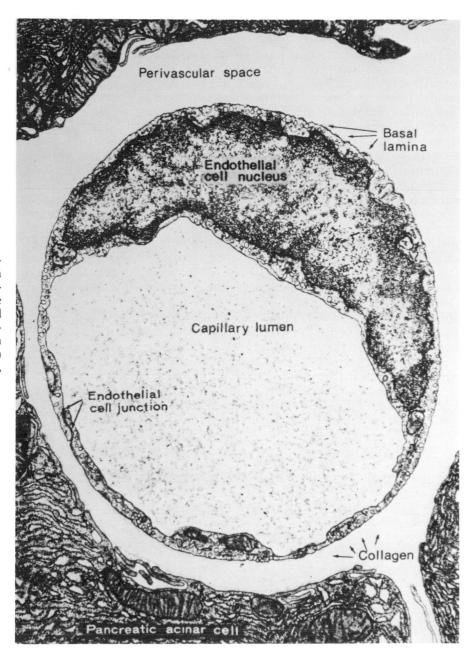

FIGURE 12–4. Electron photomicrograph of a typical capillary from guinea pig pancreas. The entire circumference is made up of a single endothelial cell. There is a thin basal lamina and a few associated collagen fibrils. No pericyte is present in this cross-section. (Reprinted from Bolender, R.: J. Cell Biol., *61*:269, 1974.)

recognized. Continuous capillaries have a complete endothelial lining with apparent tight intercellular junctions (found in muscle, nerve, and connective tissue). Fenestrated capillaries have interjunctional clefts or pores (found in pancreas, intestine, and endocrine glands). These pores represent only 0.02 per cent of the capillary surface. Some capillaries may be surrounded by undifferentiated mesenchymal cells, the pericytes, of uncertain function, but they are presumed to be contractile and to control flow.

VENOUS STRUCTURE AND FUNCTION

The venous system is a large reservoir that contains up to three quarters of the blood volume. Several capillaries join to form a venule, which is 15 to 20 μm in diameter. Although venules are larger than capillaries, their structure is not much different. The venules are quite permeable and hence play an important role in tissue exchange. Running along with the arteries, although more numerous, the veins gradually increase in size and decrease in number as they channel blood back to the heart. All veins large enough to be visible contain smooth muscle elements in their walls. Larger veins have an intima, media, and adventitia, but the layers are less distinct than in arteries (Fig. 12–5). The muscular and elastic tissue is not as well developed as it is in arteries of equivalent caliber, but the connective tissue is more prominent. The thickness of the muscular layer is related to the hydrostatic pressure within the vein; therefore, more dependent veins have thicker walls.

Veins of medium caliber, particularly those of the extremities, have bicuspid similunar valves that ensure a unidirectional flow of blood toward the heart. Located in areas where major tributaries join the vein, these valves consist of delicate thin connective tissue, with a plane of closure typically parallel to the skin. There is a dilation of the vein, a valve sinus, on the cardiac side of each valve just above the attachment of its cusps, which prevents contact between the leaflets and the vein wall when the valve is open. It is at this point, as a consequence of stasis, a hypercoagulable state, or injury, that thrombus may first form as the initial event in venous thrombosis. Flow through intact venous valves is unidirectional and directs blood from the peripheral toward the central veins, and from the superficial to the deep venous systems via venous perforators. However, in the feet, hands, and forearms, perforators direct blood flow

in the opposite direction—from the deep to the superficial veins. This notable exception is believed to play a role in thermoregulation. Interestingly, large internal veins, such as the vena cava, common iliac, hepatic, renal, mesenteric, splenic, and portal, are valveless.

Venous pressure dynamics are important to the understanding of the pathophysiology of some venous diseases and the tests used to diagnose them. Normally, venous pressure is low in the recumbent position (10 to 12 mm Hg), but rises upon standing, reaching 90 to 100 mm Hg at the foot (Fig. 12–6). There is a minute gradient (2 to 3 mm Hg) between the superficial and deep venous systems that ensures flow from the superficial to deep veins. Even in normal individuals, as much as 15 to 20 per cent of the blood volume may be lost by standing still due to fluid extravasation from the increased hydrostatic pressure, resulting in a drop in cardiac output. This hypovolemia may contribute to the syncope seen in military recruits who engage in prolonged standing at attention. The contraction and relaxation of muscles within the confined fascial compartments of the lower extremities compress the veins and help pump venous blood back to the heart. This muscle pump functions as a peripheral heart and provides up to one third of the energy required for the circulation of the blood. Therefore with ambulation, venous

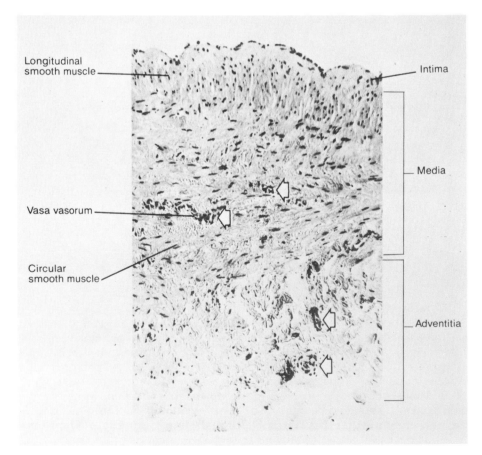

Longitudinal smooth muscle

Intima

Media

Vasa vasorum

Circular smooth muscle

Adventitia

FIGURE 12–5. Wall structure of a large vein (saphenous vein). Vasa vasorum (*arrows*) entend a fair distance into the media. The muscular media contains an inner longitudinal layer of smooth muscle in addition to its thick outer circular layer of smooth muscle. (Reprinted from Cormack, D.H.: Ham's Histology, 9th ed. Philadelphia, J.B. Lippincott Co., 1987. Figure 16–24, p. 445.)

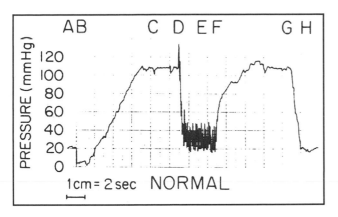

FIGURE 12–6. Pressure recorded from a dorsal vein of the foot of a normal person. *A*, supine; *B*, begin to assume standing position; *C*, resting, standing; *D*, begin exercise; *E*, repetitive dorsiflexion of foot; *F*, cease exercise; *G*, begin to assume supine position; *H*, resting, supine. (Adapted from Johnson, G., Jr.: Chronic venous insufficiency of the lower extremity: An overview. *In* Foley, W.T. (ed.): Advances in the Management of Cardiovascular Disease. Chicago, Year Book Medical Publishers, Inc., 1980.)

pressure at the ankle falls from 90 to 100 mm Hg to 25 to 30 mm Hg. In normal individuals with intact valves, it takes a minimum of 25 to 30 seconds after cessation of exercise for the pressures to return to their high baseline levels (Figure 12–7A). These relationships form the basis of such tests of venous insufficiency as ambulatory venous pressure measurement and photoplethysmography (PPG), in which a recovery to baseline in less than 22 seconds ("short recovery times") is indicative of valvular insufficiency (Fig. 12–7B). In addition, such tests may suggest significant venous obstruction when exercise fails to achieve the expected pressure drop ("congestive pattern"). In either case, venous hypertension is the physiologic hallmark of chronic venous insufficiency, which is most commonly the result of deep venous thrombosis, with destruction of multiple valves. This venous hypertension progresses to the development of interstitial edema and extravasation of protein (fibrin), which interferes with diffusion and results in local hypoxia and venous ulceration (the Browse hypothesis).

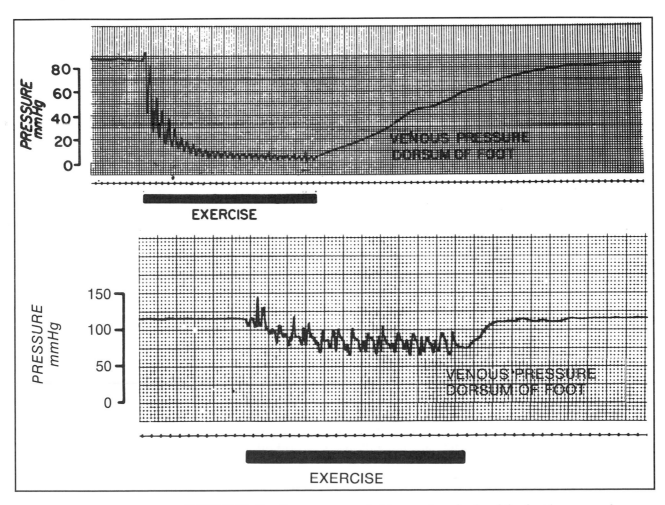

FIGURE 12–7. Pressures recorded from a dorsal vein of the foot in a normal person (*A*) and patient with venous valvular incompetence (*B*). (From Strandness, D.E., Jr., and Sumner, D.S.: Hemodynamics of Surgeons. New York, Grune & Stratton, 1975.)

In contrast to the lower body, the hydrostatic pressure is zero in the neck and is negative intracranially, accounting for the risk of air embolism during intracranial operations.

LYMPHATIC STRUCTURE

The lymph capillaries parallel the blood capillaries in most tissues, the major exceptions being the central nervous system, cartilage, bone, and bone marrow. This is an open drainage system, with the lymph capillaries originating blindly in the interstitial spaces. The lymph capillaries feed into the larger lymphatic vessels that coalesce to form the thoracic and right lymphatic ducts. These then enter the subclavian veins on each side near their junction with the internal jugular veins. On their way to join the venous circulation, lymphatic channels course through numerous lymph nodes (about 1000 in humans) that act as filters, trapping bacteria and other particulate matter. Like veins, lymphatics contain valves that promote unidirectional flow toward the larger ducts in the neck. This largely passive lymphatic circulation is maintained by such processes as tissue pressure, muscle contractions, respiratory movements, and arterial pulsations.

Lymph, made up of water, electrolytes, and protein, serves mainly to conserve plasma proteins lost through the blood capillary walls and as a filtration system through the lymph nodes to scavenge foreign material, bacteria, and antigenic substances. In the gastrointestinal tract, lymph flow contributes to the transport of absorbed nutrients, especially fat, into the circulation.

BASIC HEMODYNAMICS

The factors influencing blood flow in living organisms are extremely complex. A number of equations have been borrowed from the field of hydrodynamics in an attempt to describe quantitatively the flow of blood and its determinants (Table 12–4). Many of these equations, however, only apply to nonpulsatile laminar flow of Newtonian fluids in long cylindrical tubes with rigid walls. Blood, a nonhomogeneous suspension, is a non-Newtonian fluid, its flow pattern is pulsatile, and blood vessels are tapering conduits with elastic walls and numerous branches. Because of all these exceptions, hemodynamic equations are approximations at best. However, keeping in mind their limitations, they can be extremely useful in understanding the factors determining flow and how it is altered by various lesions affecting the circulation.

Laminar Flow, Shear Stress, Rate, and Viscosity

Laminar flow refers to a flow pattern in which infinitely thin, concentric layers or "laminae" of fluid slide past each other (Fig. 12–8). The force per unit area tending to impede this sliding movement is called the shear stress. The shear rate describes the relative velocity between two adjacent layers of the fluid and is the longitudinal displacement per second (in cm/sec) divided by the distance between layers (in cm). Its unit is therefore cm/sec per cm, or sec-1. Shear stress is proportional to shear rate, and the proportionality factor is the viscosity (η). In other words, viscosity (η) is the ratio of shear stress to shear rate:

$$\eta = \frac{\text{Shear stress}}{\text{Shear rate}} \qquad \text{(Eq. 1)}$$

Where η is expressed in dyne sec cm^{-2}, shear stress in dyne/cm^2, and shear rate in sec.$^{-1}$ Hence,

$$\text{shear stress} = \eta \times \text{Shear rate.} \qquad \text{(Eq. 2)}$$

A fluid is said to be Newtonian if its viscosity is independent of shear rate. Like many colloidal suspensions, blood at low levels of shear rate (below 100 sec-1) is not a Newtonian fluid, since its viscosity is not constant. These abnormally low shear rates are only encountered in situations of near stagnant flow such as shock, and are associated with increased viscosity, mainly as a result of rouleaux formation.

Viscosity is a major factor influencing flow. Whole blood has a variable viscosity ranging from 2 to 15 times that of water. The primary determinant of blood viscosity is the hematocrit, with viscosity increasing exponentially with increasing hematocrit (Fig. 12–9A).

Viscosity varies inversely with temperature. Both blood and water are 2.5 times more viscous at 0°C than at 40°C. At body temperature, viscosity increases by 2 per cent for every 1°C drop in temperature. This is of clinical importance when hypothermia is used in surgery or is encountered as a result of cold exposure or immersion in their influence on viscosity.

Plasma proteins, particularly fibrinogen, are of lesser but significant importance.

In larger vessels (larger than 0.5 mm in diameter), viscosity is independent of vessel diameter. However in the microcirculation, as the smaller arteries and arterioles are reached, apparent viscosity decreases with decreasing diameter (Fig. 12–9C). This phenomenon, known as the Fahraeus-Lindqvist effect, is partially explained by the alignment of red blood cells in the center of the flow as they move through very small vessels (axial accumulation and streaming). This alignment results in a cell-free marginal zone along the vessel wall consisting of the less viscous plasma. This effect is lost at the level of the 4 mm capillaries, where apparent viscosity increases

TABLE 12–4. IMPORTANT FORMULAS IN VASCULAR HEMODYNAMICS

Reynold's number

(1) $\text{Re} = \dfrac{\rho \cdot v \cdot D}{\eta}$

ρ = density in gm/cm^3
v = velocity in cm/sec
D = diameter in cm
η = viscosity in dynes·sec/cm^2

(2) $\text{Re} = \dfrac{4 \cdot \rho \cdot Q}{\pi \cdot D \cdot \eta}$

ρ = density in gm/cm^3
Q = flow in cm^3/min
D = diameter in cm
η = viscosity in dynes·sec/cm^2

For blood, turbulence is likely if Re > 1000.

Viscosity

(3) $\eta = \dfrac{\text{Shear stress}}{\text{Shear rate}}$

in dynes/cm^2
in sec^{-1}

Poiseuille's law

(4) $Q = \dfrac{\pi \cdot \Delta P \cdot r^4}{8 \cdot \eta \cdot L}$

Q = flow in cm^3/sec
ΔP = pressure gradient in dynes/cm^2
r = radius in cm
η = viscosity in dyncs·scc/cm^2
L = length in cm

Ohm's law

(5) $Q = \dfrac{\Delta P}{R}$

Q = flow in cm^3/sec
ΔP = pressure gradient in mm Hg
R = resistance in mm Hg·min/ml

Hence resistance

(6) $R = \dfrac{\Delta P}{Q}$

Can use it clinically to derive systemic vascular resistance (SVR) and pulmonary vascular resistance (PVR):

(7) $\text{SVR} = \dfrac{\text{MAP} - \text{CVP}}{\text{CO}} \times 80$

MAP = mean arterial pressure in mm Hg
CVP = central venous pressure in mm Hg
CO = cardiac output in mL/min
80 = constant to convert SVR units to dynes·sec/cm^{-5}

(8) $\text{PVR} = \dfrac{\text{MPAP} - \text{PCWP}}{\text{CO}} \times 80$

MPAP = mean pulmonary arterial pressure
PCWP = pulmonary wedge pressure
CO = cardiac output in mL/min
80 = constant to convert SVR units to dynes·sec/cm^{-5}

Compliance

(9) $C \dfrac{\Delta V}{\Delta P}$

ΔV = volume change in cm^3
ΔP = pressure change in mm Hg

Doppler equation

(10) $\Delta f = \dfrac{2 \cdot f_o \cdot V \cdot \cos \theta}{C}$

Δf = frequency shift in cycles/sec (Hz)
f_o = transmitted frequency in Hz
V = flow velocity in cm/sec
θ = angle between sound beam and direction of flow
C = velocity of sound in tissue in cm/sec

f_o and C are constants, therefore

(11) $\Delta f \; \alpha \; V \cdot \cos \theta$

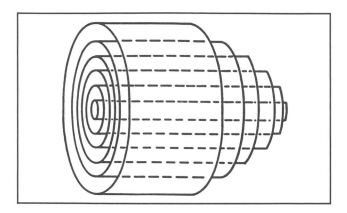

FIGURE 12–8. Concentric laminae of fluid in tube with circular cross-section. Flow is fully developed and steady. Laminae at center of tube move more rapidly than those near periphery. Velocity profile is parabolic. (Reprinted from Strandness, D.E., Jr., and Sumner, D.S.: Hemodynamics for Surgeons. New York, Grune & Stratton, Inc., 1975.)

(Fig. 12–9C) because of the force required to deform the now larger red cells and squeeze them through the capillary.

Shear stress as a function of the viscosity and shear rate increases with higher blood velocity and viscosity. Wall shear stress is a measure of the tangential drag force acting at the blood-vessel interface. In mammals, arterial wall shear stress normally ranges between 10 and 20 dynes/cm². Arterial wall shear stress appears to act as the signal regulating the adaptive responses of the vessel wall to changes in its hemodynamic parameters. Indeed, there is evidence that such processes as the adjustment of luminal diameter and the endothelial secretion of certain vasoactive agents and various proteins can be regulated by shear stress. Atherosclerotic plaques seem to localize preferentially in areas of low shear stress. Acute elevations in shear stress may also contribute to endothelial injury, especially in high-velocity vessels, such as the aorta, and may be a factor in the development of aortic dissection. The use of beta blockers, of crucial importance in the medical management of this condition, is aimed at reducing arterial wall shear stress.

The Relationship of Flow, Pressure, and Resistance

Although it is applicable to the flow of blood only as an approximation, Poiseuille's law is a very helpful illustration of the various parameters determining flow and how they relate to each other:

$$Q = \frac{\pi \cdot \Delta P \cdot r^4}{8 \cdot \eta \cdot L} \qquad \text{(Eq. 3)}$$

where Q = flow in cm³/sec, ΔP = pressure gradient

in dynes/cm² · r = radius in cm, η = viscosity in dynes. sec/cm², and L = length in cm.

This equation shows the relative contributions of various determinants of flow. It is evident that even small changes in caliber result in marked flow altera-

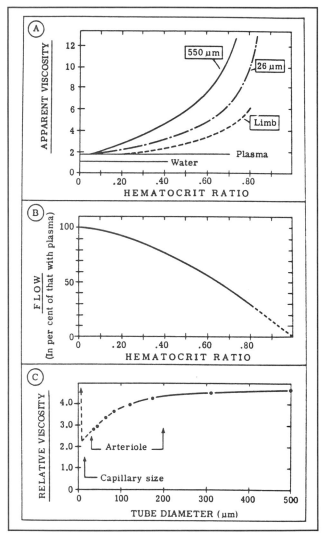

FIGURE 12–9. *A,* Effect of the concentration of erythrocytes (hematocrit ratio) on the apparent viscosity of blood perfused through tubing of various diameters and an isolated dog hind limb. The hematocrit ratio has a smaller effect on viscosity if the blood flows through small, 26-μm diameter tubes than if the flow is through larger, 550-μm glass tubes. (Data from Frey-Wyssling, (ed.): Deformation and Flow in Biological Systems. New York, Interscience 1952.) There is even less effect when blood flows through a hind limb. (Data from Whittaker and Windon. J. Physiol., *78*:357, 1933. *B,* As the hematocrit ratio of blood is increased, the flow of blood through isolated tissue decreases, other factors being constant. (Derived from data of Whittaker and Winton. J. Physiol., *78*:357, 1933. *C,* The effect of tube diameter on the relative viscosity of blood. (Data from Fahraeus and Lindqvist.: Am. J. Physiol., *96*:565, 1931. Reprinted from Selkurt, E.E.: Physiology, 4th ed. Boston, Little, Brown, and Co. 1976. Figure 11–2, p. 258.)

tions since flow is proportional to the fourth power of the radius. One can readily appreciate the detrimental effects of high viscosity and conduit length.

Ohm's law of electrical circuits can be borrowed to define the relationship between flow, pressure gradient, and resistance in the circulation as a whole or in regional beds.

$$Q = \frac{\Delta P}{R} \qquad \text{(Eq. 4)}$$

where Q = flow in cm^3/sec, ΔP = pressure gradient in mm Hg, R = resistance in mm Hg·min/cm^3. Hence, resistance is

$$R = \frac{\Delta P}{Q} \qquad \text{(Eq. 5)}$$

Hemodynamic resistance cannot be measured directly, but can be calculated using simultaneous measurements of flow and pressure gradient. Indeed, it is Ohm's law that is used clinically to derive systemic vascular resistance (SVR) and pulmonary vascular resistance (PVR) when obtaining hemodynamic profiles in critically ill patients. In the systemic vascular bed, the overall pressure gradient (ΔP) is the difference between mean arterial pressure and central venous pressure, whereas the flow is (Q) the cardiac output. Thus, systemic vascular resistance (SVR) is

$$SVR = \frac{MAP - CVP}{CO} \times 80 \qquad \text{(Eq. 6)}$$

where MAP = mean arterial pressure in mm Hg, CVP = central venous pressure in mm Hg, CO = cardiac output in mL/min, and 80 = constant to convert SVR units to dynes · sec/cm^{-5}.

For the pulmonary vascular bed, the pressure gradient is the difference between the mean pulmonary artery pressure and the left atrial pressure. In clinical practice, the pulmonary artery capillary wedge pressure is used to estimate left atrial pressure. The flow remains the same, i.e., the cardiac output:

$$PVR = \frac{MPAP - PCWP}{CO} \times 80 \qquad \text{(Eq. 7)}$$

where MPAP = mean pulmonary arterial pressure, PCWP = pulmonary wedge pressure, CO = cardiac output in mL/min, and 80 = constant to convert SVR units in dyne/sec/cm.$^{-5}$

Parabolic (Laminar) Flow

In a normal vessel, blood ordinarily assumes a smooth parabolic flow profile. The maximal velocity is found at the center of flow, whereas the flow at the wall of the blood vessel is nil (Fig. 12–10). The velocity gradient from the center to the blood-intimal interface (where it is maximal) is due to shear forces or viscous drag. In this laminar, or streamlined flow, fluid elements remain in distinct laminae. Under certain circumstances, turbulent flow may develop, with the generation of swirls and eddies. The significance of turbulent flow is that part of the driving energy is lost in the swirls and eddies as heat. Therefore, for a given pressure gradient, less flow is achieved under turbulent conditions than with laminar flow. The likelihood of turbulent flow can be estimated using Reynold's number (Re), a unitless ratio determined as follows:

$$Re = \frac{\rho \cdot v \cdot D}{\eta} \qquad \text{(Eq. 8)}$$

where ρ = density in gm/cm^3, v = velocity in cm/sec, D = diameter in cm, and η = viscosity in dynes. sec/cm^2.

Linear velocity (v) is the volume flow (Q) divided by the cross-sectional area $\pi \cdot r2$ or $\pi D2/4$. So replacing (v) by its expression in terms of flow gives the following equation:

$$Re = \frac{4 \cdot \rho \cdot Q}{\pi \cdot D \cdot \eta} \qquad \text{(Eq. 9)}$$

where ρ = density in gm/cm^3, Q = flow in cm^3/min, D = diameter in cm, and η = viscosity in dynes· sec/cm^2.

The higher the value of Reynold's number, the greater the tendency for turbulence to develop. At Reynold's numbers of 200 to 400, turbulence may occur at branch points, but at values exceeding 1000 turbulence occurs even in a normal vessel. The above equation illustrates the factors responsible for the generation of turbulent flow: areas of stenosis (lower values of D), anemia (lower values of η), and exercise (higher values of Q) all increase Reynold's number. In addition to these factors, turbulence may be caused by sudden changes in vessel size, such as at bifurcations, or by irregularities in the vessel wall created by atherosclerotic plaque.

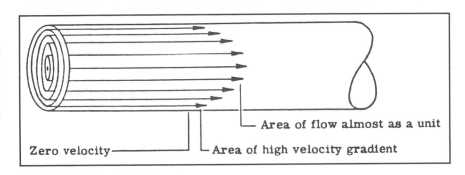

FIGURE 12–10. The velocity profile of the flowing stream is parabolic, with the highest velocity in the center and no flow at the wall. (Reprinted from Selkurt, E.E.: Physiology, 4th ed. Boston, Little, Brown, and Co., 1976. Figure 11–1, p. 256.)

Zero velocity —

Area of high velocity gradient

Area of flow almost as a unit

The law of LaPlace relates the tension of the wall of a blood vessel to the intraluminal pressure and radius. Its derivation is described in Figure 12–11.

$$T = P \times r \qquad \text{(Eq. 10)}$$

This law explains why the capillaries, with their small radius, can withstand the relatively high internal pressures compared to their fragile 1-mm thick walls. It also explains the increasing tendency for aortic aneurysm rupture associated with larger size, as high wall tensions develop even at normal arterial pressures.

Velocity in the Major Arteries and Contact Times

As shown in Table II–2, the initial velocity of blood flow is approximately 33 cm/sec as it passes through the aortic valve. It decreases gradually to 0.03 cm/sec in the capillary bed, a reduction of approximately 1000:1. Blood normally reaches the tissues within 10 seconds after oxygenation, but this interval may be shortened to 2 to 3 seconds. Blood remains in the capillary bed only 1 to 3 seconds, a surprisingly short time for exchange.

The pulse pressure is the difference between the systolic and diastolic pressures, and it is determined mainly by the ratio of the stroke volume to the arterial compliance. Vascular compliance is defined as the increase in vessel volume per incremental increase in pressure. In other words, the greater the volume increase that a vessel can accommodate for a given increment in pressure, the more compliant it is (Table 12–4). The decreased compliance of atherosclerotic vessels results in higher systolic and lower diastolic pressures, thereby widening the pulse pressure. Abnormal pulse pressure waves may also occur with a patent ductus arteriosus or aortic valvular insufficiency. The pulse pressure is related to the temporary increment in blood volume in the large conducting arteries that occurs during the ejection phase of systole (the stroke volume) since the runoff through the capillary bed is at a constant rate during the entire cardiac cycle. If the stroke volume increases or there is a decrease in total peripheral resistance or an increase in mean circulatory filling pressure, the pulse pressure increases. If there is an increase in heart rate with a constant cardiac output, pulse pressure decreases because of a smaller stroke volume. The pattern of left ventricular ejection, (e.g., the relative length of systole) can influence the pulse pressure by varying the amount of time the blood has to run off through the peripheral circulation.

The velocity of transmission of the pressure pulse—peripheral arterial pressure curve—is much higher than the actual velocity of blood flow, being approximately 15 times the actual blood velocity in the aorta (300 to 500 cm/sec) and as high as 100 times that in the distal arteries (1500 to 4000 cm/sec). The velocity of the transmitted wave is proportional to the stiffness of the arterial wall and inversely proportional to the viscosity of the blood. It generally increases with age as the aorta loses its elasticity and can be up to three times faster than normal in hypertension and arteriosclerosis. As the pressure pulse reaches the distal arteries it distends them, and because compliance is lower in the smaller arteries, the pressure wave rebounds and is augmented. This explains the higher systolic and lower diastolic pressures found in the stiffer peripheral arteries in comparison to the more elastic aorta. At the arteriolar level, the degree of reflection depends on vascular tone. It is maximal with maximal vasoconstriction and diminishes with vasodilation. It is the pulse wave that is felt when palpating a distal artery.

Measurement of Flow Velocity

The development of Doppler flow velocity measurement is based on the principle described in the nineteenth century by the Austrian physicist, Christian Johan Doppler. It states that, when a sound wave of a given frequency hits a moving object, the frequency of the reflected sound is "shifted" from the transmitted frequency by an amount proportional to the velocity of the moving object. Moreover, the fre-

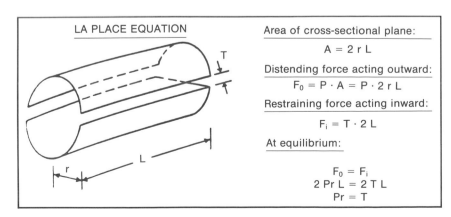

LA PLACE EQUATION

Area of cross-sectional plane:

$$A = 2\,r\,L$$

Distending force acting outward:

$$F_0 = P \cdot A = P \cdot 2\,r\,L$$

Restraining force acting inward:

$$F_i = T \cdot 2\,L$$

At equilibrium:

$$F_0 = F_i$$
$$2\,Pr\,L = 2\,T\,L$$
$$Pr = T$$

FIGURE 12–11. Derivation of the Laplace equation. (Reprinted from Selkurt, E.E.: Physiology, 4th ed. Boston, Little, Brown, and Co., 1976. Figure 11—4, p. 263.)

quency increases if the object is moving toward the sound source and decreases if the object is moving away from it. This frequency shift is referred to as the Doppler shift and is described by the Doppler equation:

$$\Delta f = \frac{2 \cdot f_o \cdot V \cdot \cos \Theta}{C} \qquad \text{(Eq. 11)}$$

where Δf = frequency shift in cycles/sec (Hz), f_o = transmitted frequency in Hz, V = flow velocity in cm/sec, Θ = angle between the sound beam and the direction of flow, and C = velocity of sound in tissue in cm/sec.

Since f_o and C are constants for a given probe, the frequency shift is proportional to the velocity of the moving object and to the cosine of the angle between the sound beam and the direction of flow:

$$\Delta f \; \alpha \; V \cdot \cos \Theta. \qquad \text{(Eq. 12)}$$

The Doppler probe contains two piezoelectric crystals. One serves as a transmitter and emits ultrasound at a specific frequency, which is generally set between 2 to 10 MHz depending on the depth of tissue penetration required. The signal reflected by moving red cells in the vessel is detected by the second crystal. The degree of shift in frequency is represented as audible sound, and changes in frequency are detected as changes in the pitch of that sound (Fig. 12–12). From the above equation, one can predict that no shift will be detected if the blood is stationary ($V=0$) or if the probe is held at a right angle to the axis of the vessel ($\Theta=90°$) (Fig. 12–13). When combined with ultrasound imaging of the vessel to determine the cross-sectional area of the vessel, it is theoretically possible to measure volume flow; however, because of unresolved technical problems, this is not yet clinically practical. Nonetheless, the Doppler flowmeter has proven to be a useful tool for measuring extremity blood pressure, especially in the obstructed circulation when used with an occlusive cuff. The Doppler signal may be bidirectional, detecting flow toward or away from the probe or may be unidirectional and unable to distinguish direction. The Doppler may be continuous or pulsed, the latter permitting measurement of flow velocity in a more discrete area, and may be directed to the center of the lumen using real-time B mode ultrasound imaging (the duplex scanner) to determine peak velocity and turbulent flow.

SENSORY ORGANS OF ARTERIES

The carotid bodies are 3 mm × 5 mm flattened organs in the wall of the common carotid bifurcation. They are innervated by the carotid sinus branch of the glossopharyngeal nerve (nerve of Hering) and by sympathetic components from the vagus and glossopharyngeal nerves. The glomus

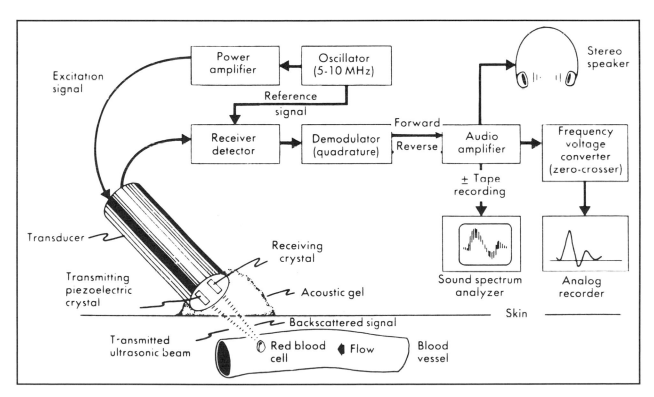

FIGURE 12–12. Components of CW Doppler ultrasonic velocity detector. (Reprinted from Bernstein, E.F. (ed.): Noninvasive Diagnostic Techniques in Vascular Disease, 3rd ed. St. Louis, C.V. Mosby Co., 1985. Figure 4–1, p. 20.)

cells in the carotid bodies are probably chemoreceptors that are stimulated by hypoxia, hypercapnia, or increased hydrogen ion concentration and have some role in the regulation of respiration. Similar chemoreceptor organs are in the aortic bodies, which are distributed around the aortic arch. The carotid sinuses are slight dilations of the common carotid artery bifurcation, which contain nerve endings stimulated by stretching. These baroreceptors, through the nerve of Hering and the hypoglossal to the medulla, inhibit baseline sympathetic impulses. Stretching of the carotid sinus produces significant vasodilation in the skeletal muscle mass, which is the largest vascular bed; this vasodilation is a major component of blood pressure regulation. Less sensitive

baroreceptors are located in the aortic arch. Cardiopulmonary baroreceptors contribute to the regulation of local resistance tone and urine output. Stimulation of these receptors inhibits vasopressin, angiotensin, and aldosterone release. The effect is to increase blood volume by increasing water resorption and salt retention.

CAPILLARIES

Transport across the capillary from the luminal to the abluminal surface is the subject of intense research and is certainly one of the most fundamental events in biology. Cells, especially monocytes, move readily through the capillary barrier by diapedesis between capillary junctions, the process being under the control of chemotactic stimuli. Simple diffusion is controlled by osmotic gradients and moves water and small water- or fat-soluble molecules across the endothelial lining. This is the primary mechanism for exchange of gases, nutrients, and waste products between tissue cells and the blood. Because diffusion is so unrestricted and rapid, the concentration gradient across the capillary wall is a function of the delivery rate of blood flow.

Capillary permeability is generally greater at the venous end of the capillary than the arterial end. The exchange of oxygen and other simple molecules is directly related to surface area. The process of diffusion is described by Fick's law:

$$dQ/dt = D \cdot A \cdot dc/dx \qquad (Eq.\ 13)$$

where Q equals the quantity of a substance moved per unit time (t), D is the free diffusion coefficient for a given molecule, A is the cross-sectional area of diffusion over a distance (x), and dc/dx is the solute concentration gradient. Available surface area must match the delivered volume of blood. When there is an increased demand, capillary recruitment follows.

Receptor-specific active transport may occur selectively by pinocytosis or transcytosis. The movement of macromolecules and lipid-insoluble substances may occur by a number of mechanisms. The permeability of microvessels is modulated apparently by the endothelial cells, although in some instances the basement membrane may be the actual barrier between the capillary lumen and the interstitial space. A variety of factors control luminal to abluminal movement, including flow rate, electrical charge, size of particles, and molecular configuration.

The sinusoids are irregular, rather large vascular channels lined with endothelium. Their shape conforms to the interstices of the organ they supply (liver, spleen, bone marrow, adenohypophysis, renal cortex). The endothelium is more active in endocytosis, and the sinusoids have often been grouped together as the reticuloendothelial system.

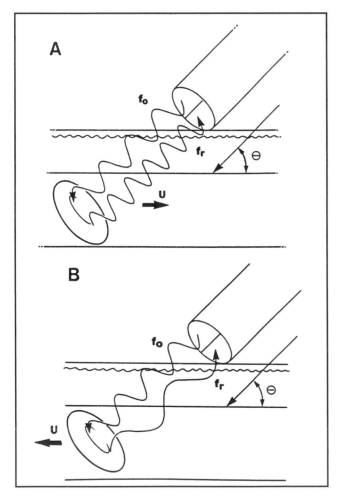

FIGURE 12–13. Doppler shifts produced by red blood cell moving toward probe (*A*) and away from probe (*B*). Transmitted frequency (f_o) is same in both examples, but backscattered frequency (f_r) is increased when cell moves toward probe and reduced when cell moves away. Velocity of red blood cell is represented by U, and the angle at which sound beam intersects velocity vector is indicated by Θ. (Reprinted from Kempczinski, R.F., and Yao, J.S.T.: Practical Noninvasive Vascular Diagnosis. Chicago, Year Book Medical Publisher, Inc., 1982. Figure 2–4, p. 27.)

Starling's Law

The movement of water between the capillary lumen and interstitial space is controlled by the net effect of the intraluminal hydrostatic pressure and the relative osmotic pressure, a phenomenon first described by Starling in 1896. The entering pressure into the capillary bed is approximately 30 mm Hg and the exiting pressure approximately 10 to 15 mm Hg. These pressures are not constant. An increase in arterial or venous pressure increases the capillary hydrostatic pressure; a drop in either decreases filtration pressure. A rise in arteriolar resistance or closure of precapillary sphincters reduces hydrostatic pressure. Increased venous resistance increases pressure. The interstitial fluid pressure may actually be slightly negative, increasing the total pressure gradient across the capillary.

The net positive osmotic pressure of blood, which draws water intravascularly, is produced largely by the plasma proteins, especially albumin (65 per cent), since small molecules (electrolytes) move freely across the membrane and are in equilibrium.

When hydrostatic pressure exceeds the retention effect of osmotic pressure, there is a filtration of fluid into the interstitial space. When the osmotic pressure is greater water is resorbed into the vascular circulation. The small amount of plasma protein that escapes from the capillaries and the excess water that is not resorbed are returned by the lymphatic network to the circulation.

In addition to these pressure effects, the movement of fluid across the capillary is further determined by capillary area, viscosity of the filtrate, and wall thickness, with viscosity and wall thickness exerting a hindering effect. These factors define the capillary filtration coefficient, which is a measure of capillary permeability and surface area. The factors controlling fluid movement are important in response to pathologic events, such as hemorrhage, when the reduced pressure causes absorption of interstitial fluid to restore blood volume, and hypoalbuminemia, in which reduced osmotic pressure contributes to loss of intravascular fluid into the interstitial space.

REGULATION OF BLOOD FLOW

The acute control of regional blood flow is determined by changes in oxygen requirement (the oxygen or nutrient demand theory) or by the local accumulation of metabolic byproducts or signals (the vasodilator theory). Among the putative substances are carbon dioxide, lactic acid, adenosine or adenosine phosphate compounds, hydrogen ions, and prostaglandins. An alternate and possibly coexisting mechanism is that the concentration of oxygen or local nutrients affects the degree of contraction of the smooth muscle cells. The fibers of these cells in the precapillary sphincter control either the degree of flow through the capillary or the number of capillaries that are open.

Autoregulation is the response of local flow to an acute decrease or increase in arterial perfusion pressure when the tissue metabolic rate is constant. It may be controlled by the metabolic mechanisms already noted. An additional myogenic mechanism may be functional (Bayliss hypothesis). The increased arterial pressure may cause stretching of the vascular smooth muscle cell, which responds by contracting and decreasing flow. This may be functional primarily at the precapillary sphincter level. Autoregulation in the kidneys and brain is unique. The concentration of solutes in the renal tubule may control flow through feedback to the juxtaglomerular apparatus. In the brain, an increase in carbon dioxide or hydrogen ion produces a rapid increase in cerebral blood flow.

Nervous and humoral influences (extrinsic factors) on regional capillary bed flows are less important under ordinary circumstances. The peripheral arteries are mainly under sympathetic control, usually with little parasympathetic influence. The sympathetic innervation is by both the sympathetic chain and spinal nerves. The sympathetics innervate all vessels except the capillaries and precapillary sphincters (Fig. 12–14). The metarterioles are variously supplied. The sympathetics carry both vasoconstrictor and vasodilator fibers, the former being more important. The vasoconstrictor center is located in the anterolateral portion of the upper medulla and lower pons. The vasodilator area, the neurons of which inhibit the vasoconstrictor area, is in the lower medulla. The degree of sympathetic activity sets the vasomotor tone and can be influenced by many higher brain centers, which either increase the vasoconstrictor center activity or decrease it by stimulation of the vasodilator center. Norepinephrine is the sympathetic vasoconstrictor transmitter substance. Simultaneous sympathetic stimulation of the adrenal medullae causes release into the circulation of norepinephrine and epinephrine, both of which generally produce vasoconstriction. However, epinephrine in low concentrations may produce vasodilation in skeletal muscle through its beta receptor effect. The sympathetic cholinergic vasodilator system appears to have minimal importance, although in skeletal muscle it may serve to produce an anticipatory increase in blood flow at the onset of exercise. In the salivary glands, parasympathetic stimulation produces vasodilation, possibly mediated by bradykinin. Where continued flow of blood is vital, such as to the brain and heart, intrinsic control predominates, whereas in the skin and splanchnic beds extrinsic factors prevail.

Several patterns of generalized response to central nervous system commands are recognized. The mass action effect of the vasoconstrictor center appears to

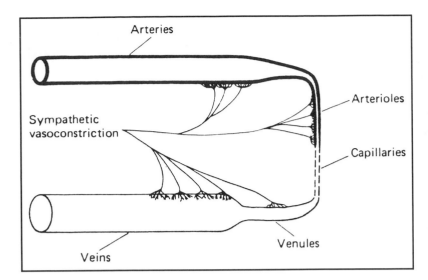

FIGURE 12–14. Sympathetic innervation of the systemic circulation. (Reprinted from Guyton, A.C.: Textbook of Medical Physiology, 7th ed. Philadelphia: W.B. Saunders Co., 1986. Figure 20–7, p. 238.)

prepare the circulation for an overall increased blood flow by (1) increasing resistance in most parts of the circulation; (2) decreasing the capacity of the venous reservoir, thereby forcing blood into the heart; and (3) stimulating the heart to manage the increased cardiac output. The alarm or defense pattern, produced by hypothalamic stimulation, is the mass action effect with the addition of vasodilation in the muscles and a generalized excitement and psychic attentiveness. The motor pattern produced by stimulation of the motor cortex results in selective vasoconstriction of most nonmuscle beds, thereby raising blood pressure and cerebral perfusion, probably from strong stimulation of the hypothalamic vasodilator center.

The humoral control of the circulation is mediated by circulating epinephrine and norepinephrine, the renin-angiotensin system, and vasopressin, which are all strong vasoconstrictors. Known vasodilators include bradykinin and histamine, which also increase capillary permeability. Serotonin and prostaglandins may vasodilate or constrict, depending on the specific conditions in a given vascular bed. An increased calcium ion concentration causes vasoconstriction, whereas increased potassium or magnesium produces vasodilation by virtue of their effect on smooth muscle contraction. Hypernatremia and hyperglycemia cause arteriolar dilation, probably because of the increased osmolality.

Long-term changes in flow, which may be required because of a substantial increase in blood pressure or chronic hyperactivity of a tissue, are mediated by changes in the vascularity of tissue; that is, the number and size of vessels. These changes may be brought about partly through the effect of angiogenisis factors.

There is some variation in the control of specific regional vascular beds. Most notable is the cerebral circulation, which has minimal neural regulation and functions almost entirely by autoregulation. Normal cerebral blood flow averages 55 mL/min/100 gm of brain. Flow can be maintained at that level over a wide pressure range from significant hypotension to moderate hypertension. Variations within the brain may be dependent on the level of activity of specific regions; for example, exercise of an arm produces increased flow in the appropriate contralateral motor cortex. The control of autoregulation in the brain is not well understood, although flow is very sensitive to carbon dioxide levels. At least three local factors—pH, K^+, and adenosine—have autoregulatory effects. Autoregulation can be abolished by chemically induced vasodilation, such as with acetazolamide, or in cases of significant head injury.

In contrast, there is little autoregulatory function in the intestinal circulation, but rather strong neural control, which is almost entirely sympathetic. There is, however, a pronounced functional (as opposed to reactive) hyperemia after eating; the increased flow is produced by several locally vasoactive substances, including gastrin and cholecystokinin, and certain absorbed foods, such as glucose and fatty acids, that mediate increased local blood flow.

ENDOTHELIAL CELL BIOLOGY

In 1860, Virchow described the vascular endothelium as "a membrane as simple as any that is ever met within the body." Once dismissed as merely a passive interface between the bloodstream and the tissues, the endothelium is increasingly being recognized as an important modulator of such diverse processes as blood vessel development and remodeling, control of coagulation and platelet activation, thrombolysis, regulation of vascular tone, leukocyte migration, wound healing, immune response and graft rejection, tumor invasion, and atherogenesis. This modulation occurs through the secretion of a myriad of biologically active substances that include enzymes, vasoactive agents, mitogens, hemostatic and fibrinolytic agents, chemotactic factors, and matrix proteins (Table 12–5). The complexities of endothelial functions and endothelial interactions with blood and its elements are only beginning to be unraveled.

Endothelial cells form a monolayer of about 1000 square meters in surface area that constitutes the primary interface between the bloodstream and all extravascular tissue. Endothelial cells (Fig. 12–4) are polygonal, 10 to 15 μm wide, and 25 to 50 μm long with a thin glycoprotein layer on their luminal surface and some short microvilli. Cellular processes may extend through fenestrae in the elastica interna to form communicating junctions with smooth muscle cells of the media (myoendothelial junctions). Capillary endothelial cells contain actin and myosin and can alter their shape, thereby altering the intercellular spaces as well. Endothelial cell turnover is normally slow, and the cells are rarely found in division. Indeed, "contact inhibition" is a characteristic property of endothelial cells.

The endothelium is an intricate selective permeability barrier that has regional variations. A tighter permeability barrier exists in the brain and has been found in the eye and thymus. In the brain, the diminished permeability appears to be related to the presence of fewer transport vesicles and tighter endothelial junctions.

The main aspects of endothelial function to be discussed are those relating to hemocompatibility/ hemostasis, flow regulation, growth control, and immune function, all of which have direct relevance to normal and pathologic physiology. Endothelial functions are dynamic in nature and can change depending on the prevailing situation. Under normal conditions, endothelial cells express a program of functions aimed at promoting the fluidity of blood and enhancing blood flow—endogenous anticoagulants, antiplatelet and fibrinolytic factors, vasodilators. Injury or inflammation can trigger the expression of a different set of functions geared toward promoting hemostasis and tissue repair— procoagulants, platelet activators, vasoconstrictors, growth factors.

The delicate balance between hemocompatibility and hemostasis is maintained through several opposing mechanisms. Endothelial hemocompatibility (or thromboresistance) is achieved via numerous mechanisms, including the synthesis and expression of plasminogen activator, thrombomodulin, protein S, heparinoids, antithrombin III, membrane ADPase, and prostacyclin; the inactivation of circulating thrombin, adenosine nucleotides, and serotonin; and the provision of binding sites for plasmin. Hemostasis, on the other hand, is promoted through the synthesis of von Willebrand factor, basement membrane components, factor V, tissue plasminogen activator inhibitor; the expression of tissue factor (thromboplastin); and the provision of binding sites for coagulation factors Va, IXa, and Xa. Contact between blood and a tissue factor procoagulant is required to launch the extrinsic coagulation pathway. Traditionally, this contact was believed to require discontinuity in the endothelium and exposure of the subendothelial connective tissue. However, with the demonstration that endothelial cells themselves can produce tissue factor-like procoagulant in response to endotoxin, tumor necrosis factor, and interleukin-1, endothelial denudation is not a prerequisite to extrinsic pathway activation. This may account for hypercoagulable states associated with malignancies and consumptive coagulopathies associated with severe sepsis.

As an example of dual hemostatic control and because of its tremendous importance, the thromboxane/prostacyclin system that regulates, in part, vascular tone and blood vessel/platelet interactions is examined in detail in this section. Eicosanoid metabolism starts with arachidonic acid, which is the most common fatty acid present in cellular phospholipids. It is the precursor of all bisenoic prostaglandins and is liberated from membrane phospholipids by activation of phospholipases. It is available in the diet directly or by desaturation and chain elongation of dietary linoleic acid. Arachidonic acid is then acted upon by a cyclo-oxygenase and a hydroperoxidase that convert it to prostaglandin G_2 and then prostaglandin H_2. It is beyond this point in the pathway that cells show selectivity in their metabolism of prostaglandin H_2 to different biologically active pros-

TABLE 12–5. ENDOTHELIAL CELL PRODUCTS

Hemostatic/Fibrinolytic

Heparinoids	Tissue factor
Thrombomodulin	Von Willebrand factor
Protein S	TPA inhibitor
Antithrombin III	Thrombospondin
Plasminogen activator	Factor V

Vasoactive

Bradykinin	Histamine
Prostacyclin	Thromboxane
Endothelium-derived relaxing factor	Endothelin

Mitogens

Interleukin-1
PDGF A and B chains
Endothelial cell growth factor

Extracellular Matrix

Collagen
Fibronectin
Laminin
Glycosaminoglycans

Miscellaneous

Angiotensin-converting enzyme
Class I and II HLA antigens
Nucleotidases

tanoids, depending on their nature and function (Fig. 12–15).

Prostacyclin (PG I2) is the main metabolite of arachidonic acid in vascular endothelium, whereas thromboxane A_2 is the main arachidonic acid derivative in platelets. Thromboxane A_2 is a powerful platelet aggregator and vasoconstrictor. Prostacyclin is an endothelial autacoid, a local hormone with actions limited to the area of its release. Measured plasma levels are too low for it to have significant biologic activity. It is the most potent endogenous inhibitor of platelet aggregation known, as well as a potent vasodilator and a stimulus for platelet disaggregation. It acts by increasing platelet phospholipase and cyclo-oxygenase, thus shutting off platelet thromboxane synthesis. Prostacyclin increases cyclic AMP in a negative feedback control for its own production. It also acts on red blood cells, increasing their deformability. After systemic administration, its effects disappear within 30 minutes. In blood, at 37° C and neutral pH, prostacyclin has a half-life of 2 to 3 minutes. Several substances have been found to stimulate prostacyclin release, including arachidonic acid, interleukin-1, bradykinin, serotonin, and thrombin. It has been shown that, under normal conditions, at the intimal surface the prostacyclin/thromboxane ratio is in favor of prostacyclin 5 to 10 : 1. This is responsible, at least in part, for maintaining endothelial thromboresistance and hemocompatibility. This balance, however, is easily altered in situations of endothelial injury or in certain pathologic states.

Deficiency in prostacyclin production has been implicated or suspected in various disease states, including the hemolytic uremic syndrome, thrombotic thrombocytopenic purpura, sudden infant death syndrome, pre-eclampsia, and hypertension. Interesting studies have examined the production of prostacyclin in diabetes and have shown blood vessels from diabetic patients to produce less prostacyclin than controls. Serum from diabetics causes less stimulation of prostacyclin synthesis by cultured endothelial cells compared to normal serum. The decreased prostacyclin secretion by blood vessels from diabetic rats can be reversed with chronic insulin administration.

Lipid peroxides, which are present in athermatous plaques, have been shown to inhibit prostacyclin production in vascular tissue. Prostacyclin generation has been found to be lower in atherosclerotic arteries compared to normals. These findings point to a possible deleterious alteration in the prostacyclin/thromboxane A_2 ratio in areas of atheromatous plaques that would predispose to thrombosis. The platelet-inhibitory effects of prostacyclin make it an important modulator of atherogenesis through regulation of smooth muscle cell proliferation. Furthermore, prostacyclin increases cholesterol metabolism in smooth muscle, suppresses cholesterol accumulation by macrophages, and inhibits growth factors that thicken vascular walls. The beneficial effects of aspirin on cardiovascular disorders are thought to be mediated in part by the profound and irreversible inhibitory effects of aspirin on platelet thromboxane production and its transient suppressive effects on prostacyclin.

Endothelial enhancement of blood flow is achieved through the release of endothelial-derived relaxing factor, prostacyclin, adenosine, and angiotensinase (degrades angiotensin II), as well as the uptake and degradation of serotonin and epinephrine. Endothelial-derived relaxing factor (EDRF) has been identified as nitric oxide, which is synthesized from the amino acid L-arginine. EDRF release is stimulated by acetylcholine, bradykinin, and such mechanical stimuli as increased shear stress and pulsatile flow. Nitric oxide not only induces relaxation of vascular smooth muscle cells but also inhibits platelet aggregation. These effects are probably responsible for the antihypertensive effects of nitroglycerine and nitroprusside. Since nitric oxide production is increased in sepsis, the vasodilation of hyperdynamic shock may be caused by excess nitric oxide production.

Endothelial-induced vasoconstriction results from the synthesis of endothelin 1, a potent local peptide vasoconstricting factor, and angiotensin-converting enzyme, as well as the uptake and degradation of bradykinin. Endothelin 1, the release of which is stimulated by thrombin and epinephrine, is the most potent endogenous vasoconstrictor known. It has ten times the potency of angiotensin II. Its actions are opposed by prostacyclin and nitric oxide.

Endothelial cells exhibit the A and B blood groups antigens, as well as class I histocompatibility antigens (present on most cells). The expression of class II histocompatibility antigens was considered a property of bone-marrow-derived cells only and is required in the processing of foreign antigens for presentation to cytolytic T cells. However, endothelial cells can also be induced to express class II histocompatibility antigens after exposure to gamma in-

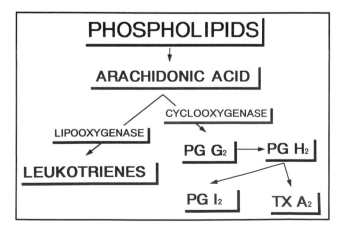

FIGURE 12–15. Thromboxane/prostacyclin system.

terferon and can become targets for cytolytic T cells. This property has serious implications for transplantation, as well as mechanisms of endothelial injury. Endothelial cells also elaborate endothelial leukocyte adhesion molecules (ELAMs) in response to IL-1 and tumor necrosis factor (TNF). These ELAMs promote adhesion of monocytes, PMNS, and lymphocytes to the endothelium and hence direct effector cells of the immune and inflammatory response to areas of local injury or inflammation, a crucial step in the development of atherosclerosis.

Inflammatory mediators, such as IL-1, can tip the balance between anticoagulant and procoagulant functions of the endothelium in favor of thrombosis and coagulation. Indeed, both interleukin-1 and tumor necrosis factor (TNF) promote tissue factor expression by intact endothelium (activating the extrinsic system) and enhance the activity of TPA inhibitor and the release of platelet-activating factors by endothelial cells. They also decrease the activity of tissue plasminogen activator and thrombomodulin activity. Interestingly, IL-1 is produced by endothelial cells themselves when subjected to injurious stimuli, such as endotoxin, TNF, and thrombin, thus amplifying the response.

PATHOGENESIS OF ATHEROSCLEROSIS

Atherosclerosis, through its manifestations as coronary artery disease, stroke, and peripheral vascular disease, remains the leading cause of death in the United States and western Europe and a significant source of morbidity and disability. It is now believed to arise from aberrations in vessel wall biology resulting from "injury" to the endothelial lining of blood vessels.

Smooth muscle intimal migration and proliferation have emerged as key events in the development of the advanced lesions of atherosclerosis. In the late 1970s, endothelial cells (ECs) were first shown to produce substances that stimulate smooth muscle cells (SMCs) to multiply. Since then there has been an explosion of interest in EC growth factors and their regulation. EC-derived mitogens have been implicated in a variety of pathologic processes (tumor development, desmoplastic response to tumors, liver cirrhosis, rheumatoid arthritis, myelofibrosis), as well as atherogenesis and the development of neointimal hyperplasia. Numerous studies have documented a significant increase in endothelial growth factor production in response to injurious stimuli of various types. Evidence in the literature suggests that this boost in mitogenic activity is due to increased production of mitogens by injured cells in response to the injury, rather than by release from an intracellular storage pool caused by loss of cellular integrity. Despite the obvious teleologic wisdom of such a proliferative response to injury in the acute setting, it has

proven devastating in long-term situations of toxin abuse (tobacco, cholesterol) or iatrogenic insult (bypass surgery).

Not surprisingly, the most widely accepted theory on atherogenesis, "the response to injury hypothesis," has recently been revised to include endothelial cell mitogens as major protagonists in the sequence of events leading to formation of the occlusive plaques. These growth factors have been demonstrated to have potent chemoattractant and vasoconstrictor properties, in addition to their mitogenic potential. They have therefore been implicated in the pathogenesis of atherosclerosis through their effects on smooth muscle cells in the media of blood vessels. These mitogens are currently believed to attract smooth muscle cells to the intimal and subintimal areas and to induce smooth muscle proliferation leading to subintimal thickening and plaque development.

There are a spectrum of changes in injured endothelium ranging from alterations in cell surface constituents to increased turnover to denudation; many of these may have no morphologic manifestations. Visible endothelial dysfunction or retraction is not necessary for the onset of atherogenesis. Activation of endothelial cells or macrophages can trigger the release of growth factors to provide the mitogenic stimulus for SM cells. Thus, the concept of endothelial injury as an initiator of atherogenesis does not necessarily imply endothelial denudation, with the consequent attachment and activation of platelets, which was believed to be a prerequisite for the onset of events resulting in the formation of atheromatous plaques. With the currently available evidence that endothelial cell mitogen production is amplified in situations of nonlethal injury, it is easy to see how even subtle forms of endothelial injury or "activation" can result in the subintimal cellular build-up that is characteristic of early atheromatous plaques.

Injury can be triggered by a host of factors, including hypercholesterolemia, injury from toxins or viruses, and mechanical injury. Hypercholesterolemia may induce a subtle form of endothelial injury. Increased numbers of cholesterol molecules on the membranes of ECs alters their cholesterol/phospholipid ratio, resulting in increased membrane viscosity. This might account for the endothelial retraction observed over fatty streaks in hypercholesterolemic animals and can cause increased attachment of monocytes to endothelial cells. Low density lipoprotein that is exposed to macrophages is oxidized and becomes toxic to cultured cells. Hypercholesterolemia can also cause lipid accumulation by SMCs, increased platelet aggregation, and macrophage transformation into foam cells.

Atherogenesis is an extremely complex process that evolves from the interaction among four cell types: endothelial cells, monocytes, platelets, and smooth muscle cells. All four principal cells involved in atherosclerosis can release chemoattractants and growth factors that include platelet-derived growth factor (PDGF). These circuitous intercellular interactions are mediated through chemical, mechanical, and cellular mechanisms.

ECs have profound effects on monocytes and SMCs through their production of vasoactive substances, growth factors, and growth inhibitors. The contributions of the endothelium to the genesis of atherosclerosis presuppose the presence of viable, albeit perturbed ECs. Indeed, there is a wide body of circumstantial data pointing to functional alterations resulting from sublethal injury to ECs as a key element in the development of atherosclerosis and fibrointimal hyperplasia.

The important role of monocytes in the development of atherosclerosis has been substantiated in numerous animal studies involving hypercholesterolemic primates, swine, rabbits, rats, and pigeons. Attachment of monocytes to ECs is one of the earliest cellular interactions that occur in hypercholesterolemia. Even in vitro, monocytes preferentially adhere to injured or regenerating ECs in culture. Leukocytes produce leukotriene B4, one of the most potent chemoattractants known. In addition, activated macrophages can secrete growth factors for fibroblasts, SMCs, and endothelium, such as a mitogen identical to PDGF, alpha 2 macroglobulin, which binds to and regulates PDGF, and fibroblast growth factor (FGF), a potent mitogen for connective tissue (CT) cells and ECs. Also, macrophages can injure neighboring cells by forming toxic substances, such as superoxide anion, lysosomal hydrolases, and oxidized lipids.

It is likely that even subtle forms of endothelial injury can promote platelet adherence and release of granule contents. Platelets contain mitogens (epidermal growth factor, PDGF), platelet factor IV, beta-thromboglobulin, and products of the lipooxygenase pathway that can be chemotactic to monocytes and even SMCs. Studies have shown that, if platelets are absent from sites of experimental endothelial injury, the intimal proliferative lesions that usually accompany such injury do not occur.

Smooth muscle cells, present in even the earliest of lesions, have receptors for low density lipoprotein (LDL), growth factors (including PDGF), and a variety of chemotactic factors. When stimulated, they proliferate, produce enormous amounts of CT matrix, and accumulate lipids. They also secret PDGF, resulting in autocrine and paracrine stimulation.

The fatty streak is the earliest lesion of atherosclerosis and is commonly found in children. It is a flat, lipid-rich lesion consisting of macrophages and some SMCs (Fig. 12–16). Fatty streaks seen early in life (as early as 10 years of age) occupy the same anatomic sites that fibrous plaques do at older ages. The fibrous plaque is the advanced lesion, consisting of increased intimal SMCs surrounded by CT matrix and variable amounts of intracellular and extracellular lipid. On the luminal surface it is covered by a dense fibrous cap of SM and connective tissue (Fig.

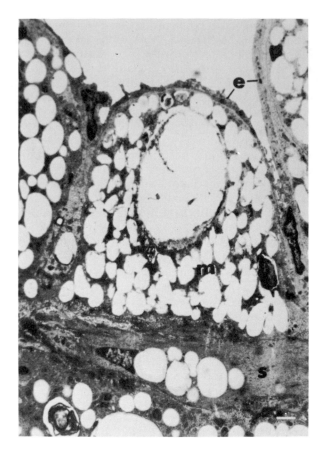

FIGURE 12–16. Transmission electron micrography of an advanced fatty streak from a monkey that was made hypercholesterolemic for 2 months (x5000). The markedly stretched and thinned endothelium (e) (to a thickness of 0.1 μm or less), although intact, covers a highly convoluted and irregular surface of lipid-filled macrophages or foam cells (m). In the depth of a crevice, an endothelial cell appears to fold on itself. Occasional lipid-laden smooth muscle cells (s) are present beneath the macrophages. (Reprinted from Faggiotto, A., Ross, R., and Harker, L.: Studies of hypercholesterolemia in the nonhuman primate. I. Changes that lead to fatty streak formation. Arteriosclerosis, 4:323–40, 1984. Figure 12, p. 335.)

12–17). Beneath the cap of SMCs and connective tissue, fibrous plaques are highly cellular lesions consisting of SMCs and macrophages that contain lipid droplets. Deep in this cell-rich region there is an area of necrotic debris, cholesterol crystals, and calcification. SMCs from fibrous plaques show a markedly diminished proliferative response to mitogenic stimulation compared to those from the media of the same artery, suggesting that they have already undergone numerous population doublings in response to some mitogenic influence (similar to senescent cells in culture).

Animal studies of atherogenesis have been conducted on three main models: hypercholesterolemic primates, hypercholesterolemic swine, and watanabe heritable hyperlipidemic rabbits. Such animal mod-

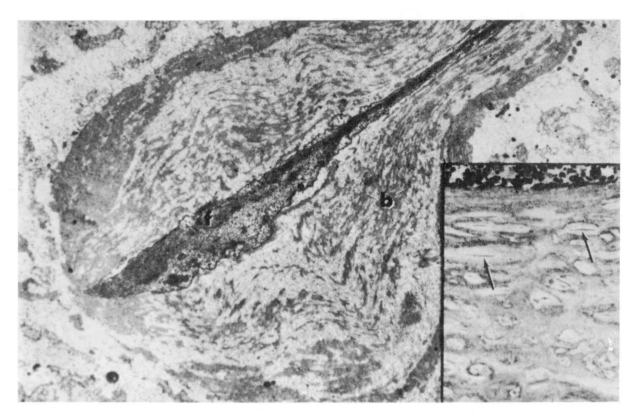

FIGURE 12–17. Electron micrography of cells of a fibrous plaque in the superficial femoral artery of a 62-year-old man (x6500; inset, x 105). The insert shows the numerous flat, pancake-shaped cells (*arrows*) surrounded by dense connective tissue that make up the fibrous cap that covers the plaque. One of these cells (main figure) shows that they look like smooth muscle because of their content of myofilaments (f) and are surrounded by concentric layers of amorphous material resembling basal lamina (b). The cells stain intensely with a monoclonal antibody to actin that is specific for smooth muscle (not shown). Notice that the numerous lamellae of basal lamina follow the contours of the cell. (Reprinted from Ross, R., Wight, T.N., Strandness, E., and Thiele, B.: Human atherosclerosis. I. Cell constitution and characteristics of advanced lesions of superficial femoral artery. Am. J. Pathol., *114*:79–93, 1984. Figure 2a, p. 82.)

els provide an insight into the sequence of morphologic changes that result in the development of atheromatous plaques and allow some correlations between these changes and the underlying humoral events to be made.

The first detectable change, seen within days of a hypercholesterolemic diet, is increased monocyte adhesion to the endothelium (Fig. 12–18). This is followed by monocyte migration to the subendothelial area where they localize and accumulate lipids, primarily in the form of cholesterol esters, forming foam cells. The accumulation of subintimal foamy macrophages represents the development of the first lesion of atherosclerosis: the fatty streak. In a matter of months, this is followed by separation of endothelial cell junctions overlying fatty streaks in areas of branches and bifurcations. The endothelial cell retraction exposes the subendothelial foam cells to the circulation (Fig. 12–19). Many of these cells are swept away, exposing the CT base on which they sat.

This leads to platelet adhesion and degranulation (Fig. 12–20), followed by migration of SMCs from the media to the intima through fenestrae of the elastic lamina. There, they proliferate and produce enormous amounts of connective tissue matrix elements, resulting in an intimal proliferative lesion containing SMCs, monocytes, and connective tissue fibers: the fibrous plaque.

A number of growth factors and inhibitors are formed in arterial walls and may be of importance in atherogenesis. For example, fibroblast growth factor (FGF) can be secreted by macrophages, SMCs, and ECs. FGF is a powerful SMC mitogen, but also stimulates EC growth and angiogenesis (development of vasa vasora from the adventitia to nourish the atherosclerotic plaque).

Platelet-derived growth factor (PDGF) is responsible for approximately one third of the growth-promoting activity produced by cultured endothelial cells. However, because of its central role in the gen-

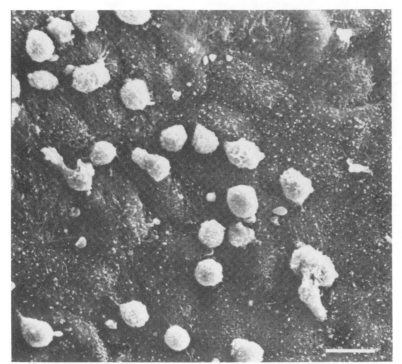

FIGURE 12–18. Electron micrograph demonstrating leukocytes adherent to the endothelium after 12 days on an atherogenic diet. Adherent leukocytes (mostly monocytes) were found scattered in patches at all levels of the aortic tree. Some of the cells appear spread on the surface, whereas most are rounded in appearance. (Reproduced from Faggiotto, A., Ross, R., and Harlan, L.: Studies of hypercholesterolemia in the nonhuman primate. I. Changes that lead to fatty streak formation. Arteriosclerosis, *4*:323–340, 1984. Figure 5A, p. 330.)

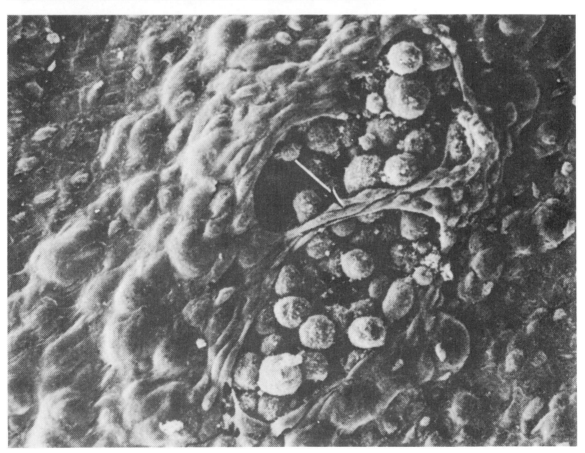

FIGURE 12–19. Scanning electron micrograph of the surface of a fatty streak in a pigtail monkey (x600). The endothelium has retracted over a portion of the lesion, exposing underlying lipid-laden macrophages. A bridge of endothelial cells (*arrow*) is present over the center of the region of exposed macrophages. Such areas of endothelial retraction were commonly observed over fatty streaks in the iliac arteries after 5 months of induced hypercholesterolemia in monkeys. (Reprinted from Ross, R.: The pathogenesis of atherosclerosis. An update. N. Engl. J. Med., *314*:488–500, 1986. Figure 4, p. 490.)

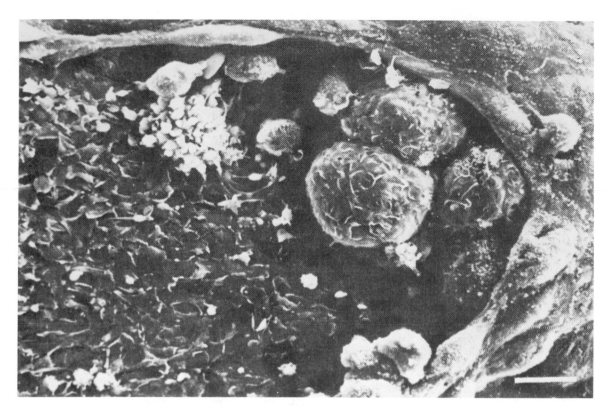

FIGURE 12–20. In this fatty streak endothelial dysjunction and contraction have apparently occurred to expose the lesion. Many of the exposed macrophages have presumably been shed into the circulation, thereby exposing the connective tissue to which platelets have attached, adhered, and spread. They have formed a small thrombus below the upper endothelial edge. A few macrophages remain partially covered by the edge of the endothelium that covers the remainder of the lesion. Bar = 10 μm. (Reprinted from Faggiotto, A., and Ross, R.: Studies of hypercholesterolemia in the nonhuman primate. II. Fatty streak conversion to fibrous plaque. Atherosclerosis, 4:341–356, 1984. Figure 5B, p. 347.)

esis of atherosclerosis, intimal hyperplasia, and numerous pathologic processes and because it has been purified and sequenced, it deserves special mention.

Discovered in 1974, PDGF is a cationic glycoprotein (28,000 to 32,000 daltons) and a heterodimer of two chains linked by disulfide bonds, the reduction of which leads to loss of mitogenic activity. It has both chemotactic and mitogenic effects on SMCs and is active in the picomolar range when purified. Notably, it is a potent vasoconstrictor; on a molar basis, much more so than angiotensin II. It also stimulates protein and collagen synthesis in responsive cells, thereby playing a possible role in the development of cirrhosis, rheumatoid arthritis, and atherosclerosis. It can also stimulate collagenase secretion by certain cells 8 to 10 hours after their exposure to PDGF (embryogenesis, tumor invasion, cartilage destruction in arthritis). It increases prostaglandin synthesis (PG-1 and PGI2) by release of arachidonic acid (early) and by promoting cyclooxygenase synthesis (late). It induces synthesis of cholesterol and increases the number of LDL receptors.

PDGF can be secreted by many cell types other than activated platelets. It bonds with high affinity to SMCs, fibroblasts, and other cells derived from mesenchyme, with the important exception of vascular endothelium. Its production is enhanced by agents that cause slow damage to endothelial cells, including endotoxin, as well as thrombin and factor Xa. Fish oils, low density lipoprotein, and calcium channel blockers inhibit its production. Regulation is by alpha 2 macroglobulin and several other plasma proteins that inhibit the binding of PDGF to its receptors, as well as by an extremely short half-life. The in vivo half-life is less than 2 minutes, making it a local tissue mitogen, the activity of which depends on local synthesis and secretion and which is unavailable at sites distal from its release. Serum levels are undetectable.

In summary, some form of injury, subtle as it may be, results in activation of the endothelium and release of a host of biologically active substances, many of which are still poorly characterized. These have mitogenic, chemotactic, angiogenic, and vasoconstrictor effects and are loosely classified as growth factors. The subsequent or concomitant activation of platelets, monocytes, and smooth muscle cells leads to further generation by these cells of such growth factors. These induce the migration of smooth muscle cells from the media into the intima and subintimal area and their proliferation and production of connective tissue elements, such as collagen, thereby setting the stage for the development of atherosclerotic plaques (Fig. 12–21). Exactly how most risk factors traditionally associated with atherosclerosis translate into the complex cellular interactions involved in its pathogenesis remains largely unclear.

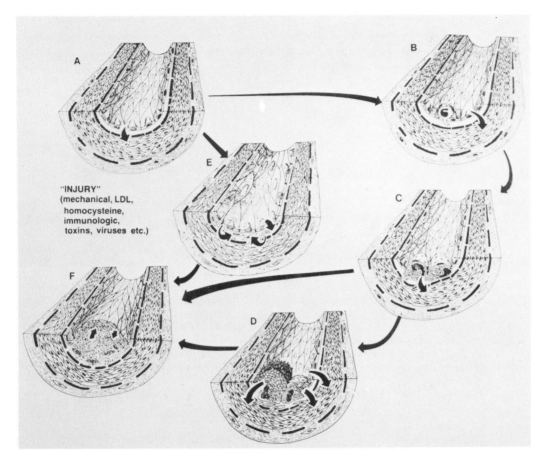

FIGURE 12–21. The revised response to injury hypothesis. Advanced intimal proliferative lesions of atherosclerosis may occur by at least two pathways. The pathway demonstrated by the clockwise (*long*) arrows to the right has been observed in experimentally induced hypercholesterolemia. Injury to the endothelium (*A*) may induce growth factor secretion (*short arrow*). Monocytes attach to endothelium (*B*), which may continue to secrete growth factors (*short arrow*). Subendothelial migration of monocytes (*C*) may result in fatty streak formation and release of growth factors, such as PDGF (*short arrow*). Fatty streaks may become directly converted to fibrous plaques (*long arrow from C to F*) through release of growth factors from macrophages or endothelial cells or both. Macrophages may also stimulate or injure the overlying endothelium. In some cases, macrophages may lose their endothelial cover, and platelet attachment may occur (*D*), providing three possible sources of growth factors: platelets, macrophages, and endothelium (*short arrows*). Some of the SMCs in the proliferative lesion itself (*F*) may form and secrete growth factors, such as PDGF (*short arrows*).

An alternative pathway for development of advanced lesions of atherosclerosis is shown by the arrows from *A* to *E* to *F*. In this case, the endothelium may be injured, but remain intact. Increased endothelial turnover may result in growth factor formation by endothelial cells (*A*). This may stimulate migration of SMCs from the media into the intima, accompanied by endogenous production of PDGF by smooth muscle, as well as growth factor secretion from the "injured" endothelial cells (*E*). These interactions could then result in fibrous plaque formation and further lesion progression (*F*). (Reprinted from Ross, R.: The pathogenesis of atherosclerosis: An update. N. Engl. J. Med., *314*:488–500, 1986. Figure 6, p. 496.)

Effects of Obstruction—Collateral Blood Flow

If a major artery is obstructed, there is a partial compensation of lost distal tissue flow by increased flow through naturally present collateral communications. What were normal outflow branch arteries beyond an obstructed artery now become inflow vessels through micro- or macro-connections to an outflow branch artery proximal to the obstruction. The opening of these connections, through which ordinarily there is little or no flow, appears to occur as a result of both the pressure gradient and the metabolic mechanisms described earlier. Although these collateral channels remain a relatively high resistance bed because of their small diameter, the collaterals may enlarge gradually in size (and possibly in number) to permit substantial total flow beyond the obstruction.

Aneurysms

Aneurysms are a localized dilation of a vessel and may be saccular, involving only a portion of the circumference, or fusiform. At times, diffuse dilation of the conducting arteries, arteriomegaly, may be seen. The commonest aneurysms are "atherosclerotic," and over 80 per cent are located in the infrarenal aorta. Although gene expression is typically delayed until the sixth decade of life or later, there is strong evidence that there is an inherited predisposition to aneurysm formation. Environmental factors, particularly smoking and hypertension, may contribute to their development. There are incompletely understood biochemical events occurring in the arterial wall that account for the initial development, subsequent growth, and rupture of aneurysms. Abnormal collagen and excessive proteolytic activity (collagenase, elastase) have been implicated, or possibly a loss of normal antiproteolytic activity. The law of Laplace, relating increasing wall tension to increasing diameter, partially explains the propensity for larger aneurysms to rupture.

Arteriovenous Fistulas

Arteriovenous fistulas are congenital or acquired connections between the arterial and venous circulation. They may occur anywhere from the largest vessels (aortocaval fistula) down to small or extensive angiomatous lesions at the precapillary-capillary level. Larger fistulas, with high flow, produce venous hypertension and distal edema and may result in "high output" congestive failure. At times, in the more diffuse angiomas, microthrombosis and a consumptive coagulopathy may develop with thrombocytopenia.

Arterial Stenosis

As arterial constriction develops, no significant hemodynamic effect is produced until an approximate 50 per cent diameter stenosis occurs, which represents a 75 per cent cross-sectional obstruction (area of circle = pi × radius squared). Unfortunately, most plaques are quite eccentric, so that multiplanar views are required with angiography to assess accurately the degree of obstruction. For this reason, duplex scans, by recording peak velocity, which is related to the degree obstruction, are at times a better physiologic measurement (especially with carotid disease). Long segment stenosis may produce a greater pressure drop than a short segment, because of increased resistance and turbulence. Although segmental pressures, as measured by the Doppler technique, may quantitate the degree of obstruction, direct transluminal measurement of the pressure gradient across the stenosis may be required. This technique is accurate when withdrawing from proximal to distal to the stenosis, but is less so when withdrawing from distal to proximal, because the catheter partially (or at times completely) occludes the residual lumen when attempting to record the distal pressure.

BIBLIOGRAPHY

1. Berne, R.M., and Levy, M.N.: Cardiac Physiology, 2nd ed. St. Louis, C.V. Mosby Co., 1988.
2. Berne, R.M., and Levy, M.N. (eds.): Physiology, 2nd ed. St. Louis, C.V. Mosby Co., 1988.
3. Fawcell, D.W.: Textbook of Histology. Philadelphia, W.B. Saunders Co., 1986.
4. Green, J.F.: Fundamental Cardiovascular and Pulmonary Physiology, 2nd ed. Philadelphia, Lea & Febiger, 1987.
5. Guyton, A.C.: Textbook of Medical Physiology, 7th ed. Philadelphia, W.B. Saunders Co., 1986.
6. Selkurt, E.E.: Physiology, 4th ed. Boston, Little, Brown, and Co., 1976.
7. Kelly, D.E., Wood, R.L., and Enders, A.C.: Bailey's Textbook of Microscopic Anatomy, 18th ed. Baltimore, Williams & Wilkins, 1984.
8. Patton, H.G., Fuchs, A.E., Hille, B., Scher, A.M., and Steiner, R. Textbook of Physiology. Philadelphia: W.B. Saunders Co., 1989.
9. Moncada, S.: Prostacyclin and arterial wall biology. Arteriosclerosis, 2:193–207, 1982.
10. Moncada, S., and Vane, J.R.: Pharmacology and endogenous roles of prostaglandin endoperoxides, thromboxane A_2 and prostacyclin. Pharmacol. Rev., 30:292–331, 1979.
11. Oates, J.A., Fitzgerald, G.A., Branch, R.A., et al.: Clinical implications of prostaglandin and thromboxane A_2 formation (first of two parts). N. Engl. J. Med., 319:689–698, 1988.
12. Oates, J.A., Fitzgerald, G.A., Branch, R.A., et al.: Clinical implications of prostaglandin and thromboxane A_2 formation (second of two parts). N. Engl. J. Med., 319:761–767, 1988.
13. Vane, J.R., Anggard, E.E., and Botting, R.M.: Regulatory functions of the vascular endothelium. N. Engl. J. Med., 323:27–36, 1990.
14. DiCorletto, P.E., and Bowen-Pope, D.F.: Cultured endothelial cells produce a platelet-derived growth factor-like protein. Proc. Natl. Acad. Sci. USA, 80:1919–1923, 1983.

15. Fox, P.L., and DiCorletto, P.E.: Regulation of production of a platelet-derived growth factor-like protein by cultured bovine aortic endothelial cells. J. Cell Physiol., *121:*298–308, 1984.

16. Harlan, J.M., Harker, L.A., Reidy, M.A., et al.: Lipopolysaccharide-mediated bovine endothelial cell injury in vitro. Lab. Invest., *48:*269, 1983.

17. Mason, R.A., Hui, J.C.K., Campbell, R., and Giron, R.: The effects of endothelial injury on smooth muscle cell proliferation. J. Vasc. Surg., *5:*389–392, 1987.

18. Ross, R., and Glomset, J.A.: The pathogenesis of atherosclerosis. N. Engl. J. Med., *295:*369–377 and 420–425, 1976.

19. Ross, R.: The pathogenesis of atherosclerosis: An update. N. Engl. J. Med., *314:*488–500, 1986.

13

GASTROINTESTINAL PHYSIOLOGY

ANTHONY O. UDEKWU

Pathology is the accomplished tragedy; physiology the basis on which our treatment rests.

EDWARD MARTIN (1859-1938)

The alimentary canal is a mucous-membrane-lined muscular tube with an enormous surface area across which the internal human interfaces with the external world. In addition to the traditional functions of aboral propulsion of food; the digestion and absorption of proteins, carbohydrates, and fats; and elimination of waste products, the alimentary tract is now known to have important endocrine and immunologic functions.

THE ESOPHAGUS

The esophagus begins at the upper esophageal sphincter, the striated muscle sphincter that anatomically separates the hypopharynx from the esophagus. It ends at the lower esophageal shincter, a physiologic sphincter separating the tubular esophagus from the saccular stomach at or just below the esophageal hiatus of the diaphragm. The esophagus proper is 20 to 25 cm long.

Swallowing begins voluntarily, but is then under reflex control. It occurs in three phases: (1) a voluntary stage characterized by contraction of the muscles of the floor of the mouth and tongue that propels the food bolus into the hypopharynx; (2) automatic, synchronized contraction of the pharyngeal constrictor mechanism and laryngeal elevators that introduces the food bolus to the upper esophageal sphincter; and (3) an involuntary propulsion of the food bolus down the length of the esophagus and into the stomach.

The pharyngeal phase is a complex process that involves the reflex inhibition of respiration. The upper esophageal sphincter is 2.5 to 4 cm in length, with a mean resting pressure between 20 and 60 mm Hg. It is closed at rest and is composed of the cricopharyngeus muscle, the posterior one third of the cricoid cartilage, and the upper esophageal circular muscle fibers. Closure of the upper esophageal sphincter is best explained by tonic contraction of the cricopharyngeus muscle, which produces anteroposterior approximation of the sphincter walls. The upper esophageal sphincter opens during swallowing, vomiting, eructation, and gagging. Coordinated and sequential contraction of the upper, middle, and lower pharyngeal constrictor muscles is followed 200 to 300 msec later by relaxation of the upper esophageal sphincter to allow passage of the food bolus and, 500 to 1200 msec later, a return of pressures to and above normal within the upper esophageal sphincter (Fig. 13–1). Innervation of the upper esophageal sphincter is predominantly from the vagus, with smaller contributions from the glossopharyngeal and accessory nerves. Central coordination of deglutition and upper esophageal sphincter control appears to reside in the dorsal vagal nuclei and nucleus ambiguus (medulla and lower pons). Lack of coordination of the relaxation of the upper esophageal sphincter, as the peristaltic waves sweeping through pharyngeal constrictors raise intrapharyngeal pressures, may play a role in the pathogenesis of pharyngoesophageal (Zenker's) diverticulum.

Esophageal pressure in the normal resting subject is equal to intrathoracic pressure, varying from +2 mm Hg to −2 mm Hg. Primary esophageal peristalsis is the rapid (4 to 8 seconds) propulsion of a swallowed food bolus from the upper esophagus into the stomach by a coordinated primary peristaltic

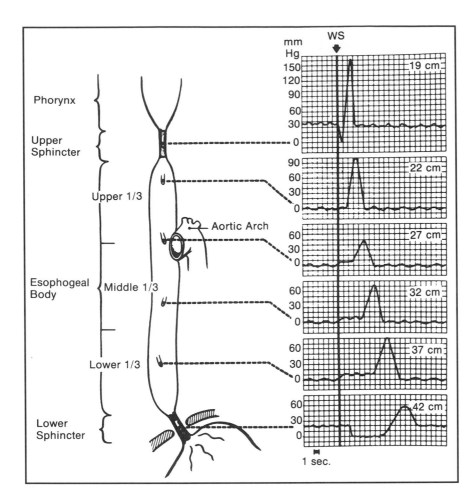

FIGURE 13–1. Esophageal pressures at rest and after a wet swallow as summarized by Dodds. (Reprinted from Dodds, W.J.: Instrumentation and methods for intraluminal esophageal manometry. Arch. Intern. Med. *136*:520, 1976.)

wave. The duration of the wave varies from 1.5 seconds in the upper esophagus to 7 seconds in the lower esophagus and is associated with pressure elevations in the range of 40 to 80 mm Hg. Propagation of the peristaltic wave is more rapid in the midportion of the esophagus than at either end. Afferent vagal impulses originating in the esophagus may modulate the configuration and rate of propagation of the primary peristaltic waves. Local afferent stimuli include bolus size, consistency, and pH. Propagation of a pressure wave varies from 1 to 5 cm/sec, and the duration of the pressure wave complex is inversely related to the speed of propagation.

Incomplete emptying distends the esophagus and stimulates the production of secondary peristalsis. These "stripping" waves (6 to 8/min) empty the esophagus or retained material (including refluxed gastric contents) and are largely independent of the normal mechanisms of swallowing. Secondary peristaltic waves are inhibited by the initiation of a second primary wave above the level of distension. Tertiary esophageal contractions (nonperistaltic) occur normally, probably reflecting local reflexes within the myenteric plexus. Usually, such simultaneous, nonperistaltic, nonpropagated waves are most prominent in the distal third, but can occur along the entire length of the esophagus.

Although its anatomic definition is unclear, a physiologic lower esophageal sphincter normally acts to prevent reflux of highly acidic gastric contents into the lower esophagus. The lower esophageal sphincter is a functional area of high pressure interposed between the thoracic esophagus with its normally negative resting pressure and the intra-abdominal stomach with its positive intraluminal pressure.

Various anatomic factors, including the "diaphragmatic pinchcock," a circular anatomic sphincter, a flap valve, or an angle, have been suggested as explanations for the lower esophageal sphincter, which itself extends for a variable length from the esophageal hiatus to the true stomach. Reported normal mean resting pressures of the lower esophageal sphincter are 13 ± 5 to 26 ± 9 mm Hg. The intra-abdominal esophagus is subjected to the same external pressures as the stomach, and by virtue of its smaller radius, it need only contribute a small additional pressure by increased wall tension to effectively prevent the reflux of gastric contents into the lower esophagus. Intrinsic tone is regulated primarily by vagal cholinergic means that cause contraction, but a complex endocrine control is suggested by Tables 13–1 and 13–2.

Abnormalities of the lower esophageal sphincter, when measured manometrically, do not always correlate well with the presence or absence of abnormal gastroesophageal reflux. Table 13–1 lists various factors that have been associated with alterations in lower esophageal sphincter pressure. If the intrinsic tone of the lower esophageal sphincter is diminished, its competency is dependent on a segment of intra-abdominal esophagus that functions as a barrier to reflux only when intra-abdominal pressure is equal to or greater than intragastric pressure. Thus, the length of the intra-abdominal segment of esophagus determines its ability to act as a barrier to reflux. The shorter the intra-abdominal segment, the higher the intrinsic sphincter pressure required to prevent reflux. It appears that the major determinants of lower esophageal sphincter competency under physiologic conditions in humans are dependent upon intra-abdominal pressure acting on an intra-abdominal segment of the esophagus upon which is superimposed varying levels of intrinsic tone. Thus, occasional reflux occurs in all people, and the acid is cleared by secondary esophageal contractions.

Achalasia of the esophagus is an esophageal motor disorder characterized by failure of relaxation of the lower esophageal sphincter to allow passage of a food bolus, and an absence of coordinated motor activity in the proximal esophagus. This disorder has

TABLE 13–1. FACTORS DECREASING LOWER ESOPHAGEAL SPHINCTER PRESSURE

AGENT	MECHANISM
Atropine	Anticholinergic
Propantheline	
Dicyclomine	
Isoproterenol	Beta adrenergic stimulation
Carbuterol	
Salbutamol	
Phentolamine	Alpha adrenergic blockade
Prostaglandins	Adenylate cyclase activation
E$_1$, E$_2$, A$_2$, I$_2$	
Secretin	Direct muscle action
VIP	
CCK	Stimulation of inhibitory neurons
Calcium channel blockers	
Fatty meal	CCK release
Others	
Chocolate	Progesterone
Peppermint	Meperidine
Ethanol	Morphine
Tobacco	Lidocaine

Reprinted from Postlethwait, R.W.: Physiology. *In* Surgery of the Esophagus. Norwalk, CT, Appleton Century Crofts, 1986, p. 602.

TABLE 13–2. FACTORS INCREASING LOWER ESOPHAGEAL SPHINCTER PRESSURE

AGENT	MECHANISM
Acetylcholine	Cholinergic stimulation
Bethanechol	
Methacoline	
Norepinephrine	Alpha adrenergic stimulation
Phenylephrine	
Bombesin	Norepinephrine release
Edrophonium	Anticholinesterase
Eserine	
Neostigmine	
Gastrin	? Acetylcholine release
Motilin	
Metoclopramide	? Muscarinic receptor facilitation
Prostaglandin F$_2$	
Protein meal	? Gastrin release
Gastric alkalinization	
Histamine	H-2 receptor
Glucagon	Preganglionic parasympathetic
Doperidone	

Reprinted from Postlethwait, R.W.: Physiology. *In* Surgery of the Esophagus. Norwalk, CT, Appleton Century Crofts, 1986, p. 602.

been related anatomically to the degeneration of intramural parasympathetic ganglia. Achalasia is frequently successfully treated by hydrostatic dilation of the lower esophageal sphincter, but in approximately 25 percent of cases, surgical disruption of the sphincter (myotomy) is required. Some patients with chest pain of noncardiac origin have been demonstrated to exhibit abnormal patterns of esophageal motility, including diffuse esophageal spasm (corkscrew esophagus), and frequent tertiary contractions. Correlation between motility abnormalities and symptomatology is imperfect, but some patients have a salutary response to pharmacologic agents known to alter esophageal motility.

THE STOMACH

The stomach is a saccular organ that acts as a temporary receptacle for food, initiating proteolytic digestion, and regulates the discharge of chyme into the duodenum for further digestion. In addition, the stomach serves a vital function in micronutrient metabolism through the secretion of intrinsic factor, essential for vitamin B$_{12}$ absorption.

The stomach has been subdivided into many regions anatomically. From a physiologic perspective, however, only two major zones exist—the body (including the fundus) and antrum—with clearly differing structures and functions.

Gastric storage may exceed 1000 mL. Intragastric pressure remains low until this limit is exceeded, a phenomenon mediated by the intrinsic mechanical properties of a stomach wall, as well as by stretch inhibition of basal vagal tone.

Gastric Digestion and Absorption

Only minor protein digestion occurs within the stomach under normal circumstances, its major functions being mechanical change rather than chemical. Water and certain simple organic compounds (i.e., alcohol), as well as poisons, such as cyanide or arsenic, are absorbed from the stomach under normal circumstances. Fluids proceed rapidly along the lesser curvature "fast track" in the empty stomach and are emptied more rapidly than solids or semisolids.

Gastric Emptying

Gastric motility is initiated by a pacemaker located in the fundus/cardia. Varied patterns of muscular activity mix ingested food with gastric secretions (mixing waves) and propel gastric chyme into the duodenum (peristaltic waves). The fundus is basically a storage area without effective propulsive activity. Propulsive activity is largely confined to the antrum. Gastric emptying is determined by the balance between pyloric resistance and antral peristalsis. The pylorus acts like a sphincter that responds to constricting signals (cholinergic and alpha adrenergic) and relaxing signals (neurotransmitters, secretin, and possibly vasoactive intestinal polypeptide). Factors that enhance gastric emptying include gastric distension and release of the antral hormone gastrin. Duodenal acidification and fat within the duodenal bulb diminish the rate of gastric emptying. The specifics of these interactions are not completely understood, but may be related to the secretion of gastric inhibitory polypeptide or secretin.

Regulation of Gastric Secretion

The secretion of gastric juice is a tightly regulated physiochemical process, culminating in the secretion of a mixture of parietal cell (H^+ 150-170 mEq/L, Cl^- 165-170 mEq/L, K^+ 7 mEq/L) and nonparietal cell (pepsinogen, Na^+ 144-150 mEq/L, Cl^- 90-105 mEq/L, K^+ 3.0-5 mEq/L) secretions. Clearly, gastric secretion is directly related to changes in mucosal blood flow.

Gastric secretion occurs at a relatively constant rate independent of stimulation of food ingestion (interdigestive secretion), with modulated peaks of secretion provoked by meals (prandial secretion). Three main agonists, both neural (acetylcholine) and humoral (histamine, gastrin), are responsible for the augmented acid secretory rate associated with meals.

Multiple, *distinct* parietal cell receptors, when occupied by transmitters of either neural or humoral origin, are responsible for increased secretion. This concept explains the facilitation of secretion produced by multiple and/or sequential stimuli. The ability of H-2 blocking agents to reduce acid secretion by all agonists argues strongly for the participation of histamine in the mechanism of all agonists. Both the adenylate cyclase and Ca^{++} second intracellular mechanisms are involved.

Neural Control. The bulk of sensory and motor innervation of the stomach is carried within the vagi. Gastric vagal afferents terminate predominantly in the nucleus of the tractus solitarius. Gastric vagal efferents originate in the medial subnucleus of the dorsal motor nucleus of the vagus with probable contributions from the nucleus ambiguus.

Gastric neurons in the dorsal vagal motor nucleus possess extensive dendritic connections that penetrate the nucleus tractus solitarius, providing an anatomic basis for monosynaptic vagovagal interactions, as well as the telencephalic influence on gastric secretion.

Gastric vagal neurons are activated by the paraventricular nucleus and lateral hypothalamic nuclei. The details of intracerebral neurotransmission are not completely understood, but it is thought that thyrotropin-releasing hormone (TRH) increases gastric secretion by a vagovagal stimulation mechanism. Corticotropin-releasing factor (CRF) is thought to contribute to the gastric response to stress. Peripheral mediation is by vagal muscarinic cholinergic nerves. The binding of acetylcholine to parietal cell receptors opens Ca^{++} channels into the cytosol, permitting the influx of calcium ion that results in the secretion of gastric juice.

Humoral Control of Acid Secretion. Stimulation of gastric acid secretion is the major action of the antral hormone gastrin. Gastrin is a 17 amino acid linear peptide with a molecular weight of 2100 that is found in several longer peptide chains (big gastrin) and at least one smaller form (mini-gastrin). Big gastrin is the major circulating form of gastrin in the human. Biologic activity is conferred by the four C-terminal amino acids and has been reproduced synthetically as pentagastrin.

Gastrin in physiologic concentrations has stimulatory effects on gastric acid secretion. Other effects are increased pepsinogen secretion and augmented mucosal blood flow. At doses above physiologic levels, gastrin exhibits marked trophic activity on the stomach, in addition to its properties as a secretagogue.

Gastrin is secreted into the blood by G cells in the pyloric glands of the antral mucosa and in the proximal small intestine. G cells release gastrin in response to gastric distension, amino acids (phenylalanine, tryptophan), certain foods (e.g., milk), and antral alkalinity. Gastrin secretion is tightly controlled by biofeedback inhibition; an antral pH of less than 1.5

TABLE 13–3. MAJOR MECHANISMS FOR STIMULATION OF GASTRIC ACID SECRETION

PHASE	STIMULUS	PATHWAY	STIMULUS TO PARIETAL CELL
Cephalic	Chewing, swallowing, etc.	Vagus nerve to 1. Parietal cells 2. G cells	Acetylcholine, gastrin
Gastric	Gastric Distension	Local and vagovagal reflexes to 1. Parietal cells 2. G cells	Acetylcholine, gastrin
Intestinal	Protein digestion products	Intestinal G cells, intestinal endocrine cells	Gastrin, Entero-oxyntin

Adapted from Johnson, L.R. (ed.): Gastrointestinal Physiology, 2nd ed. St Louis, C.V. Mosby Co., 1981; adapted from Grossman M.I.—original source. Reprinted in Kutchai, H.S.: The gastrointestinal system: Gastrointestinal secretions. *In* Berne, R.M., and Levy, N.M. (eds.): Physiology, 2nd ed. St. Louis, C.V. Mosby Co., 1988, p. 700.

essentially shuts off further gastrin secretion. Local neurotransmitters (gamma amino butyric acid, and bombesin) within the gastric wall likely modulate gastrin responses to intragastric stimuli. Somatostatin in physiologic doses also acts to decrease gastrin release.

Inhibition of Secretion. The predominant inhibitor of gastric secretion is intragastric acid, which diminishes gastrin secretion from the antral G cells. Active duodenal inhibition of gastric secretion is triggered by the presence of acid in the duodenal bulb. It is not clear whether local neural reflexes or gastric inhibitory polypeptide plays the dominant role in duodenal inhibition; a dual mechanism is currently favored.

The major mechanisms of gastric acid secretion are listed in Tables 13–3 and Table 13–4.

Cephalic Phase. The thought, smell, taste, or presence of food in the mouth results in central (telencephalic) vagal stimulation via the nucleus tractus solitarius. The end result is muscarinic (acetylcholine-mediated) stimulation of parietal cells and chief cells, causing a rise in gastric secretory rate. Acetylcholine release in antral mucosa also causes gastrin release, resulting in further acid secretion.

Gastric Phase. The entry of food into the stomach causes gastrin release and a consequent increase in secretion. This effect is potentiated by local vagovagal reflexes that produce muscarinic stimulation of the parietal cell, as well as of antral G cells. As antral acidification progresses, gastrin release diminishes and eventually stops altogether.

Intestinal Phase. The release of acid chyme into the duodenum slows gastric emptying and further enhances gastric secretion of acid and pepsinogen. Amino acids have been postulated as mediators of the intestinal phase of gastric secretion.

Hypergastrinemia. The sole utility of serum gastrin estimation lies in the diagnosis and management of the Zollinger-Ellison syndrome. Normal basal gastrin levels are less than 150 pg/mL. Basal levels above 500 pg/mL are considered diagnostic of the Zollinger-Ellison syndrome. Table 13–5 lists other conditions that are sometimes associated with hypergastrinemia.

Measurement of Gastric Secretion. Clinically, gastric secretion is measured by collecting basal- and pentagastrin-stimulated gastric juice from a fasting subject utilizing a nasogastric tube. Results are expressed in volume and milliequivalents of acid secretion per hour. Basal acid output varies between 4 to 6 mEq/h and tends to be higher in men than in women. Maximal acid outputs are in the 30 to 40 mEq/h range and again are somewhat higher in

TABLE 13–4. MAJOR MECHANISMS FOR INHIBITION OF GASTRIC ACID SECRETION

REGION	STIMULUS	MEDIATOR	INHIBITION OF GASTRIN RELEASE	INHIBITION OF ACID SECRETION
Antrum	Acid (pH < 3.0)	None, direct	+	
Duodenum	Acid	Secretin, bulbogastrone, nervous reflex	+	+
			+	+
Duodenum and jejunum	Hyperosmotic solutions, fatty acids, monoglycerides	Unidentified enterogastrone, gastrin inhibitory peptide, cholecystokinin	+	+
				+

Adapted from Johnson, L.R. (ed.): Gastrointestinal Physiology, 2nd ed. St Louis, C.V. Mosby Co., 1981; adapted from Grossman M.I.—original source. Reprinted in Kutchai, H.S.: The gastrointestinal system: Gastrointestinal secretions. *In* Berne, R.M., and Levy, N.M. (eds.): Physiology, 2nd ed. St. Louis, C.V. Mosby Co., 1988, p. 700.

TABLE 13–5. CAUSES OF HYPERGASTRINEMIA

Condition	Mechanism
Zollinger-Ellison syndrome	Gastrinoma
Vagotomy	Loss of vagal inhibition
Pernicious anemia	Loss of acid inhibition
Antral exclusion	Lack of acid inhibition
Chronic renal failure	Decreased catabolism
Pyloric obstruction	

men than in women. The significant overlap between normal and disease states has limited the application of these measurements to the differential diagnosis of acid-peptic disease of the stomach and duodenum. The presence of achlorhydria, however, makes a diagnosis of duodenal ulcer unlikely.

Effects of Surgery on Gastric Physiology. Truncal vagotomy increases basal plasma gastrin levels, decreases the cephalic phase of gastrin release (vagal mediated), and has variable effects on the food-stimulated gastrin response. Vagotomy and antrectomy result in decreased basal and stimulated plasma gastrin levels. Proximal gastric vagotomy increases the gastrin response to vagal stimulation, with a decrease in the cephalic phase of gastric acid secretion and a variable response to food-stimulated gastrin secretion. Postvagotomy hypergastrinemia is probably produced by a combination of G cell hyperplasia (a late effect), as well as diminished acid secretion (compensatory).

Other Gastric Secretions. Agents that stimulate acid secretion from the parietal cell also stimulate the chief cells to secrete pepsinogen. In addition, acid itself stimulates the chief cells and furthermore activates pepsin by cleaving acid-labile linkages in the precursor proenzyme pepsinogen. Pepsin may act on 20 percent of gastric proteins, but is permanently inactivated in the neutral duodenal environment.

PHYSIOLOGY OF THE SMALL INTESTINE

The major function of the human small intestine is the absorption of nutrients, including vitamins, electrolytes, and water. Appropriate functioning of the small intestine is vital to human existence.

Intestinal Motility

Motility describes movement of the intestinal wall, but for clinical purposes, this movement is frequently equated with the aboral transport of luminal content. Yet, it is important to remember that motility and aboral propulsion are not always one and the same. Considerable variability exists in patterns of intestinal motility, and some caution must be applied when ascribing clinical abnormalities to one pattern of motility or the other.

During the interdigestive phase, the motility of the small intestine is characterized by the presence of periodic propagated aboral peristaltic contractions that have been named the migrating motor complex. These occur at intervals of approximately 90 minutes and are also known as phase III of the interdigestive myoelectrical cycle. These migrating motor complexes are often preceded by a briefer period of less regular peristaltic activity (phase II); they end in a brief transition phase (phase IV) of irregular waning myoelectrical activity and finally (phase I) a phase of quiescence. The next migrating motor complex begins at approximately the time that the preceding one ends.

Activity fronts or migrating motor complexes typically originate high in the stomach and propagate aborally, ending in the distal ileum; however, they can originate lower in the gastrointestinal tract. Few migrating motor complexes are propagated through the entire length of the ileum. Most typically wane at the midileal level.

Oral feeding produces a consistent inhibition of the migrating motor complex and results in irregular, generally nonpropagating contractions distributed through most of the small intestine. Some contractions may be coordinated, with proximal and distal contractions resulting in limited segmental motion of luminal contents during digestion. This postprandial motility pattern generally persists for 3 to 4 hours after a test meal, but varies with the ingested material. Lipids appear to produce the most sustained inhibition of the migrating motor complex. Discrete clustered contractions (phasic and trained contractions predominantly in the jejunum) and prolonged propagated contractions (isolated, rapidly propagated contractions most marked in the terminal ileum) are additional motility patterns found in humans. These patterns of motility are of uncertain physiologic or clinical significance. Both appear to be related to the rapid aboral transport of luminal content.

Intestinal motility is controlled by the autonomic nervous system, local peptides, and neurotransmitters. Denervation of the human small intestine, although at least initially associated with a diminished frequency of generation of migrating motor complexes, does not produce consistent long-term disturbance of function.

The interactions between motility and luminal transit and absorption are not entirely clear. Interdigestive migrating motor complexes are thought perhaps to have an important "housekeeper function" in ridding the intestinal lumen of cellular debris, bacteria, and unabsorbed food material. Postprandial intestinal motor activity, although disorganized and not clearly propagated, does nonetheless result in consistent aboral propulsion of chyme. Absorption, generally a very efficient process, does not appear to be affected by changes in intestinal motility, except at nonphysiologic extremes. This finding has important implications regarding the use of the enteral feeding route in patients with postoperative alterations of intestinal motility.

Small intestinal motility patterns are temporarily abrogated by general anesthesia and laparotomy. The frequency of migrating motor complexes does diminish in response to laparotomy, but usually returns to normal within 6 to 24 hours. The decrease in motor activity has not been well correlated with abnormalities in aboral propagation of luminal content or nutrient absorption, perhaps accounting for the success with which early jejunal enteral feeding has been employed in postoperative patients. The production of postoperative ileus is thought to be related to the endogenous catecholamines released as part of the metabolic response to the injury, suggesting a possible role for sympathetic blocking agents in the prevention of postoperative disturbances in gastrointestinal function.

The effect of anesthetic agents upon intestinal motility has generally been exaggerated. However, a predictable disturbance of *gastric* tone follows most operations performed under general anesthesia for periods of up to 24 hours and contributes to the significant incidence of postoperative nausea and emesis. Peritonitis or intra-abdominal abscesses may have more important and sustained effects on the transit of intestinal luminal contents, with sustained periods of hypomotility lasting for days or perhaps even weeks. In usual circumstances, however, these effects bear little relation to the effects of routine laparotomy on intestinal motility.

Endocrine control of gastrointestinal motility is thought to be closely related to the endogenous peptide motilin, which has been shown to produce migrating motor complexes after intravenous administration. This substance is produced mainly in the duodenal muscularis. Other peptides known to influence intestinal motility include cholecystokinin, somatostatin, and pancreatic polypeptide. In physiologic conditions, it is likely that interactions between all these peptides are important in their regulation of intestinal motor function.

Vagotomy quite frequently results in diarrhea. This may be related to persistence of the interdigestive phase motility patterns during the postprandial state.

Interruption of the continuous myoelectrical circuit of the intestine by segmental resection produces a block to propagation of migrating motor complexes, as well as other forms of propagated intestinal motility. This effect is temporary, and the resultant clinical effects of intestinal resection and anastomosis are insignificant, provided that significant intestinal length is not sacrificed.

The production of sounds by the gastrointestinal tract varies considerably from individual to individual. Most "bowel sounds" are produced by gastric emptying into the duodenum and the emptying of small intestinal contents into the cecum across the ileocecal valve. Migrating motor complexes (occurring every 60 to 90 minutes) also may produce prominent intestinal sounds. The absence of bowel sounds can hence be due either to disturbance of normal motility or sampling error in the clinical setting. On the other hand, vigorous bowel sounds, especially if accompanied by rushes and cramps, can be important supportive evidence of a mechanical intestinal obstruction.

Digestion and Absorption

The small intestine is a huge semipermeable membrane with important functions, both absorptive and secretory (Table 13–5). It is charged with the complex task of the absorption of materials sufficient for the nutritional support of the human organism, as well as the reabsorption of the endogenous fluids—salivary, gastric, biliary, pancreatic, and intestinal—that are responsible for the digestion of food. The reserve of the small intestine for absorption indicates a rather impressive degree of overengineering by Nature. Certain functions, however, are restricted to anatomically discrete areas of the intestinal tract and are not easily replaced by other portions of the GI tract; this fact must be kept in mind when intestinal resection or disease is part of the clinical picture.

In a very general sense, absorption of materials across the intestinal mucosal barrier may be either active or passive. Usually, the flux of water across the intestinal mucosal barrier follows that of solutes, whether the flux be secretory or absorptive. Patterns of absorption and secretion vary from segment to segment of the intestine, but the net effect is near-complete absorption of nutrients and a net absorption of 1 to 2 L/day of exogenous fluid.

Water and Electrolyte Absorption. Three mechanisms are responsible for electrolyte absorption and secretion: (1) passive diffusion, (2) solvent drag, and (3) active transport. Passive diffusion, most prominent in the jejunum, is the simple diffusion of electrolytes along a chemical or electrical potential gradient through channel proteins or between cells. This process is dependent on a highly permeable membrane, with an abundance of pericellular pathways, low electrochemical resistance, and high water permeability.

Solvent drag is electrolyte absorption secondary to the flow of water. It is characteristic of the proximal small intestine and is analagous to the movement of electrolytes and water in the proximal convoluted tubule of the kidney. The majority of glucose-stimulated sodium absorption is probably due to this mechanism.

Energy-dependent active transport mechanisms set up the electrochemical gradients that permit net absorption against apparent chemical or electrical gradients. The most important active transport mechanism involves the sodium-potassium ATPase pump, located at the basolateral membrane of the cell, which actively transports sodium from the interior of the cell into the intercellular spaces, and K^+ from the interstitial tissue into the cell. This transport has two effects: (1) luminal sodium flows into the cell, and (2) the intercellular spaces become hyperosmolar (so that water passes between the cells) and positively charged (so that Cl^- passes from the lumen between cells into the interstitial space and HCO_3^- passes from the cell into the interstitial space). The apical small intestinal epithelium also has a Na^+-H^+ pump in which the passage of sodium into the cell pumps H^+ into the lumen. The excess HCO_3^- in the cell then passes along its electrochemical barrier into the interstitial space. Carrier-mediated glucose-amino acid electrolyte absorption is a second important mechanism of active transport in the proximal small intestine, resulting in near-complete sodium absorption. These reactions are schematically summarized in Figure 13–2.

Most electrolyte absorption in the distal small intestine is probably accomplished by the sodium-hydrogen and chloride-bicarbonate ion exchange processes. The net effect of small intestinal water and electrolyte absorption is the production of a fluid that is slightly lower in sodium than in plasma and is considerably depleted of chloride, with a high bicarbonate content. Every 24 hours, 800 to 1300 mL of this chyme are delivered to the right colon, where water and sodium absorption is completed by the Na^+-K^+ ATPase active transport mechanism in which the flow of water into the intercellular space is magnified. The activity of this electrogenic sodium pump is aldosterone dependent, resulting in the absorption of sodium in exchange for potassium across the colonic epithelium. The sodium absorption enhances water absorption, and the ultimate volume of water lost daily in the feces is generally less than 200 mL.

Carbohydrate Digestion and Absorption. Carbohydrates are a major energy source, constituting 30 to 40 percent of the typical Western diet. The two major forms are polysaccharides and disaccharides. Polysaccharides consist of amylose and amylopectin. Cellulose, the other major dietary polysaccharide, is not digested in the human intestinal tract, but rather contributes to the bulk content of the feces.

Carbohydrate digestion begins with salivary amylase, and carbohydrate absorption is generally completed within the proximal 1 to 1 1/2 meters of small intestine. Salivary and pancreatic amylases are highly efficient enzyme systems that produce digestion of starches to oligosaccharides within minutes of their arrival in the duodenal lumen. Amylose and amylopectin consist of alpha-1,4 straight chain glucose molecules. Amylopectin, in addition, has side chains originating from alpha-1,6 branch points. Both salivary and pancreatic alpha amylase hydrolyze the alpha-1,4 glucose-glucose links of dietary starches, but do not hydrolyze alpha-1,4 linkages adjacent to chain terminations. The end result of amylose digestion consequently is a mixture of alpha-1,4 disaccharides (maltose) and trisaccharides (maltotriose) as final linear breakdown products. In addition, alpha amylase does not hydrolyze 1,6 branch links, resulting in the production of polysaccharide units called alpha-limit dextrins, consisting of five to eight glucose units.

Completion of carbohydrate digestion and absorption is dependent on surface oligosaccharidases (Fig. 13–3). These enzymes may be classified as alpha glucosidases (glucoamylase, sucrase, and beta galactosidase). These surface enzymes are produced by and retained by the membranes of the enteric brush border. They are highly efficient enzyme systems that hydrolyze oligosaccharides at rates exceeding membrane transport capabilities. Hence, hydrolysis is not the rate-limiting step for carbohydrate absorption. The one exception to this rule is lactase, which is relatively inefficient in the hydrolysis of lactose.

Oligosaccharidases are present at birth in the human small intestine. Increases in intake are gradually accompanied by increased levels of surface oligosaccharidases, resulting in complete digestion and absorption.

Over three fourths of ingested carbohydrate is eventually broken down to and absorbed as glucose. Because glucose and other monosaccharides are molecules too large to be absorbed by simple diffusion, they require specific transport mechanisms. This absorption process is probably dependent on a membrane transport protein in the brush border

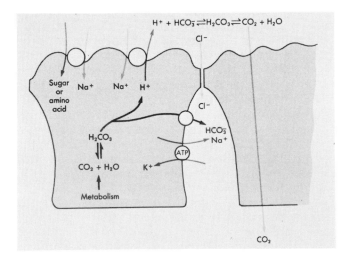

FIGURE 13–2. A summary of major ion transport processes that occur in the jejunum. (Reprinted from Kutchai, H.E.: The gastrointestinal system: Digestion and absorption. *In* Berne, R.M., and Levy, M.N.: Physiology, 2nd ed. St. Louis, C.V. Mosby Co., 1988, p. 727.)

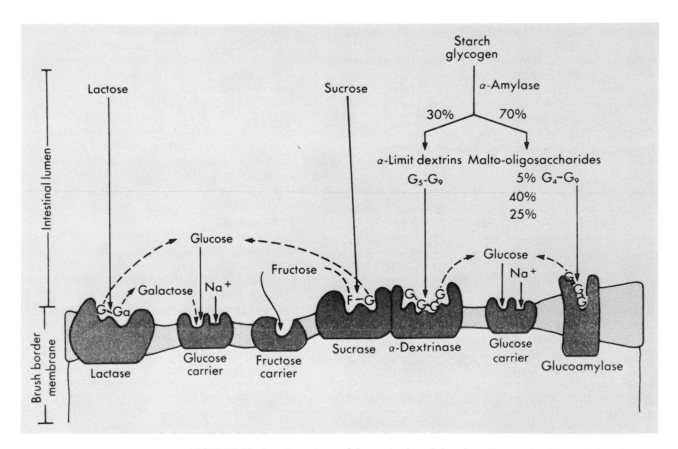

FIGURE 13–3. Functions of the major brush border oligosaccharidases. The glucose, galactose, and fructose molecules released by enzymatic hydrolysis are then transported into the epithelial cell by specific transport carrier proteins. G, Glucose; Ga, galactose; F, fructose. (Reprinted from Gray, G.M.: N. Engl. J. Med., *292*:1225, 1975—original reference. Reprinted in Kutchai, H.C.: The gastrointestinal system: Digestion and absorption. *In* Berne, R.M., and Levy, M.N. (eds.): Physiology, 2nd ed. St. Louis, C.V. Mosby Co., 1988. Fig 44–2, p. 719.)

membrane. Glucose absorption at the brush border is coupled to the active extrusion of sodium from the cell at the basolateral cell membranes, which is mediated by the sodium-potassium ATPase pump. The pump sets up an electrochemical gradient along which sodium then travels. The energy supplied by this gradient is sufficient for the carrier protein to transport both sodium and glucose into the cell. Fructose transport is unique in that its absorption is a carrier-protein-mediated, energy-independent mechanism.

Deficiencies in carbohydrate absorption and digestion are relatively uncommon in surgical practice. For practical purposes, even in marked pancreatic insufficiency, maldigestion of starch does not occur because of the great excess of pancreatic amylase secreted. Secondary deficiencies in oligosaccharidases can accompany such diseases as celiac sprue, as well as other diseases resulting in generalized mucosal flattening.

Protein Digestion and Absorption. Despite the presence of pepsin in the stomach, only a small amount of protein digestion takes place in that organ. Pancreatic proteases (Table 13–6) are responsible for the majority of protein digestion. They are dependent on activation by enterokinase, an enzyme produced by the duodenal mucosa. Enterokinase cleaves the proenzyme trypsinogen to trypsin, which in turn activates chymotrypsin and procarboxypeptidase. All these enzymes act to hydrolytically digest peptide links so that 50 per cent of protein absorption is completed in the duodenum.

Residual long protein chains are broken down by the endopeptidases, which are integral enzymes of the brush border of the duodenal and small intes-

TABLE 13–6.   PANCREATIC PROTEASES

Endopeptidases	Trypsin
	Chymotrypsin
	Elastase
Exopeptidases	Carboxypeptidase A
	Carboxypeptidase B

tinal epithelium. These endopeptidases consist of amino-peptidases, dipeptidases, and dipeptidyl amino-peptidases. Peptide chains are then further digested to amino acids and dipeptides for absorption. Some small peptides may be absorbed intact for intracellular hydrolysis (glycine and proline; Fig. 13–4).

Peptide absorption in the human is an active process that is ATP and sodium dependent. This process is highly efficient, resulting in rapid absorption, especially of dipeptides, which may be a more efficient nutrient source for elemental enteral feedings than fully hydrolyzed amino acids. The absorption of amino acids varies, depending on the chemical structure. All mechanisms, however, are energy and sodium dependent and use support transport proteins in a similar manner to glucose absorption. In this enzyme-linked carrier protein mechanism, dipeptides and tripeptides are preferentially transported. Transmembrane transport of amino acids is the rate-limiting step of protein absorption. Two thirds of the products of protein digestion are oligopeptides. Protein digestion is complete at the midjejunal level. Protein absorption can be efficiently accomplished at most levels of the small intestine, reflecting the rarity of clinically significant protein malabsorption states, even with extensive intestinal resection. Some undigested proteins are absorbed by endocytosis.

Fat Digestion and Absorption. The process of fat digestion and absorption is fairly complex and is dependent on the appropriate coordination of pancreatobiliary secretions, as well as surface epithelial cell function within the jejunoileum. Several unique biochemical processes are central to the appropriate absorption of fat (Fig. 13–5).

Fat in the duodenum stimulates the secretion of cholecystokinin and secretin, resulting in stimulation of pancreatic secretion and gallbladder emptying. Cholecystokinin and secretin are released by endocrine cells of the duodenum in proportion to the fat load. The major stimulus to secretin stimulation is duodenal acidification. Severe duodenal disease may inhibit the stimulation of pancreatic and biliary secretion. Vagotomy results in variable, but significant decreases in pancreatic secretions. Pancreatic juice contains several lipolytic enzymes, the most important of which are pancreatic lipase, cholesterol esterase, and phospholipase A_2. Lipase in an alkaline environment hydrolyzes triglycerides to a monoglyceride and two fatty acids. Phospholipase A_2 results in the similar digestion of phospholipids.

Bile salts are important for the emulsification of the fats. After initial digestion, micelles are formed, the single most important step in fat absorption. In this process the fatty acids, monoglycerides, phospholipids, and cholesterol are enveloped in a bilayer bile salt disc in which the hydrophobic region of the

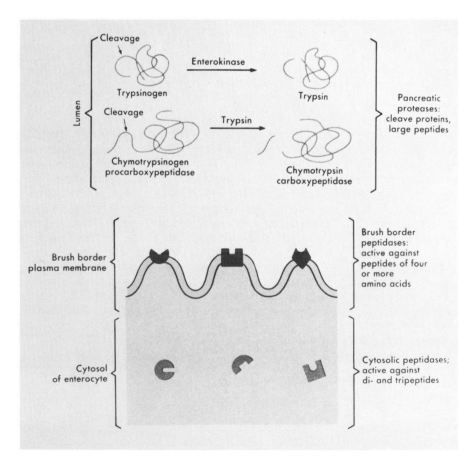

FIGURE 13–4. The major proteases and peptidases present in the lumen of the small intestine, on the brush border plasma membrane, and in the cytosol of enterocytes of the small intestine. (Reprinted from Kutchai, H.C.: The gastrointestinal system: Digestion and absorption. *In* Berne, R.M., and Levy, M.N. (eds.): Physiology, 2nd ed. St. Louis, C.V. Mosby Co., 1988, p. 722.)

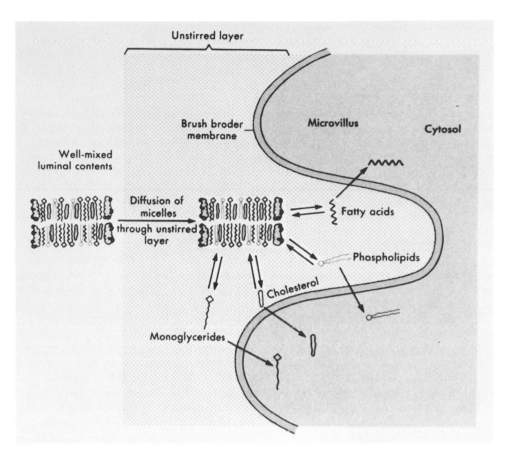

FIGURE 13–5. Lipid absorption in the small intestine. Mixed micelles of bile acids and lipid digestion products diffuse through the unstirred layer and among the microvilli. As digestion products are absorbed from free solution by the enterocytes, more digestion products partition out of the micelles. (Reprinted from Kutchai, H.C.: The gastrointestinal system: Digestion and absorption. *In* Berne, R.M., and Levy, M.N. (eds.): Physiology, 2nd ed. St. Louis, C.V. Mosby Co., 1988, p. 739.)

bile salt molecule is directed inward and the hydrophilic portion of the molecule remains in contact with the aqueous environment of the intestinal luminal content. Once in contact with the brush border, diffusion of the nonpolar lipids across the lipid membrane is rapid and requires no energy. The structure of the micelle may enhance diffusion through the normal nonstirred aqueous interface between intestinal lumen and brush border membrane of the intestinal cell (Fig. 13–5).

After absorption of the lipid contents, triglyceride resynthesis and re-esterification of cholesterol occur within the cytoplasm of the intestinal epithelial cells, probably in the smooth endoplasmic reticulum with the aid of a lipid-binding protein. The final step in triglyceride absorption is chylomicron formation, in which small amounts of cholesterol are added to the resynthesized triglycerides and are subsequently covered by an envelope of phospholipids and newly synthesized lipoproteins that is crucial for the transport across the basolateral cell membrane. Chylomicrons are too large for capillary absorption, but can pass into the lacteals and via the thoracic duct to the bloodstream.

Shorter fatty acid triglyceride combinations (medium chain triglycerides) can often be absorbed intact across the luminal membrane. These substances are often more easily and more completely digested by pancreatic lipase and are especially useful in the management of patients with clinical deficiencies of fat digestion and absorption.

In general, an excess of bile salt is delivered to the intestine. Reabsorption is then required to maintain the bile salt pool. This reabsorption predominantly occurs in the distal ileum after fat absorption is complete; the distal ileum is the intestinal limb of the enterohepatic circulation of bile salts. Major ileal resection may exceed the liver's ability to compensate for intestinal bile salt losses by increased synthesis, with consequent depletion of the bile salt pool. The result is an increase in the amount of bile salts lost in the feces (normally, 500 mg/day) and a secretory diarrhea produced by colonic irritation by fatty acids.

Mineral Absorption. Calcium is absorbed predominantly from the duodenum and jejunum in a process that is vitamin D dependent. Ca^{++} binds to a specific transport protein on the brush border, is transferred to a cytosolic calcium-binding protein, and then passes out the lateral-basal membrane via either a Ca^{++} ATPase or a Na^{+}-Ca^{++} transport system. Vitamin D_3, which acts like a hormone to increase protein production, increases all these protein-dependent mechanisms. Major proximal intestinal resection may temporarily result in significant calcium malabsorption. With time, however, ileal adaptation may result in more efficient calcium absorption, provided that transit times are not too rapid. Calcium malabsorption rarely accompanies serious fat malabsorption because calcium salts precipitate under such circumstances.

The major site of iron absorption is the duodenum (Fig. 13–6). Total body stores of iron, by mechanisms that are incompletely understood, regulate the absorption of iron. Iron tends to form insoluble salts in the intestinal lumen so that the effective dissolution of iron is an important prerequisite to absorption. Solubility is enhanced by gastric or ascorbic acid and is impaired by phytates, certain forms of dietary fiber, or phosphates. In general, ferrous iron is absorbed better than ferric iron. Figure 13–6 summarizes the process. Iron is bound to a secreted form of transferrin, and then the complex is endocytosed. After endocytosis, both the receptor and the transferrin are recycled (Fig. 13–6). Iron may be stored locally in the intestinal cell as ferritin or released into the general circulation where it binds once more to a transferrin in the plasma. Iron bound to ferritin in the epithelial cell is lost when the cell desquamates.

Magnesium absorption occurs in the distal small intestine, predominantly by passive diffusion. Clinical states associated with marked decreases in intestinal transit times can result, if prolonged, in significant disturbances in magnesium absorption.

Zinc, copper, and selenium are other important trace elements absorbed in the small intestine. The details of the dynamics of absorption of these trace elements are not well understood, but zinc and copper absorption probably occur through similar and possibly competing transport mechanisms (since oral zinc therapy can result in diminished copper absorption). Increased fecal losses of zinc can occur in steatorrhea and exudative diarrheal states and with increased fiber or phosphate intake.

Vitamin Absorption. Fat-soluble vitamins are absorbed, as are lipids, by free passage into epithelial cells after these form micelles in duodenum and jejunum. Some are re-esterified in the epithelial cell where they enter the chylomicrons and pass into the lacteals. Therefore, assuming adequate intake, deficiencies only occur when there are bile salt deficiencies.

Water-soluble vitamins require slightly more complex absorption processes. Folic acid (polypteroyl glutamate) is hydrolyzed into monoglutamate before absorption by folate deconjugase in the intestinal brush border. Absorption occurs by a carrier-mediated system followed by reduction and methylation to methyltetrahydrofolate within the intestinal mucosal cell. Severe generalized intestinal mucosal disease can result in deficiencies of folate digestion and absorption. Sulphasalazine (frequently used in the treatment of inflammatory bowel disease) therapy has been associated with folate deficiency, which

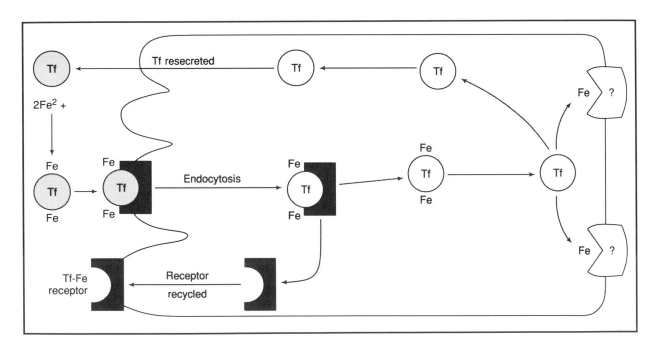

FIGURE 13–6. A current view of the mechanism of iron absorption by the epithelial cells of the small intestine. A form of transferrin (Tf) is secreted into the lumen where it binds Fe^{++}. The Fe_2-Tf complex is taken up by receptor-mediated endocytosis, and the receptor and the Tf are recycled. Iron is transported across the basolateral membrane by a poorly understood process and appears in portal blood bound to the plasma form of transferrin. (Reprinted from Kutchai, H.C.: The gastrointestinal system: Digestion and absorption. *In* Berne, R.M., and Levy, M.N. (eds.): Physiology, 2nd ed. St. Louis, C.V. Mosby Co., 1988, p. 733.)

is presumed to be secondary to competitive inhibition of folate transport and metabolism. The ileum is the major site of vitamin C absorption, which is an energy-dependent, sodium carrier-mediated process.

Vitamin B_{12} absorption requires gastric pepsin digestion of complexes of vitamin B_{12} with ingested dietary protein, followed by binding to gastric intrinsic factor. The intrinsic factor-vitamin B_{12} complexes bind to ileal receptors predominantly in the most distal 100 cm of ileum, where absorption is mediated by an energy-dependent process dependent on both ionic calcium and neutral intraluminal pH. Bacterial vitamin B_{12} cannot be absorbed because it is not bound to intrinsic factors.

Summary

Great physiologic reserve allows surgical resection of major portions of the small intestine with only limited disturbance of absorptive function. Certain substances (iron, vitamin B_{12}, and bile salts) are absorbed most efficiently in discrete segments of the small intestine (Table 13–7), and deficiencies may result from even limited disease or resection of those areas.

TABLE 13–7. ABSORPTION IN THE SMALL INTESTINE

	DUODENUM	JEJUNUM	ILEUM
Water	+	+++	++
Sodium	+	+++	++
Potassium	+	+++	+
Chloride	+	++	+++
Fats	++	+++	+
Proteins	++	+++	+
Carbohydrates	++	+++	+
Bile salts	0	0	+++
Fat-soluble vitamins*	+	+++	+
Water-soluble vitamins			
Vitamin B_{12}	0	0	+++
Folic acid	+	+++	++
Ascorbic acid	?	+	+++
Minerals			
Iron	+++	++	0
Calcium	++	+++	+
Magnesium	+	++	++
Zinc†	0	+	++

* Vitamin K (endogenously produced fraction) absorbed in colon.
† Based on animal studies.

Reprinted from Wilson, J.A.P., and Owyang, C.: Physiology of digestion and absorption. *In* Nelson, R.L., and Nyhus, L.M. (eds.): Surgery of the Small Intestine. Norwalk, CT, Appleton & Lang, 1987, p. 22.

COLONIC PHYSIOLOGY

The colon is a 1.5 meter long, predominantly intraperitoneal organ. Its major functions include absorption of water and electrolytes and the storage of nonabsorbed fecal material for evacuation at the convenience of the human organism. The colon is innervated by preganglionic parasympathetic vagal fibers, as well as by parasympathetic pelvic fibers, both of which cause increases in motility that are manifested predominantly as segmenting contractions. Sympathetic nervous innervation occurs via the inferior and superior mesenteric plexus, as well as the hypogastric plexus. Sympathetic nervous stimulation results in inhibition of colonic motility. Approximately 1000 cc of fluid chyme is delivered to the right colon daily, yet only 100 to 200 ml/day of water are excreted in the feces. The colon slowly moves the fecal mass aborally at rates of 5 to 10 cm/hr, with the interposition of one to three daily mass movements in which coordinated, propagated colonic activity results in the sustained aboral transport of fecal material. The control of colonic motility is predominantly dependent on its intrinsic neural plexus. The importance of this plexus is evident in patients with Hirschsprung's disease in which its absence results in tonic contraction and a consequent functional obstruction to fecal transit.

Several local and distant reflexes affect colonic function. Colocolic reflexes act locally so that distension of the colon results in a reflex tonic inhibition of contraction of other segments mediated by local adrenergic reflex arcs. The gastrocolic reflex is a somewhat more distant reflex in which gastric distension results in increased motility. It is produced by increases in parasympathetic tone modulated by the secretion of gastrin and cholecystokinin.

Acute illness, sleep, or general anesthetics may have profound effects on colonic function. Laparotomy is known to inhibit colonic function, with a return to normal taking 48 to 72 hours. Being the slowest portion of the gastrointestinal tract to recuperate from the effects of general anesthesia and abdominal surgery, the return of normal colonic function (the passage of flatus and/or bowel movement), *in general,* signifies the return of consistent aboral peristalsis and hence prompts the resumption of oral alimentation. Abnormal motility on the basis of deranged local reflexes may play an important role in the pathogenesis of colonic pseudo-obstruction (Ogilvie's syndrome). Resections of major portions of the intraperitoneal colon usually result in minimal derangement of colonic function due to the great physiologic reserve and the ability of adjacent colonic segments to compensate. Right hemicolectomy does, however, result in predictable increases in stool volume because of the slight diminution in the colon's water-absorptive capacity. As a general rule, the ability to compensate decreases with age.

Diverticular disease of the colon has been hypothesized to be caused by abnormalities in colonic circular muscle function that result in sustained segmental colonic hypertension and consequent mucosal herniation. Although muscular hypertrophy is a pathognomonic feature of diverticular disease of the colon, a direct cause-and-effect relationship has never been clearly documented. It is interesting, however, that considerable overlap exists between patients with functional disorders of the colon (in whom abnormal, sustained contractions in response to various stimuli have been demonstrated) and patients with symptomatic diverticular disease of the colon.

MICROBIOLOGY OF THE GASTROINTESTINAL TRACT

The human gastrointestinal tract is sterile at birth. However, within a few hours of birth, the oral and anal orifices become colonized with bacteria prevalent in the infant's environment. The ingestion of food, commencing within the first 24 hours of birth, results in progressive colonization of the gastrointestinal tract. Over the next several days, a more consistent and stable microflora invades and establishes itself. The breast-fed infant has a largely Gram-positive microflora, predominantly *Lactobacillus bifidis*. Formula-fed infants have a more complex microflora, with a heavy predominance of facultative Gram-negative organisms, as well as some anaerobes, resembling the stool of older children.

The normal stomach contains few if any retrievable bacteria, except in patients with gastrointestinal hemorrhage, gastric outlet obstruction, diminished gastric acidity, or malignancy. The majority of upper gastrointestinal pathogenic bacteria are sensitive to penicillins and first-generation cephalosporins. Bacterial counts in the oropharynx and esophagus in general are fairly high, with 10^4 to 10^7 bacteria/mL accounting for the devastating clinical effects of perforation and uncontrolled leakage into tissue planes from either of these sources.

In general, the upper small intestine is secondarily colonized from the oropharynx and esophagus, with a slight predominance of anaerobic organisms (*Peptostreptococcus, Fusobacterium, Bacteroides melaninogenicus, Bacteroides oralis, Peptococcus, Eikenella corrodens*). Bacterial counts vary between 10^2 to 10^3/mL in the presence of normal gastric acidity.

In the more distal small intestine, there is a slight predominance of aerobic organisms (*Escherichia coli, Klebsiella, Enterobacter, Streptococcus faecalis*), but significant numbers of anaerobes are also present (*Bacteroides fragilis, Peptostreptococcus, Clostridium*). Anaerobic bacteria achieve even more prominence in the microflora of the colon, with bacterial counts in the region of 10^8 to 10^{12} bacteria/mL of aspirate/gram of stool.

In the presence of acute intestinal obstruction, there is a marked increase in the number of both aerobic and anaerobic organisms that can be recovered from the intestinal lumen, both proximal and distal to the site of obstruction. Bacterial translocation from the intestine may account for cryptogenic sepsis that is not infrequently seen in patients succumbing to multiple system organ failure in the intensive care unit. Bacterial translocation seems to be a normal phenomenon, but relatively few bacteria survive phagocytosis by phagocytes in the lamina propria or liver. Systemic illness or bacterial overgrowth increases the number of bacteria that survive. Normal motility of the entire gastrointestinal tract serves a housekeeping function, maintaining a balance between intraluminal enteric pathogens and the host.

The use of perioperative antibiotic therapy for patients undergoing elective gastrointestinal surgery can be based scientifically on the above information. Obviously, surgery of the oropharynx, esophagus, and the obstructed or diseased small intestine; the patient with gastrointestinal hemorrhage, gastric malignancy, or previous gastric surgery; and all operations on the intraperitoneal colon would stand to benefit from the administration of perioperative antibiotics. In a similar sense, measures aimed at reducing the numbers of viable intraluminal pathogens (for example, mechanical or antibiotic preparation of the intestinal tract) may help the surgeon achieve a salutary reduction in perioperative infectious complications. More study will be required to determine whether "sterilization" of the gastrointestinal tract in critically ill patients will diminish the incidence of multiple system organ failure based on bacterial translocation.

ANORECTAL PHYSIOLOGY

The levatores ani fuse in the midline to form the pelvic floor. The most important component of this muscle is the puborectalis, which functions with the internal anal sphincter muscle, fusing partially with this muscle as it loops around the anorectal junction. The anal canal is the only part of the lower gastrointestinal tract with a somatic innervation, the integrity of which is important in the maintenance of continence.

The surgical anal canal begins at the cephalic border of the puborectalis muscle and ends at the perianal skin. It is surrounded by two concentric muscular tubes, the inner internal sphincter that is autonomically innervated smooth muscle and the somatically innervated external anal sphincter. The external anal sphincter has been subdivided into three portions: the superficial, the deep, and the subcutaneous sphincters. Functionally these three segments cannot be separated easily. The internal anal sphincter is a continuation of the circular muscle layer of the rectum innervated by the autonomic nervous system; it is responsible for sustained tonic contraction (sympathetic mediated) that is episodically interrupted by relaxation (parasympathetic mediated) to allow defecation. The normal human rectum is empty at rest, but in conditions of rapid stool transit and abnormalities of colonic motility resulting in stasis or anal sphincter dysfunction (for example, spasm resulting from perianal trauma or inflammation), it can take on a reservoir function.

Anal continence is dependent on many factors, including the anorectal high-pressure zone, the anorectal angle created by the puborectalis sling, rectal compliance, normal anorectal sensory mechanisms, colonic transit time, stool volume and consistency, rectal motility, and anal canal motility. The anorectal high-pressure zone is dependent on both extrinsic and intrinsic pressure. Extrinsic pressure is provided by increases in intra-abdominal pressure, which tend to compress the distal rectum in an anteroposterior orientation, acting as a flap valve. Intrinsic pressures are due to the normal tonic contraction of the internal sphincter muscle and require an intact autonomic nervous system. Normal tone in the puborectalis sling produces a marked anteroposterior angulation at the anorectal junction, contributing dramatically to continence.

Rectal capacity is fairly low, with urgency developing at approximately 200 mL of distension and incontinence above volumes of 400 mL, when produced acutely. The normal rectum is protected from distension by the valves of Houston, the angulation of the rectosigmoid junction, and the slow rate of delivery of stool to the rectum.

Anorectal reflex mechanisms are not intrinsic to the rectum itself, but rather are based in the response to distension of the levator ani musculature, as well as the somatic innervation of the anal canal. The normal rectoanal reflex results in increasing relaxation of the internal anal sphincter with increasing degrees of rectal distension. It is mediated by stretch receptors in Meissner's and Auerbach's plexus and is consequently absent in patients with Hirschsprung's disease. Lesser degrees of rectal distention can result in increasing tone in the internal anal sphincter, known as the rectoanal contractile reflex, but ultimately beyond a certain threshold of rectal distension, relaxation with a urge to defecate supervenes. The rectoanal inhibitory and contractile reflexes are important in the discrimination of flatus and solid and liquid stool, so important to normal everyday life, and is dependent on an intact spinal reflex. Inhibition of the internal sphincter allows small samples of rectal content to descend into the upper portion of the somatically innervated anal ca-

nal. Continence is then maintained by contraction of the external anal sphincter, allowing discrimination between gas and liquid and solid stool and consequent discrete elimination of flatus or inhibition of the defecatory process until socially convenient.

In the presence of large volumes of liquid stool, as in diarrheal states, temporary fecal incontinence may supervene despite normal pelvic musculature and innervation. This incontinence is presumably due to rectal overload, secondary to high stool volumes, and is similar to that associated with fecal impaction. Complete rectal prolapse is frequently associated with incontinence, and both abnormalities probably share a common pathophysiologic factor: weakness of the pelvic floor musculature.

Anatomic disruptions of part or all of the sphincter mechanism result in varying degrees of incontinence. In general, complete disruption of the internal anal sphincter results in complete incontinence for flatus and stool. Preservation of one quarter to one third of the length of the normal internal anal sphincter may be enough to maintain continence, a fact employed successfully in the application of internal anal sphincterotomy to anorectal pathology. Clinical assessment of anorectal function includes defecography, anorectal manometry, and pelvic floor myography. These tests have not achieved wide clinical applicability, mainly due to difficulty in interpretation of the results because of the wide overlap between different pathologic conditions.

HORMONES OF THE ALIMENTARY TRACT

Clinical and basic science research in the second half of this century has firmly established the existence and role of several peptide hormones in the normal and abnormal function of the alimentary tract. A thorough understanding of their physiology is a prerequisite to the successful surgical therapy of digestive disease. Although complex interactions during the digestive sequence have been proposed, it is most practical to examine the physiology of these hormones separately.

Gastrin

Secreted by G cells of the gastric antrum, this 34 amino acid peptide is liberated from its prepro-hormone by a series of enzymatic cleavages. A smaller peptide, G-17 (small gastrin), has identical biologic effects and is the most abundant molecular form of gastrin in the antrum. The secretion of gastrin is a result of a variety of intraluminal, hormonal, and vagal influences. Amino acids and small peptide fragments within the gastric lumen are the primary stimulants of gastrin release under physiologic conditions. The pH of the gastric antral contents also modulates gastrin release, with inhibition below a pH of 3 and stimulation in conditions associated with chronic elevations of antral pH (pernicious anemia, atrophic gastritis). Free intragastric calcium ions also stimulate gastrin release. Elevated basal and postprandial serum gastrin levels postvagotomy occurring within hours of denervation suggest a predominantly inhibitory tonic vagal effect on gastrin release. Vagal stimulation results in gastrin release, probably mediated via a gastrin-releasing peptide within the antral mucosa. Somatostatin inhibits both gastrin release and the action of gastrin on the oxyntic cell. Other peptides secreted by the upper small intestine may have effects on gastrin release.

The two primary actions of gastrin in normal subjects are stimulation of parietal cell HCl secretion and regulation of growth of the oxyntic mucosa (Table 13–8). G-17 and G-34 are equally potent in the stimulation of HCl secretion. This increase in acid secretion is dependent on activation of specific membrane-bound gastrin receptors, which in turn activate an intracellular calcium messenger system. Local concentrations of histamine and acetylcholine have important influences on the function of this system; both to exaggerate the secretagogue effect. These effects are probably intracellular since known inhibitors of parietal cell function have no apparent effect on gastrin binding to the cell membrane receptors. Gastrin has important trophic effects on the mucosa of much of the intestinal tract. These effects are most prominent in the stomach, but the widespread mucosal atrophy that follows antrectomy underlines its role in other parts of the intestinal tract.

Cholecystokinin

Cholecystokinin (CCK), a 33 amino acid peptide hormone secreted from the duodenum and proximal small intestine, has several physiologic actions on the structure and function of the pancreatobiliary

TABLE 13–8. PHYSIOLOGIC EFFECTS OF GASTRIN ON GASTROINTESTINAL FUNCTION

STOMACH
↓ Gastrin-mediated HCl and pepsin secretion
↓ Vagal-mediated HCl and pepsin secretion
↓ Basal and stimulated gastrin release
PANCREAS
↓ Protein absorption
↓ Insulin/glucagon secretion
↓ DNA, RNA, and protein synthesis
INTESTINE
↓ Protein absorption
↓ H$_2$O/electrical secretion
↓ Motility
HORMONES
↓ Release of gastrointestinal hormones

TABLE 13–9. ACTIONS OF CHOLECYSTOKININ

PRIMARY (Proven)
Gallbladder contraction
Relaxation of sphincter of Oddi
Stimulation of pancreatic enzyme secretion
Increased intestinal motility
SECONDARY (Probable)
Inhibition of gastric emptying
Inhibition of gastric secretion
Regulation of pancreatic growth
Regulation of satiety

system, gastroduodenal secretion, and intestinal blood flow. These actions are summarized in Table 13–9. The primary effects of CCK are to increase pancreatic enzyme secretion and stimulate gallbladder emptying. Stimulation of CCK release is produced by the presence of fat within the duodenal lumen. Only long-chain fatty acids (>9 carbon) dispersed in micelles exert this effect. Other nutrients—amino acids, and to a lesser extent, glucose—also cause CCK release when present in the proximal small intestine. Deficient production of CCK is present in patients with extensive destruction of the mucosa of the upper small intestine as seen in celiac disease. The contribution of this deficient production to the malabsorption seen in this disease entity is not clear, but secretion of CCK returns to normal with successful treatment.

Secretin

Secretin, a 27 amino acid linear peptide, is secreted by argyrophil S cells of the duodenum and jejunum. Acidification of the duodenum provokes the release of secretin in proportion to the length of intestine in contact with acidic chyme. Food itself probably plays a minor role in the release of secretin. No clear evidence exists for vagal-mediated secretin release in humans, but secondary changes in the rate of pancreatic and biliary secretion after vagotomy may decrease secretin release.

The primary biologic effect of secretin is to cause an increase in production of pancreatic juice that is rich in bicarbonate. In isolation, secretin has minor effects on the rate of pancreatic enzyme secretion, but in combination with CCK it causes a dramatic enhancement of the CCK-mediated increase in enzyme secretion. Most water and bicarbonate secretion is from the ductal tissue of the pancreas. In pharmacologic doses secretin causes hypertrophic changes in the pancreas associated with increased weight and RNA. Secretin also increases bile flow and bicarbonate content. It is unlikely that secretin has an important influence on gastric function under physiologic conditions other than a modest decrease in the rate of gastric emptying.

Somatostatin

This 14 amino acid peptide produced by D cells of the stomach, pancreas, and small intestine is also present in the autonomic myenteric plexus and has unique physiologic actions on the stomach, pancreas, and small intestine. The recent commercial production of a long-acting somatostatin analogue has allowed the application of the physiologic effects of this peptide hormone to everyday surgical practice. The paracrine effects of somatostatin play an important role in the regulation of gastric secretion and glucose homeostasis. Somatostatin secreted in response to a meal appears to attenuate the increase in gastric acid and pepsin secretion. Its influence on glucose conditions may be a tonic inhibition of glucagon release from the pancreatic islet cells. Somatostatinomas, rare endocrine tumors of the pancreas, predictably produce hypochlorhydria, steatorrhea, weight loss, and impaired glucose tolerance.

Gastric Inhibitory Polypeptide

This 42 amino acid peptide produced by the K cells of the small intestine is released in response to oral or intravenous glucose loading and appears to exert its physiologic effect by enhancing pancreatic insulin release. No clear evidence of a physiologic role in the modulation of gastric secretion or motility has as yet emerged despite its name.

Motilin

The basal myoelectric activity of the small intestine is characterized by periodic peristaltic waves originating in the upper gastrointestinal tract and propagated aborally; these are called migrating motor complexes. The release of motilin from the duodenum and jejunum prompted by luminal acidification results in two- to threefold increases in plasma motilin levels that coincide with the initiation of migrating motor complexes at 60 to 90 minute intervals. The presence of fat or a mixed meal in the duodenum inhibits motilin release. Thus, motilin is a prominent modulator of the interdigestive myoelectric activity of the gut, but probably plays no role in postprandial motility patterns. Motilin is a linear peptide of 22 amino acid residues.

Other Gut Hormones

Many other biologically activity peptides are found in varying concentrations in gut mucosa and serum, but have not been shown to have physiologic roles in the structure and function of the GI tract. As knowledge of their actions expands, it is possible that physiologic roles for neurotensin, pancreatic polypeptide enteroglucagon, and peptide YY may be assigned.

BIBLIOGRAPHY

1. Postlethwait, R.W.: Physiology. Surgery of the Esophagus, 2nd ed. Norwalk, CT, Appleton-Century-Crofts, 1986, p. 591.
2. Schoen, H.S., Morris, D.W., and Cohen, S.: Esophageal peristaltic force in man. Response to mechanical and pharmacologic alterations. Am. J. Dig. Dis. 22:589, 1977.
3. Hellemans, J., and Vantrappen, G.: Physiology. In Vantrappen, G., and Hellemans, J. (eds.): Diseases of the Esophagus. New York, Springer, 1974, pp. 40–102.
4. Laughton, W.B., and Powley, T.L.: Localization of the efferent function in the dorsal motor nucleus of the vagus. Am. J. Physiol., 252:R13, 1987.
5. Walsh, J.H.: Peptides as regulators of gastric acid secretion. In Berne, R.M. (ed.): Annual Review of Physiology. Palo Alto, CA, Annual Review, 1988.
6. Borody, T.J., and Phillips, S.F.: Motility of the small intestine. In Nelson, R.L., and Lyhus, L.M. (eds.): Surgery of the Small Intestine. Norwalk, CT, Appleton & Lang, 1987, pp. 29–36.
7. Smith, J., Kelly, K.A., and Weinshilboum, R.M.: Pathophysiology of postoperative ileus. Arch. Surg., 112:203, 1977.
8. Gray, G.M.: Carbohydrate digestion and absorption. New. Engl. J. Med., 292:1225, 1975.
9. Malagelada, J.R., Go, V.L.W., and Summerskill, W.H.J.: Altered pancreatic and biliary function after vagotomy and pyloroplasty. Gastroenterology, 66:22, 1974.
10. Wilson, J.A.P., and Owyang, C.: Physiology of digestion and absorption. In Nelson, R.L., and Nyhus, L.M. (eds.): Surgery of the Small Intestine. Norwalk, CT, Appleton & Lang, 1987, p. 21.
11. Shafik, A.: A new concept of the anatomy of the anal sphincter mechanism and the physiology of defecation. I: The external anal sphincter: A triple-loop system. Invest. Urol., 12:412, 1975.
12. Parks, A.G.: Anorectal incontinence. Proc. Roy. Soc. Med., 68:681, 1975.

14

THE LIVER AND BILIARY TREE

TODD K. HOWARD *and* TIMOTHY R. BILLIAR

ANATOMIC CONSIDERATIONS

The external anatomy of the liver does not reflect the arrangement of functional units within the liver. The functional division of the right and left lobes of the liver is based on the right and left branches of the portal vein and hepatic artery (Fig. 14–1). This division occurs along a line from the hepatic hilum, through the bed of the gallbladder, and posteriorly to the vena cava. Based on subdivision of the portal vein and hepatic artery, the right lobe is further divided into four segments (V, VI, VII, VIII): anterior-superior, anterior-inferior, posterior-superior, and posterior-inferior (Fig. 14–1). Similarly, the left lobe is divided into three segments (II, III, IV): medial, superior-lateral, and inferior-lateral. The caudate lobe (I) has unique arterial and venous anatomy derived from brances of both the right and left hepatic artery and portal vein. The hepatic venous drainage follows a similar pattern, with the right hepatic vein draining the right lobe, the middle hepatic vein draining primarily the medial segment of the left lobe, as well as portions of the right lobe, and the left hepatic vein draining the lateral segments of the left lobe (Fig. 14–2). Several medium and small hepatic veins drain from the right lobe directly into the vena cava. Similarly, the caudate lobe has separate drainage into the vena cava.

On a microscopic level, the liver architecture has traditionally been based on a lobule centered around hepatic venule. Surrounding the venule are radiating cords of hepatocytes. Arranged around the periphery of the lobule are the portal triads consisting of the hepatic arteriole, portal venule, and bile duct. The portal venule and hepatic arteriole empty together into the hepatic sinusoids that bathe the hepatic cords and subsequently empty into the hepatic venule. Hepatologists now consider that the functioning unit ("hepatic acinus") consists of the central portal triad containing the terminal portal venule

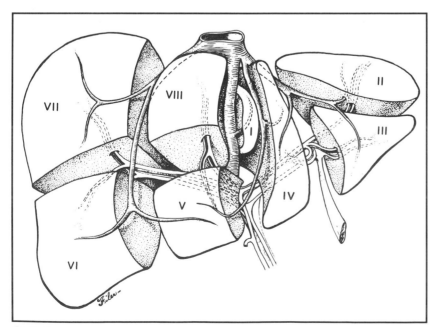

FIGURE 14–1. Subdivisions of the right lobe. (Reprinted from Iwatsuki, S., Sheahan, D.G., and Starzl, T.E.: The changing face of hepatic resection. Curr. Prob. Surg. *26*(May):291, 1989. Figure 2.)

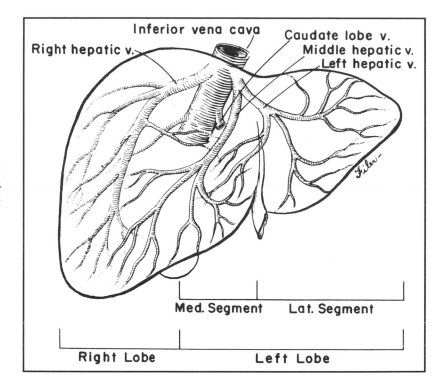

FIGURE 14–2. Hepatic venous drainage. (Reprinted from Iwatsuki, S., Sheahan, D.G., and Starzl, T.E. The changing face of hepatic resection. Curr. Prob. Surg. *26* (May):297, 1989. Figure 7.)

and hepatic arteriole and that flow is outward along the sinuses to multiple terminal hepatic venules (Fig. 14–3).

The liver is composed of three major types of cells. About 50 per cent of the cells in the liver are hepatocytes. They make up about 80 per cent of the liver volume. Endothelial cells that live in the hepatic sinusoids make up just over half of the nonhepatocyte cells, whereas Kupffer cells, the largest collection of tissue macrophages in the body, represent 40 per cent of the nonhepatocyte cell population. Lipocytes (Ito cells), fibroblasts, neurons, and bile duct cells make up the small remaining portion of the hepatic cellular mass.

The hepatocytes perform the major metabolic and excretory functions of the liver. They are arranged in cords or plates of one cell thickness and are surrounded by the sinusoids (Fig. 14–4). The function of any individual hepatocyte depends upon the position of the cell within the lobule and the proximity of the cell to the blood supply. Based on these functional differences, hepatocytes can be divided into three zones. Zone 1 hepatocytes lie in closest proximity to the periportal region and are the first hepatocytes exposed to the various substrates delivered to the liver by the portal vein and hepatic artery. Accordingly, these cells contain the highest concentration of enzymes involved in glycogenesis and gluconeogensis. Cells in this area also produce the majority of the proteins and are responsible for protein metabolism. In contrast, cells in the periportal area (zone 3), an area with decreased oxygen tension, are equipped for glycolysis and lipogenesis.

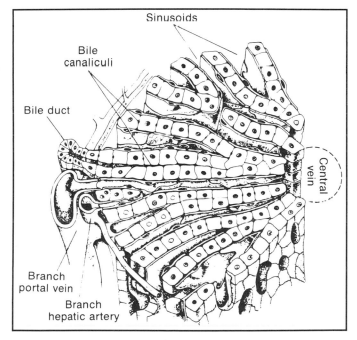

FIGURE 14–3. A hepatic lobule. A central vein is located in the center of the lobule, with plates of hepatic cells disposed radially. Branches of the portal vein and hepatic artery are located on the periphery of the lobule, and blood from both perfuses the sinusoids. Peripherally located bile ducts drain the bile canaliculi that run between the hepatocytes. (Redrawn from Bloom, W., and Fawcett, D.W.: A Textbook of Histology, 10th ed. Philadelphia, W.B. Saunders Co., 1975. *In* Berne, R.M., and Levy, M.N. (eds.): Physiology, 2nd ed. St. Louis, C.V. Mosby Co. 1988. Figure 43–27, p. 708.)

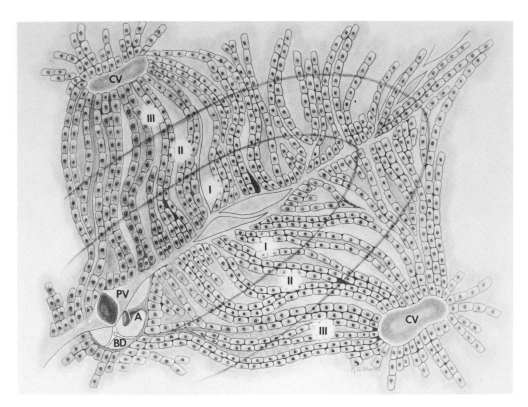

FIGURE 14–4. Location of hepatocyte zones within the liver acinus. Abbreviations: A—artery; BD—bile duct; CV—central vein; PV—portal vein.

Ureagenesis also occurs in zones 2 and 3. The enzymes responsible for gluconeogenesis are much more abundant in the periportal region than in the centrilobular area. These functional differences may be related to the concentration of the various substrates arriving via the hepatic artery and portal vein. As the blood passes from portal to central regions, substrates may be removed and metabolic products added to the sinusoidal blood. These substrates and metabolic products may induce the synthesis of enzyme systems within the hepatocyte and regulate the function of the cells within the lobule. The hepatocytes replicate rapidly, and it is estimated that the entire cell mass of the liver could be replaced every 50 days. This characteristic accounts for the rapid growth of the hepatic remnant after major liver resections.

Kupffer cells lie within the sinusoids, giving them immediate access to the perfusing blood. They are phagocytic cells and participate in antigen processing and presentation. They represent a major portion of the reticuloendothelial system and the nonspecific immune response. In this capacity, they may also modulate the immune response by sequestering gut-derived antigens and thereby modulating immune responses to them. The hypergammaglobulinemia of chronic liver diseases may result from shunting of gut-derived antigen away from the Kupffer cells and into the mainstream of the immune system, allowing a more vigorous response to them.

The endothelial cells of the liver constitute the specialized capillary bed of the hepatic sinusoidal sysem. They do not form a continuous cellular layer; instead, the gaps between the cells are wide, and the cytoplasm is fenestrated. Thus, the sinusoids are usually porous and allow the migration of most large molecules into the space of Disse between the endothelial cells and the hepatocytes. No oncotic pressure difference can be maintained between the sinusoid and the space of Disse. The net filtration across the sinusoid is consequently about thirty times that seen in a normal muscle capillary bed. Mass flow into the space of Disse is accordingly very sensitive to hydrostatic pressure, and elevated sinusoidal pressure, as seen in cirrhosis or the Budd-Chiari syndrome, results in dramatic increases in net filtration. This fluid is removed by the hepatic lymphatics that exit the liver via the porta hepatis and via the hepatic capsule to the diaphragmatic lymphatics.

Between adjoining hepatocytes, the bile canaliculus forms the origin of the biliary system (Fig. 14–4). The canaliculus is separated from the space of Disse by tight junctions between hepatocyte membranes. The plasma membrane of hepatocyte that forms the canaliculus contains many microvilli and is active in the production of bile. Passing along the plates of hepatocytes, the canaliculi drain into ductules within the portal triads at the periphery of the lobule. From this point the bile ducts follow the portal vein and hepatic artery retrograde to the hilum of the liver where the hepatic duct is formed.

BLOOD FLOW

Total hepatic blood flow is approximately 20 per cent of the cardiac output. The liver receives nutritive blood flow from two sources: the hepatic artery and the portal vein. Hepatic arterial blood supplies about one third of the total hepatic blood flow and about half of the oxygen consumed by the liver. The portal vein supplies the remaining two thirds of hepatic blood flow. These relationships are dependent upon normal hemodynamics and can change dramatically in response to the alteration of normal flow patterns. For example, occlusion or thrombosis of the portal vein results in substantial increases in hepatic arterial flow. Similarly, ligation of the hepatic artery increases the portal flow. These changes are mediated by neurohumoral and local metabolic events.

That normal liver parenchyma is able to survive without hepatic arterial flow is demonstrated by the tolerance of the liver of hepatic artery ligation. Compensatory increase in flow via the portal vein will supply adequate oxygen for hepatocellular function because the O_2 needs of the liver are constant. The centrilobular areas of the liver are ordinarily relatively hypoxic because of their distance from portal venous and hepatic arterial branches. When oxygen-poor portal blood is the only source of flow to the organ, temporary dysfunction and mild increase in serum levels of aminotransferases occur as the normally hypoxic centrilobular areas undergo some degeneration. More severe injury or infarction occurs if hepatic artery flow is interrupted in a diseased liver, particularly in the cirrhotic liver with impaired or reversed portal flow.

The drop of pressure across the sinusoidal bed is only 2 to 3 mm so that increases in hepatic vein pressure (as in congestive heart failure) are transmitted to the sinusoids, markedly increasing transsinusoidal fluid loss. Ascites then results.

The biliary system, particularly the gallbladder, is dependent upon arterial flow since no portal branches supply the major bile ducts or the gallbladder. Collateral arterial flow from the pancreaticoduodenal artery via the common bile duct can supply sufficient arterial blood to prevent necrosis of the gallbladder in the event of hepatic artery occlusion or ligation. Simultaneous injury to the common duct and the hepatic artery would be expected to result in serious ischemia or necrosis of the proximal bile ducts and gallbladder. The tenuous arterial supply to these structures partly accounts for the tendency of reconstructions of the bile duct to stricture. In addition, relative ischemia of the biliary system in the setting of arterial occlusion may predispose to bacterial invasion of the biliary tree.

METABOLISM

The liver is the center of the body's metabolic machine and is critical to the metabolism of carbohydrate, protein, and fat. In addition, it secretes bile, stores vitamin and iron, degrades hormones and hemoglobin, and inactivates drugs and toxins.

Carbohydrate

The liver plays a central role in glucose homeostasis. It is responsible for the storage of glucose during periods of excess supply (feeding) and the release of glucose when exogenous glucose is not available (fasting). As in other tissues, the glucose, once absorbed, is phosphorylated. Because glucokinase, the enzyme responsible for the phosphorylation of glucose in the liver, is less avid than hexokinase, the enzyme responsible for phosphorylation in other tissues, it allows the liver to produce and release glucose while other tissues are removing it from the blood. The position of the liver in the portal circulation gives it preferential access to glucose during feeding, compensating for the diminished avidity of glucokinase and allowing the liver to remove approximately 50 per cent of the glucose presented in the portal vein during feeding.

Glucose is absorbed from the gut and enters the liver via the portal blood. Glucose absorbed by the hepatocyte is converted directly to glycogen for storage up to a maximum of about 65 grams of glycogen per kilogram of liver tissue. Excess glucose is converted to fat. Glycogen is also produced in muscle, but is not available for use by other tissues.

Liver glycogen is the principal source of glucose during the early fasting state. Glucose produced in the liver is required for the normal function of brain and red blood cells. Other tissues can utilize fatty acids during the fasting state. After 48 hours of fasting, liver glycogen is exhausted, and protein, mobilized primarily from muscle, is converted by the liver to glucose.

Lactate, produced during anaerobic metabolism or in the red cells, is metabolized only in the liver. Ordinarily it is converted to pyruvate and subsequently back to glucose. This glucose is then available for use by other tissues. This shuttling of glucose and lactate between liver and peripheral tissues is carried out in the Cori cycle. The brain does not participate in this cycle, and a continuous supply of glucose for the brain must come at the expense of muscle protein, primarily alanine. In prolonged fasting, the requirement for glucose is decreased, and fat and ketones become the primary source of calories for the brain. Even in starvation, however, there is continued need for small amounts of glucose and the steady utilization of muscle protein for its production.

In liver disease the metabolism of glucose is frequently deranged. Portal hypertension may produce large portosystemic shunts in which the exposure of portal blood to functioning hepatocytes is decreased so that abnormal glucose tolerance results. The oral glucose tolerance test is more frequently abnormal than the intravenous glucose tolerance test, suggesting that shunting of glucose absorbed from the gut is more important than the inability of hepatocytes to process glucose in this form of glucose intolerance. Decreased exposure of hepatocytes to insulin because of shunting of pancreatic venous blood also changes the balance of hepatocyte function toward the production of glucose. Shunting of the portal blood that contains insulin secreted by the pancreas also results in increased peripheral insulin levels. The combination of increased peripheral insulin with glucose intolerance is not suggestive of diabetes in the cirrhotic patient.

Hypoglycemia is rare in chronic liver disease since the synthetic capacity of hepatocytes is great even in the cirrhotic liver. In fulminant hepatic failure, however, there is extensive hepatocyte loss, and hypoglycemia may supervene as gluconeogenesis fails.

The alcoholic may also develop hypoglycemia when no exogenous glucose is available during chronic alcohol intoxication. When alcohol is metabolized, it produces NADH, which inhibits gluconeogenesis by preventing the entry of amino acids, lactate, and glycerol into the gluconeogenetic pathway. Once the supply of glycogen is depleted, hypoglycemia will develop if high levels of NADH continue to inhibit gluconeogenesis. Although the normal supply of glycogen is adequate for 48 hours of fasting, the alcoholic frequently has poor dietary habits and inadequate reserves of glycogen and may develop hypoglycemia after shorter periods of fasting.

Lipids

There are three sources of free fatty acid available to the liver: fats absorbed from the gut, fat liberated from the adipocytes in response to lipolysis, and fatty acid synthesized from carbohydrate or amino acids. These fatty acids are esterified with glycerol to form triglyceride. The export of triglyceride is dependent upon the synthesis of very low density lipoprotein (VLDL). If the supply of precursors of triglyceride exceeds the capacity of the liver to synthesize and export VLDL, the triglyceride accumulates within the hepatocytes, with the characteristic findings of fatty change seen on biopsy. These findings do not necessarily indicate disordered hepatocyte function,

but rather an imbalance in lipid supply and VLDL production and most commonly result from disorders outside the liver. Excess supply is the basis of fatty liver seen in obesity, steroid use, pregnancy, diabetes, and total parenteral nutrition. Inhibition of protein synthesis by such drugs as tetracycline or such toxins as carbon tetrachloride may result in fatty change because of the inability to produce lipoproteins for export. Simple protein malnutrition or marked protein-calorie imbalance may result in fatty change when the lipid available for export exceeds the supply of protein precursors for lipoprotein synthesis.

The fatty infiltration of the liver seen in alcohol abuse is the result of several abnormalities. First, alcohol is a source of calories that are converted to Acetyl-CoA and are available for fat synthesis. Second, NADH produced in the metabolism of alcohol inhibits fatty acid oxidation and shifts metabolism toward triglyceride synthesis and esterification. Finally, chronic alcoholism may, because of malnutrition, inhibit the synthesis of VLDL.

Fatty infiltration per se is not indicative of damage. Nor does the persistence of fat in the hepatocytes result in permanent damage. Once the primary abnormality responsible for the accumulation of fat is reversed, full recovery of hepatic function is possible. Although some hepatocellular disruption may occur if fat accumulation is severe, permanent damage and cirrhosis do not occur, and the course of fatty liver is usually benign.

Beta oxidation of fatty acid in the liver produces ketone bodies for oxidative metabolism in peripheral tissues. Ketone bodies (beta-hydroxybutyric acid and aceto-acetic acid) provide energy in the fasting state and reduce the requirement for protein catabolism and gluconeogenesis, thus preserving muscle mass. The rapid loss of muscle mass in chronic liver failure may in part be due to failure of ketone production and the ensuing rapid catabolism of lean muscle mass during fasting.

Protein Metabolism

The metabolism of amino acids in the process of gluconeogenesis has been outlined earlier.

The liver is the site of synthesis of many of the serum proteins. In particular, albumin and most coagulation factors and lipoproteins are among the serum proteins synthesized in the liver. Albumin is the most abundant serum protein. In addition to its oncotic effects, albumin binds many substances and is responsible for the transport of bilirubin, pyridoxal phosphate, fatty acid, thyroxine, cortisol, testosterone, tryptophan, copper, zinc, nickel, cadmium, calcium, and other molecules. Furthermore, many drugs are avidly bound to albumin, falsely expanding their apparent volume of distribution. Albumin synthesis accounts for 11 to 15 per cent of total hepatic protein synthesis and may reach 11 mg/gm of liver tissue/day. Synthesis of albumin is influenced by nutritional status; hormones, including thyroxine, insulin, glucagon, and cortisol; cytokines produced in sepsis; and the effects of osmotic pressure on the hepatocyte.

Dramatic changes in both the types and amounts of plasma proteins produced by the liver take place in inflammatory states. This reaction of the liver, known as the acute phase response, occurs in response to hormone-like factors released from wounds remote from the liver or during sepsis. The acute phase response is characterized by a sudden and transient increase in the production of several proteins. This is associated with measurable increases in the circulating levels of the protein; these increases of ten reach several 100-fold over baseline (Table 14–1). The greatest increases in humans are seen in C-reactive protein and serum amyloid A. The synthetic rate for other plasma proteins, such as albumin, decreases. The acute phase proteins have a wide range of biologic activity, including inhibition of proteases, blood clotting, opsonization of bacteria and debris, modulation of the immune response, and binding of heavy metals. In general, it is thought that the ultimate functions of the acute phase reactants are to localize and limit tissue damage while enhancing microbial clearance. These actions are accomplished by counteracting the numerous proteases released at a site of active inflammation, promoting clot formation and opsonizing bacteria and tissue debris.

The primary hormonal signal for induction of the hepatic acute phase response in humans is interleukin-6 (IL-6). Glucocorticoids are also important, but appear to have only a permissive effect and do not stimulate the acute phase response alone. In humans, interleukin-1 (IL-1) and tumor necrosis factor (TNF) do not stimulate increases in specific acute phase reactants, but may be responsible for the decrease in some of the negative acute phase reactants, such as albumin. The primary action of IL-1 and TNF is probably to stimulate IL-6 production by fibroblasts and endothelial cells, thus amplifying the IL-6 signal. In addition to fibroblasts and endothelial cells in wounds, infiltrating monocytes/macrophages are the primary sources of IL-6 in localized wounds.

In sepsis, circulating monocytes and hepatic macrophages (Kupffer cells) and endothelial cells are the most likely sources of IL-6.

Vitamin Metabolism

The liver is responsible for the modification of most vitamins into their active co-enzyme form. The water-soluble vitamins include riboflavin, niacin, pyridoxine, cyanocobalamin, ascorbic acid, biotin, thiamine, folic acid, and pantothenic acid. These co-enzymes participate in a broad variety of metabolic processes. The deficiency states are well described, but one should be aware of possible deficiency complicating hepatic dysfunction. In addition to modification, the liver is responsible for the storage and excretion of vitamins and their metabolites, and acute hepatic necrosis may result in elevated levels of several vitamins.

Fat-soluble vitamins A, D, E, and K are dependent on bile production for absorption from the GI tract. The vitamins appear in thoracic duct lymph 2 to 6 hours after oral administration and are subsequently taken up quickly by the hepatocytes. Vitamin A is also stored and metabolized to active form in the parenchymal cells. A role for the storage of vitamin A in Ito cells has been suggested. Vitamin D, actually a hormone rather than a vitamin, undergoes the first step of metabolism, 25-hydroxylation, in the liver. Deficiency of vitamin D due to malabsorption and atered metabolism in liver disease can be associated with severe osteomalacia and pathologic fractures. Vitamin K also undergoes metabolism in the liver.

Alcohol interferes with the absorption and metabolism of most of the water-soluble and all of the fat-soluble vitamins. Chronic alcoholism can be expected to produce a generalized vitamin deficiency state, as well as malnutrition.

Hepatic Metabolism in Sepsis

Significant changes in hepatic metabolism and substrate utilization occur in the liver in sepsis. In early sepsis, glycogenolysis is the predominant

TABLE 14–1.   HUMAN HEPATIC ACUTE PHASE REACTANTS

SYNTHETIC RATE INCREASES (RATE)			
10- to 1000-fold	*2- to 10-fold*	*≤ 2 fold*	SYNTHETIC RATE DECREASES
C-reactive protein Serum amyloid A	Fibrinogen haptoglobin α_1 proteinase inhibitor α_1 acid glycoprotein α_1 antichymotrypsin	C_3 C_1 inactivator ceruloplasmin(?) α_2 antiplasmin	Albumin Prealbumin Transferrin Inter-2-anti-trypsin α_1 lipoprotein

feature. It is followed by increased gluconeogenesis as the liver attempts to produce greater amounts of glucose for use in the periphery. These changes are thought to be regulated at least in part by hormones, such as glucagon. Associated with these changes in the liver are a decrease in amino acid uptake in the muscles and concomitant increases in protein breakdown. Amino acids liberated from muscle are taken up by the liver where they are used to synthesize acute phase proteins or as substrate for glucose production. The amino acid alanine appears to be preferentially used as a substrate for glucose. Glucose is converted to lactate in the peripheral tissues and returned to the liver where it is converted to glucose via the Cori cycle. Fat metabolism is characterized by a shift from ketogenesis and toward lipogenesis. Within the liver carbohydrate carbons are converted to fat via malonyl-CoA. In late sepsis, there is a progressive decrease in gluconeogenesis, and hypoglycemia typically develops in the premorbid state. The factors that regulate the early changes in hepatic metabolism in sepsis and the conditions that contribute to the eventual decline in hepatocellular metabolic capacity have not yet been delineated.

RETICULOENDOTHELIAL SYSTEM

The liver is the site of the largest collection of fixed macrophages in the body. Kupffer cells have a dual origin. In resting states, most are derived from the bone marrow in the form of circulating monocytes. In inflammation, some local proliferation probably takes place. Kupffer cells are constantly turning over and appear to have a half-life of about 5 weeks. The Kupffer cells lie entirely within the sinusoids, but are in close contact with the hepatocytes because of the fenestrations in the endothelium of the sinusoids. They thus represent the only large collection of macrophages in constant contact with the bloodstream. The primary functions of these macrophages are phagocytosis of foreign or abnormal material. It is likely that they also process this material for recognition by lymphocytes as lymphatic tissue is not part of the normal liver. The Kupffer cells almost certainly act as modulators of hepatocyte function by means of cytokine secretion in response to circulating septic stimuli.

The Kupffer cells possess specific receptors for both complement (C_3b) and the Fc portion of IgG and IgM. These receptors facilitate attachment to and phagocytosis of circulating organisms opsonized by complement and immunoglobulins. Although complement activation alone can be a sufficient opsonin for phagocytosis in certain circumstances, immunoglobulin is generally more effective in this regard. If opsonization is adequate, organisms are rapidly cleared by the liver. Defects in opsonization, such as depletion of complement or defective production of immunoglobulin, result in decreased hepatic clearance and preferential sequestration of organisms in the lung and spleen. Certain encapsulated virulent organisms, such as encapsulated pneumococci, which may be resistant to opsonization, are also more dependent on splenic clearance. The ability of the liver to clear most organisms when opsonized may help explain why postsplenectomy sepsis is rarely seen in splenectomized individuals with otherwise normal immune function and who are capable of clearing most organisms via the Kupffer cells.

Reticuloendothelial system dysfunction can be seen in individuals with compromised hepatic blood flow, which may partly explain the predisposition to sepsis seen in cirrhotic patients. As blood is shunted around the liver and portal flow decreases, the efficiency of antigen clearance by the Kupffer cells is impaired. Not only is there increased susceptibility to sepsis but also antigen that may otherwise be sequestered by the liver is shunted into the systemic circulation where an exaggerated immune response may be generated. This action may explain the generalized increase in antibody levels seen in cirrhotic patients.

The Kupffer cells have many of the characteristics of macrophages, and like macrophages their functions are under the regulation of cytokines and other hormonal systems. For example, their function is downregulated after splenectomy or by gut decontaminations—sources of lymphocyte cytokines and gut endotoxin, respectively. Gamma interferon is the most important known regulatory interleukin for macrophages and Kupffer cells. Kupffer cells, like other macrophages, are sources of IL-1, IL-6, TNF, and PGE_2, especially after being activated by gamma interferon. Thus, Kupffer cells *receive* signals from the spleen, gut lymphoid tissue, and absorbed microbial products and send signals that regulate the metabolism of hepatocytes.

HEPATIC SECRETION

Bile consists of an electrolyte solution containing bile acids, lecithin, cholesterol, bile pigments (from tetrapyrrole), and protein. Bile has two components: the hepatocellular (bile salts, bile pigments, water, and a plasma filtrate of electrolytes) and ductal (watery fluid rich in bicarbonate). The hepatocellular compound is stimulated by cholecystokinin; the ductal component is stimulated by secretin.

Bile acids are synthesized by the hepatocyte from cholesterol and make up 90 per cent of the nonelectrolyte components of bile. Two to four polar groups are located on one surface of each steroid nucleus, with the remainder being nonpolar and insoluble in water. Cholic acid and chenodeoxycholic acid are the bile acids synthesized by the human liver. Conjugation with glycine or taurine is essential for hepatic excretion and ileal reabsorption of bile salts. The conjugated bile acids are generally excreted as salts. Once in the gut, bile salts participate in the formation of micelles required for the absorption of fatty acids, fat-soluble vitamins, and other lipid-soluble substances. After fat absorption, the conjugated bile acids are reabsorbed and cleared by the liver for excretion. This enterohepatic circulation of bile salts allows the entire pool of 3 to 4 grams to be recycled six to ten times each day while only about 100 mg is lost in the stool in each cycle. About 20 per cent of the total bile acid pool is lost in the stool daily. If bile salts are deconjugated by intestinal bacteria or ileal function is poor or absent, reabsorption of bile salts is impaired, so that larger quantities are lost and must be replaced by hepatic synthesis. When hepatocyte function is poor, uptake of bile salts from the portal blood is reduced, blood levels are increased, and less bile salts are available for excretion into the intestine. Postprandial blood bile salt levels are a sensitive test for hepatocyte dysfunction.

Bile acids have a cholesterol nucleus. The primary bile acids are cholic acid and chenodeoxycholic acids, which are more soluble than cholesterol by virtue of their added hydroxyl and carboxyl groups. Secondary bile acids (deoxycholic acid and lithocholic acid) are formed by gut bacteria after which they are absorbed and secreted from the liver as part of the enterohepatic circulation. Both types are normally secreted as conjugates of taurine and glycine, which are even more soluble and therefore primarily exist as salts with cations (mostly Na^+).

Bile acids and salts owe their fat-emulsifying function to their amphipathic structure in which the cholesterol nucleus and the hyperphilic domains are on opposite sides of the molecule. Therefore, at concentrations above a critical level (critical micelle concentration), bile acids will go into micelles exclusively—not into solution. Bile concentrations greatly exceed the critical micelle concentration.

Cholesterol and lecithin comprise the remaining 10 per cent of the nonelectrolytes in the bile. Lecithin is amphipathic as are bile salts, can participate in the formation of micelles in the gut, and can increase the amount of cholesterol in micelles. Cholesterol is essentially insoluble in water and precipitates and crystallizes in the bile whenever a critical concentration is exceeded. In normal persons, such conditions may occur occasionally throughout a typical day, but in those who form cholesterol gallstones, such an abnormal condition may persist for many hours during the day and allow the growth of stones.

Bile excretion begins with the bile canaliculus situated between adjacent hepatocytes (Fig. 14–3). Bile salts are excreted here, as are many organic compounds and electrolytes. Water passively follows these compounds into the canaliculus. Bile flow is primarily dependent upon bile salt excretion and is modified by the action of the bile ducts that can actively excrete into or remove fluid and electrolyte from the bile. Further modification occurs within the gallbladder where more fluid and electrolyte are removed.

In addition to bile salts, a wide variety of other substances are excreted into bile. Bilirubin and urobilinogen are byproducts of heme metabolism that are excreted in bile and produce the characteristic bile color. Numerous antibiotics are excreted in the bile, including penicillins, cephalosporins, tetracycline, and streptomycin. Adrenal and sex steroids are also excreted in the bile. Many of the substances excreted in the bile are reabsorbed in the small bowel and undergo enterohepatic circulation. When hepatocellular function is impaired, extraction of these substances from portal blood is poor, and they may appear in increased amounts in the peripheral blood or in the urine; for example, urobilinogen. In addition, several substances of diagnostic interest are excreted in the bile, including HIDA, PIPIDA, and indocyanine green.

COAGULATION

Coagulation factors I, VII, IX, and X are synthesized primarily in the liver and are dependent upon vitamin K for their synthesis. Of these, only fibrinogen (factor I) is synthesized exclusively in the liver. Factors V, IX, and XIII are synthesized in the liver, as well as in other tissues, and are not dependent upon hepatic function for the maintenance of adequate levels. In a deficiency state, the prothrombin time is most sensitive to liver dysfunction. When replacing coagulation factors with fresh-frozen plasma (FFP), one should bear in mind that factor VII has the shortest half-life at 5 hours. Other factors persist longer, with a half life of 1 to 5 days. Because of the short half-life of factor VII and the large volume of plasma required to provide adequate levels of coagulation factors (approximately 20 per cent of the normal level), bolus infusion is preferred to continuous infusion of FFP to prevent bleeding in patients with hepatic insufficiency.

In cholestatic disorders, hepatocellular function can be normal while bile production or excretion is defective. The resulting fat malabsorption can impair the absorption of vitamin K and result in coagulopathy. This defect appears similar to hepatocellular dysfunction on standard clinical tests (PT and PTT), but responds rapidly to administration of vitamin K.

The liver also participates in the regulation of coagulation both by degrading plasminogen activator and by prompt inactivation of clotting factors once the cascade is initiated. For this reason, in patients with hepatic insufficiency, coagulation, once initiated, may persist and result in disseminated intravascular coagulation. This consumption of coagulation factors may exacerbate synthetic deficiency. The presence of fibrin split products in the serum may suggest a substantial contribution of persistent inappropriate coagulation to the coagulopathy.

The serum levels of glycosyl transferases, including sialotransferase, are increased in patients with hepatocellular disease. Hence, fibrin monomers in patients with liver disease may have increased the net negative charge on the molecule and may inhibit polymerization of fibrin. Whether this chemical abnormality contributes to abnormal coagulation in liver disease is unknown.

PATHOPHYSIOLOGY OF PORTAL HYPERTENSION

A variety of disorders may produce elevated pressure within the portal venous system or in an isolated segment thereof. The site of obstruction may be prehepatic, intrahepatic, or posthepatic. Although this classification is anatomically simple, the functional disturbances found in portal hypertension are more dependent upon the site of obstruction to flow relative to the hepatic sinusoid. The sinusoid is the site of molecular exchange within the liver and thus is the crucial point at which hepatocellular function and fluid exchange can be disturbed by alterations in hemodynamics. Portal hypertension can be subdivided on this basis into presinusoidal, sinusoidal, and postsinusoidal. Many hepatic diseases produce obstruction to blood flow at more than one site.

Hypertension within the splanchnic venous bed encourages the development and dilation of collateral venous pathways. The resulting varices may become the site of brisk bleeding, particularly in the esophagus and gastric cardia. Such bleeding is exacerbated by coagulopathy that may result from hepatocellular dysfunction. These collateral pathways may also allow substances that would normally be cleared by the liver to escape into the systemic circulation. Again, hepatocellular dysfunction may exacerbate such shunting by reducing the rate of clearance from the systemic circulation. This shunting may play a role in many of the disturbances resulting from cirrhosis, including encephalopathy, coagulopathy, and immune dysfunciton; these are discussed elsewhere in this chapter.

In addition to hemorrhage, venous hypertension in the splanchnic bed can result in splenic enlargment and hematologic derangements of hypersplenism. Abnormal pooling of blood within the spleen produces alterations in splenic architecture and decreased survival of circulating elements. Generally, there is a reduction in leukocytes, erythrocytes and platelets, but no severe hematologic disor-

der. If, however, there are other factors operative, such as vitamin deficiency or rapid loss of cellular elements by hemorrhage, hematologic deficiency may become severe.

The most common cause of portal hypertension in adults is intrahepatic obstruction resulting from cirrhosis. The obstruction to venous flow is both sinusoidal and postsinusoidal and can produce both variceal hemorrhage and ascites, depending upon the relative contribution of sinusoidal and postsinusoidal obstruction. The physiology of this disorder is quite different from portal vein thrombosis, which produces about 50 per cent of cases of portal hypertension in the pediatric population. In that condition, sinusoidal pressure is normal, and hepatocellular function is well preserved. Consequently, ascites is rare, and portal shunting and varices are the predominant findings. Even more localized portal venous hypertension can be seen with splenic vein thrombosis wherein only part of the splanchnic venous system is exposed to elevated pressure. In that condition, esophageal varices and hypersplenism are common without other symptoms. Simple posthepatic obstruction, such as is seen with Budd-Chiari syndrome, results in marked hepatomegaly, ascites, and the sequelae of splanchnic venous hypertension.

ASCITES

In most cases of cirrhosis one locus of increased resistance to blood flow is at the hepatic veins and venules. The resulting hepatic outflow block produces hypertension throughout the portal system. Ascites is a common result of increased hydrostatic pressure at the hepatic sinusoid. The sinusoid is nearly completely permeable to protein. As a result, the protein content of interstitial fluid is 95 per cent that of sinusoidal plasma. Therefore, the hydrostatic pressure gradient alone determines the flow of fluid across the sinusoidal membrane and into the space of Disse. Small increments in sinusoidal pressure produce large increases in trans-sinusoidal flow and hepatic lymph production. The capacity of the hepatic lymphatic system to return fluid to the vascular system is considerable and may be as high as 20 L/day. When this capacity is exceeded by lymph production, the fluid will escape into the peritoneal cavity. The accumulation of fluid will continue until the pressure transmitted from the abdominal cavity to the hepatic interstitium reduces the flow of lymph to match the capacity for removal.

In contrast, many mechanisms work to reduce the flow of fluid across the intestinal capillary bed in the presence of portal hypertension. Only about 60 per cent of increased portal pressure is transmitted to the intestinal capillary bed. At the same time, capillary permeability decreases. In addition, increases in interstitial fluid increase interstitial hydrostatic pressure, which opposes the further transudation of fluid. Ascites is not a common finding in patients with extrahepatic portal hypertension, in which only the intestinal capillary bed is exposed to elevated hydrostatic pressure.

HEPATORENAL SYNDROME

Renal dysfunction is common in hepatic failure, and there are many potential causes in the patient with a failing liver. Hepatorenal syndrome (HRS) represents only a subset of these cases. It is characterized by progressive azotemia associated with oliguria, urine that is essentially free of sodium, and an unremarkable urinary sediment. Moderate or tense ascites and some degree of encephalopathy are present in nearly all patients with HRS. The azotemia and oliguria of HRS are functional in nature. This is demonstrated by the rapid return of function in kidneys transplanted from a donor with HRS into a recipient without liver disease or when a patient with HRS receives a functioning liver transplant. Antemortem arteriography demonstrates severe spasms of the renal vessels and redistribution of blood flow away from the cortex. These changes appear in the postmortem state.

Aberrations in the neurohumoral system, possibly in response to decreased effective circulating volume, may produce the redistribution of blood flow seen in HRS. These derangements include increased sympathetic tone as a consequence of hypotension resulting from peripheral vasodilation, and increased renin and angiotensin activity. Endotoxin, also a potent renal vasoconstrictor, is shunted into the systemic circulation in portal hypertension and may contribute to abnormal renal blood flow. Alterations in the production of prostaglandins in renal parenchyma probably also play a significant role in HRS. Drugs inhibiting the production of prostaglandins, such as nonsteroidal anti-inflammatory drugs, may induce renal failure in patients with hepatic insufficiency by altering the balance of vasodilatory and vasoconstrictive prostaglandins produced in the kidney.

The clinical picture in HRS of marked sodium retention and oliguria closely parallels that seen in prerenal azotemia. In addition, contraction of effective circulating volume as seen with vigorous diuresis, bleeding, or sepsis often precedes the onset of HRS. The differentiation of HRS from prerenal azotemia or acute tubular necrosis depends on the demonstration of functioning tubules (UNA less than 10), "adequate" intravascular volume, failure to respond to fluid loading. Clear differentiation may be difficult, and a mixture of disorders may be seen. Furthermore, those factors that are reported to precipitate HRS typically involve manipulation of the intravascular volume in an effort to treat ascites or edema. Alternatively, HRS may be precipitated by disorders producing decreased effective circulating volume, such as sepsis or bleeding.

Recovery of function in true HRS is quite unusual, and therapeutic efforts should be directed toward treatment of other causes of renal failure that may be present simultaneously. If other causes are excluded, treatment of the renal failure and attendant complications is all that is possible. Paracentesis or peritoneovenous shunting to reduce intraabdominal pressure and low-dose dopamine are unproven therapeutic maneuvers intended to improve renal function in HRS. Dialysis will provide temporary support during renal failure. Hepatic transplantation is curative.

THE GALLBLADDER AND BILIARY TREE

Most bile secreted by the liver passes into the gallbladder because the tone of the sphincter of Oddi is so high. The gallbladder has an average capacity of 35 mL and, to hold the secretion of bile by the liver, concentrates hepatic bile 5 to 20 times by means of active transport of sodium. Chloride, bicarbonate, water, and K^+ follow passively along the osmotic and electrochemical gradient.

The gallbladder empties into the duodenum soon after food is ingested. Cholinergic fibers of the vagal nerve both induce gallbladder contraction and relaxation of the sphincter during this cephalic and gastric phase. When fat or essential amino acids reach the duodenum, cholecystokinin is released from the duodenal mucosa and induces gallbladder contraction and sphincter relaxation. Gastrin is a much weaker cholecystagogue. Vasoactive intestinal polypeptide (VIP) inhibits gallbladder contraction, and VIP-containing nerve fibers are present in the gallbladder wall.

The normal pressure within the biliary system is less than 10 cm of H_2O. Elevated pressures within the bile ducts, as seen in obstruction from stones or tumor, can result in hepaticovenous reflux of bile. Obstruction and subsequent infection with bacteria are prerequisites for the development of ascending cholangitis. At pressures greater than 20 cm H_2O, bacteria escape into the lymphatics, whereas at pressures exceeding 25 cm, bacteria easily escape into the blood. Pressures above 37 cm H_2O exceed the secretory capacity of the hepatocytes, and bacteria are forced into the liver parenchyma. Studies in humans have shown that intraductal pressures greater than 30 cm H_2O are associated with cholangitis.

BIBLIOGRAPHY

1. Rappaport, A.M.: Physioanatomic considerations. *In* Schiff, L., and Schiff, E.R. (eds): Diseases of the Liver, 6th ed. Philadelphia, J.B. Lippincott Co., 1987, pp. 1–46.
2. Popper, H., and Shaffner, F. (eds.): Progress in Liver Disease. Philadelphia, W.B. Saunders Co., 1990.
3. Heinrich, P.C., Castell, J.V., and Andus, T.: Interleukin-6 and the acute phase response. Biochem. J., *265*:621–636, 1990.
4. Corless, J.K., and Middleton, H.M.: Normal liver function: A basis for understanding hepatic disease. Arch. Intern. Med., *143*:2291–2294, 1983.

15

PHYSIOLOGY OF THE EXOCRINE PANCREAS

KENNETH K.W. LEE *and* SAMUEL J. DURHAM

The pancreas is a small organ, weighing approximately 5 gm in the newborn, 85 gm in adult females, and 100 gm in adult males. Despite its small size, it has great clinical significance both in sickness and in health. Under normal circumstances the pancreas has important exocrine functions that aid in the digestion of food and important endocrine functions that aid in glucose and cellular metabolism. In sickness, the pancreas may be affected by acute and chronic inflammatory processes, or undergo neoplastic changes that are often incurable.

EMBRYOLOGY AND HISTOLOGY

The pancreas appears during the fifth week of gestation as endodermal dorsal and ventral evaginations of the developing gut tube at the level of the liver. Both anlage contain central ducts; the dorsal duct communicates directly with the duodenum, whereas the ventral duct is variably related to the common bile duct. At about 7 weeks of gestation, asymmetric growth of the gut rotates the ventral anlage and places it in apposition with the dorsal anlage. The two components fuse, giving rise to the mature form of the gland with its characteristic relationship to the second portion of the duodenum (Fig. 15–1). The dorsal anlage, having grown more rapidly than the ventral anlage, becomes the tail, the body, and a portion of the head of the pancreas, while the ventral anlage becomes the uncinate process and the remainder of the pancreatic head. Attachment of the ventral pancreas to the duodenum prior to rotation may result in an extramural constricting band of pancreatic tissue. This condition, known as annular pancreas, presents as duodenal obstruction early in life and requires surgical correction. An intramural constricting ring of pan-

creatic tissue may also occur and is hypothesized to result from abnormal differentiation of the gut.

The dorsal and ventral ductal elements undergo fusion and produce the main pancreatic duct of Wirsung. In approximately 70 per cent of cases the dorsal duct remains patent beyond the site of ductal fusion, forming the accessory duct of Santorini. This accessory duct may itself fuse with the main pancreatic duct or may enter into the duodenum separately through an accessory pancreatic papilla. In 5 to 10 per cent of cases the dorsal and ventral ducts fail to fuse, producing a condition referred to as pancreas divisum. In this instance, drainage of the dorsal and ventral portions of the pancreas remains separate, and most of the pancreatic exocrine secretion drains via the accessory papilla and the accessory duct (Fig. 15–2). The significance of this variation in pancreatic ductal anatomy remains uncertain. The relatively small size of the accessory duct and papilla in comparison to the duct of Wirsung and the main papilla has led to the suggestion that pancreas divisum predisposes to inadequate drainage of the dorsal pancreas, and that this in turn predisposes to the development of pancreatitis.

The enzyme-secreting unit of the exocrine pancreas, the acinus, is detectable by 12 to 14 weeks of gestation. The acini consist of spherical or tubular clusters of cells that are the terminal elements of a branching network of ductules or are situated along the course of the ductules, and they comprise approximately 80 per cent of the pancreatic mass. The acinar cells are tall pyramidal or columnar cells that rest upon a basal lamina with their apices oriented toward the ductal lumen. The location of their cellular organelles exhibits polarity that reflects the synthetic and secretory function of these cells. Close to the basal lamina, abundant rough endoplasmic reticulum is found. The Golgi complex is situated more centrally, and near the luminal aspect of the cells are

257

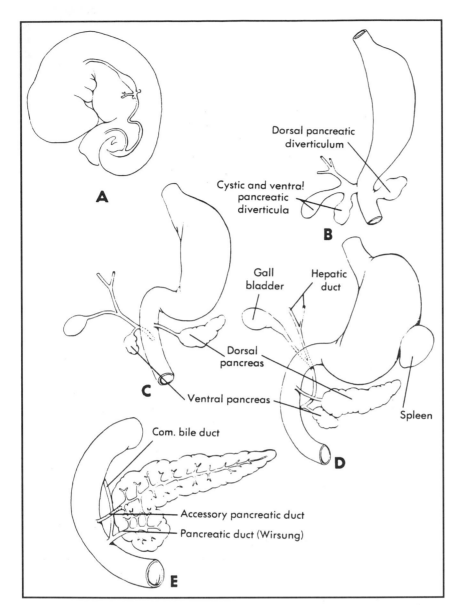

FIGURE 15–1. Embryologic development of the pancreas demonstrating rotation and fusion of dorsal and ventral anlage. *A:* 30 days; *B:* 30 days; *C:* 33 days; *D:* 36 days; *E:* Definitive (mature) relationships. (Reprinted from Gray, S.W., and Skandalakis, J.E.: Embryology for Surgeons. The Embryological Basis for the Treatment of Congenital Defects. Philadelphia, W.B. Saunders Co., 1972, p. 264.)

found two forms of secretory granules, condensing vacuoles and zymogen granules. Analysis of the content of both forms of secretory granules indicates that they contain the full array of secreted enzymes, although the relative amounts of each enzyme present may vary from granule to granule.

In the fasted state, zymogen granules may occupy as much as 20 per cent of the intracellular volume. In response to appropriate stimuli, zymogen granules are discharged into the ductal lumen and the acinar cells may become entirely depleted of these granules. Release of the granules occurs through the process of exocytosis, in which the zymogen granule membrane fuses with the apical membrane of the cell. This process is not fully understood; however, abundant contractile proteins are found near the zymogen granules in the apices of the acinar cells and may have a role in exocytosis.

Adjacent acinar cells are tightly bound to one another by means of specialized junctions. These junctions prevent entrance of secreted enzymes into the intracellular space. Lining the acini and interdigitated between the acinar cells are the centroacinar cells, which constitute the initial portion of the intralobular ductal system. The intercalated ducts lead outward from the acini to the intralobular ducts. These in turn lead to the interlobular ducts, which course together with nerves and blood vessels and finally drain into the main pancreatic ducts. Together the ductal elements comprise approximately 4 per cent of the pancreatic mass.

In contrast to the acinar cells, the centroacinar cells and the cells of the intercalated and intralobular ducts do not display highly developed synthetic and secretory apparatuses. Rough endoplasmic reticulum is rare, and condensing vacuoles and zymogen

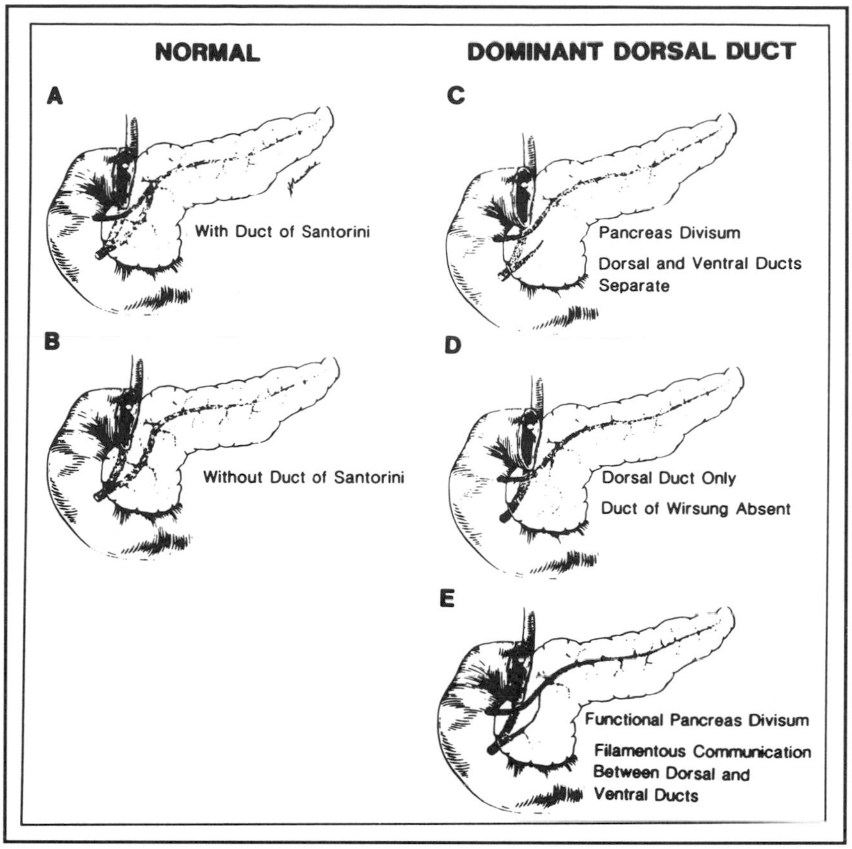

FIGURE 15–2. Variations in pancreatic ductal anatomy. Abnormal fusion of the dorsal and ventral ducts may result in drainage of the bulk of the pancreas via the dorsal duct and accessory papilla. (Reprinted from Warshaw, A.L., Simeone, J.F., Schapiro, R.H., and Flavin-Warshaw, B.: Evaluation and treatment of the dominant dorsal duct syndrome (pancreas divisum redefined). Am. J. Surg. *159*:60, 1990.)

granules are absent. Carbonic anhydrase, the enzyme necessary for bicarbonate production, can be localized to these cells, reflecting their role in water and bicarbonate secretion. Secretory granules containing mucoproteins and a more prominent rough endoplasmic reticulum can be found, however, in the cells of the interlobular and main pancreatic ducts. The function of these mucoproteins is uncertain but is likely to be protective.

Interspersed among the lobules of acini are endocrine cells arranged in islets of Langerhans. In the human pancreas approximately 1 million islets are present, constituting approximately 2 per cent of the total pancreas. In contrast to acinar cells, which may synthesize multiple enzymes, individual cells within the islets appear to be dedicated to the production of a single hormone. Insulin-producing B cells are most abundant, comprising 50 to 80 per cent of the islet cell mass. Glucagon-producing A cells comprise 5 to 20 per cent of the islet cell mass and are more common in the dorsal pancreas, whereas pancreatic polypeptide-producing cells, comprising 10 to 35 per cent of the islet cell mass, are more common in the ventral pancreas. D cells produce somatostatin and comprise only 5 per cent of the islet cells.

In addition to their afferent arteriolar blood supply, acinar cells may also have a second blood supply that links them to nearby islet cells. Blood leaving the islets travels through a portal circulation that leads to adjacent acini. In this manner, the hormones synthesized and released by the islet cells may have local effects upon the exocrine pancreas in addition to their systemic effects.

EXOCRINE PANCREAS

Functions of the Exocrine Pancreas

The exocrine pancreas has two interrelated functions: secretion of bicarbonate-rich fluid, and synthesis and secretion of digestive enzymes.

Secretion of Bicarbonate-Rich Fluid

Chyme entering the intestine may have a pH in the 1 to 2 range, at which several pancreatic enzymes are denatured and inactivated and others are minimally active. Secretion of bicarbonate alkalinizes the chyme, helping to protect the duodenal mucosa from gastric acid while achieving a pH at which most pancreatic enzymes are optimally active and bile salt solubility is enhanced. The total volume of fluid secreted by the pancreas in a day is 1500 to 2000 ml. The synthetic capacity of the pancreas is enormous; in 24 hours, 6 to 20 gm of protein are secreted into pancreatic juice, of which approximately 90 per cent is composed of digestive enzymes produced by acinar cells. On a weight basis, therefore, the pancreas produces more protein than any other organ.

Micropuncture studies of the pancreatic ductal system and such treatments as a copper-free diet, which leads to atrophy of acinar tissue, have confirmed that centroacinar and intralobular duct cells produce a bicarbonate-rich aqueous fluid. This fluid is clear, colorless, and of low viscosity, and remains isotonic with plasma irrespective of its rate of flow. In normal individuals the maximum flow rate is 4 to 5 ml/minute, but this rate is reduced with parenchymal destruction or ductal obstruction. The concentrations of the principal anions, bicarbonate and chloride, vary reciprocally with each other and are flow dependent. At high flow rates the bicarbonate concentration is high, approaching 150 mEq/liter, and chloride concentration is low, whereas at low flow rates the opposite is true, with bicarbonate concentration falling as low as 30 mEq/liter. The principal cations, sodium and potassium, are present in concentrations similar to those of extracellular fluid and show no flow rate dependence.

Two processes give rise to the variations in bicarbonate and chloride concentration: mixing of fluid produced by acinar cells with fluid produced by ductal cells, and passive diffusion of bicarbonate across the duct epithelium in exchange for chloride (Fig. 15–3). Acinar cells, in addition to their secretion of digestive enzymes, also secrete fluid that has a plasmalike composition low in bicarbonate and high in chloride, whereas the fluid secreted by ductal cells has high bicarbonate and low chloride concentrations. Mixing of acinar fluid with ductal fluid is an important determinant of the final composition of pancreatic juice. Under conditions of high flow the relative contribution of ductal fluid is increased, resulting in a higher bicarbonate concentration, whereas at lower flow rates the relative contribution of acinar fluid is increased, resulting in a lower bicarbonate concentration.

The second flow-dependent process influencing the anion composition of pancreatic juice is the diffusion of bicarbonate and chloride along their electrochemical gradients, the net result of which is exchange of intraductal bicarbonate for intracellular chloride. Low flow rates allow for more complete equilibration and greater diffusion, giving rise to lower bicarbonate and higher chloride concentrations. At high flow rates anion exchange is limited and a higher concentration of bicarbonate is maintained.

Secretion of bicarbonate by ductal cells occurs against the electrochemical gradient of bicarbonate and is therefore energy requiring. The mechanism of secretion is not known, but may involve either active forward (cell to duct lumen) transport of bicarbonate, or active backward (cell to interstitium) transport of protons. In one proposed model, car-

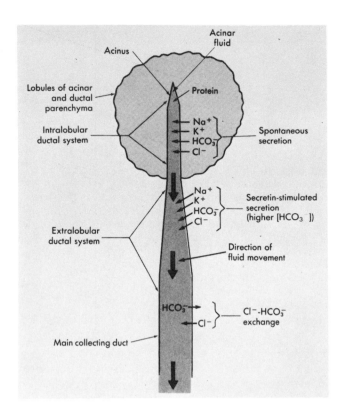

FIGURE 15–3. The electrolyte composition of pancreatic juice is dependent upon acinar and ductal cell secretion, and exchange of bicarbonate and chloride across the ductal epithelium. (Redrawn from Swanson, C.H., and Solomon, A.K.: A micropuncture investigation of the whole tissue mechanism of electrolyte secretion by the in vitro rabbit pancreas. J. Gen. Physiol. *62*:26, 1973.)

bon dioxide diffuses into the duct lumen and is hydrated to form carbonic acid (H_2CO_3), which dissociates to yield H^+ and HCO_3^- (Fig. 15–4). The proton is transported actively into the cell by means of a Na^+/H^+ adenosine triphosphatase (ATPase) pump located at the luminal membrane. The resulting sodium concentration gradient drives a second Na^+/H^+ pump that then transports the proton into the interstitium. In a second proposed model, intracellular carbon dioxide undergoes hydration and dissociation, yielding H^+ and HCO_3^-. Bicarbonate enters the duct lumen along its resulting electrochemical gradient, while the proton is actively transported across the basolateral membrane by means of coupled Na^+/H^+ and Na^+/K^+-ATPase pumps. A third model proposes that HCO_3^- is actively transported into the cell at the basolateral membrane and then enters the duct along its electrochemical gradient. In each of these models, water follows along the osmotic gradient established by the secreted solute, thereby maintaining the isotonicity of ductal fluid.

Synthesis and Secretion of Digestive Enzymes

Synthesis and secretion of digestive enzymes is the second important function of the exocrine pancreas.

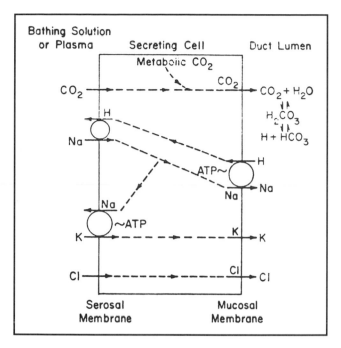

FIGURE 15–4. Proposed mechanism of bicarbonate secretion. Bicarbonate is formed intraluminally by dissociation of carbonic acid into bicarbonate and H^+. The proton is discharged into the interstitium by Na^+/H^+-ATPase and Na^+/H^+ pumps situated at the luminal and basolateral membranes, respectively. (Reprinted from Swanson, C.H., and Solomon, A.K.: Micropuncture analysis of the cellular mechanisms of electrolyte secretion by the in vitro rabbit pancreas. J. Gen. Physiol. *65*:22, 1975, p. 32.)

A number of enzymes have been isolated and identified in human pancreatic juice (Table 15–1). Several of these are proteases active in the digestion of proteins and peptides, reducing them to oligopeptides and amino acids that can be directly transported by enterocytes or further digested by brush border enzymes. Trypsin, chymotrypsin, and elastase each act upon internal peptide bonds and are therefore classified as *endo*peptidases. These enzymes share some homology and have at their active sites a serine residue that undergoes successive acylation and deacylation, and that can be blocked by binding of diisopropylfluorophosphate. The substrate specificity of each enzyme is determined by the presence of additional bonding groups at the catalytic site.

Trypsin (precursor trypsinogen) hydrolyzes arginine and lysine peptide bonds. Present at the catalytic site of trypsin is a negatively charged aspartyl group to which the positive charges of arginine and lysine bind. The enzyme occurs in anionic and cationic forms that have molecular weights of approximately 25,000, and like other pancreatic enzymes acts optimally in a slightly alkaline (pH 7.5 to 8.5) environment.

Chymotrypsin (precursor chymotrypsinogen) occurs in two variants, Λ and B, weighing 24,000 and 27,000 daltons, respectively. Lining the catalytic site of chymotrypsin are hydrophobic residues that interact preferentially with hydrophobic substrates such as the aromatic amino acids phenylalanine, tryptophan, and tyrosine, and to a lesser extent leucine and methionine. Hydrophilic residues such as glutamine, glutamate, aspartate, asparagine, arginine, and lysine are excluded from the catalytic site. Elastase (precursor pro-elastase), named for its ability to hydrolyze the protein elastin, also occurs in two variants, elastase 1 and 2, weighing 29,300 and 25,000, respectively. The catalytic site of these enzymes contains valine and threonine residues at its entrance. These are hypothesized to limit access to the catalytic site to smaller amino acids such as serine, glycine, and alanine.

Carboxypeptidase A and B (precursor procarboxypeptidase A and B) are *exo*peptidases that cleave the carboxy-terminal amino acid from peptide chains. Unlike the serine proteases, these enzymes contain a zinc atom at their active sites. Carboxypeptidase A acts upon neutral and aromatic carboxy-terminal amino acids (phenylalanine, tyramine, tryptophan) whereas carboxypeptidase B acts upon arginine and lysine carboxy-terminal amino acids.

Several enzymes active in the digestion of lipids are synthesized by acinar cells and secreted into pancreatic juice. Lipase, a 48,000-dalton glycoprotein, is active in the digestion of triglycerides. Through its action, the ester linkages at carbons 1 (C1) and 3 (C3) are hydrolyzed, yielding two fatty acid molecules and one β-monoglyceride. Because lipase is water soluble and its substrate is water insoluble, lipase activity is limited to the interface between the fat and water phases and requires satisfactory adsorption of lipase to the substrate surface. Bile salts form micelles with the products of triglyceride digestion and thereby facilitate their diffusion to the brush border, but interfere with the adsorption of lipase to triglyceride droplets and thereby inhibit its activity. This inhibition is overcome by colipase, a small protein (9900) that is also synthesized by the pancreas and secreted in pancreatic juice and acts as a cofactor for lipase. Colipase is believed to complex with bile salts and lipase and to promote adherence of lipase to triglyceride droplets, thereby permitting its digestive action.

An additional carboxyl esterase with less substrate specificity than lipase has also been isolated from pancreatic juice. This enzyme is active upon both water-soluble and water-insoluble substrates and has its activity enhanced by bile salts. It may be active in the metabolism of cholesterol esters.

The pancreas also synthesizes and secretes an A_2 type of phospholipase that hydrolyzes phospholipids, an important component of cell membranes. Pancreatic phospholipase A_2 (precursor prophospholipase A_2) weighs about 14,000 and requires cal-

TABLE 15–1. PANCREATIC ENZYMES AND ZYMOGENS

Enzyme, Zymogen	Function of Enzyme	Molecular Weight	pH Optimum	pI	Carbohydrate
EC 3.4.21.4	Hydrolysis of proteins; Arg and Lys peptide bonds	Zymogens		Zymogens	
Trypsin(ogen) 1 Anionic		25,006	7.5–8.5	4.7	–
Trypsin(ogen) 2 Mesotrypsin		25,000	8.25	5.95	
Trypsin(ogen) 3 Cationic		23,438	7.5–8.5	6.6	–
EC 3.4.21.1	Hydrolysis of proteins; Phe, Tyr, Trp peptide bonds	Zymogens		Zymogen	
Chymotrypsin(ogen) A		24,000	8	7.2	–
Chymotrypsin(ogen) B		27,000	8	7.2	–
EC 3.4.21.11	Cleavage of peptide bonds adjacent to aliphatic amino acids (elastin)	Enzymes		Zymogens	
(Pro)elastase 1 (Pancreatopeptidase E)		29,300	7.5–10.5	7.6	
(Pro)elastase 2		25,000	7.5–10.5	9.5	
Kallikrein(ogen)	Cleavage of kininogen to active kinin	Enzyme 35,000	8	Enzyme 3.9–4.1	+
EC 3.4.17.1	Cleavage of carboxyl-terminal Phe, Tyr, and Trp residues	Zymogen		Zymogens	
(Pro)carboxypeptidase A1		46–47,000	7.5–8	6.22–6.72	–
A2		Enzyme 34,000	7.5–8	4.6–4.7	
B1	Cleavage of carboxyl-terminal Arg, Lys residues	Zymogen 47,000		Zymogens 6.2	–
B2		Enzyme 34,000	7.65	6.7	–
EC 3.1.1.4	Hydrolysis of fatty acid esters at 2-position of 1,2-diacylglycerophosphocholines	Zymogen 14,000		Zymogen 7.5	–
(Pro)phospholipase A_2 (Phosphatide 2-acylhydrolase)		Enzyme ~14,000	6	Enzyme 8.7	–
EC 3.1.1.3 Lipase Triacylglycerol acylhydrolase	Hydrolysis of C_1 and C_3 glycerol ester bonds	48,000	8–9	5.8	+
Colipase I and II	Cofactor for lipase	9,900	—	6.1 / 5.8	+
EC 3.1.27.5 RNase	Hydrolysis of phosphate ester bonds in RNA	15,000	8.2	7.25–7.82	+ / –
DNase I	Hydrolysis of phosphate ester bonds in DNA	33–38,000	7–7.5	3.9–4.3 / 4.79–4.86	–
EC 3.1.1.1 Nonspecific carboxylesterase (Carboxyl ester hydrolase)	Hydrolysis of water-soluble and insoluble esters	54,000 / 100,000	7.4 / 8	4.65	+
EC 3.2.1.1 Amylase (α-1,4-glucan-4-glucanohydrolase)	Hydrolysis of α-1,4-glycosidic bonds in starches	50,000	7.5–8	7.1 / 6.5	+

Reprinted from Rinderknecht, H: Pancreatic secretory enzymes. *In* Go, V.L.W., Brooks, F.P., DiMagno, E.P., Gardner, J.D., Lebenthal, E., and Scheele, G.A.: The Exocrine Pancreas. Biology, Pathobiology, and diseases. New York, Raven Press, 1986, p. 164.

cium ion for activity. It hydrolyzes the C2 ester bond of phosphatidylcholines (lecithins), producing a fatty acid and a lysophosphatidylcholine. Lysophosphatidylcholines possess strong detergent properties that can disrupt cell membranes. The pancreas additionally secretes a lysophospholipase that hydrolyzes the remaining acyl group from lysophosphatidates.

Starch comprises more than half of the carbohydrate ingested by humans and occurs in two forms. Amylose is the unbranched form of starch and consists of glucose residues linked together by α-1,4-glycosidic bonds. Amylopectin is the branched form of starch and differs from amylose by the additional presence of α-1,6-glycosidic bonds. Both forms of starch are hydrolyzed by amylase, a glycoprotein synthesized by the pancreas and having a molecular weight between 50,000 and 56,000. Amylase, like phospholipase A_2, requires calcium ions for its activity. It hydrolyzes internal α-1,4-glycosidic linkages to produce maltose (two glucose residues), maltotriose (three glucose residues), and α-dextrins (short branched polysaccharides). Maltose and maltotriose are further hydrolyzed by the intestinal brush border enzyme maltase, while α-dextrins are hydrolyzed by α-dextrinase. Amylase, together with lipase, has found further clinical usefulness as an indicator of pancreatic inflammation and injury.

Other enzymes identified in pancreatic juice include ribonuclease and deoxyribonuclease, which hydrolyze phosphate ester bonds in RNA and DNA, respectively, and kallikrein, which activates kinins.

Inappropriate activation of pancreatic enzymes

may lead to injury of the pancreas and indeed has been postulated as an important factor in the pathogenesis of pancreatitis. Several mechanisms exist to prevent this problem, of which the most important is synthesis of proteases and phospholipase A_2 in inactive precursor forms. Under normal circumstances none of these enzymes can be isolated in active form from within the pancreatic ductal system. Activation occurs within the intestine and requires hydrolysis of a peptide bond by trypsin (Fig. 15–5), which is itself activated by two mechanisms. Release of the amino-terminal octapeptide, Ala-Pro-Phe-$(Asp)_4$-Lys-, converts trypsinogen, the precursor form of trypsin, to active trypsin. Trypsin itself undergoes activation by two mechanism. Trypsinogen may undergo activation at a low rate by spontaneous release of its amino-terminal octapeptide. Because the specificity of trypsin is for lysine or arginine peptide linkages, the active enzyme can then catalyze further conversion of trypsinogen to trypsin. The enzyme's activity, however, is not specific for the amino-terminal octapeptide bond, and the enzyme may concurrently digest trypsinogen molecules. The balance between activation and digestion is determined by the pH and calcium level. At higher pH (8) and low calcium levels (less than 1 mM), as are found in the pancreatic duct, digestion of trypsinogen by trypsin is favored, whereas at lower pH (6) and calcium levels greater than 1 mM, as are found in the duodenum, activation of trypsinogen is favored. The second and predominant mechanism of trypsinogen activation occurs in the duodenum and involves the enzyme

enterokinase. Enterokinase is present in duodenal mucosa and fluid and has specific activity for the amino-terminal oligopeptide of trypsinogen (Fig. 15–6). Enterokinase is six times more powerful and 2000 times faster than trypsin in its ability to activate trypsinogen.

Inhibitors of trypsin also prevent inappropriate activation of pancreatic enzymes. The pancreas synthesizes and secretes a polypeptide containing a -Lys-Ile- site that bonds covalently with the active site of trypsin to produce a stable, enzymatically inactive complex. This bonding is reversible, resulting in recovery of enzyme function. Other protease inhibitors such as α_1-antitrypsin and α_2-macroglobulin limit the destructive potential of the small quantities of pancreatic proteases normally released into the general circulation.

Regulation of Pancreatic Secretion

Pancreatic secretion of bicarbonate and enzymes is subject to hormonal control. Indeed, the action of a circulating mediator, or hormone, was first proposed by Bayliss and Starling in 1902 to explain their observations that (1) pancreatic secretion could be stimulated by instillation of acid into the duodenum but not intravenously and (2) a substance extracted from the mucosa of the proximal small bowel could stimulate pancreatic secretion when administered intravenously. These observations led Bayliss and Starling

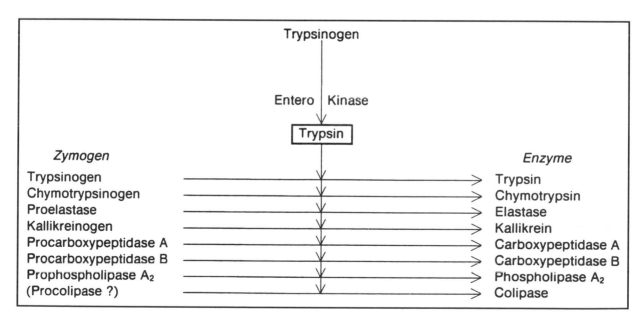

FIGURE 15–5. Activation of pancreatic enzymes results from the action of trypsin, which is itself activated by means of autoactivation or the action of enterokinase. (Reprinted from Rinderknecht, H.: Pancreatic secretory enzymes. *In* Brooks, F.P., DiMagno, E.P., Gardner, J.D., Lebenthal, E., and Scheele, G.A.: The Exocrine Pancreas: Biology, Pathobiology, and Disease. New York, Raven Press, 1986, p. 165.)

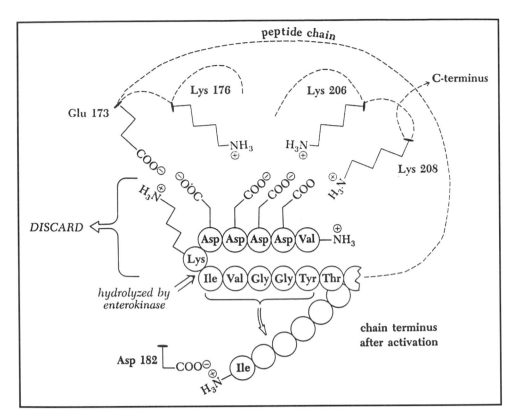

FIGURE 15–6. Cleavage of the amino (NH_3^+)-terminal oligopeptide of trypsinogen by enterokinase results in conformational changes and yields enzymatically active trypsin. (Reprinted from McGilvery, R.W., and Goldstein, G.W.: Biochemistry: A Functional Approach. Philadelphia, W.B. Saunders Co., 1983, p. 338.)

to postulate the existence of the circulating hormone secretin.

Secretin is a 27-amino acid peptide that is the most potent stimulus for pancreatic bicarbonate secretion, and a weak stimulus for pancreatic enzyme secretion. The principal stimulus for secretin release is the delivery of titratable acid into the duodenum with reduction of pH to 4 to 4.5. Recently, it has also been demonstrated that products of fat digestion stimulate secretin release independent of pH when placed into the proximal intestine. Extensive experimental and clinical data demonstrate that entry of acidic chyme into the proximal intestine stimulates release of secretin, that secretin stimulates pancreatic secretion of bicarbonate-rich fluid, and that the postprandial secretion of bicarbonate is at least in part attributable to increases in circulating secretin. In the fasting state secretin levels are very low. Intraduodenal infusion of acid or ingestion of a normal meal causes increases in serum secretin levels that correlate well with the secretion of bicarbonate (Fig. 15–7 and 15–8), whereas reduction in the amount of acid delivered to the intestine by means of gastric aspiration, type 2 histamine (H_2) receptor blockade, or administration of antacids reduces secretin release and bicarbonate secretion. Administration of exogenous secretin in doses that reproduce

postprandial serum levels stimulates bicarbonate secretion, and administration of antisecretin serum reduces bicarbonate output in dogs by about 80 per cent.

The second classic pancreatic hormone, cholecystokinin (CCK), was first described by Ivy and Goldberg in 1928 as a stimulator of gallbladder contraction and pancreatic protein secretion. In the gastrointestinal tract, CCK is found in the mucosa of the small intestine in concentrations that are greatest in the duodenum and gradually diminish toward the distal ileum. Several bioactive forms of CCK, all derived from post-translational cleavage of the precursor peptide preproCCK, have been identified; CCK-8 and CCK-33, however, are most important physiologically. Bioactivity of any of these peptides requires the amino-terminal octapeptide -Asp-Tyr(SO_3)-Met-Gly-Trp-Met-Asp-Phe-NH_2. Basal levels of CCK are low, but increase five- to tenfold following ingestion of a meal. Secretion of CCK is stimulated primarily by protein and fat, and to a lesser extent by acid. Breakdown products of fat and protein, such as free fatty acids, short peptides, and amino acids, which result from the action of pancreatic digestive enzymes, are particularly effective stimulators of CCK release. Recent evidence suggests that trypsin and possibly other pancreatic

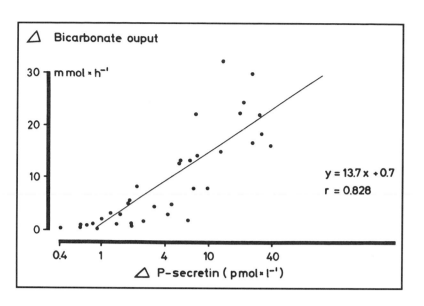

FIGURE 15-7. Increases in pancreatic bicarbonate secretion are correlated with changes in plasma secretin levels. (Reprinted from Schaffalitzky de Muckadell, O.B., Fahrenkrug, J., Watt-Boolsen, S., and Worning, H.: Pancreatic response and plasma secretin concentration during infusion of low dose secretin in man. Scand. J. Gastroenterol. *13*:309, 1978.)

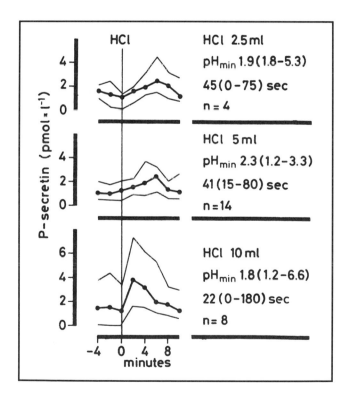

FIGURE 15-8. Concentration of secretin in plasma after an intraduodenal injection of 2.5, 5, or 10 ml of 0.1 molar HCl. The dose of acid, minimal intraduodenal pH, duration of pH spike, and number of injections are shown in the right panel. Medians and total range ($n=4$) or 95 per cent confidence limit of the median ($n=14$ and n = 8). (Reprinted from Schaffalitzky de Muckadell, O.B., Fahrenkrug, J., and Rune, S.J.: Physiological significance of secretin in the pancreatic bicarbonate secretion. Scand. J. Gastroenterol. *14*:82, 1979.)

proteases are important regulators of CCK release. A trypsin-sensitive peptide that stimulates CCK release has been identified in the proximal small intestine. In the presence of trypsin, this peptide is degraded and stimulation of CCK release is lost. Exogenous CCK given in doses sufficient to achieve postprandial levels results in pancreatic enzyme secretion. Further evidence for a physiologic role for CCK rests in the inhibition of postprandial pancreatic enzyme secretion following administration of anti-CCK serum.

The stimulatory action of secretin is potentiated by CCK. Bicarbonate secretion following simultaneous administration of secretin and CCK exceeds the response to either given separately and the sum of the separate responses (Fig. 15–9). Available evidence suggests that enzyme secretion following CCK administration is similarly augmented by secretin.

Several other hormones or peptides have been shown to influence pancreatic secretion, although their physiologic roles have not been confirmed. Gastrin shares amino-terminal homology with CCK and is a weak stimulus for pancreatic enzyme secretion. Vasoactive intestinal peptide (VIP) shares homology with secretin and stimulates water and bicarbonate secretion when given intravenously. VIP levels do not rise postprandially, however, and current evidence suggests a role for VIP as a neurotransmitter rather than a circulating mediator. Pancreotone, a polypeptide derived from ileal and colonic mucosa, inhibits secretin- and CCK-stimulated pancreatic secretion and may mediate the inhibition of pancreatic secretion that follows instillation of free fatty acids into the distal ileum.

Several islet cell products have also been shown to influence pancreatic exocrine function. This influence may be exerted via release into the general circulation (endocrine interaction), or via release

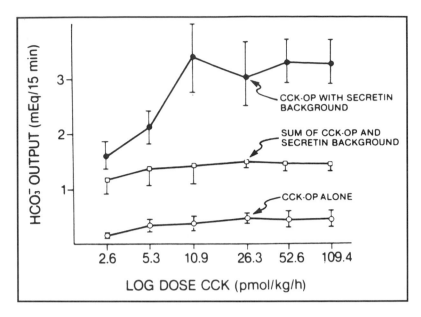

FIGURE 15–9. The pancreatic bicarbonate output in response to the graded log dose of cholecystokinin-octapeptide (CCK-OP) with or without secretin background in a dose of 0.03 CU/kg/hour (2.8 pmol/kg/hour). A *solid circle* represents the bicarbonate output produced by simultaneous infusion of secretin and varying doses of CCK-OP. An *open square* represents the calculated sum of bicarbonate output produced by two individual hormones. An *open circle* represents the bicarbonate output produced by varying doses of CCK-OP alone. Each point with vertical bar represents a mean ± SE of five subjects. (Reprinted from You, C.H., Rominger, J.M., and Chey, W.Y. Potentiation effect of cholecystokinin-octapeptide on pancreatic bicarbonate secretion stimulated by a physiologic dose of secretin in humans. Gastroenterology *85*:42, 1983.)

into the intrapancreatic portal circulation (paracrine interaction). Experimentally, insulin potentiates the action of CCK, whereas glucagon inhibits both CCK- and secretin-stimulated secretion. Pancreatic polypeptide is released in response to a meal, duodenal acidification, or CCK, secretin, or gastrin, and inhibits basal as well as stimulated bicarbonate and enzyme secretion. Somatostatin, produced by D cells, inhibits secretin release as well as the response of the pancreas to exogenous or endogenous hormones. These inhibitory properties have led to interest in the use of somatostatin analogues in the treatment of various pancreatic disease states.

Pancreatic exocrine function is also subject to neural regulation. Vagal stimulation, either direct or reflexively induced as with administration of insulin, increases enzyme and bicarbonate secretion and in some studies potentiates the action of hormones upon the pancreas. Muscarinic cholinergic agonists elicit a similar response and can be shown to bind to acinar receptors, resulting in enzyme secretion (see earlier discussion). The responses to vagal stimulation and cholinergic agonists can both be largely blocked by atropine. Vagotomy reduces basal secretion and the response to either intraduodenal infusions or meals, and may alter the response of the pancreas to secretory hormones.

The effects of vagal stimulation are, however, partially resistant to blockade by atropine, indicating that a noncholinergic mechanism is also active. Current evidence suggests that VIP may mediate the bicarbonate secretory response to vagal stimulation. VIP-containing nerves can be identified in the pancreas, and release of VIP from these nerves can be detected following vagal stimulation. Exogenous VIP stimulates pancreatic water and bicarbonate secretion, and the concentration of VIP in pancreatic venous effluent rises following vagal stimulation in

parallel with bicarbonate secretion. Further, the response to vagal stimulation can be inhibited by anti-VIP serum.

The mechanisms by which these secretagogues act upon the pancreas have been best studied for acinar cells. Binding of CCK, gastrin, bombesin, cerulein, and muscarinic cholinergic agonists to acinar cells activates phospholipase C, resulting in production of inositol triphosphate and diacylglycerol. Inositol triphosphate causes release of Ca^{2+} from intracellular stores and a rapid rise in intracellular Ca^{2+} concentrations. Intracellular Ca^{2+} binds to calmodulin and then activates various protein kinases necessary for synthesis and release of pancreatic exocrine enzymes. Diacylglycerol activates a separate protein kinase leading to synthesis and release of pancreatic enzymes.

Binding of secretin and related peptides such as VIP to acinar cells does not result in increased intracellular Ca^{2+}, but rather causes activation of adenylate cyclase and an increase in intracellular cyclic adenosine monophosphate (AMP). Cyclic AMP in turn activates a protein kinase distinct from the Ca^{2+}-activated protein kinases by binding to its regulatory subunit. Further intracellular events are not known. Little is known pertaining to the mechanism of hormone action upon pancreatic ductal cells, but current evidence suggests that the action of secretin upon these cells is also mediated through adenylate cyclase activation and elevation of cyclic AMP levels. The mechanism by which CCK acts upon ductal cells and potentiates the effects of secretin is unknown.

Digestion

Pancreatic secretion of enzymes, bicarbonate, and water occurs between meals, during the interdigestive period, as well as after meals, during the digestive period. Basal secretion of enzymes during the interdigestive period is 10 to 15 per cent of maximal levels achieved with CCK stimulation, and basal secretion of bicarbonate is 1 to 2 per cent of maximal levels achieved with secretin stimulation. Basal secretion is both intrinsic and acetylcholine dependent, since basal secretory activity is evident in the isolated perfused pancreas and is reduced by atropine. Cyclical changes in secretory activity are also observed during the interdigestive period; these changes correlate with motility and migrating motor complex activity. Four phases are defined: I—absence of motor activity; II—irregular increasing contractions; III—regular contractions; and IV—irregular contractions leading to inactivity. Pancreatic secretion is not detected during phase I, but gradually increases during phase II and reaches peak interdigestive levels shortly before the onset of phase III. During phases III and IV secretory activity decreases until phase I quiescence is reached. Enzyme secretion is maximal during the late phase II, whereas peak bicarbonate secretion occurs at the start of phase III.

The postprandial response of the exocrine pancreas is conveniently divided into three phases: cephalic, gastric, and intestinal. The cephalic phase of pancreatic secretion results from the sight or smell of appetizing food, and can be provoked by sham feeding. When acid is prevented from entering the duodenum, enzyme secretion increases to approximately 50 per cent of maximum with little accompanying increase in bicarbonate output. Allowing acid to enter the duodenum increases enzyme secretion to 90 per cent of maximum and stimulates bicarbonate secretion. Circulating CCK cannot be detected and atropine blocks the response to sham feeding, indicating that the acid-independent response is cholinergically mediated. Gastrin has also been suggested as a mediator of the cephalic phase, but in human studies gastrin levels do not change significantly and are unaffected by atropine pretreatment, arguing against such a role. The role of VIP fibers in the cephalic phase has not been fully investigated.

The gastric phase of pancreatic secretion commences with entrance of a food bolus into the stomach and is characterized by secretion of enzyme-rich, bicarbonate-poor fluid. Gastric distention stimulates enzyme secretion through vagal cholinergic mechanisms that can be inhibited by either atropine or vagotomy. Balloon distention experiments suggest that separate oxynto(fundic)pancreatic and antropancreatic reflexes exist. Earlier studies indicated that secretion during the gastric phase of pancreatic secretion was small, but recent studies in humans have shown that gastric distention can stimulate a pancreatic response comparable to a maximal CCK stimulus. This response is similar for distending solutions containing dextrose alone, dextrose with bovine serum albumin, and dextrose containing amino acids, suggesting that gastric distention and not the composition of the distending solution principally determines the pancreatic response.

Although gastrin shows homology with CCK and has an important role in gastric acid production, its role in the gastric phase of pancreatic secretion is less important. Gastrin is a weak stimulator of pancreatic secretion, having one third to one tenth the potency of CCK. Little or no change in gastrin levels can be detected with gastric distention, and exogenous gastrin sufficient to stimulate maximal gastric acid output causes only minor stimulation of pancreatic secretion. The most important role of gastrin as it pertains to pancreatic secretion is probably to stimulate secretion of gastric acid, which, upon entering the duodenum, stimulates secretin release and bicarbonate secretion.

The entrance of food into the duodenum and proximal intestine initiates the intestinal phase of post-prandial pancreatic secretion. Gastric activity strongly influences this phase by modification of chyme (acidification, peptic digestion) and by regulation of nutrient delivery to the intestine. As opposed to the cephalic and gastric phases of secretion in which little bicarbonate secretion occurs, bicarbonate as well as digestive enzyme secretion occur during the intestinal phase. As noted previously, bicarbonate secretion is primarily stimulated by secretin released in response to the delivery of titratable acid, and to a lesser extent peptides, amino acids, and calcium ions, into the duodenum. Secretin activity is potentiated by CCK and acetylcholine. Neural mechanisms may also mediate some bicarbonate secretion via VIP containing nerve fibers.

Delivery of food into the duodenum and proximal intestine stimulates enzyme secretion which is about 70 per cent of the maximum achieved with exogenous CCK. The response is dependent upon several factors including the type of food entering the intestine. Products of fat digestion provide a potent stimulus for secretion, as do products of protein digestion; free fatty acids of C8 or greater length, monoglycerides, peptides, and amino acids, especially methionine, valine, and phenylalanine, are particularly effective stimuli. Carbohydrates elicit lower and shorter secretory responses than either fat or protein. The area of intestine exposed to the food, and the presence of other substances such as bile acids, also influence the intestinal phase of secretion. For example, increased bile acid concentrations enhance absorption of lipid emulsions, resulting in decreased intestinal exposure to the secretory stimulus and decreased secretion. Bile acids inhibit the response to amino acids, but when individually instilled stimulate enzyme and bicarbonate secretion.

Enzyme secretion is mediated by hormonal and neural mechanisms. As previously noted, abundant evidence supports a physiologic role for CCK as the principal hormone mediator. Denervation experiments and latency studies suggest that one-half of the enzyme response to duodenal infusion of nutrients is mediated through cholinergic neural pathways, and that the initial enzyme response is neurally mediated. In contrast, similar experiments suggest that the initial bicarbonate response is hormonally mediated.

Mechanisms by which pancreatic secretion is inhibited or down-regulated have not been fully determined. Bicarbonate secretion is subject to feedback inhibition, as secretion neutralizes intraduodenal acid and eliminates the major stimulus of secretin release. Evidence that intraluminal enzymes evoke similar feedback inhibition is less clear. Exogenous enzyme preparations can inhibit pancreatic enzyme secretion, but requires dosages for in excess of maximal physiologic levels. Nevertheless, this mechanism of inhibiting pancreatic secretion has been applied in the treatment of chronic pancreatitis. The significance of neural pathways and mediators such as pancreatone and islet cell products in inhibiting pancreatic secretion have not been defined.

Tests of Pancreatic Function

A variety of tests have been developed to evaluate pancreatic exocrine function (Table 15–2). Direct tests measure the secretion of water, bicarbonate, or enzymes in response to exogenous hormone (secretagogue), whereas indirect tests measure secretion in response to endogenous hormone released by meal ingestion or intraluminal infusion. Samples are collected either by duodenal intubation or cannulation of the pancreatic duct. Direct tests commonly have employed secretin alone or in combination with CCK or other enzyme secretagogues such as cerulein. The standard indirect test is the Lundh test, in which a 300-ml test meal containing 6 per cent fat, 5 per cent protein, and 15 per cent carbohydrate is instilled into the duodenum, after which the duodenal contents are periodically aspirated and collected. Secretory responses to standard protocols have been determined in normal volunteers; direct and indirect tests both assume that secretory capacity is altered in disease states.

Other tests have been developed in an effort to obviate difficulties associated with specimen collection. Substrates of pancreatic enzymes that, when metabolized, yield easily recovered, measurable byproducts have been added to standard test meals. For example, N-benzoyl-L-tyrosyl-p-aminobenzoic acid is hydolyzed by chymotrypsin to generate p-aminobenzoic acid, which can be recovered from the urine. Radiolabeling of pancreatic enzymes by administration of radiolabeled amino acids may provide an additional means of measuring pancreatic secretion. Radioimmunoassays also permit measurement of circulating and excreted enzymes following pancreatic stimulation.

Finally, stool analysis is a useful and simple, albeit unesthetic, method of evaluating pancreatic function. With exocrine insufficiency, microscopic analysis may reveal undigested meat fibers or fat globules. Fecal nitrogen and fat can also be determined quantitatively, as can fecal trypsin and chymotrypsin activity.

TABLE 15–2. NORMAL RANGE OF VALUES FOR TESTS OF PANCREATIC EXOCRINE FUNCTION

Secretin test[a]
  Volume (ml/80 min): 117–392
  HCO_3^- concentration (mEq/L): 88–137
  HCO_3^- output (mEq/80 min): 16–33
Secretin + CCK[a]
  Volume (ml/80 min): 111–503
  HCO_3^- concentration (mEq/L): 88–144
  HCO_3^- output (mEq/80 min): 10–86
  Amylase output (units/80 min): 441–4038
Lundh test[b]
  Mean tryptic activity (IU/L): 61

[a] Modified from Dreiling, D.A., Janowitz, H.D., and Perrier, C.V.: Pancreatic Inflammatory Disease. A Physiologic Approach. New York, Hoeber Medical Division, Harper & Row, Publishers, 1964.

[b] Value from Mottaleb, A., Kapp, F., Noguera, E., Kellock, T.D., Wiggins, H.S., and Waller, S.L.: The Lundh test in the diagnosis of pancreatic disease: a review of five year's experience. Gut 14:835, 1973.
Reprinted from Meyer, J.H.: Pancreatic physiology. In Sleisenger, M.H., and Fordtran, J.S.: Gastrointestinal Disease. Pathophysiology, Diagnosis, Management. Philadelphia, W.B. Saunders Co., 1989.

BIBLIOGRAPHY

1. Anagnostides, A., Chadwick, V.S., Selden, S.C., and Maton, P.N.: Sham feeding and pancreatic secretion. Evidence for direct vagal stimulation of enzyme output. Gastroenterology 87:109–114, 1984.
2. Go, V.L.W., Brooks, F. P., DiMagno, E.P., Gardner, J.D., Lebenthal, E., and Scheele G. A. (eds.): The Exocrine Pancreas. Biology, Pathobiology, and Diseases. New York, Raven Press, 1986, chap. 1, 2, 9, 10, 12, 14, 15, 18, 20, 21, and 22.
3. Kuipers, G.A.J., Van Nooy, I.G.P., De Pont, J.J.H.H.M., and Bonting, S.L.: The mechanism of fluid secretion in the rabbit pancreas studied by means of various inhibitors. Biochim. Biophys. Acta 774:324–331, 1984.
5. Lankisch, P.G.: Exocrine pancreatic function tests. Gut 23:777–798, 1982.
6. Lu, L., Louie, D., and Owyang, C.: A cholecystokinin releasing peptide mediates feedback regulation of pancreatic secretion. Am. J. Physiol. 256:G430–G435, 1989.
7. Meyer, J.H.: Pancreatic physiology. In Sleisenger, M.H., and Fordtran, J.S. (eds.): Gastrointestinal Disease. Pathophysiology. Diagnosis, Management. Philadelphia, W.B. Saunders Co., 1989, pp 1777–1788.
8. Schaffalitzky de Muckadell, O.B., and Fahrenkrug, J.: Secretion pattern of secretin in man: Regulation by gastric acid. Gut 19:812–818, 1978.
9. Swanson, C.H., and Solomon, A.K.: Micropuncture analysis of the cellular mechanisms of electrolyte secretion by the in vitro rabbit pancreas. J. Gen. Physiol. 65:22–45, 1975.

10. Warshaw, A.L., Simeone, J.F., Schapiro, R.H., and Flavin-Warshaw, B.: Evaluation and treatment of the dominant dorsal duct syndrome (pancreas divisum redefined). Am. J. Surg. *159*:59–66, 1990.

11. Williams, J.A.: Regulatory mechanisms in pancreas and salivary acini. Annu. Rev. Physiol. *46*:361–375, 1984.

12. You, C.H., Rominger, J.M., and Chey, W.Y.: Potentiation effect of cholecystokinin-octapeptide on pancreatic bicarbonate secretion stimulated by a physiologic dose of secretin in humans. Gastroenterology *85*:40–45, 1983.

16

PHYSIOLOGY OF THE KIDNEY, URETERS, AND BLADDER

ROBERT R. BAHNSON

FUNCTIONAL ANATOMY

The functional unit of the kidney is the nephron, of which there are approximately one million per kidney. Each nephron is made up of a filter called the glomerulus and a tubule that acts as the receptacle for the filtrate. The glomerulus (Fig. 16–1) is actually a globe-shaped interconnected loop of capillaries that arise from the afferent arteriole and that project into a hollow capsule called Bowman's capsule. The portion of the capsule in contact with the glomerulus is not in contact with the opposite side, and the space between them is referred to as Bowman's space. It is here that the protein-free filtrate from plasma first collects. By electron microscopy the filtration membrane is a three-layered structure composed of the capillary endothelium, the basement membrane, and the epithelial foot processes of cells (podocytes) lining Bowman's capsule. Within the glomerular capillary network is the mesangial cell. These cells have phagocytic properties and also contain myofilaments that can contract in response to various stimuli.

The tubule (Fig. 16–2A) is a luminal structure of several segments, all of which are lined by epithelial cells. The first portion, the proximal convoluted tubule, subsequently gives rise to the loop of Henle, which is composed of thin descending, thin ascending, and thick ascending limbs (Fig. 16–3). The tubule then passes back between the arterioles supplying the glomerulus and forms the macula densa (Fig. 16–4). The distal convoluted tubule is next, and it empties into the last segment of the tubule, which is termed the collecting duct.

Nephrons are supplied with blood by afferent arterioles. These arborize into the individual glomerular capillary tufts and then coalese into a second efferent arteriole. This arteriole also branches to form peritubular capillaries in intimate contact with the tubules (Fig. 16–2B).

Based upon their location, two structurally distinct nephrons have been identified. Ninety per cent of the nephrons are cortical, located near the periphery of the kidney cortex with a short loop of Henle (Fig. 16–2B). The remaining 10 per cent are juxtamedullary nephrons located near the junction of the cortex and medulla with a long loop of the Henle descending deeply into the medulla.

A final anatomic structure of importance is the juxtaglomerular apparatus (Fig. 16–4). It is composed of the macula densa (the specialized tubular cells between the loop of Henle and distal tubule), mesangial cells, and granular (juxtaglomerular) cells of the smooth muscle of the afferent arteriole. These granular cells are the source of renin, which helps regulate blood pressure.

BASIC RENAL PHYSIOLOGY

The kidney's involvement in bodily homeostasis is substantial. In addition to its regulation of fluids and electrolytes, it also contributes to waste elimination and acid-base balance, regulates blood pressure, and secretes hormones. With the exception of the latter two processes, all of the other functions are dependent upon three physiologic properties: glomerular filtration, tubular reabsorption, and tubular secretion.

270

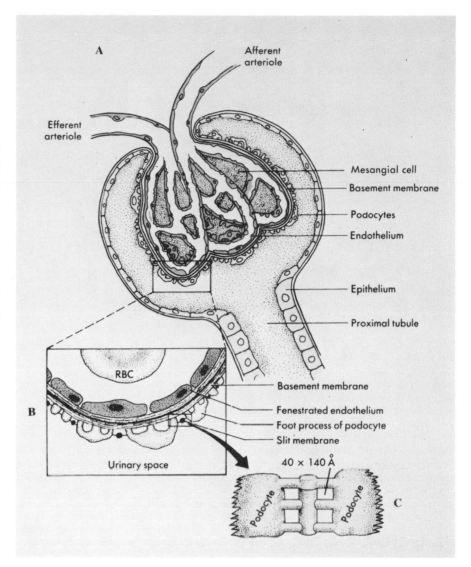

FIGURE 16–1. Anatomy of the mammalian glomerulus. The dark color represents endothelium, and the light color represents epithelium. *A,* Cross-section through a single glomerulus. Note that the glomerular capillaries form an invagination into a capsule of epithelial cells (Bowman's capsule). The surface of Bowman's capsule covers the glomerular capillaries in the form of specialized epithelial cells (podocytes). *B,* Expanded view of the filtration membrane of the glomerulus. *C,* View of one of the slip membranes rotated 90 degrees and viewed en face. (Reprinted with permission from Duling, B.R.: The kidney: Components of renal function. *In* Berne, R.M., and Levy, N.M. (eds.): Physiology, 2nd ed. St. Louis, C.V. Mosby Co., 1988. Chapter 45, p. 752.)

Glomerular Filtration

Glomerular filtration, like all capillary systems, obeys Starling's hypothesis: net filtration pressure is the sum of the opposing hydraulic and colloid osmotic (oncotic) pressures across a capillary membrane. Thus, the filtration pressure (FP) is calculated by this equation:

$$FP = (P_{GC} + BC) - (P_{BC} + GC) \quad \text{(Eq. 1)}$$

where P_{GC} = hydraulic pressure of glomerular capillary, BC = oncotic pressure of Bowman's capsule, P_{BC} = hydraulic pressure of Bowman's capsule, and GC = oncotic pressure of glomerular capillary.

Because the filtrate in Bowman's capsule during normal renal function contains virtually no protein, the equation can be simplified to

$$FP = P_{GC} - P_{BC} - GC \quad \text{(Eq. 2)}$$

In the first portion of the glomerular capillary, the hydraulic pressure is the driving force favoring fil-

tration. As plasma nears the end of the glomerular capillary, the rising oncotic pressure of the plasma, owing to the loss of filtered water, is sufficient to overcome the glomerular capillary hydrostatic pressure, and the net filtration pressure is virtually zero.

Glomerular capillaries are freely permeable to water and small molecular solutes up to a molecular weight of 7000. They are selectively permeable to larger molecules and are relatively impermeable to larger molecules, such as plasma proteins. In disease states the glomerular filtration membrane can be altered so that protein appears in the urine. Alternatively, low molecular weight proteins not normally present in plasma may be filtered if present in large quantities, e.g., myoglobin from muscle damage, and hemoglobin from hemolysis.

Other factors in addition to filtration pressure influence the rate of filtration from the glomerulus. The glomerular filtration rate (GFR) depends upon the filtration pressure, the hydraulic permeability of

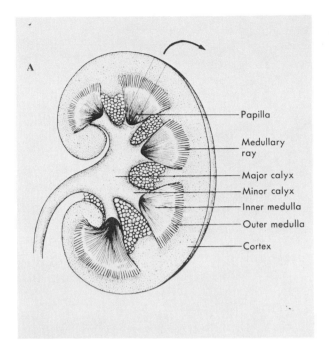

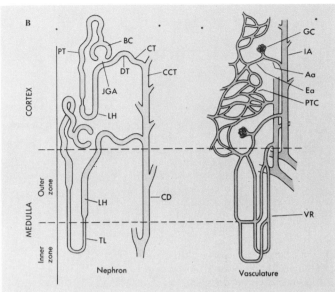

FIGURE 16–2. Anatomy of the nephrons and vasculature of the mammalian kidney. *A*, Sagittal section through the kidney showing gross anatomic relations. The outer, stippled portion of the kidney is known as the *cortex*. The inner, striated portion is referred to the *medulla*. *B*, The segment from the renal pyramid shown by the lines in *A* is enlarged to illustrate the relations among nephrons from cortical and juxtamedullary regions. The vascular and tubular anatomies are drawn to the same scale, and if desired, a transparent copy of the tubular anatomy can be made to overlay the vascular anatomy. There are two populations of nephrons, the cortical and the juxtamedullary. Note that only juxtamedullary nephrons possess long, thin loops, which penetrate into the interstitium of the medullar (TL). It should also be noted that the ascending thick limb of the loop of Henle returns to the afferent arteriole of the glomerulus from which the nephron originated. This site is the origin of the distal convoluted tubule, and the tubular structures in combination with the arterioles form the *juxtaglomerular apparatus* (JGA). The nephron continues from the distal convoluted tubule via a short *connecting tubule* (CT) to empty into the cortical collecting duct (CD) and finally forms a papillary collecting duct (not shown), which empties into the ducts of Bellini. PT, proximal tubule; BC, Bowman's capsule; LH, loop of Henle; TL, thin limb; IA, interlobular artery; Aa, afferent arteriole; Ea, efferent arteriole; PTC, peritubular capillary; CG, glomerular capillary; VR, vasa recta. (Reprinted with permission from Duling, B.R.: The kidney: Components of renal function. *In* Berne, R.M., and Levy, N.M. (eds.): Physiology, 2nd ed. St. Louis, C.V. Mosby Co., 1988. Chapter 45, p. 750.)

the glomerular membrane, and the surface area available for filtration.

$$GFR = \text{Hydraulic permeability} \times \text{surface area} \times FP \quad \text{(Eq. 3)}$$

The product of hydraulic permeability and surface area is known as the filtration coefficient (Kf).

$$GFR = Kf \times FP \quad \text{(Eq. 4)}$$

Since FP is determined by ($P_{GC} - P_{BC} - GC$), any change in Kf, P_{GC}, P_{BC}, or GC can directly alter the GFR. The Kf can change in glomerular disease or in response to chemical mediators that relax or constrict the mesangial cells. P_{GC} reflects renal arterial pressure, afferent arteriolar resistance, and efferent arteriolar resistance. P_{BC} is increased by any process that obstructs the flow of filtrate along the tubule or urinary collecting system. Finally, systemic plasma protein concentration determines GC at the beginning of the glomerular capillary. Table 16–1 summarizes the factors that directly influence the GFR.

Tubular Reabsorption

During a 24-hour period, roughly 180 L of plasma is filtered into Bowman's capsule, and all but 1 to 2 L/day is reclaimed by the second basic renal physiologic function of tubular reabsorption. Many filtered substances contained within the tubular lumen, including water, sodium, glucose, and urea, can be

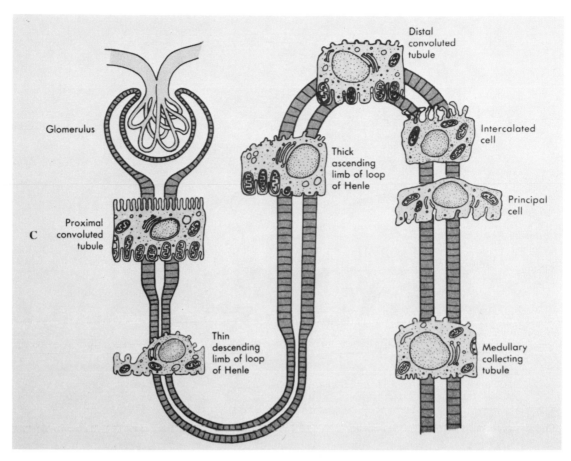

FIGURE 16–3. The histology of the cells of the various segments of the tubule. (Reprinted with permission from Duling, B.R.: The kidney: Components of renal function. *In* Berne, R.M., and Levy, M.N. (eds.): Physiology, 2nd ed. St. Louis, C.V. Mosby Co., 1988, Chapter 45, p. 751.)

reclaimed by the peritubular plasma. Movement of these molecules involves at least four separate transport mechanisms: (1) small nonpolar substances may be transported by simple diffusion; (2) facilitated diffusion involves a carrier, but does not require energy unless two or more substances are co-transported, i.e., a situation in which two substances move across a membrane in the same direction; one moving with and the other against an electrochemical gradient; (3) active transport also involves a carrier, but since the substance is generally moving against an electrochemical, gradient energy is required; (4) finally, endocytosis, which is also energy dependent, may be utilized to reclaim filtered substances.

The reabsorptive capacity of the renal tubule for a given substance per unit of time is not unlimited. As seen in diabetic patients with hyperglycemia, the transport maximum (T_M) for reabsorption of filtered glucose (375 mg/min) can be exceeded so that glucosuria results. A maximal tubular transport exists for virtually all filtered substances.

Tubular Secretion

Tubular secretion, as does glomerular filtration, adds substances to the plasma filtrate. The very same processes responsible for tubular reabsorption function in a similar fashion, albeit in the opposite direction, for tubular secretion; namely, simple diffusion, facilitated diffusion, active transport (secretion), and excytosis. Secretory processes are particularly important for both potassium and hydrogen.

MEASUREMENT OF RENAL FUNCTION

The most frequently used technique in modern medical practice to estimate glomerular filtration rate is clearance. Glomerular filtration rate (GFR) is, by definition, the volume of plasma filtered per unit time. The formula that describes GFR is

$$GFR = \frac{U_x V}{P_x} \qquad \text{(Eq. 5)}$$

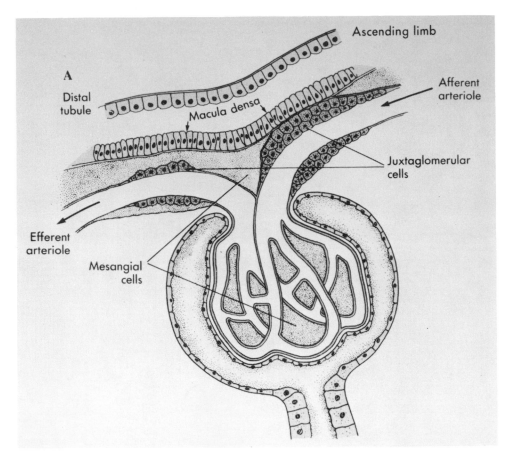

FIGURE 16–4. Renin-angiotensin system. The juxtaglomerular apparatus is composed of the macula densa (specialized cells of the distal tubule) and modified smooth muscle (the juxtaglomerular cells located primarily on the afferent arteriole). The mesangial cells (Goormaghtigh cells) are outside the glomerulus. (Reprinted with permission from Duling, B.R.: The kidney: Integrated nephron function. *In* Berne, R.M., and Levy, M.N. (eds.): Physiology, 2nd ed. St. Louis, C.V. Mosby Co., 1988. Chapter 47, p. 786.)

where U_x = urinary concentration of substance x, V = volume of urine per unit time, and P_x = plasma concentration of substance x.

In order for such a clearance formula to be valid, substance x must possess the following four properties:

1. It must be freely filtered at the glomerulus.
2. It cannot undergo tubular reabsorption.
3. It cannot be secreted by the tubules.
4. It can be neither synthesized nor metabolized by the tubules.

Inulin, a carbohydrate, is such a substance, but it is inconvenient to use clinically. Instead, GFR is estimated by calculating the clearance of creatinine, an endogenous breakdown product of muscle creatine. Clearance of a substance is defined as the volume of plasma from which that substance is completely cleared by the kidneys per unit time. In the case of inulin, clearance equals GFR because it is completely "cleared" from the plasma by glomerular filtration and is neither reabsorbed nor secreted by the tubules. Creatinine, however, is secreted in minute amounts by the tubules so that clearance of creatinine slightly overestimates GFR. Because the breakdown of creatine is relatively constant, a single serum creatinine measurement is sufficient to calculate clearance along with a timed urine collection.

The serum creatinine in most instances is an excellent barometer of renal function because a steady-state relationship exists between serum creatinine and GFR. However, it is imprecise as a single measurement, and as shown by Figure 16-5, in the middle of the curve, large decreases in the clearance (GFR) may produce only small changes in serum creatinine.

Renal plasma flow (RPF) can be estimated by measuring the clearance of an organic anion para-aminohippurate (PAH). PAH is filtered at the glomerulus, and at low plasma concentrations, all of the PAH that escapes glomerular filtration undergoes tubular secretion. Thus, PAH is completely cleared

TABLE 16–1. SUMMARY OF DIRECT GFR DETERMINANTS AND FACTORS THAT INFLUENCE THEM

DIRECT DETERMINANTS OF GFR $GFR = K_1 \cdot (P_{GC} - P_{BC}\, \pi_{GC})$	MAJOR FACTORS THAT TEND TO INCREASE THE MAGNITUDE OF THE DIRECT DETERMINANT
K_1*	↑ glomerular surface area due to relaxation of glomerular mesangial cells Result: ↑ GFR
P_{GC}*	↑ renal arterial pressure ↓ afferent arteriolar resistance (afferent dilation) ↑ efferent arteriolar resistance (efferent dilation) Result: ↑ GFR
P_{BC}*	↑ intratubular pressure due to obstruction of tubule or extrarenal urinary system Result: ↓ GFR
π_{GC}*	↑ systemic plasma oncotic pressure (sets π_{GC} at beginning of glomerular capillaries) ↓ total renal plasma flow (sets rate of rise of π_{GC} along glomerular capillaries) Results: ↓ GFR

* K_1 = filtration coefficient; P_{GC} = glomerular-capillary hydraulic pressure; P_{BC} = Bowman's capsule hydraulic pressure; π_{GC} = glomerular-capillary oncotic pressure. A reversal of all arrows in the table will cause a decrease in the magnitudes of K_1, P_{CG}, P_{BC}, and π_{GC}.

Adapted with permission from Vander, A.J.: Renal Physiology, 3rd ed. New York, McGraw-Hill Co., 1985, p. 29.

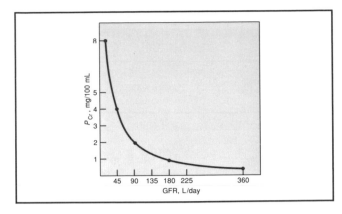

FIGURE 16–5. Steady-state relationship between GFR and plasma creatinine assuming no creatinine is secreted. (Reprinted with permission from Vander, A.J.: Renal Physiology, 3rd ed. New York, McGraw-Hill Publishing Co., 1985, p. 56).

The degree of net tubular reabsorption or secretion of a substance can be assessed by calculating fractional excretion, the fraction of the filtered mass of a substance that is actually excreted. The formula for fractional excretion (FE) is

$$FE_x = \frac{U_x\, V}{(GFR)\, P_x} \qquad (Eq.\ 6)$$

where U_x = urinary concentration of X, V = urine volume, and P_x = plasma concentration of x.

If FE_x is less than 1, then the mass of X excreted is less than the mass of X filtered, and net reabsorption of X has occurred (Table 16–2). (If FE_x = .25, then 75 per cent of filtered X has been reabsorbed.) Conversely, if FE_x is greater than 1, then secretion of X is occurring. (If FE_x = 1.5, then 50 per cent more X was excreted than filtered.)

ELIMINATION OF WASTE AND FOREIGN CHEMICALS

The kidneys are an integral component of the body's waste disposal system. Byproducts of metabolism and catabolites of exogenous chemicals are transported by the processes of glomerular filtration, tubular reabsorption, and tubular secretion. Most of these substances are organic compounds, such as proteins, peptides, amino acids, urea, urate, and weak acids or bases. Proteins with molecular weight less then 7000 are freely filtered at the glomerulus. With proteins above MW7000, the glomerular filtration barrier begins to act as a sieve and becomes virtually impenetrable for plasma albumin. The proximal tubule acts primarily by endocytosis to reclaim proteins and peptides that are filtered. This is an active transport process that exhibits a transport maximum or T_M—the maximal amount of material

from the plasma as it flows through the kidney. In fact, a small amount of total RPF (10 to 15 per cent) supplies nonsecreting cells of the kidney (e.g., peripelvic fat) so that the clearance of PAH is called the effective RPF, which represents 85 to 90 per cent of total RPF.

These physiologic principles are used clinically in the assessment of renal disorders with radiopharmaceuticals. Effective RPF can be determined by single bolus or continuous intravenous infusion of I^{131} ortho-iodohippurate (Hippuran). GFR can be calculated quickly and easily with technetium-99 m (Tc-99m) diethylenetriamine penta-acetic acid (DPTA), which is principally excreted in the urine by glomerular filtration. This technique is also exceedingly useful for noninvasive determination of differential (split) renal function.

TABLE 16–2. LABORATORY TESTS FOR DISCRIMINATION OF PATIENTS WITH AZOTEMIA AND OLIGURIA

Test	Prerenal (Hypovolemia)	Intrarenal (Acute Renal Failure)
Urine specific gravity	> 1.020	1.010
BUN: serum creatinine	> 15:1	10:1
Urine sodium (U_{NA}) (mEq/L)	< 20	> 40
Urine osmolality (mosm/kg H_2O)	> 500	< 350
Urine to plasma osmolality	> 1.5	1.0
Urine to plasma urea nitrogen	> 8	< 3
Urine (U_{cr}) to plasma (P_{cr}) creatinine	< 40	X20
Renal failure index: U_{Na}	< 1	> 1
U_{cr}/P_{cr}	< 1	> 1
Fractional excretion of filtered sodium: $\dfrac{U_{Na} \cdot U_{cr} \cdot 100}{P_{Na} \cdot U_{cr}}$		

per unit of time that the renal tubule can transport; it is relatively specific and can be inhibited. For example, cystinuria, an inborn error of metabolism, is characterized by a deficient reabsorption of the amino acids cystine, ornithine, lysine, and arginine. Urea, the primary product of protein catabolism, is somewhat different because it is freely filtered at the glomerulus, but the net excretion of this substance is governed primarily by the diffusion gradients within the kidney parenchyma.

Special mention must be made of the renal handling of weak acids and bases because most drugs used in medical interventions are either weak organic acids or bases. Depending upon the pK of the substance and the pH of the tubular fluid or plasma, weak acids and bases exist as polar ions or nonpolar molecules. In acidic solutions the diffusible form of weak acids is generated, and in basic solutions the diffusible form of a weak base is present. This distinction is important because the renal tubular epithelium is mainly a lipid barrier, and nonpolar molecules diffuse more readily across a lipid membrane than do charged substances.

Since the pH of urine in a normal individual ranges from 5 to 7, the luminal fluid is relatively acidic and favors the generation of the nonpolar,

diffusible form of a weak acid. Passive reabsorption of the weak acid then occurs. Conversely, the nondiffusible or charged form of the weak base is generated, and passive secretion of the weak base occurs. In clinical practice, the excretion of a therapeutic drug can be prevented or enhanced by urinary acidification or alkalinization. For example, acetylsalicylic acid (aspirin) is passively reabsorbed from the tubular lumen in an acid urine that favors the diffusible form of aspirin. Alkalinization of the urine results in the formation of the negatively charged acetylsalicylate, which results in the net tubular secretion of aspirin. Thus, a cornerstone of therapy for aspirin overdose is administration of bicarbonate to alkalinize the urine.

REGULATION OF SYSTEMIC BLOOD PRESSURE AND RENAL HEMODYNAMICS

The kidneys are important organs for regulating arterial blood pressure. They directly control sodium and water balance and therefore are critical for the maintenance of normal cardiac output. Furthermore, they function as endocrine organs in the renin-angiotensin system that is an important regulator of systemic arterial blood pressure and local renal hemodynamics. Renin is a proteolytic enzyme secreted by the granular cells of the juxtaglomerular apparatus (Fig. 16–4). Secretion is stimulated by decreased perfusion pressure, decreased sodium concentration of fluid in the distal tubule, increased beta (most likely beta-1) sympathetic outflow, and some prostaglandins. The half-life of renin is short (10 to 20 minutes), and it is metabolized primarily in the liver.

Once in the plasma, renin catalyzes the cleavage of a decapeptide, angiotensin I, from a plasma protein, angiotensinogen, which is produced in the liver and is present in the plasma in high concentration. Angiotensin I is biologically inactive, but in the presence of converting enzyme (also called kininase) it is cleaved to an octapeptide, angiotensin II. Converting enzyme is found in plasma, vascular endothelium, and the lung, and it can be inhibited by captopril or enalapril. Angiotensin II is a potent arteriolar and weak venous vasoconstrictor, a promoter of sodium retention from the ascending portion of the loop of Henle, and a strong stimulator of aldosterone production and secretion. Aldosterone is produced in the zona glomerulosa of the adrenal cortex and increases plasma volume by promoting sodium retention. Angiotensin II can be competitively antagonized by saralasin. Renin release is subject to feedback inhibition by increased intravascular volume or sodium, increased renal blood pressure and by angiotensin II levels.

REGULATION OF RENAL BLOOD FLOW

Autoregulation

The kidneys themselves are subject to precise hemodynamic regulation and for good reason. The total blood flow to the kidneys (1.1 L/min) in an average adult is 20 to 25 per cent of the total cardiac output (5 L/min). Assuming a hematocrit of 45, the total renal plasma flow is 605 mL/min. Since the GFR is 125 mL/min, 20 per cent of the plasma is filtered into Bowman's capsule—the so-called filtration fraction.

Blood flow to the kidney, as in any other organ, is determined by this equation:

$$RBF = \frac{R_{map} - R_{vp}}{R_r} \qquad (Eq.\ 7)$$

where R_{map} = renal mean arterial pressure in renal artery, R_{vp} = venous pressure in the renal vein, and R_r = resistance in the renal artery. The major determinant of resistance is the radii of the arterioles within the kidney, and the degree of arteriolar smooth muscle contraction is most responsible for determining the radius.

The blood flow to the kidney is relatively constant despite fluctuations in systemic mean arterial pressure. The phenomenon of autoregulation is operative when the mean arterial pressure is between 80 and 180 mm Hg and similarly maintains a constant GFR over this range of pressure (Fig. 16–6). The major regulatory site is the afferent arteriole. Afferent arteriolar resistance increases (arterioles constrict) when systemic arterial pressure rises, blunting the transmission of increased pressure to the glomerulus. Conversely, it decreases (arterioles relax) when pressure falls.

Two physiologic mechanisms are thought to be responsible for autoregulation. The first is the myogenic mechanism, which is simply a stretch response of the arteriolar wall. Increased stretch from increased pressure results in arteriolar smooth muscle contraction; diminished stretch from hypotension yields arteriolar smooth muscle relaxation. The second mechanism is tubuloglomerular feedback. Increased arterial pressure produces increased renal blood flow and glomerular filtration rate, which in turn increase the delivery of fluid through the tubular lumen. This increase is detected by the macula densa and the juxtaglomerular apparatus, which release vasoconstrictors that increase afferent arteriolar resistance. Tubuloglomerular feedback is less important in the response to diminished arterial pressure, although decreased tubular flow probably reduces the release of vasoconstrictors from the juxtaglomerular apparatus.

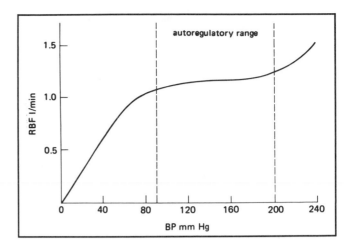

FIGURE 16–6. Autoregulation of renal blood flow (RBF). A similar pattern holds for the glomerular filtration rate. (Reprinted with permission from Vander, A.J.: Renal Physiology, 3rd ed. New York, McGraw-Hill Publishing Co., 1985, p. 72).

Systemic Regulation

Although autoregulation blunts the renal hemodynamic effects of changes in mean arterial pressure, other systemic responses to these changes do have an influence on renal blood flow. The most important of these responses are the sympathetic renal nerves, angiotensin II, and the prostaglandins. For the purpose of discussion one can use the example of hypotension caused by hemorrhage to illustrate the effects of these systemic responses.

The sympathetic response to decreased arterial blood pressure is mediated via baroreceptors located in the carotid sinus and aortic arch. Increased renal sympathetic activity produces afferent and efferent arteriolar constriction, which decreases renal blood flow and, to a lesser extent, the glomerular filtration rate. This renal vasoconstriction contributes to a rise in systemic vascular resistance that restores mean arteriolar pressure to normal. Angiotensin II also constricts afferent and efferent arterioles, but in addition causes contraction of glomerular mesangial cells. This decreases the Kf, which contributes to a decrease in glomerular filtration rate. Prostaglandins, specifically PGE_2 and PGI_2, produced by the kidney in response to renal nerve stimulation or angiotensin II, are vasodilators that act principally upon the afferent arteriole. Thus, in the example of hypotension caused by hemorrhage, the reduction of renal blood flow and glomerular filtration rate produced by decreased blood pressure, increased activity of renal sympathetic nerves, and angiotensin II is effectively counterbalanced by autoregulation and the prostaglandins, PGE_2 and PGI_2.

BASIC RENAL PROCESSES FOR HANDLING SODIUM, CHLORIDE, AND WATER

The kidney is the most important regulator of total body water and sodium. As mentioned previously, this is a critical determinant of cardiac output and consequently arterial blood pressure. The excretion of sodium, chloride, and water is intimately coupled. All three substances are freely filtered at the glomerulus, and none undergoes tubular secretion. Sodium undergoes active tubular reabsorption via a sodium-potassium-dependent ATPase pump located at the basilar membrane between the tubular epithelial cell and the interstitial fluid. As sodium is pumped into the interstitium and out of the cell, the osmolarity of the tubular lumen is lowered (increased concentration of water) and the osmolarity of the interstitium is increased (decreased concentration of water). Thus, an osmotic gradient is created that results in the absorption of water from the lumen across the epithelial cell into the interstitial fluid by simple diffusion. In a similar fashion, chloride reabsorption is favored by a concentration gradient that is created by the movement of water. Therefore, the active reabsorption of sodium creates an osmotic gradient that results in passive reabsorption of both chloride and water. In addition, as positively charged sodium ions move into the interstitial fluid, the tubular lumen becomes relatively negatively charged, creating an electrical gradient favoring chloride reabsorption. The amount of water reabsorbed is also influenced by the permeability of the tubular epithelium. Although the proximal tubule is quite permeable, the distal convoluted tubule is virtually impermeable. The collecting duct permeability varies, depending upon physiologic regulation by antidiuretic hormone (ADH).

ADH, or vasopressin, actually exerts its effect upon the luminal membrane of the collecting duct tubular epithelium. ADH binds to a receptor on the basolateral membrane and activates adenylate cyclase, which catalyzes the formation of cyclic AMP. This second messenger, in some unknown fashion, increases the permeability of the collecting duct epithelium, and water reabsorption is facilitated. ADH secretion also promotes renal synthesis and release of prostaglandins that act as negative feedback inhibitors by blocking the generation of cyclic AMP.

The concentration of urine takes place in those loops of Henle that occupy the medulla. Its control rests with the medullary countercurrent system. In this system the salt concentration and osmolarity of the tubular fluid increases as a result of differential permeability of the descending and ascending tubules to water. The descending limb is permeable to water so that water is absorbed passively as sodium is absorbed actively. In the ascending loop, sodium and chloride are actively transported out of the lumen into the interstitium, but the ascending loop is now impermeable to water, so that water does not follow the movement of sodium. The medullary interstitium then becomes hyperosmolar. As a consequence, tubular fluid is concentrated as it flows down the descending limb and diluted as it flows up the ascending limb. It reaches its greatest concentration at the tip of the loop, in the medullary portion of the kidney. In humans, this value is approximately 1400 mosm/L, which is also the maximal urinary concentration the human kidney can produce. (Only about 600 mosm of this hypertonicity is due to salt; 600 more is due to urea.) However, since the tubular fluid leaves the cortical collecting tubule isosmotic to plasma (300 mosm/L), the final concentration of the urine occurs in the medullary collecting tubule. The interstitium in the medulla is hyperosmolar, and water is reabsorbed from the collecting duct under ADH influence along an osmotic gradient. Thus, the principal function of the medullary countercurrent system is the establishment of highly concentrated interstitium that permits a concentrated urine to be made in the collecting ducts.

The kidney has an obligatory daily excretion of urea, sulfate, and other waste products that amounts to 600 mosm/day. Since its maximum concentrating ability is 1400 mosm/L, the water required for excretion of normal byproducts of metabolism is

$$\frac{600 \text{ mosm/day}}{1400 \text{ mosm/L}} = 0.429 \text{ L/day} \qquad \text{(Eq. 8)}$$

This represents the minimal water requirement per day to maintain kidney function.

Regulation of Salt and Water Balance

The total extracellular fluid volume depends primarily upon the mass of extracellular sodium. This is a critical concept that underscores the importance of sodium regulation for maintenance of normal cardiovascular function. Regulation of extracellular sodium is accomplished primarily by altering the degree of renal sodium excretion. Since there is no sodium secretion in the tubules, excretion represents the difference between the filtered sodium and that which is reabsorbed by the tubules. Filtered sodium is determined by the plasma sodium concentration and the glomerular filtration rate. Since plasma sodium concentration changes very little in physiologic states, glomerular filtration rate and sodium reabsorption are the prime determinants of sodium excretion.

Three major factors determine the glomerular filtration rate. The first and most important is change in vascular volume, which is detected by baroreceptors in the carotid sinus, aortic arch, veins, and atria. A decrease in blood pressure results in sympathetic stimulation of the renal arterioles, producing vasoconstriction, a diminished glomerular filtration rate, and reduced loss of sodium (volume). The second factor is change in plasma protein concentration that alters the oncotic pressure in the glomerulus. Increased oncotic pressure (plasma protein concentration) as a result of diarrheal fluid loss, for example, reduces net filtration pressure and the GFR. Finally, the Kf can be influenced by catecholamines and angiotensin II. Both substances reduce Kf and subsequently the glomerular filtration rate by producing mesangial cell contraction.

These mechanisms are relatively crude and inadequate for fine tuning. Quantitatively, sodium reabsorption is far more important than the glomerular filtration rate in determining total sodium excretion. In a manner similar to autoregulation of renal blood flow, one of the regulatory processes for sodium reabsorption—termed glomerular tubular balance—blunts the ability of major changes in the glomerular filtration rate to produce large changes in sodium excretion. Although the phenomenon cannot be explained completely, it results in sodium reabsorption that varies directly with the glomerular filtration rate. Thus, large increases or decreases in the filtered load of sodium are managed by simultaneous increases or decreases in tubular reabsorption.

Clearly, however, aldosterone, a mineralocorticoid produced in the adrenal cortex, has the greatest single influence on tubular reabsorption of sodium (Fig. 16–7). Aldosterone exerts its effects in the distal tubules and collecting ducts, and approximately 2 per cent of the total filtered sodium is under its regulatory control. Lest this amount seem insignificant, bear in mind that total filtered sodium in a normal individual approximates 26,100 mmol/day. Therefore, aldosterone controls the reabsorption of 522 mmol/day of sodium, which amounts to roughly 30 gm/day of sodium chloride.

Aldosterone itself is subject to several regulatory mechanisms, including plasma sodium and potassium concentrations, plasma ACTH concentration, and plasma angiotensin II concentration. Changes in plasma sodium concentration or plasma potassium concentration are sensed by osmoreceptors in the adrenal so that secretion of aldosterone increases with decreased sodium concentration or increased potassium concentration and decreases if sodium concentration increases or potassium concentration decreases. ACTH is a trophic hormone primarily responsible for regulating cortisol; however, at high concentrations it is also stimulatory for aldosterone. The most potent and important controller of aldosterone is angiotensin II. Since the major regulator of angiotensin II is renin, factors that govern the release of renin simultaneously influence the release of angiotensin II.

Other known regulatory factors for sodium reabsorption include atrial natriuretic factor; hydraulic pressure in the renal interstitium; redistribution of renal blood flow; direct tubular effects of renal nerves, circulating epinephrine, and angiotensin II; and intrarenal humoral agents, such as prostaglandins, kinins, and dopamine. Certain commonly used

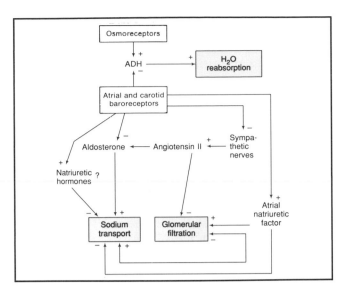

FIGURE 16–7. Regulation of volume and osmolality. Compare the single factor relating ADH and osmolarity with the complex web of interactions concerned with volume control. Atrial natriuretic factor is probably only one of several natriuretic factors. The dark color shows receptors; the light color shows altered function. (Reprinted with permission from Duling, B.R.: The kidney: Regulation of the composition of extracellular fluid. *In* Berne, R.M., and Levy, N.M. (eds.): Physiology, 2nd ed. St. Louis, C.V. Mosby Co., 1988. Chapter 48, p. 795.)

medications, such as cortisol and estrogens, have sodium-retentive properties, whereas progestational agents and parathyroid hormone promote sodium excretion.

Although extracellular water is controlled primarily by factors regulating extracellular sodium, a second mechanism controlling water excretion is also important. Antidiuretic hormone profoundly influences the permeability of the distal tubule and collecting duct to water. Baroreceptors located in arteries, veins, and the left atrium provide afferent input to the supraoptic and paraventricular nuclei of the hypothalamus that produce ADH, which migrates down the supraoptic hypophyseal tract to be released into capillaries of the posterior pituitary. Increased atrial pressure inhibits ADH release, whereas decreased atrial pressure is stimulatory.

In addition to baroreceptors, osmoreceptors in the hypothalamus and liver sense alterations in body fluid osmolarity and induce renal compensation by free water clearance. This is not to be confused with clearance as described earlier. Rather, it refers to the volume of pure water that would have to be added or removed from urine to make it isosmotic with plasma. The formula for calculating free water clearance is

$$C_{H_2O} = \frac{V - U_{osm} V}{P_{osm}} \qquad \text{(Eq. 9)}$$

where V = urine volume per unit time, U_{osm} = urine osmolarity, and P_{osm} = plasma osmolarity. A positive value means that water free of solute was eliminated in the urine, whereas a negative valve indicates that free water was reabsorbed.

Thus, two major control mechanisms exist for ADH release from the hypothalamus. To a much smaller extent, angiotensin II also promotes ADH release, and as is well known to most surgeons, ethanol is a powerful inhibitor of ADH release.

In addition to these internal regulatory processes, thirst and salt appetite also govern body sodium and water balance. the stimulus for water ingestion is most likely from the same baroreceptors and osmoreceptors responsible for the release of ADH. The regulation of salt intake is less well understood since the average American dietary intake of 10 to 15 gm/day of sodium far exceeds the amount required for normal function (less than 0.5 gm/day).

REGULATION OF POTASSIUM BALANCE

Approximately 95 percent of total body potassium is intracellular, and this maintains a normal electrical resting membrane potential. Excessive movement of potassium out of cells lowers the membrane potential and increases cell excitability, whereas influx of potassium into cells hyperpolarizes them and reduces cellular excitability. Thus, potassium is critical for the normal propagation of neural impulses and stimulation of muscle and must be regulated closely. The control mechanisms are located primarily in the kidney. However, any factor that influences the ratio of extracellular to intracellular potassium also contributes to potassium homeostasis. In this regard, it is recognized that epinephrine, insulin, aldosterone, and alkalosis stimulate potassium uptake by cells, whereas acidosis is associated with a movement of potassium out of the cells.

In the kidney, potassium is completely filtered at the glomerulus and can undergo both tubular reabsorption and secretion. Clearly, reabsorption is the dominant mechanism since only 10 to 15 percent of filtrated potassium is excreted in the urine. Most of potassium reabsorption occurs in the proximal tubule and the ascending limb of the loop of Henle and is not subject to significant physiologic regulation. Nearly all of the renal regulatory mechanisms are located in the final portion of the distal tubule and the initial collecting tubule where potassium is regulated.

Potassium secretion in the distal tubule and collecting tubule is dependent upon a sodium-potassium ATPase pump that transports potassium from the interstitium across the basolateral tubular membrane into the cell. This process creates a high intracellular potassium concentration and results in diffusion of potassium into the tubular lumen along a concentration gradient. The luminal membrane of the tubular epithelium is highly permeable to potassium as it contains specific ion channels for potassium movement.

The regulation of potassium secretion is accomplished by homeostatic control of both the sodium-potassium ATPase pump and the permeability of the luminal membrane to potassium. If a high plasma concentration of potassium exists, the basolateral sodium-potassium ATPase pump is stimulated, and increases cellular accumulation of potassium occurs. This increases the chemical gradient favoring movement of potassium out of the tubular cells into the lumen, thereby increasing the excretion of potassium. Simultaneously, the adrenal cortex senses the increased potassium concentration in plasma and releases aldosterone. Aldosterone stimulates the cellular uptake of potassium (coupled with the reabsorption of sodium described earlier) by stimulating the sodium-potassium ATPase pump and increasing the permeability of the tubular membrane to potassium. Both of these factors result in increased potassium secretion.

If a low plasma concentration of potassium is present, such as in the diarrheal state, the sodium-potassium ATPase pump is inhibited by inhibiting the secretion of aldosterone; potassium conservation results.

Changes in potassium secretion also occur indirectly when acidosis, alkalosis, or an altered pattern of sodium excretion is present. Alkalosis that is associated with a movement of potassium into cells results in an increased distal tubular (cellular) potassium concentration that favors potassium secretion. The opposite effect occurs to a lesser degree in acidosis.

When increased sodium excretion occurs as a consequence of saline infusion, excessive salt intake, osmotic diuresis, or diuretic drugs that act on the proximal tubule or loop of Henle, potassium excretion is increased as well. All of these situations reduce renal tubular potassium reabsorption and result in an increased rate of fluid delivery to the distal tubule. this dilutes the luminal fluid in the distal tubule and favors the secretion of potassium along a concentration gradient. In the opposite situation, when sodium conservation is present, a decreased delivery of fluid to the distal tubule can inhibit potassium secretion.

REGULATION OF ACID-BASE BALANCE

The maintenance of fluid and electolyte balance is almost exclusively under renal control. The kidneys are also intimately involved in the regulation of acid-base balance, but they share this responsibility with the respiratory system. This interrelationship exists because the hydrogen ion balance of the body is heavily influenced by buffering, and the most important physiologic buffer is the $H_2O + CO_2$ $H^+ + HCO_3^-$ system. The two critical components of this buffer, CO_2 and HCO_3^-, are regulated by the respiratory system and the kidneys, respectively. Buffering is critical for balancing the generation and elimination of hydrogen ions that result from physiologic processes. Sources of hydrogen ion are oxidative metabolism (CO_2), protein catabolism (H_2PO_4 H_2SO_4), gastrointestinal secretions, and urine. Metabolism of the average American diet releases 40 to 80 mEq/day of hydrogen ion.

The kidneys maintain hydrogen ion balance via two different mechanisms: by varying the amount of reabsorption of filtered bicarbonate and by adding new bicarbonate to the peritubular plasma. Of these two mechanisms, the first is quantitatively more important in maintaining acid-base balance. However, both variation is bicarbonate reabsorption and addition of new bicarbonate to plasma are actually determined by the extent of tubular hydrogen ion secretion.

To understand bicarbonate reabsorption, recall that hydrogen ion is secreted into the tubular lumen via counter-transport with sodium. The hydrogen ion within the tubular cell is generated from carbonic acid breakdown to hydrogen ion and bicarbonate. The carbonic acid is formed (in the presence of carbonic anhydrase) when water combines with carbon dioxide, which diffuses into the cell from peritubular plasma. The secreted hydrogen ion combines with the filtered bicarbonate to form carbonic acid, which then breaks down to form water and carbon dioxide in the presence of carbonic anhydrase in the tubular membrane. Water and carbon dioxide either diffuse into the plasma or combine in the renal tubular cell to generate hydrogen ion and bicarbonate (Fig. 16–8).

The addition of new bicarbonate to plasma is also intimately intertwined with hydrogen ion secretion. Essentially, it occurs as a result of hydrogen ion excretion via two different urinary buffering systems. In the first system, a reaction in the tubular lumen with filtered phosphate forms phosphoric acid, which is excreted in the urine. Thus, the bicarbonate generated in the tubular cell by carbonic acid breakdown enters the plasma and represents a net gain of bicarbonate, instead of a recapture of a filtered bicarbonate. In a similar fashion, ammonia, which is synthesized in the renal tubular cells from deamidation and deamination of glutamine and is secreted into the tubular lumen, combines with secreted hydrogen ion to form ammonium, which is eliminated in the urine. At urinary pH, which seldom exceeds 7.4, virtually all ammonia accepts a hydrogen ion to form ammonium (pK for ammonia/ammonium reaction is 9.2). This is an important example of the concept of non-ionic diffusion or diffusion trapping. Ammonia synthesized by the tubules is nonpolar and highly lipid soluble so it moves freely across the tubular membrane into the lumen. The ammonium formed by the addition of hydrogen ion is charged and lipid insoluble; therefore, it is trapped in the tubular lumen. At urinary pH, ammonia converts quickly to ammonium so the tubular concentration of ammonia is low, and a concentration gradient favoring diffusion from cell to lumen is maintained.

The renal contribution to acid-base balance can be summarized by discussing the fate of secreted hydrogen ion. It can combine with filtered bicarbonate in which case bicarbonate is reabsorbed, or it can combine with filtered phosphate or secreted ammonia. In the latter process hydrogen ion is actually excreted in the urine, and new bicarbonate is added to the plasma, thereby alkalinizing it. Thus, in normal physiologic states, the 40 to 80 mEq/day of hydrogen ion generated by metabolism must be excreted in the urine. As a consequence, all filtered bicarbonate must be reabsorbed and 40 to 80 mEq/day of new bicarbonate must be added to the plasma. This is accomplished by excreting 40 to 80 mEq of hydro-

FIGURE 16–8. General mechanisms by which filtered bicarbonate is reabsorbed. In studying this figure, begin with the carbon dioxide entering the cell from the peritubular plasma. Not shown in the figure are two facts that apply only to the proximal tubule: (1) the breakdown of H_2CO_3 to CO_2 and H_2O in the lumen is also catalyzed by carbonic anhydrase, which is present in the luminal membrane, and (2) most of the hydrogen ion is secreted into the lumen via countertransport with sodium. (Reprinted with permission from Vander, A.J.: Renal Physiology, 3rd ed. New York, McGraw-Hill Publishing Co., 1985, p. 165.)

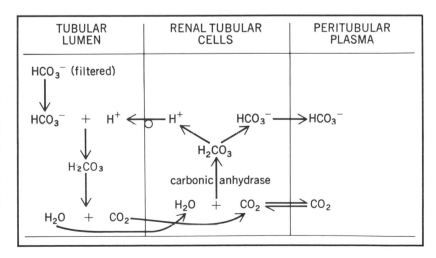

gen ion buffered by phosphate or ammonia in the urine. Renal adaptation to pathologic states of imbalance involves changes in the amounts of bicarbonate reabsorption and acid secretion. In the case of alkalosis, decreased secretion of hydrogen ions by the kidneys limits the absorption of filtered bicarbonate, and in acidotic states new bicarbonate is added to the plasma when excess hydrogen ion is excreted in the urine buffered by phosphate or ammonia. Since roughly 75 percent of filtered phosphate is reabsorbed and unavailable for buffering, ammonia is quantitatively the more important urinary buffer.

It is possible to quantitate the individual contributions of these processes to the acid secretion rate. The amount of acid secreted that combines with filtered bicarbonate can be calculated by measuring the amount of bicarbonate reabsorption as follows:

$$\text{Filtered bicarbonate} = \text{GFR} \times P_{HCO_3}$$
$$\text{Excreted bicarbonate} = U_{HCO_3} \times V$$
$$\text{Reabsorbed bicarbonate} = \text{Filtered } HCO_3 -$$
$$\text{Excreted } HCO_3$$
$$\text{(Eq. 10)}$$

Except for the hydrogen ion that combines with ammonia, that which is excreted in the urine with phosphate and organic buffers can be calculated by taking a sample of urine and measuring the amount of sodium hydroxide required to bring the urine to a pH of 7.4. The number of milliequivalents of sodium hydroxide equals the number of milliequivalents of hydrogen ion that combined with phosphate and organic buffers and is known as the titratable acid. The reason that ammonia does not contribute to titratable acidity is because the pK of ammonia/ammonium reaction is 9.2. Titration to pH 7.4 will result in little if any dissociation of hydrogen ion from ammonium. Thus, a separate measurement of ammonium excretion is required to calculate the sum total of tubular hydrogen ion secretion. Normal daily values are approximately

- HCO_3 reabsorption 4300 mEq.
- Titratable acid 20 mEq.
- NH_4 excretion 40 mEq.

Many factors govern the kidneys' rate of hydrogen secretion, which in turn regulates the body's pH. As previously noted for sodium, there is glomerulotubular feedback for hydrogen ion, and secretion of hydrogen ion varies direcly with the GFR. Far more important is the P_{CO_2} of arterial blood: a direct relationship exists with the rate of hydrogen ion secretion. CO_2 diffuses easily across cell membranes, and an increased P_{CO_2} of arterial blood leads to a like increase in the P_{CO_2} of tubular cells. Recall that diffusion of CO_2 into the tubular cell creates an elevation of intracellular hydrogen ion that then stimulates the rate of hydrogen ion secretion.

Thus, the kidneys are able to compensate for pH changes of respiratory acidosis and alkalosis that accompany pulmonary insufficiency (CO_2 retention)

and hyperventilation, respectively. In respiratory acidosis, the elevated plasma CO_2 diffuses into the renal tubular cell, resulting in increased hydrogen ion secretion. As a consequence all the filtered bicarbonate is reclaimed, and the excess secreted hydrogen ion is excreted in the form of titratable acid or ammonium. In respiratory alkalosis the diminished plasma CO_2 reduces renal tubular cell hydrogen ion secretion. This in turn leads to a reduction in bicarbonate reabsorption and increased excretion of bicarbonate.

In metabolic acidosis the plasma bicarbonate is low, and the amount of filtered bicarbonate is reduced proportionally. Therefore, the kidney needs to secrete less hydrogen ion to accomplish total bicarbonate reabsorption. The remaining hydrogen ion forms titratable acid and contributes new bicarbonate to plasma. In metabolic alkalosis the increased plasma bicarbonate leads to such an increase in filtered bicarbonate that not all of it is reabsorbed and no titratable acid can be formed. Thus, bicarbonate is lost in the urine and pH decreases toward normal.

In addition to changes in pH, other factors can influence hydrogen ion secretion. Salt depletion stimulates not only sodium reabsorption but also hydrogen ion secretion. By itself, salt depletion does not lead to a primary metabolic acidosis, but it can interfere with the kidneys' ability to compensate for a metabolic alkalosis from another cause. Aldosterone stimulates hydrogen ion secretion in the distal tubules and collecting ducts. Potassium depletion also stimulates hydrogen ion secretion. Recall that aldosterone stimulates potassium ion secretion, and excess aldosterone can cause hypokalemia. In a patient with aldosterone excess and potassium deficiency, synergistic stimulation of hydrogen ion secretion occurs, and metabolic alkalosis can develop. Clinical examples of this condition are hyperaldosteronism from an adrenal tumor and extensive use of diuretics. In the latter situation, diuretics deplete both sodium and potassium, and the low plasma sodium stimulates renin, which ultimately increases aldosterone.

REGULATION OF CALCIUM HOMEOSTASIS

Calcium homeostasis is very precise because of the importance of calcium in neuromuscular excitability. The renal influence of calcium regulation occurs in two ways: (1) it is the site of final activation of vitamin D_3 to 1,25-dihydroxy vitamin D_3 (1,25-$(OH)_2$ D_3), and (2) under the influence of parathyroid hormone (PTH), the distal tubule increases calcium reabsorption.

Vitamin D_3 is ingested in normal diets and is formed by the action of sunlight on 7 dehydrocholesterol. In the blood, vitamin D_3 is hydroxylated at position 25 by the liver and in the 1 position by the kidneys. Hydroxylation in the kidney is subject to physiologic control and is stimulated by both PTH and decreased plasma phosphate. The importance of the kidney in vitamin D_3 activation is emphasized by the inability of renal failure patients to synthesize $1,25\text{-}(OH_2) D_3$ when given large amounts of vitamin D.

Roughly 60 percent of serum calcium is filtered at the glomerulus. Over 95 percent of the filtered calcium is reclaimed. Current estimates are that 60 percent of the filtered load is reabsorbed in the proximal tubule, 20 percent by the loop of Henle, 10 percent by the distal convoluted tubule, and 5 percent by the collecting system. In the proximal tubule, calcium reabsorption is tightly coupled with sodium transport. Factors that enhance sodium reabsorption (salt or volume depletion) similarly increase calcium reabsorption, and those that diminish reabsorption (saline diuresis) tend to decrease calcium reabsorption. In the distal nephron, calcium reabsorption is dissociated from sodium reabsorption. In this location calcium transport is active, against an electrochemical gradient, and is regulated by PTH in response to systemic needs.

RENAL PHARMACOLOGY

Since the kidneys are intimately involved in the maintenance of fluid and electolyte balance and blood pressure regulation, pharmacotherapy can be used to correct disturbances of fluid and electrolyte homeostasis and the cardiovascular system. The most important classes of drugs are the diuretics and antagonists of the renin-angiotensin system.

Diuretics are drugs that act direcly upon the kidneys to promote loss of excess extracellular fluid and electrolytes. Although the mechanism of action for each of the seven major groups of diuretics is slightly different, they all act by decreasing the tubular reabsorption of salt water. The diuretics are usually classified according to their chemical structure and their site of action in the tubules (Table 16–3).

Xanthines, organic mercurials, and carbonic anhydrase inhibitors are seldom if ever used, but are discussed here because of their historical or mechanistic importance. Thiazides, high-ceiling or loop diuretics, potassium-sparing diuretics, and osmotic diuretics are used frequently in clinical practice and are presented in greater detail.

Xanthines are probably the first known diuretic of which theophylline is the prototype. Caffeine, a related drug, enjoys widespread nonprescription usage. Xanthines inhibit Na^+ reabsorption at the proximal convoluted tubule and also increase cardiac output and, in turn, the GFR. Organic mercurials probably act by inhibiting active chloride ion transport in the ascending limb of the loop of Henle. As a result, Na^+ reabsorption is diminished. These agents

TABLE 16–3. CLASSIFICATION OF DIURETICS

By Structure	By Major Site of Action
Osmotic diuretics } Xanthines }	Proximal tubule
Carbonic anhydrase inhibitors	
High-ceiling or loop diuretics	Ascending limb of loop of Henle
Organic mercurials	Distal tubule
Potassium-sparing diuretics	
Thiazides	

require parenteral administration and are both nephrotoxic and cardiotoxic. Carbonic anhydrase inhibitors were the first orally active, nonmercurial diuretic drugs. These drugs, which rely on an unsubstituted sulfonamide group for their activity, act by decreasing bicarbonate reabsorption in the proximal tubule. To maintain ionic balance, chloride is retained, which ultimately produces a hyperchloremic acidosis. Acetazolamide is still used to treat glaucoma.

Benzothiadiazides (thiazides) were discovered serendipitously in the search for synthetic compounds that produced carbonic anhydrase inhibition. Although they retain the sulfamyl group, the essential group(s) for activity is a halogen adjacent to the sulfonamide group on the benzene ring.

The primary mechanism of action of thiazides is an inhibition of chloride reabsorption at the distal protion of the ascending limb or the distal tubule. There are several nonthiazide compounds (chlorthalidone, quinethazone, metolazone) that act in a similar fashion. In the kidney, due to the distal reabsorption of calcium, thiazides also reduce the excretion of calcium. This is useful for treating urinary stone formers with "renal leak" hypercalciuria. Thiazides also have mild diabetogenic potential and can elevate serum uric acid.

High-ceiling or loop diuretics are the most effective agents available for producing a diuresis. Drugs in this group include furosemide, bumetanide, and ethacrynic acid. Their major site of action is the thick ascending portion of Henle's loop, and the mechanism of action is inhibition of the active reabsorption of Na^+. These agents are particularly potent and can block reabsorption of up to 40 per cent of the filtered load of Na^+ and Cl^-. Ototoxicity has been noted with loop diuretics and apparently is dose related and more common in patients with pre-existing renal insufficiency.

Potassium-sparing diuretics include the aldosterone antagonist spironolactone and the nonsteroidal potassium-sparing drugs, triamterene and amiloride. Aldosterone and other mineralocorticoids bind to a specific receptor in the cytoplasm of the distal tubule called aldosterone-binding protein. The hormone-receptor complex is translocated to the nucleus and directs protein synthesis, which regulates distal Na$^+$ reabsorption and K$^+$ secretion. Spironolactone competes for the aldosterone receptor and produces a mild natriuresis associated with a decreased K$^+$ elimination. Spironolactone can be effective only if mineralocorticoids are present. Triamterene and amiloride are physiologic antagonists and are active even in the absence of aldosterone. They both appear to decrease Na$^+$ reabsorption in the mineralocorticoid-independent portion of the distal tubule. Reduction in Na$^+$ reabsorption reduces the gradient that normally facilitates passive K$^+$ secretion. Potassium-sparing diuretics are low in potency and are most often utilized in combination with other diuretics, such as thiazides, to prevent hypokalemia.

Osmotic diuretics are compounds that are not reabsorbed by the tubule and thus contribute to the osmotic pressure of the tubular fluid. They create an obligatory loss of water for their excretion and also promote Na$^+$ loss. Mannitol, a six-carbon sugar, is the prototypical osmotic diuretic and is primarily used to promote urine flow during acute oliguria. It can also be used to hasten the elimination of nephrotoxic agents, such as the antineoplastic drug cisplatin.

Antagonists of the renin-angiotensin system are now widely employed for the treatment of both hypertension and heart failure. Teprotide, captropril, enalopril, and lisinopril are all inhibitors of peptidyldipeptide hydrolase (converting enzyme), which converts the relatively inactive decapeptide angiotensin I to the very active octapeptide angiotensin II.

These drugs reduce blood pressure in patients with renovascular disease and in those with essential hypertension. They also enhance cardiac output in patients with congestive heart failure by reducing ventricular preload and afterload. These drugs are contraindicated in patients with bilateral renal artery stenosis or unilateral renal artery stenosis in a solitary kidney.

Saralasin is an angiotensin II receptor blocker that decreases blood pressure in patients with renovascular hypertension, end-stage renal disease and malignant hypertension. It has been proposed as an aid to diagnose patients with angiotensin-dependent hypertension.

LABORATORY STUDIES OF RENAL FUNCTION

The practicing surgeon is often required to evaluate patients with disorders of renal function. The first manifestation of renal disease is often azotemia with or without oliguria. An elevated BUN and serum creatinine and reduced urine output are non-specific and require further investigation for diagnosis and appropriate therapy. Generally, the cause can be attributed to prerenal (hypovolemia), intrarenal (acute renal failure), or postrenal (obstruction) factors.

The patient with prerenal azotemia due to decreased renal perfusion pressure usually shows physical signs of volume depletion, such as postural hypotension, decrease skin turgor, and dry mucous membranes. Laboratory tests that point to the presence of prerenal azotemia include a urine with high specific gravity (greater than 1.020), a BUN to serum creatinine ratio of over 15 : 1, and changes in urinary sodium, creatinine, urea nitrogen, and osmolality as outlined in Table 16–2. In addition, examination of the urinary sediment shows no evidence of the coarse granular casts seen in acute renal failure. If azotemia and diminished urine volume are a result of acute renal failure, the urine specific gravity is similar to that of plasma (1.010), the urine sediment often shows hyaline casts, and the serum BUN creatinine ratio is usually 10 : 1. It is important to note that urinary indices (listed in Table 16–2) are invalid if the patient has received potent diuretic therapy in an attempt to treat acute azotemia.

Patients with postrenal azotemia may often have laboratory values that mimic those observed in acute renal failure. However, the obstruction to the flow of urine in this group of patients can be uncovered by physical examination, bladder catheterization or irrigation, and ultrasonography.

PHYSIOLOGY OF THE RENAL PELVIS AND URETER

The calyces, infundibula, renal pelves, and ureters are all part of the upper urinary collecting system. Their sole function is the transport of urine from the kidneys to the urinary bladder for storage.

Propulsion of urine begins with pacemaker activity located in multiple sites at the border of the minor calyces and the major calyx. At normal rates of urine flow, these pacemakers produce approximately six calyceal contractions per minute and propel urine through the infundibula into the renal pelvis. Transmission of the electrical impulse is usually blocked at the ureteral pelvic juntion (UPJ), and it remains closed during renal pelvic filling. Ultimately, when renal pelvic pressure rises, urine is discharged into the upper ureter, which is in a collapsed state. Once the urine is expelled, renal pelvic pressure declines to baseline, and the cycle repeats itself. The closed UPJ is most likely protective for the kidney since ureteral contractile pressures are higher than renal pelvic pressures. In the proximal ureter, electrical activity gives rise to peristaltic contraction waves that occur at the rate of two or six per minute. As urine from the pelvis fills the collapsed proximal ureter, a contraction wave is initiated and pushes the urine bolus in front of it. These peristatic waves produce pressures of 20 to 60 cm H_2O that are sufficient to overcome resting ureteral pressure of 0 to 5 cm H_2O and propel urine antegrade into the bladder.

As urine flow increases, the frequency of peristalsis and the bolus volume increase proportionally, However, at extremely high flow rates, urine is transported as a continuous column of fluid instead of a series of boluses. If urine transport is inefficient because either too much fluid per unit time enters the ureter or too little fluid exits the ureter per unit time, stasis occurs and dilation results. Any degree of obstruction will cause more dilation at high urine flow rates, but it is important to note that even a nonobstructed ureter can impede antegrade transport if flow rates are high enough. Dilation of the ureter also diminishes the effectiveness of ureteral transport because it limits the contractile pressures that can be generated according to the law of Laplace. At the ureterovesical junction (UVJ), the pressure within the urine bolus must exceed the bladder pressure in order for urine to enter the bladder. If the UVJ does not relax, however, during urine passage, the distal ureter retracts within its sheath, which lessens UVJ resistance. Increased UVJ resistance due to either increased bladder pressure or UVJ obstruction will result in inefficient urine transport unless the pressure within the urine bolus rises appropriately. Recall that dilation of the ureter may substantially limit the ability to strengthen contractile pressure.

PHYSIOLOGY OF THE BLADDER

The bladder has only two physiologic functions: the storage and emptying of urine (Table 16–4). The process of micturition, however, is quite complex. Normal bladder function requires (1) a compliant bladder that fills without a concomitant rise in pressure at low volumes, (2) a competent bladder neck, (3) a sensation of a desire to void when bladder capacity is reached, (4) inhibition of the micturition reflex by cortical activity until an appropriate time, (5) faciliatation of emptying by cortical pathways when voiding is desired, and (6) coordination between detrusor contraction and bladder neck relax-

TABLE 16–4.   STAGES OF NORMAL MICTURITION CYCLE

	ACTIVITY
Bladder filling	Alpha sympathetic nerves keep outlet closed; beta sympathetic fibers allow filling without rise in intravesical pressure (compliance).
Perception of desire to void	At critical volume (cystometric capacity), pelvic parasympathetic fibers send signal via Bradley's loop II to micturition center in midbrain; signal is relayed through loop I to cortex and person perceives desire to void.
Postponement	Cortical inhibition occurs, and voiding is delayed.
or	
Site appreciation, locomotion, posturing	Person seeks place to void.
Initiation	Signal via Bradley's loop I
Contraction	Signal via Bradley's loop II is sent to detrusor muscle and parasympathetic efferent fibers.
and	
Outlet relaxation	Signal is sent via Bradley's loop III.
Bladder emptying*	

*Normally, this step can be inhibited by voluntary contraction of the striated sphincter muscle and suppression of detrusor contraction via loop III.

Adapted with permission from Badlani, G.H., Foley, C.J., and Snyder, J.A.: Evaluation of urinary dysfunction in the elderly. Semin. Urol., 5:88, 1987.

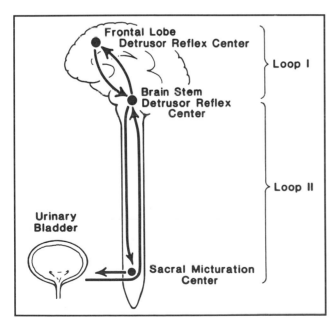

FIGURE 16–9.   Neural pathway for micturition control: loops I and II. (Reprinted with permission from Badlani, G.H., Foley, C.J., and Snyder, J.A.: Evaluation of urinary dysfunction in the elderly. Semin. Urol, 5:88, 1987.)

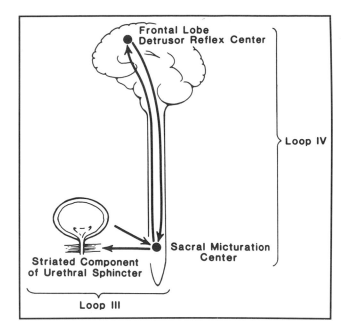

FIGURE 16–10. Neural pathway for micturition control: loops III and IV. (Reprinted with permission from Badlani, G.H., Foley, C.J., and Snyder, J.A.: Evaluation of urinary dysfunction in the elderly. Semin. Urol., 5:88, 1987.)

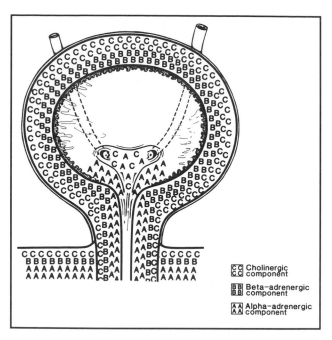

FIGURE 16–11. The urinary bladder: receptor distribution in the bladder and the outlet. ▨ Cholinergic component; ▨ beta-adrenergic component; ▨ alpha-adrenergic component. (Reprinted with permission from Badlani, G.H., and Smith, A.D.: Pharmacotherapy of voiding dysfunction in the elderly. Semin. Urol., 5:121, 1987.)

ation to permit complete bladder emptying. Table 16–4 and Figures 16–9 and 16–10 provide an overview of this process and demonstrate the involved neural pathways.

In clinical practice, disorders of urine storage and emptying often require therapy. This requires a basic understanding of the neuropharmacology of the

bladder and bladder neck. These structures are composed almost entirely of smooth muscle and are innervated by the parasympathetic and sympathetic divisions of the autonomic nervous system. The parasympathetic nerves originate in the sacral (S2,3,4) portions of the cord. The preganglionic fibers (pelvic nerves) synapse near the bladder, and

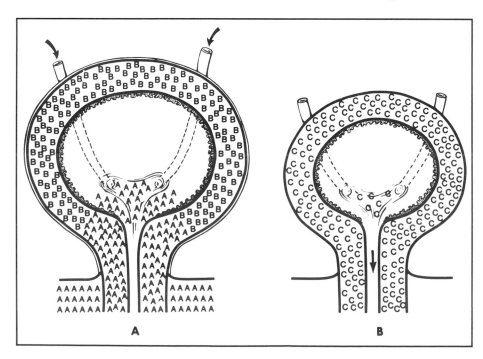

FIGURE 16–12. The urinary bladder: A, Filling (sympathetic) phase; B, emptying (parasympathetic) phase. (Reprinted with permission from Badlani, G.H., and Smith, A.D.: Pharmacotherapy of voiding dysfunction in the elderly. Semin. Urol., 5:121, 1987.)

the neurotransmitter at this level is acetylcholine. The short postganglionic fibers also have acetylcholine as the neurotransmitter. The sympathetic nerves from the thoracolumbar cord (T10 to L2) have short preganglionic fibers that terminate in ganglia of the paravertebral sympathetic chain. The neurotransmitter is acetylcholine. The relatively long postganglionic fibers travel through the presacral plexus and arborize as the hypogastric nerves that innervate the bladder and bladder neck. The neurotransmitter at the neuromuscular junction is norepinephrine, but beta adrenergic receptors predominate in the fundus of the bladder while alpha receptors densely populate the bladder neck (Fig. 16–11) Stimulation of beta receptors leads to relaxation of the body of the bladder, which promotes urine storage, as does alpha stimulation, which closes the bladder neck to maintain continence during filling (Fig. 16–12A). Cholinergic stimulation (Fig. 16–12B) promotes bladder contraction, and emptying is facilitated by simultaneous inhibition of sympathetic activity. Thus, the pharmacotherapy of voiding dysfunction uses drugs designed to promote storage (anticholinergics, alpha agonists) or facilitate emptying (cholinergics, alpha antagonists).

BIBLIOGRAPHY

1. Vander, A.J.: Renal Physiology, 3rd ed. New York, McGraw-Hill Publishing Co. 1985.
2. Berndt, W.O, and Stitzel, E.: Water, electrolyte metabolism, and diuretic drugs. *In* Craig, C.R., and Stitzel, R. E. (eds.): Modern Pharmacology. Boston, Little, Brown, and Company, 1990.
3. Schrier, R.W., and Gottschalk, C.W.: Diseases of the Kidney, 4th ed. Boston, Little, Brown, and Company, 1988.
4. Brenner, B.M., and Rector, F.C. Jr.: The Kidney, 3rd ed. Philadelphia, W.B. Sauders Co., 1986.
5. Leslie, B.R., and Vaughan, E.D. Jr.: Normal renal physiology. *In* Walsh, P.C., Gittes, R.F., Perlmutter, A.D., and Stamey, T.A. (eds.): Campbell's Urology, 5th ed. Philadelphia, W.B. Saunders Co., 1986.
6. Weiss, R.M.: Physiology and pharmacology of the renal pelvis and ureter. *In* Walsh, P.C., Gittes, R.F., Perlmutter, A.D., and Stamey, T.A. (eds.): Campbell's Urology, 5th ed. Philadelphia, W.B. Saunders Co., 1986.
7. Bradley, W.E.: Physiology of the urinary bladder. *In* Walsh, P.C., Gittes, R.F., Perlmutter, A.D., and Stamey, T.A. (eds.): Campell's Urology, 5th ed. Philadelphia, W.B. Sauders Co., 1986.

17

PHYSIOLOGY OF THE THYROID

CHARLES G. WATSON

The thyroid gland in adults is a 15- to 20-gm bilobulated gland, straddling the anterior aspect of the proximal trachea, and responsible for the synthesis and release of levothyroxine (T_4), triiodothyronine (T_3), and calcitonin. Embryologically the thyroid first appears at 3 weeks of age as an ectodermal proliferation in the midline floor of the pharyngeal gut. Proliferation results in a diverticulum that descends in the midline (thyroglossal duct) and then develops into a bilobed structure that, by the seventh week, receives branchiogenic material from the fourth pharyngeal pouch (the ultimobranchial bodies). The thyroglossal duct then disappears, although remnants may persist in the form of ectopic thyroid, thyroglossal duct cysts, or a pyramidal lobe (in 30 per cent of adult thyroids).

Each thyroid lobe is subdivided by fibrous extensions of its capsule into lobules that in turn are subdivided into individual follicles. Each follicle is a sphere consisting of a single layer of epithelial (follicular) cells enclosing a space filled with colloid (viscous thyroglobulin solution). Half of a follicle's surface interfaces with capillaries, and the capillary network expands with follicular hyperplasia. The prominent vascularity reflects the robust metabolic activity of the follicular cell. Lymphatic networks exist, but are less apparent histologically and drain into both cervical and mediastinal collecting systems. There is histologic evidence of both sympathetic and parasympathetic innervation, the functional roles of which are unclear. Parafollicular cells derived from the lateral (ultimobranchial) thyroid anlagen are by and large clustered between follicles, with a few cells appearing in the wall of a follicle.

The two functional cellular components of the thyroid gland, the follicular and parafollicular cells, synthesize and secrete hormones with distinctly different chemical composition and peripheral effects. The two hormones, thyroid hormone (follicular cells) and calcitonin (parafollicular cells), are considered separately.

THYROID HORMONE

The synthesis, storage, release, circulatory transport, and peripheral utilization of thyroid hormone involve a complex array of biochemical and physiologic reactions, many of which are well understood. The bioactive thyroid hormones are thyroxine (3, 5, 3', 5'-tetraiodothyronine) or T_4 and 3, 5, 3'-triiodothyronine or T_3. Reverse T_3 (rT_3) or 3, 3', 5'-triiodothyronine has negligible biologic activity and is rapidly metabolized.

The synthesis of thyroid hormones is absolutely dependent upon the bioavailability of iodide. The major dietary sources of iodide are iodized bread, iodized salt, and dairy products. "Contaminating" sources include various medications, radiologic contrast agents, and disinfectants. The minimal daily requirement of iodide is 75 μg and the average American diet contains 500 μg a day, ingested in both inorganic and organically bound forms. Dietary iodides are efficiently absorbed from the gastrointestinal tract, circulate with a pool size of 250 μg, and are actively extracted by both thyroid and kidney; the renal extraction matches more or less the dietary iodide intake. The thyroid iodide pool approximates 8000 μg, 1 per cent of which is turned over on a daily basis. The transport of iodide into the follicular cell via an iodide "pump" or "trap" is an energy-dependent process capable of achieving a 20- to 40-fold concentration gradient across the follicular cell membrane. The iodide gradient is increased even further under the influence of TSH stimulation and in the face of dietary iodide deprivation. The effect of TSH upon iodide transport is blunted by increasing intracellular iodine concentrations and is inhibited altogether in the presence of certain anions, most notably perchlorate and thiocyanate.

The other prerequisite for thyroid hormone synthesis is the availability of thyroglobulin, which is synthesized within the rough-surfaced endoplasmic reticulum of the follicular cell and extruded by exo-

288

cytosis into the follicular lumen under the stimulation of thyroid-stimulating hormone (TSH). Thyroglobulin is a large, complicated, soluble polypeptide with a molecular weight of 660,000; it contains many tyrosine residues within its matrix. Iodination of these tyrosine residues takes place outside the cell within colloid. In the presence of thyroperoxidase and hydrogen peroxide, iodide is oxidized to a higher oxygen state (I^+) and then organified, binding to the tyrosine residues within the thyroglobulin matrix to form diiodotyrosine (DIT) and monoiodotyrosine (MIT). Thyroperoxidase is thought also to be responsible for catalyzing the coupling of the resulting iodotyrosines to form thyroxine (from two molecules of DIT) and triiodothyronine (from one molecule of DIT and one molecule of MIT) (Fig. 17–1). The rate of iodination of the tyrosine residues increases with increasing extracellular concentration of iodide until a maximum rate is achieved. Above a certain extracellular iodide concentration, iodination of tyrosine is inhibited (Wolff-Chaikoff effect)

from which the thyroid escapes or to which it adapts in several days. This accounts at least in part for the temporary antithyroid effect of the oral administration of excessive iodide in the preparation of hyperthyroid patients for thyroidectomy.

The most commonly used antithyroid agents are the thionamides, examples of which are methimazole and propylthiouracil. The thionamides impair the iodination of the tyrosine residues within the thyroglobulin matrix, as well as the coupling of iodotyrosines to form T_4 and T_3. The method of action is thought to be through the inhibition of thyroperoxidase. Under normal circumstances, ten times as much T_4 is produced than T_3. Thyroid hormone is stored as an iodothyronyl residue within the thyroglobulin matrix. Thyroglobulin is essential to thyroid hormone homeostasis through its (1) high capacity for hormonogenesis, (2) modulation of thyroid hormone production in response to the availability of iodide, and (3) its storage of thyroid hormone within the protective intrafollicular environment, which is

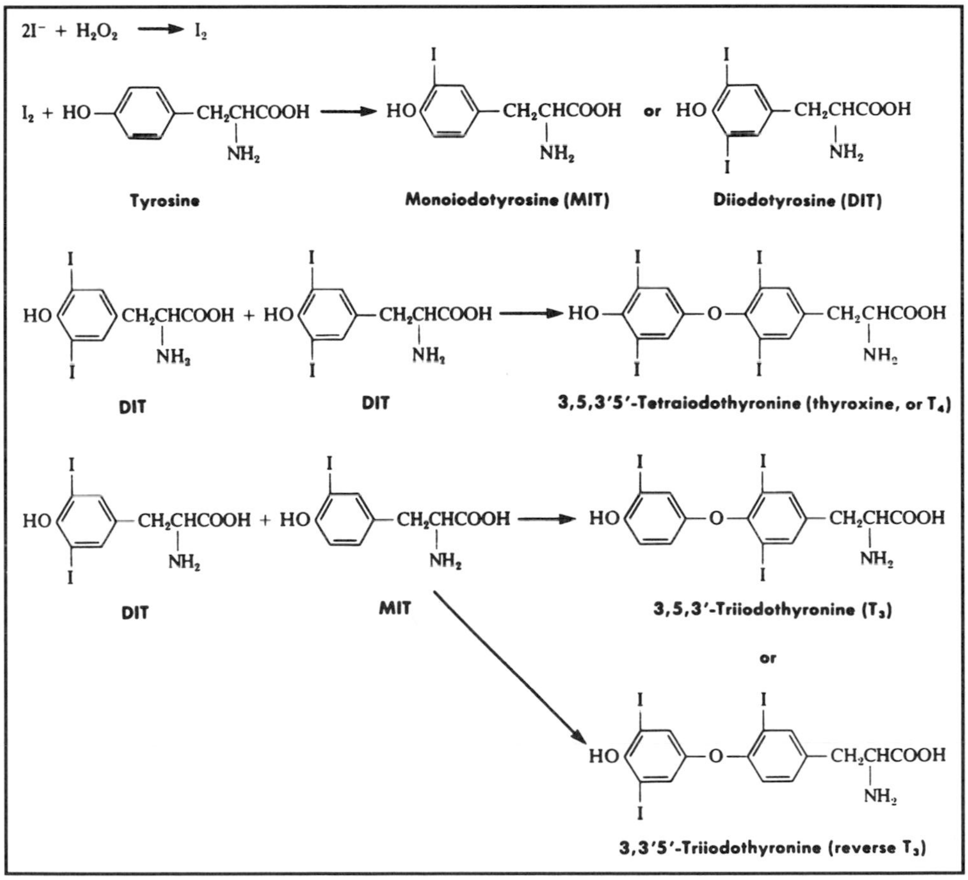

FIGURE 17–1. Outline of thyroid hormone synthesis. Tyrosine as a component of thyroglobulin is iodinated under the influence of thyroperoxidase and hydrogen peroxide. Thyroperoxidase is thought to catalyze the coupling of iodotryosines to form tetraiodothyronine and triiodothyronine. These reactions occur within the lumen of the thyroid follicle. (Modified from Genuth, S.M.: The thyroid gland. *In* Berne R.M., and Levy, M.N. (eds.): Physiology, 2nd ed. St. Louis, C.V. Mosby Co., 1988, p. 935.)

capable of maintaining a euthyroid state for 2 months in the absence of hormone synthesis.

In response to TSH, the follicular cell resorbs thyroglobulin. Within the cell, thyroglobulin is exposed to lysosomal proteases, thereby splitting off iodothyronines (T_3 and T_4), as well as iodotyrosines (MIT and DIT); the iodotyrosines are degraded further by intrathyroid deiodinases, which allow the iodide to be recycled within the follicle cell. Free thyroid hormones (iodothyronines) are released into the circulation via the basal end of the follicular cell. Under normal circumstances roughly 80 μg of T_4 and 6 μg of T_3 are produced a day (Fig. 17–2).

In the circulation, roughly 70 per cent of T_4 and T_3 are bound to thyroid hormone-binding globulin (TBG) and the remainder to albumin and prealbumin. Only 0.03 per cent of total T_4 and 0.30 per cent of total T_3 exist in plasma in their free forms. Because of the higher affinity of T_4 than T_3 for

thyroid hormone-binding proteins, T_4 is metabolized more slowly and has a longer half-life (7 days) than T_3 (1 day). The concentration of TBG may be affected by rare inherited defects and by various drugs, hormones, and disease states. Hyperestrogenism characteristically increases the concentration of TBG. In pregnancy an increased TBG is apparent by the third week, peaks late in the second and early third trimester (up to 2 1/2 times normal concentrations), and may persist for up to 4 to 6 weeks after delivery.

Though T_4 is synthesized and transported as the predominant thyroid hormone, it is in actuality a prehormone insofar as most of the circulating free T_4 and that bound to albumin are converted peripherally to T_3, with the remaining T_4 being excreted. T_3 is biologically ten times as active as T_4. Most of the peripheral conversion of T_4 occurs in the liver and kidney where it is catalyzed by the enzyme 5' de-

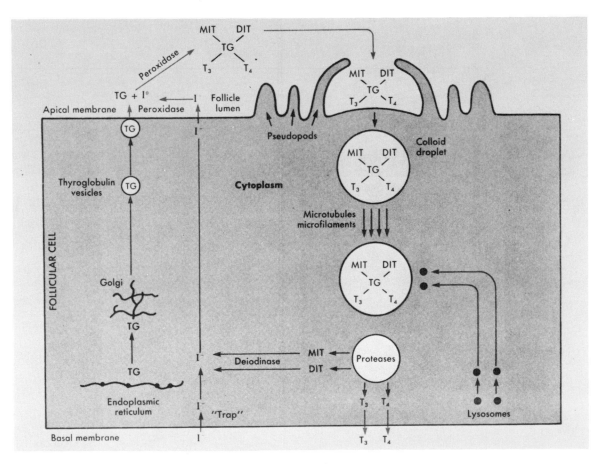

FIGURE 17–2. Thyroid hormone synthesis, transport, and release into the bloodstream. The follicular cell is the site of thyroglobulin synthesis and absorption, transport, degradation, and secretion of the thyroid hormones, T_3 and T_4. Iodide recovered from intracellular thyroid hormone proteolysis is recycled and added to the iodide pool for iodination of tyrosine residues within the intrafollicular thyroglobulin matrix. The rate of iodide uptake and thyroid hormonogenesis and release is determined by the concentration of TSH. (Modified from Genuth, S.M.: The thyroid gland. *In* Berne, R.M., and Levy M.N. (eds.): Physiology, 2nd ed. St. Louis, C.V. Mosby Co., 1988, p. 938.)

iodinase I, which releases T_3 into the circulation. The enzyme 5' de-iodinase I is inactivated by propylthiouracil (PTU) but not by methimazole. Its concentration is decreased with starvation (protein-sparing effect) and increased with increased thyroid hormonogenesis, with the resultant increased formation of T_3. In the pituitary a related but different enzyme, 5' de-iodinase II, is responsible for converting T_4 to T_3, which in turn inhibits the release of thyroid-stimulating hormone (TSH). The enzyme 5' de-iodinase II is not inhibited by PTU. Both the oral cholecystography contrast agent, iopanoic acid, and the anti-arrhythmic amiodarone inhibit 5' de-iodinase I and II, resulting in increased levels of both TSH and T_4. Iodide conservation is accomplished by (1) storage within the thyroglobulin matrix in the form of iodinated tyrosine; 2) recycling within the follicular cell after the de-iodination of MIT and DIT; and, (3) binding in the form of iodothyronine to thyroid hormone-binding proteins, therefore avoiding renal clearance and excretion.

The physiologic effects of thyroid hormone are manifold and primarily are the result of the interaction of T_3 with specific nuclear receptors. Thyroid hormone increases cellular oxygen consumption, enhances the effects of tissue growth factors, increases the rate of protein synthesis and degradation, and affects most aspects of carbohydrate metabolism. A constant supply of thyroid hormone is essential for growth and development, for maintaining normal levels of intermediary metabolism, and for the overall normal functional activity of most organs.

The metabolic effects of thyroid hormone on the heart rate, central nervous system, and motor activity superficially resemble those produced by adrenergic hormones. Evidence is available to support the ideas that the cAMP response to epinephrine in heart muscle is augmented by T_3 and that T_3 increases the number of beta adrenergic receptors in heart muscle. Beta adrenergic blockade relieves many of the physiologic manifestations of hyperthyroidism.

The rate of thyroid hormone production is dependent upon the concentration of TSH, the availability of iodide, and the integrity of the thyroid and its component follicles. TSH secretion is controlled by the hypothalamic thyrotropin-releasing hormone (TRH). The responsiveness of TSH to TRH is inversely related to the intracellular concentration of thyroid hormone (predominantly T_3). Somatostatin, dopamine, and supraphysiologic levels of adrenocorticosteroids have an inhibitory effect on TSH secretion. TSH binds to follicular cell surface receptors and induces cyclic AMP formation and a cascade of metabolic events, including iodide uptake and transport, thyroglobulin synthesis and exocytotic excretion into the follicular lumen, and thyroglobulin resorption, which results in the enhanced secretion of thyroid hormone.

LABORATORY ASSESSMENT

Several laboratory tests are available to assess both the level of thyroid function and the various causes of thyroid dysfunction. Total iodothyronine levels (both T_4 and T_3) are readily assessed by radioimmunoassay. Because the bioavailable levels of both T_4 and T_3 are a fraction of 1 per cent of the total and because the remainder is bound to circulating thyroid hormone-binding proteins (particularly TBG), TBG levels have a significant effect on the levels of total T_4 and total T_3 and the interpretation thereof. Although TBG levels may be determined by RIA, such tests are not clinically available. It is possible, however, to determine the availability of thyroid hormone-binding sites on TBG by indirect methods. One such method is the T_3-resin uptake (T_3-RU) in which a small amount of radiolabeled T_3 is equilibrated with a serum sample. During the period of equilibration, available TBG binding sites will bind a certain fraction of the radioactive additive. The serum containing the unbound radiolabeled T_3 is then absorbed onto a cation exchange resin, with the measured resin uptake being inversely proportional to the available TBG binding sites. An increased T_3-RU would reflect a decreased number of available thyroid hormone-binding sites as seen in patients with excessive production of thyroid hormone (e.g., hyperthyroidism) or in the presence of decreased concentrations of TBG. On the other hand, a decreased T_3-RU would suggest an increased number of available thyroid hormone-binding sites on TBG as seen in the face of decreased production of thyroid hormone (hypothyroidism) or with an increased concentration of TBG, i.e., hyperestrogenism. T_3-RU is expressed either as percentage uptake or the ratio of the resultant resin uptake as compared to the resin uptake of normal pooled sera.

The T_3-RU and total T_4 are then combined to calculate a unitless index referred to as the free thyroxine index (FTI). The FTI correlates reasonably well with the functional status of the thyroid under most circumstances. In the normal adult, total T_4 varies between 5 and 12 μg/dL, total T_3 between 70 and 200 ng/dL, and the normal range for FTI between 0.85 and 1.15. Increased TBG levels may result from hyperestrogenism (both endogenous and exogenous), acute and chronic active hepatitis, and inherited disorders. Diminished TBG levels are the result of exposure to excessive androgens and anabolic steroids, supraphysiologic levels of corticosteroids, chronic liver disease, chronic systemic illness, acromegaly, proteinuria, and rare hereditary disorders.

With hyperthyroidism, the synthesis and release of T_4 and T_3 are both significantly elevated, but to a much greater degree with T_3. For this reason, if the FTI in a patient with suspected hyperthyroidism is normal, a more sensitive diagnostic test would be the determination of total T_3 by RAI. The diagnosis might also be suspected by documenting decreased levels of TSH. Until recently, TSH determinations by RAI were relatively insensitive, but ultrasensitive TSH assays are now available and may be diagnostic in "early" cases of hypothyroidism (elevated TSH) and hyperthyroidism (depressed levels of TSH). Another sensitive assay to diagnose early hyperthyroidism assesses the impact of TRH on TSH concentrations by the TRH stimulation test. Five hundred micrograms of TRH are administered intravenously, and serial TSH measurements are obtained over a period of 2 hours. In the face of increased circulating levels of T_4 and T_3, the TSH response to administered TRH is "blunted" or absent.

Radioactive iodine uptake (RAIU) may provide additional information about thyroid functional derangements. A small quantity of radioiodine is administered, and 24 hours later the percent uptake by the thyroid is determined. In hyperthyroid patients in whom there is an excessive production of thyroid hormone, RAIU uptake is increased. In the hyperthyroid phase of acute thyroiditis with decreased hormonogenesis and an increased release of preformed hormone, RAIU uptake may be depressed.

In those receiving exogenous T_4 for replacement or for TSH-suppressive purposes, the FTI is elevated in up to 50 per cent of patients who are euthyroid by every other parameter. Therefore, a more reliable biochemical index of the thyroid functional state in the face of exogenous T_4 administration is the determination of T_3 by RAI.

A number of thyroid diseases appear to be mediated by immunologic mechanisms. Antibodies to thyroglobulin and to thyroid epithelial cell microsomal antigen are found in many patients with autoimmune thyroiditis of the fibrotic and lymphocytic (Hashimoto's) type. In addition, antithyroid antibodies have been found in Graves' disease stimulating the thyroid gland by interacting with TSH-binding sites. Furthermore, infiltrative ophthalmopathy present in a few patients with Graves' disease may be caused by antibodies against human eye muscle.

CALCITONIN

Calcitonin is a 32 amino acid single chain polypeptide synthesized by the parafollicular cells (C cells) found in the mammalian thyroid and submammalian ultimobranchial bodies. The C cells are neuroendocrine cells of neural crest origin that arise ventrally in the fourth branchial pouch and descend embryologically as the lateral anlagen (ultimobranchial bodies) of the developing thyroid. They are members of the class of APUD (amine precursor uptake and decarboxylase) cells and as such may participate in polyendocrine syndromes (multiple endocrine neoplasm (MEN) IIa, IIb, see Chapter 18).

There is considerable variance in the amino acid sequence from species to species, resulting in different levels of bioactivity. For example, salmon calcitonin is ten times as potent as human calcitonin in human in vivo studies.

Calcitonin is bound to cell membrane receptors, resulting in the excitation of adenylate cyclase and protein kinase. Membrane binding sites for calcitonin have been demonstrated in both osteoclasts and renal proximal tubal epithelial cells, and osteoclasts have been demonstrated to be exquisitely sensitive to calcitonin. In response to calcitonin stimulation of the osteoclast, bone resorption is inhibited, resulting in decreased serum calcium and phosphate levels. Calcitonin binding in the kidney results in increased renal losses of calcium, phosphate, and sodium, as well as increased production of $1,25\text{-}(OH_2)D_3$. The exact role of calcitonin in humans is not well understood, although it appears to be that of skeletal protection, rather than calcium homeostasis. Calcium homeostasis appears not to be affected by total thyroidectomy in humans. Elevated levels of calcitonin during pregnancy, growth, and lactation would support the concept of the skeletal protective role of calcitonin during periods of calcium stress. In the postmenopausal female, progressive bone loss coexists with decreased calcitonin concentrations and may be minimized by the administration of calcitonin.

Serum calcitonin levels are determined by radioimmunoassay. The normal basal concentration in humans is 5-100 pg/mL. Its half-life is 5 minutes. Stimuli for C cell secretion of calcitonin are calcium and various GI hormones, most notably gastrin. Serum calcitonin assays are employed clinically to diagnose a medullary (C cell) carcinoma of the thyroid (MCT) or to screen for C cell hyperplasia of MCT. In screening patients who are suspected of having MCT and relatives of patients with MCT for familial MCT or the MEN IIa and IIb syndromes, basal calcitonin levels are relatively insensitive. Therefore, all such individuals should be tested with a pentagastrin-stimulated calcitonin assay.

The clinical uses of salmon calcitonin are limited, but include (1) the treatment of the osteolytic form of Paget's disease; (2) management of severe postmenopausal osteoporosis, although the results of long-term therapy are not known; (3) management of hypercalcemia of surgically uncontrolled metastatic parathyroid carcinoma; (4) management of symptomatic hypercalcemia of pseudohyperparathyroidism (paraneoplastic disorder); and (5) management of hypercalcemia in those few patients with symptomatic and surgically uncontrolled primary hyperparathyroidism. In the last three instances, long-term management of hypercalcemia is usually not feasible because of an apparent down-regulation of calcitonin cell membrane receptors within days of onset of therapy leading to an "escape" from the calcium lowering effects of calcitonin.

BIBLIOGRAPHY

1. Breslau, N.A.: Calcium homeostasis. *In* Griffin, J.E., and Ojeda, S.R., (eds.): Textbook of Endocrine Physiology. New York, Oxford University Press, 1988, pp. 284–286.
2. Ekholm, R.: Anatomy and development. *In* DeGroot, L.J., Besser, G.M., Cahill, G.H., Jr., Marshall, J.C., Nelson, D.H., Odell, W.D., Potts, J.T., Jr., Rubenstein, A.H., and Steinberger, A.H. (eds.): Endocrinology, vol. 1. Philadelphia, W.B. Saunders Co., 1989, pp. 505–511.
3. Griffin, J.E.: The thyroid. *In* Griffin, J.E., and Ojeda, S.R. (eds.): Textbook of Endocrine Physiology. New York. Oxford University Press, 1988, pp. 222–244.
4. Ingbar, S.H.: The thyroid gland. *In* Wilson, J.D., and Foster, D.W. (eds.): Williams Textbook of Endocrinology. Philadelphia. W.B. Saunders Co., 1985, pp. 682–815.
5. Larson, P.R., Silva, J.E., and Kaplan, M.N.: Relationships between circulating and intracellular thyroid hormones: Physiological and clinical implications. Endocrinol. Rev., *2:* 87–102, 1981.
6. Lavin, T.N.: Mechanisms of action of thyroid hormone. *In* DeGroot, L.J., Besser, G.M., Cahill, G.F., Jr., Marshall, J.C., Nelson, D.H., Odell, W.D., Potts, J.T., Jr., Rubenstein, A.H., and Steinberger, E. (eds.): Endocrinology, vol. 1. Philadelphia. W.B. Saunders Co., 1989, pp. 562–573.
7. Lissitzky, S., Torresani, J., Carayon, P., and Amr, S.: Physiology of the thyroid. *In* DeGroot, L.J., Besser, G.M., Cahill, G.F., Jr., Marshall, J.C., Nelson, D.H., Odell, W.D., Potts, J.T., Jr., Rubenstein, A.H., and Steinberger, E. (eds.): Endocrinology, vol. 1, Philadelphia, W.B. Saunders Co., 1989, pp. 512–540.
8. MacIntyre, I.: Calcitonin: Physiology, biosynthesis, secretion, metabolism, and mode of action. *In* DeGroot, L.J., Besser, G.M., Cahill, G.F., Jr., Marshall, J.C., Nelson, D.H., Odell, W.D., Potts, J.T., Jr., Rubenstein, A.H., and Steinberger, E. (eds.): Endocrinology, vol. 2. Philadelphia, W.B. Saunders Co., 1989, pp. 892–901.
9. Refetoff, S.: Thyroid function tests and effects of drugs on thyroid function. *In* DeGroot, L.J., Besser, G.M., Cahill, G.F., Jr., Marshall, J.C., Nelson, D.H., Odell, W.D., Potts, J.T., Jr., Rubenstein, A.H., and Steinberger, E. (eds.): Endocrinology, vol. 1. Philadelphia, W.B. Saunders Co., 1989, pp. 590–639.
10. Refetoff, S., and Larsen, P.R.: Transport, cellular uptake, and metabolism of thyroid hormone *In* DeGroot, L.J., Besser, G.M., Cahill, G.F., Jr., Marshall, J.C., Nelson, D.H., Odell, W.D., Potts, J.T., Jr., Rubenstein, A.H., and Steinberger, E. (eds.): Endocrinology, vol. 1. Philadelphia, W.B. Saunders Co., 1989, pp. 541–561.
11. Sarne, D.H., DeGroot, L.J.: Hypothalamic and neuroendocrine regulation of thyroid hormone. *In* DeGroot, L.J., Besser, G.M., Cahill, G.F., Jr., Marshall, J.C., Nelson, D.H., Odell, W.D., Potts, J.T., Jr., Rubenstein, A.H., and Steinberger, E. (eds.): Endocrinology, vol. 1. Philadelphia, W.B. Saunders Co., 1989, pp. 574–589.

18

CALCIUM HOMEOSTASIS: THE PARATHYROIDS AND VITAMIN D

CHARLES G. WATSON

Calcium homeostasis is essential for skeletal stability and optimal cellular and organ function. Although 99 per cent of the body's calcium is complexed in the mineral phase of bone, the remaining 1 per cent in the intra- and extracellular compartments is critical for neuromuscular excitability, blood coagulability, and the regulation of intracellular metabolic activity. Plasma calcium levels are maintained in a "tight" normal range, which in most laboratories is 8.5 to 10.5 mg/dL. The normal calcium range is maintained by a delicate balance between calcium absorption from and secretion into the intestines, accretion into and loss out of the skeleton, and the filtration into and reabsorption from urine. Plasma calcium exists in three components: 50 per cent in the free or ionized form, 40 per cent or more bound to protein, and the remainder organically complexed. Albumin accounts for most of the protein binding, and for each 1.0 gm/dL reduction in albumin concentration there is a 0.8 mg/dL reduction in total calcium concentration. The albumin binding of calcium is pH-dependent, being decreased in the face of acidosis and increased with alkalosis.

The average daily calcium oral intake is roughly 1 gm, one third of which is absorbed from the intestines; half of that amount, in turn, is resecreted into the intestines, yielding a net absorption of roughly 170 mg/day of calcium. Intestinal absorption of calcium, skeletal calcium outflow, and renal excretion and reabsorption of calcium are primarily controlled by parathyroid hormone (PTH) and 1,25-dihydroxyvitamin D_3 (1,25 $(OH)_2D_3$), the physiologic activities of which are interrelated. Calcitonin plays a lesser and much less well understood role in these processes (see Chapter 17). PTH and 1,25 $(OH)_2D_3$ are considered separately here, although their mechanisms of action are highly integrated.

Embryologically, parathyroid tissue develops in the third and fourth pharyngeal pouches as early as the sixth week of gestation. The paired inferior glands arise from the third pouch and ultimately descend with the thymus toward the inferior pole of the thyroid. The paired superior parathyroids arise from the fourth pharyngeal pouch and descend a shorter distance, along with the lateral anlagen (ultimobranchial bodies) of the thyroid. Any one of the four parathyroids may fail to descend or may hyperdescend, resulting in ectopic locations in the adult ranging from retropharyngeal to anterior mediastinal (inferior parathyroids) and posterior mediastinal (superior parathyroids). The parathyroids consist predominantly of chief cells; the other two types of cells are oxyphil and clear cells. Hyperfunctioning glands consisting predominantly of each of the three cell types have been described, although chief cell pathology is the most common.

The parathyroids synthesize and secrete one hormone (PTH) and various cleavage products. PTH is a single chain polypeptide consisting of 84 amino acids with a molecular weight of 9500. The intracellular synthetic sequence of events begins with the production of preproparathormone (115 amino acids), which is cleaved to proparathormone (90 amino acids), which is further cleaved to parathormone (84 amino acids). The two precursor forms are thought to play a role in the intracellular transport of PTH, are not secreted, and are biologically inactive. The rate of PTH synthesis is thought to be more or less constant. Intracellular hydrolysis of intact PTH yields free amino acids, as well as N-terminal (1-34 PTH) and middle-carboxy terminal (mid-C, 35-84 PTH) fragments. The rate of PTH hydrolysis varies proportionally with the plasma concentration of ionized calcium; therefore PTH secretion is regulated by plasma calcium levels through a negative feedback mechanism. To a much lesser degree, PTH production is also stimulated by hypomagnesemia and increased concentrations of beta adrenergic agonists and is inhibited by increased concentrations of 1,25 and 24,25 dihydroxyvitamin D_3.

Intact PTH (1-84) is metabolized by the Kupffer cells of liver, has a circulating half-life of 2 to 4 minutes, and is hydrolyzed to N-terminal, midmolecular, and C-terminal fragments. The N-terminal fragment of PTH (1-34) is the bioactive component of PTH, its site of degradation is unknown, and it is thought to have a half-life of 2 to 4 minutes. The mid-C fragments (35-84 PTH) are biologically inactive, comprise 80 per cent of the circulating PTH immunoactivity, are eliminated only by glomerular filtration, have a circulating half-life of an hour or so, and in the face of renal failure are significantly increased in concentration.

Intact PTH affects bone and kidney primarily (Table 18–1). In bone it stimulates the resorption of calcium and, with prolonged stimulation, destabilization of bone structure. In the kidney, PTH significantly increases the reabsorption of calcium, inhibits tubular reabsorption of phosphate, and stimulates the 1-hydroxylation of 25-hydroxyvitamin D_3, which in turn enhances intestinal absorption of calcium and phosphorus. PTH exerts its cellular effects through stimulation of adenylate cyclase, thereby increasing the concentrations of cyclic AMP; cyclic AMP appears in increased concentrations in urine with excess PTH stimulation.

VITAMIN D

In many countries, various foods are fortified with vitamin D; milk is the principal example of fortified food in the United States. The principal non-dietary source of vitamin D is the photosynthetic conversion of provitamin D_3 (7-dehydrocholesterol) to previtamin D_3, which is dependent upon the ultraviolet component of sunlight. Previtamin D_3 thermally converts to vitamin D_3 at room temperature in a process requiring several days; after conversion it binds to plasma vitamin-D-binding protein and is transported to the liver where 25-hydroxylation occurs. In turn, 25-hydroxyvitamin D_3 undergoes a second hydroxylation at the 1 position in the renal tubular epithelial cell, forming 1,25-dihydroxyvitamin D_3. The rate of 1 hydroxylation is dependent upon the availability of PTH and the existing concentration of 1,25-dihydroxyvitamin D_3. In turn, 1,25-dihydroxyvitamin D_3 increases serum calcium concentration by significantly increasing intestinal absorption of calcium and by mobilizing calcium from bone. The vitamin D effects on bone are mediated through increasing the number of osteoclasts and indirectly increasing osteolytic activity, possibly by inducing the release of osteoblast-derived resorp-

TABLE 18–1. EFFECTS OF PTH ON CALCIUM METABOLISM

Bone	↑	Calcium resorption
Kidney	↑	Calcium reabsorption
	↓	PO_4 reabsorption
		Stimulation of 1-hydroxylation of 25-hydroxy vitamin D, which in turn increases intestinal absorption of calcium

tive factors. In the intestine, 1,25-dihydroxyvitamin D_3 increases the calcium and phosphorous flux through intestinal mucosal cells by mechanisms that are not well understood. Parathyroid cell receptor sites for 1,25-dihydroxyvitamin D have been demonstrated, and evidence exists for an inhibitory effect of vitamin D on PTH secretion. By stimulating PTH secretion, decreased levels of 1,25-dihydroxyvitamin D_3 are thought to contribute to the secondary hyperparathyroidism associated with chronic renal failure.

PTH and 1,25-dihydroxyvitamin D_3 are the principal regulators of calcium metabolism in the human. Their biosynthesis and target organ effects are intertwined, although their physiologic effects differ. PTH regulates calcium metabolism on a minute-to-minute or hour-to-hour basis, whereas vitamin D modulates calcium concentrations at longer intervals (day-to-day, week-to-week, etc.). The role of calcitonin in humans is not well understood as there are no known calcitonin deficiency syndromes (see Chapter 17 for details of calcitonin physiology.).

HYPERCALCEMIA

Table 18–2 lists the most commn causes of hypercalcemia with their corresponding PTH levels.

The hypercalcemia seen in 10 to 20 per cent of patients with sarcoidosis and less frequently with other granulomatous disorders is associated with excessive conversion of vitamin D to 1,25-dihydroxy-

TABLE 18–2. COMMON CAUSES OF HYPERCALCEMIA

CAUSES OF HYPERCALCEMIA	INTACT PTH
Primary hyperparathyroidism	↑
Tertiary hyperparathyroidism	↑
Familial hypocalciuric hypocalcemia	↑
Pseudohyperparathyroidism	↓
Osteolytic metastases	↓
Multiple myeloma	↓
Sarcoidosis	↓
Hypervitaminosis D	↓
Milk alkaline syndrome	↓
Hyperthyroidism	↓

vitamin D_3. The production of activated vitamin D is probably extrarenal, and the cell most likely responsible for this production is the activated macrophage.

Hypercalcemia associated with various malignancies is multifactorial. The final common pathway appears to be tumor-stimulated osteoclastic bone resorption, resulting in osteolytic bone metastases and/or hypercalcemia. Malignancies associated with hypercalcemia fall into three distinct groups: hematologic cancers, solid tumors with skeletal metastases, and solid tumors without skeletal metastases. The hypercalcemia seen with hematologic cancers has been most commonly described with myeloma, and with certain myeloma cell lines, and osteoclast-activating factor has been demonstrated. There is usually a positive correlation between tumor cell burden, magnitude of bone destruction, and the degree of hypercalcemia.

Of the solid tumors with skeletal metastases, breast cancer is by far the most common. Tumor cells interface directly with bone, and there is evidence to suggest, as part of the cell-mediated immune response to the tumor, that lymphocytes and monocytes migrate to the site of metastasis, where they release osteoclast-activating factors. The relationship of osteoclast-activating factor and tumor cell-osteoclast interaction is conjectural.

In patients with solid tumors without skeletal metastases who present with hypercalcemia (pseudo-hyperparathyroidism), depressed parathyroid hormone levels, intestinal absorption of calcium and levels of 1,25-dihydroxyvitamin D_3 argue against PTH as the mediating factor. Prostaglandins, non-PTH parathyroid hormone receptor agonists, colony-stimulating factor, and tumor-derived transforming growth factors have been suggested as possible humoral agents mediating this response.

The diagnosis of primary hyperparathyroidism is suggested by repeatedly elevated serum calcium levels and is further corroborated by a currently available highly accurate serum intact PTH assay. In 1963, Berson and Yallow developed the first radioimmunoassay (RIA) for a polypeptide hormone—namely, a PTH RIA—for which they ultimately received the Nobel Prize. It was based on an antibody to a C-terminal PTH fragment. Over the ensuing 25 years, the assay has been refined and modified to include antisera to N-terminal and midmolecular PTH fragments, and its clinical applications have greatly expanded. In general, mid-C-terminal PTH assays have taken advantage of the fact that 80 per cent of circulating PTH immunoradioactivity resides in the C-terminal fragment, maximizing assay sensitivity. Until recently, only heterologous (bovine and porcine) PTH antigens were available. Currently, human PTH has become available through recombinant DNA technology, further enabling the refinement of the assay with an increase in its accuracy.

However, all RIAs for PTH have suffered by being unable to reliably differentiate patients with pseudohyperparathyroidism from those with primary hyperparathyroidism, there being a significant assay overlap between the radioimmunoactivity of PTH-related peptide (pseudohyperparathyroidism) and PTH (primary parathyroidism). More recently, a highly sensitive two-site immunoradiometric (IRMA) assay has been developed for the quantitation of intact PTH, utilizing the sequential application of anti mid-C-terminal PTH (39-84) and anti N-terminal PTH (1-34) antibodies. An inert substance (polystyrene) is coated with anti PTH 39-84, which, on exposure to the test serum, binds with intact PTH and all C-terminal PTH fragments. A second antibody, an anti N-terminal (1-34) PTH, is radiolabeled with ^{125}I and then exposed to the anti C-terminal PTH complex. The amount of resultant bound radioactivity accurately reflects the concentration of intact PTH. The PTH-related peptide associated with pseudohyperparathyroidism bears a striking homology with the N-terminal component of human PTH, but is a 115 amino acid polypeptide. Most of the molecule is chemically and immunologically different from PTH and fails to react to the the IRMA PTH assay. The IRMA intact PTH assay has thereby a distinct advantage over previously available RIAs by clearly differentiating between primary and pseudohyperparathyroidism (Fig. 18–1).

The differentiation of pseudohyperparathyroidism from primary hyperparathyroidism can be further corroborated by determining 1,25-dihydroxyvitamin D_3 levels and the chloride-phosphate ratio. The hypercalcemia of pseudohyperparathyroidism suppresses PTH secretion, which in turn decreases the 1 hydroxylation of 25 hydroxyvitamin D by the kidney; this results in a reduced concentration of 1,25-dihydroxyvitamin D_3 in patients with pseudohyperparathyroidism. Patients with pseudohyperparathyroidism tend to be alkalotic and exhibit a chloride-phosphate ratio of less than 33. More often than not, the chloride phosphate ratio in patients with primary hyperparathyroidism is greater than 33.

The three disorders that are associated with an elevated serum calcium and an elevated IRMA intact PTH level are primary hyperparathyroidism, tertiary hyperparathyroidism, and familial hypocalciuric hypercalcemia (FHH). Because tertiary hyperparathyroidism is associated with renal failure and intact PTH values tend to be considerably higher than those seen with primary hyperparathyroidism, the differentiation between primary and tertiary hyperparathyroidism is straightforward. FHH is an uncommon hereditary disorder characterized by hypercalcemia, hyperparathormonemia, and hypocalciuria, its distinguishing feature. Patients with FHH appear to have an elevated cell membrane threshold for ionized calcuim, are hypercalcemic and hyper-

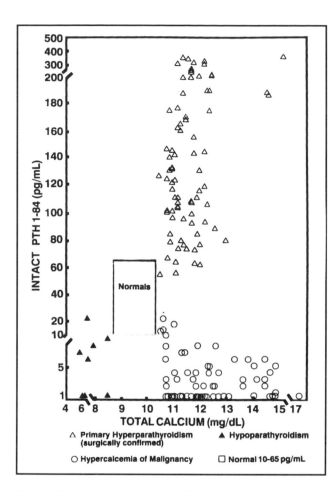

FIGURE 18–1. Intact PTH (IRMA) and total calcium in various disease states. (Reprinted with permission of Nichols Institute Reference Laboratories, San Juan Capistrano, CA 92675.)

parathormonemic for life, and remain free of the nonspecific symptoms (polydypsia, polyuria, constipation, depression, fatigability) and specific target organ involvement (nephrolithiasis, nephrocalcinosis, osteitis fibrosa, peptic ulcer disease) associated with primary hyperparathyroidism. The diagnosis of FHH is made by the documentation of a depressed 24-hour urine calcium in the face of hypercalcemia and hyperparathormonemia. The diagnosis of primary hyperparathyroidism is therefore one of exclusion, made by ruling out FHH and tertiary hyperparathyroidism in the face of an elevated calcium and elevated serum intact PTH.

Although usually a sporadic disorder, primary hyperparathyroidism may be inherited in the setting of

familial hyperparathyroidism or as a component of a polyendocrine syndrome [multiple endocrine neoplasm (MEN) Type I or Type IIA]. MEN I consists of neoplasms of the pituitary (benign) and pancreatic islets (benign or malignant) and hyperparathyroidism (usually benign). MEN IIA consists of adrenal medullary neoplasms (pheochromocytoma, usually multiple, benign or malignant), thyroid parafollicular (C cell) disorders (usually medullary carcinoma, occasionally its precursor, C cell hyperplasia), and hyperparathyroidism (usually benign). MEN IIB is identical to MEN IIA except for the absence of parathyroid disease and the presence of frequently associated submucosal neuromas throughout the GI tract, hyperplastic corneal nerves, ocular hypertelorism, and marfanoid features. The pathology of hyperparathyroidism in any one of the inherited disorders is hyperplasia, to which there are very few reported exceptions.

BIBLIOGRAPHY

1. Breslau, N.A.: Calcium homeostasis. *In* Griffin, J.E., and Ojeada, S.R. (eds.): Textbook of Endocrine Physiology. New York, Oxford University Press, 1988. Chapter 14, pp. 273–301.
2. Bringhurst, F.R.: Calcium and phosphate distribution, turnover, and metabolic actions. *In* Besser, G.M., Cahill, G.E., Jr., Marshall, J.C., Nelson, D.H., O'Dell, W.D., Potts, J.T., Jr., Rubenstein, A.H., and Steinberger, E. (eds.): Endocrinology. Philadelphia, W.B. Saunders Co., 1989. Chapter 52, pp. 805–843.
3. Holick, M.F.: Vitamin D: Biosynthesis, metabolism, and mode of action. *In* Besser, G.M., Cahill, G.F., Jr., Marshall, J.C., Nelson, D.H., O'Dell, W.D., Potts, J.T., Jr., Rubenstein, A.H., Steinberger, E. (eds.): Endocrinology. Philadelphia, W.B. Saunders Co., 1989. Chapter 57, pp. 902–926.
4. Mundy G.R., Ibbotson, K.J., D.'Souza, S.M., Simpson, E.L., Jacobs, J.W., Martin, T.J.: The hypercalcemia of cancer: Clinical implications and pathogenic mechanisms. N. Engl. J. Med., *310:* 1718–1727, 1984.
5. Reichel, H., Koefler, H.P., and Norman, A.W.: The role of the vitamin D endocrine system in health and disease. N. Engl. J. Med., *320:* 980–991, 1989.
6. Rosenblatt, M., Kronenberg, H.M., and Potts, J.T., Jr.: Parathyroid hormone: Physiology, chemistry, biosynthesis, secretion, metabolism, and mode of action. *In* Besser, G.M., Cahill, G.E., Jr., Marshall, J.C., Nelson, D.H., O'Dell, W.D., Potts, J.T., Jr., Rubenstein, A.H., Steinberger, E. (eds.): Endocrinology. Philadelphia, W.B. Saunders Co., 1989. Chapter 54, pp. 848–891.
7. Berson, S.A., Yalow, R.S., Aurbach, G.D., and Potts, J.T., Jr.: Immunoassay of bovine and human parathyroid hormone. Proc. Natl. Acad. Sci. USA, *49:* 613, 1963.
8. Nussbaum, S., Keutmann, H., Wang, C.A. Potts, J.T., Jr., and Segre, G.: Development of a highly sensitive two site immunoradiometric assay for parathyroid hormone and its clinical utility in evaluation of patients with hypercalcemia. Clin. Chem., *33:* 1364, 1987.

19

THE ADRENAL GLAND

K. ERIC SOMMERS *and* CHARLES G. WATSON

The adrenal glands comprise two distinctive organs, the medulla and cortex. Derived from embryologically different sources and secreting different hormones, the medulla and cortex appear to have little in common except an anatomic locale. However, considered as a whole, the adrenal's response to stress constitutes the fundamental host endocrine defense to injury (and operation).

The adrenal glands are situated in the retroperitoneum adjacent to the superior pole of the kidneys at about the T12 level. They receive arterialized blood from three main sources: the aorta, the renal, and the phrenic arteries. Each adrenal is drained by a single large vein that drains into the renal vein on the left and directly into the vena cavae on the right, a fact of importance in operations on the adrenals. The medulla receives preganglionic sympathetic innervation from the splanchnic nerves. Grossly, normal adrenal glands weigh between 5 to 10 gm and appear yellow. The medulla makes up approximately 10 per cent of the total gland weight.

ADRENAL CORTEX

Embryology and Histology

The adrenal cortex is derived from celomic mesoderm from which gonadal tissue also arises. The fetal adrenal is composed of two distinct layers: the inner layer, which is seen only during fetal growth and degenerates shortly after birth, and the outer layer, which goes on to develop into the adult adrenal cortex. Fetal adrenocortical secretion is composed largely of dihydroepiandrosterone, but by the time of birth, cortisol secretion predominates. Fetal cortisol levels are usually higher than maternal levels during parturition.

The mature adrenal cortex is divided histologically into three zones: glomerulosa, fasciculata, and reticularis (from capsule to medulla). The glomerulosa is chiefly concerned with mineralocorticoid se-

cretion; the size of this zone increases with salt deprivation, angiotensin stimulation, potassium loading, and, to a lesser extent adrenocorticotropin (ACTH) stimulation. The fasciculata and reticularis are primary sites of glucocorticoid synthesis, and the width of these zones is responsive to ACTH stimulation.

Hormone Biochemistry

Three classes of steroid hormones are secreted by the adrenal cortex: glucocorticoids, mineralocorticoids, and androgens. The glucocorticoid or mineralocorticoid potency of any adrenocorticoid hormone is determined by the relative affinity of the hormone for the glucocorticoid or mineralocorticoid receptors. Thus, adrenocorticoids exhibit a range of relative glucocorticoid versus mineralocorticoid potency. Table 19–1 lists the relative potency of common steroid compounds. The term "glucocorticoid" was historically used to describe the prominent effect of these compounds on carbohydrate metabolism, although a myriad of physiologic effects were subsequently ascribed to glucocorticoids. Mineralocorticoids, on the other hand, are more specific in their effects, which relate primarily to electrolyte and water regulation.

Cholesterol is the precursor of all adrenal steroids. The rate-limiting step of steroid synthesis is the side chain cleavage reaction, which removes the six carbon side chain of cholesterol at C-20. This reaction produces the precursor molecule pregnenolone, which can follow several pathways of steroid synsthesis (Fig. 19–1). The biochemical mechanism by which ACTH stimulates cortisol synthesis is not known; however, it has been postulated that ACTH, in concert with a "labile protein factor," facilitates cholesterol transport into the mitochondria where the side chain cleavage reaction occurs, thereby driving steroid production. Cyclic AMP has been proposed as the mediator of this reaction.

The rate of adrenal corticoid secretion is variable, but under basal conditions approximately 15 to 20 mg of cortisol and 50 to 200 mcg of aldosterone are

298

TABLE 19–1. PHARMACEUTICAL DERIVATIVES OF ADRENOCORTICOSTEROIDS

ORAL PREPARATIONS

USP Name	Trade Name(s)	Anti-Inflammatory Relative Potency (Cortisol = 1)	Mineralocorticoid Relative Potency (D O C = 1)	Anti-Inflammatory Mineralocorticoid
Dexamethasone	Decadron, Deronil, Dexameth, Gammacorten, Hexadrol	30.0	Mild natriuretic	∞
Betamethasone	Celestone	30.0	Mild natriuretic	∞
Triamcinolone	Aristocort, Kenacort	5.0	0	∞
Methylprednisolone	Medrol	6.0	0.02	300
Prednisone	Deltasone, Deltra, Meticorten, Paracort	4.0	0.04	100
Cortisone	Cortogen, Cortone	0.8	0.03	27
Hydrocortisone (cortisol)	Cortef, Contril, Hydrocort, Hydrocortone	1.0	0.03	33
Fludrocortisone (9α-fluorocortisol)	Cortef-F, Florinef	10.0	4.2	2.4
Deoxycorticosterone	Cortate, Decortin, Decosterone, Doca	0	1.0	0
Aldosterone	Not available	0.1	20	0.005

INTRAVENOUS PREPARATIONS		TOPICAL PREPARATIONS		SLOW-RELEASE PREPARATIONS	
USP Name	Trade Name	USP Name	Trade Name	USP Name	Trade Name
Hydrocortisone hemisuccinate	Solu-Cortef	Triamcinolone acetonide	Aristoderm Kenalog	Hydrocortisone acetate	Cortef acetate
Hydrocortisone phosphate	Hydrocortone phosphate	Fluocinolone acetonide	Synalar	Methylprednisolone acetate	Depo-Medrol
Methylprednisolone hemisuccinate	Solu-Medrol	Flurometholone	Oxylone	Deoxycorticosterone triethylacetate	Percorten
Dexamethasone phosphate	Decadron	Beclomethasone dipropionate	Vanceril		
Prednisolone phosphate	Hydeltrasol				

* In addition to these topical preparations, most of the anti-inflammatory steroids are supplied in the form of creams, aerosols, and eyedrops, for special topical use. Reprinted from Bondy, P.K.: Disorders of the adrenal cortex. *In* Wilson, J.D., and Foster, D.W. (eds.): Williams Textbook of Endocrinology, 7th ed. Philadelphia, W.B. Saunders Co., 1985, p. 843.

secreted daily. In serum, cortisol is bound by a high-affinity transport protein, corticosteroid-binding globulin (CBG), as well as by albumin, but with much lower affinity. Approximately 8 to 10 per cent of total serum cortisol is unbound. This fraction of "free" cortisol rises with increasing serum levels as serum binding sites become saturated. The physiologic range of total serum cortisol is 5 to 25 mcg/dL depending on the time of day. Unbound cortisol is the active form of the hormone and diffuses into cells where receptor binding occurs. Steroid metabolism occurs primarily within the liver where conjugation with glucuronic acid occurs. These soluble metabolites are excreted in the urine where they are measured as 17 hydroxy and 17 keto steroids. A small fraction of cortisol is excreted as free cortisol.

Steroid activity is dependent on binding to receptors in the cell cytoplasm. The glucocorticoid recep-tor is a soluble intracellular 94 kilodalton protein with one binding site per molecule, which binds the hormone in the cytoplasm and is subsequently bound to DNA in the nucleus. Steroid-receptor-DNA interaction leads in turn to messenger RNA production, and protein transcription soon follows. Thus, specific steroid hormonal action on cells and tissues is mediated by the proteins that are induced by steroid-receptor-DNA interaction.

Secretory Control Mechanisms

Cortisol secretion is under the primary control of adrenocorticotropin (ACTH), which in turn is secreted by the anterior pituitary in response to corticotropin-releasing factor (CRF). These are the elements of the hypothalamic-pituitary-adrenal axis

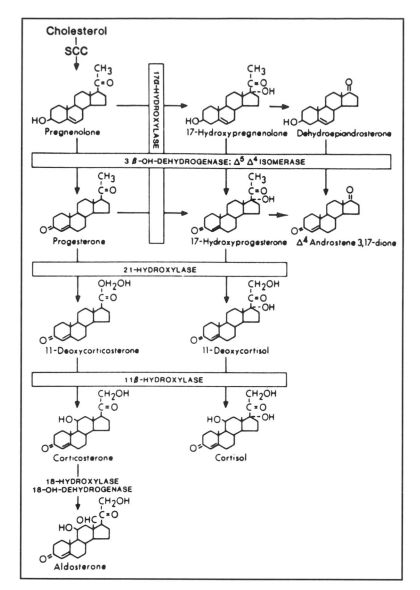

FIGURE 19–1. Pathway of biosynthesis of corticosteroids. (Reprinted from Simpson, E.R., and Waterman, M.R.: Steroid hormone biosynthesis in the adrenal cortex and its regulation by adrenocorticotropin. *In* DeGroot, L.J. (ed.): Endocrinology, 2nd ed. Philadelphia, W.B. Saunders Co., 1989. Chapter 93, p. 1544.)

(HPA). Chemically, CRF is a linear 41 amino acid peptide and ACTH is a 39 amino acid peptide released in the form of a precursor molecule, pro-opiomelanocortin (POMC). POMC gives rise to ACTH and many other cleavage products, including beta endorphin, melanocyte-stimulating hormone (MSH), enkephalin, and beta lipotrophin. Many of these and other cleavage products have been found to exert powerful neuroendocrine and immune influences.

The normal adrenocortical secretion of cortisol is characterized by two distinct features: a circadian rhythm and episodic secretion. Cortisol secretion peaks in the morning upon wakening and falls throughout the day until shortly after sleep when levels are lowest. This pattern can be changed by altering sleep-waking patterns or light-dark cycles, but only if the changes are maintained for several days. Absence of this normal diurnal cycle occurs in depression, congestive heart failure, and Cushing's syndrome.

The other unique characteristic of normal cortisol secretion is episodic secretion, an intermittent, spiking pattern of hormone secretion that gives rise to constantly fluctuating cortisol levels. These patterns are independent of environmental stimuli and are reproducible in given individuals. Neither the circadian nor the episodic secretory patterns are initiated by low cortisol levels in a positive feedback manner, and they are not affected by short-term ACTH elevations. Additionally, patients with adrenal insufficiency receiving adequate steroid replacement demonstrate similar ACTH secretory patterns. Apparently, the circadian and episodic patterns are intrinsic to the hypothalamus and are not subject to feedback control.

Stress will stimulate ACTH and cortisol secretion, as well as adrenal medullary responses. A partial list of physiologic stresses that cause ACTH secretion includes hypoglycemia, hypovolemia, pain, shock, operation, general anesthesia, burns, infection, hypothermia, dehydration, and irradiation. Some of these operate via peripheral nervous stimuli; others act via the stimulatory effect of inflammatory cytokines, such as interleukin-1 (IL-1), tumor necrosis factor, or interleukin-6 (IL-6), on the HPA. In a fashion similar to the medulla, ACTH and adrenal cortisol secretion can be attenuated or ablated if the afferent sensory input to the hypothalamus is interrupted. Thus, trans-section of afferent pathways from a painful locus, spinal cord trans-section, epidural or spinal anesthesia, and narcotic anesthesia have all been shown to abrogate ACTH secretion in response to pain. In addition to neural pathways, soluble mediators of injury induce ACTH secretion. IL-1 is a cytokine released by activated macrophages. Cortisol is known to inhibit production of IL-1 and TNF, and it has been postulated that cytokine-HPA interaction may function in a feedback fashion in immunologic or infectious processes.

In general, the ACTH response to physiologic stress correlates with the magnitude of stress. For example, multiple trauma in patients elicits maximal ACTH stimulation, whereas uncomplicated elective operations evoke only mild ACTH elevation. Similarly, minor blood loss provokes a suppressible ACTH response, whereas major hemorrhage with shock induces ACTH simulation that cannot be suppressed. Emotional stress also causes ACTH secretion. Elevated cortisol levels suppress ACTH via action on the pituitary, although negative feedback to the hypothalamus can also be demonstrated.

Aldosterone secretion is controlled by several factors, but the most important and best studied is the renin-angiotensin system. This system senses changes in volume and sodium concentration and transmits signals for aldosterone secretion via the renin-angiotensin pathway. Renin is secreted by renal juxtaglomerular cells and enzymatically cleaves angiotensinogen into angiotensin-I, a decapeptide. Angiotensin-converting enzyme (ACE), located within the pulmonary circulation, releases the octapeptide, angiotensin-II, which has two powerful physiologic effects: direct stimulation of aldosterone secretion from the zona glomerulosa and arterial vasoconstriction. A further metabolite of angiotensin-II, angiotensin-III, lacks the vasoconstrictor potency of angiotensin-II, but is equally as potent in stimulating aldosterone secretion. This separation of vasomotor from adrenal effects is thought to provide a mechanism for finer regulatory control of the relative pressor and mineralocorticoid effects of the renin-angiotensin system. Stimulation of renin secretion (and indirectly aldosterone) occurs mainly by three mechanisms: hypovolemia, decreased sodium intake, and sympathetic (beta adrenergic) stimulation, all of which act to increase renin levels and subsequently aldosterone secretion.

In addition to the renin-angiotensin system, there are several other major influences on aldosterone secretion, which are depicted in Figure 19–2. Hyperkalemia stimulates and hypokalemia inhibits aldosterone secretion. Abnormal potassium levels are apparently sensed within the aldosterone-secreting cells of the zona glomerulosa itself. Increased aldosterone levels in response to hyperkalemia are capable of overcoming renin-angiotensin inhibition by salt loading. Excretion of potassium and retention of sodium result. In addition, the atrial natriuretic peptide secreted by atrial myocytes in response to atrial distension acts directly on aldosterone-secreting cells to decrease aldosterone secretion. The peptide also acts to inhibit renin release and causes sodium excretion. ACTH is also capable of stimulating aldosterone secretion. However, the response to ACTH is inconsistent, and the physiologic importance of the relationship between ACTH and aldosterone is unknown. POMC-derived products also have been shown to stimulate aldosterone secretion.

Physiologic Hormonal Effects

Glucocorticoids have far-ranging effects on almost every tissue in the body. Cortisol-induced hyperglycemia is attributed to increased gluconeogenesis by amino acid deamination. Additionally, glucocorticoids cause mobilization of fatty acids and glycogen synthesis in the liver. Although steroids induce protein synthesis through their subcellular mechanism of action, their overall effect on body protein economy is to produce a negative nitrogen balance primarily by skeletal muscle amino acid mobilization and hepatic gluconeogenesis.

Steroids are immunosuppressives. The mechanism of immunosuppression is complex, but primarily involves cellular immunity. Glucocorticoids cause monocytopenia and lymphopenia, which primarily affects T cells. T cells responsiveness to antigen challenge is markedly attenuated. Production of IL-1 is inhibited, which interferes with antigen processing and T cell activation. Lymphocyte proliferation is retarded due to decreased production of interleukin-2 (IL-2) by lymphocytes. Clinically, the depression in cellular immunity translates into a marked predisposition for opportunistic infection.

Humoral immunity is affected less profoundly by steroids. Glucocorticoids do not affect antibody production per se in primary and secondary immune responses. However, total serum antibody levels are lower after steroid administration.

The anti-inflammatory properties of glucocorticoids occur through the stabilization of lysosomal membranes. Histamine release, as well as mast cell number and function, is decreased by glucocorticoids. Decreased histamine-induced lysosomal enzyme activation contributes to the steroid inactivation of lysosomal enzymes. Neutrophil functions,

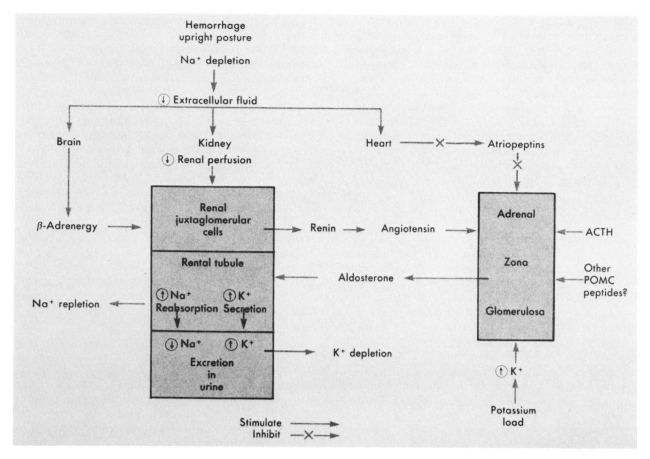

FIGURE 19–2. Aldosterone secretion is influenced by many factors and is related through the renin-angiotensin system to changes in renal perfusion and sodium status. (Reprinted from Genuth, S.M.: The adrenal glands. *In* Berne, R.M., and Levy, M.N. (eds.): Physiology, 2nd ed. St. Louis, C.V. Mosby Co., 1988. Chapter 54, p. 970.)

including migration, adherence, and phagocytosis, are all severely attenuated by glucocorticoids, although paradoxically steroids cause a relative leukocytosis. Steroids also inhibit prostaglandin synthesis by inhibiting phospholipase-A_2, an initiator of eicosanoid synthesis.

Many ion transport systems, including those of the distal nephron, sweat gland ducts, colonic mucosa, and salivary glands, are sensitive to mineralocorticoid influences. In the distal nephron, aldosterone acts to increase both sodium resorption and hydrogen ion and potassium excretion. These effects are mediated by the sodium-potassium ATPase pump, although the exact biochemical mechanism of action is unknown. Clinically, mineralocorticoid excess presents as hypernatremia, hypertension, hypokalemia, and metabolic alkalosis. Deficiency of these hormones produces the opposite effects; namely, hyponatremia, hyperkalemia, and metabolic acidosis. "Escape" from the sodium-retaining effects of aldosterone occurs after a few days in states of aldosterone hypersecretion and probably reflects the complex interrelated physiologic factors controlling

sodium and water hemostasis. This escape mechanism accounts for the lack of edema in patients with primary hyperaldosteronism.

PHYSIOLOGIC BASIS OF DIAGNOSTIC TESTS OF ADRENAL CORTICAL FUNCTION

Diagnostic Techniques: Hyperadrenalism

Hyperadrenalism, or Cushing's syndrome, is caused most often (70 per cent) by excess production of ACTH from, most commonly, a pituitary adenoma (Cushing's disease) and less commonly from an ectopic ACTH-producing malignant neoplasm. Less often, autonomous lesions of the adrenal (adenoma or carcinoma) are found. Cushing's disease results in bilateral adrenal cortical hyperplasia secondary to ACTH secretion from functioning pituitary adenomas. It is nine times more prevalent in women and produces the typical cushinoid habitus and pigmentation. Adrenocorticoid adenomas are relatively common, in up to 5 per cent of the population. In contrast, hyperadrenalism secondary to functional adenomas is relatively uncommon, representing only 20 to 30 per cent of all cases of Cushing's syndrome. Ectopic ACTH-producing tumors include tumors of the lung, pancreas, thymus, and, more rarely, thyroid (C cell), gonad, adrenal medulla, prostatic, and carcinoid tumors. The cells that produce ectopic ACTH are generally members of the amine precursor and uptake decarboxylation (APUD) system.

Establishing the diagnosis of hyperadrenalism is based on demonstrating the presence of excess serum and urinary cortisol and the loss of dexamethasone suppression of pituitary ACTH secretion. The most specific assay for hypercortisolism is the 24-hour urinary cortisol assay, with greater than 100 mcg/24 h representing hypersecretion. Urinary 17 keto and 17 hydroxy (17 OH) steroids are generally reliable assays, although they are subject to false-positive results secondary to cross-reactions with drugs. A single serum cortisol level is unreliable in establishing a diagnosis of hypercortisolism because of the normal daily variation of cortisol secretion. Furthermore, many factors influence cortisol-binding globulin levels. CBG is increased by pregnancy, estrogens, and hyperthyroidism, resulting in elevated total serum cortisol levels; hypothyroidism, liver disease, and nephrotic syndrome decrease CBG and total serum cortisone. Loss of diurnal variation by elevated 8 A.M. and 8 P.M. cortisol levels is suggestive but not confirmatory of a primary adrenal source, since the loss of diurnal variation is also seen in obesity, depression, and alcoholism.

ACTH secretion from the pituitary is suppressed by endogenous and exogenous steroids. The loss of normal ACTH suppression is highly suggestive of hypercortisolism. The overnight low-dose suppression test is widely used as a screening test. One milligram of dexamethasone is taken at 11:00 P.M., and a serum cortisol level is drawn at 8:00 A.M. the next morning. Serum cortisol levels less than 5 mcg/dL suggest normal feedback inhibition of cortisol secretion and thus eliminate hyperadrenalism as a likely diagnosis. Patients with Cushing's syndrome usually have levels greater than 20 mcg/dL. False-positive results can be seen, especially in obese patients. The formal low-dose suppression test, 0.5 mg every 6 hours for 2 days, is usually confirmatory and can be combined with a high-dose (2 mg/q 6 h/2 days) test to aid in differentiating pituitary from other causes of hyperadrenalism. Of the three major causes of hyperadrenalism—pituitary, nonpituitary/nonadrenal cortical neoplasms, and adrenal cortex—only pituitary adenomas, in approximately 50 per cent of cases, show suppression of cortisol production with the high-dose test.

Determining the cause of hyperadrenalism can be difficult. Serum ACTH levels help differentiate between most causes of hyperadrenalism. In pituitary adenoma, levels are normal or mildly elevated; in adrenal adenoma, ACTH is absent; and in ectopic ACTH-producing tumors, ACTH levels are markedly elevated. Overlap in ACTH levels between the various causes of hypercortisolism may exist, and the metyrapone test may assist in the differentiation. This test involves administering metyrapone, an inhibitor of cortisol synthesis and therefore a strong stimulus to ACTH secretion. Blocking cortisol synthesis produces an increase in 11-deoxycorticosterone production, a proximal metabolite also measured in the urine as a 17 OH corticosteroid. Levels of urinary 17 OH corticosteroids are then assayed to ascertain pituitary responsiveness to inhibition of cortisol production, being increased further in those patients with Cushing's disease and unchanged in those with the other causes of Cushing's syndrome.

Distinguishing adrenocortical adenomas from ectopic ACTH-producing tumors is based on ACTH levels, the demonstration of a known nonadrenal malignancy, CT scan evidence of an adrenal tumor, or ^{131}I-19 iodocholesterol scintography, which demonstrates metabolically hyperfunctioning adrenal tissue.

Adrenocortical hypofunction, or Addison's disease, can be either primary, due to adrenal gland unresponsiveness, or secondary, caused by lack of ACTH secretion at the pituitary level. The most common cause of Addison's disease today is exogenous steroid administration and subsequent withdrawal. Other causes include idiopathic or autoimmune hypoadrenalism, infectious disorders (e.g., tuberculosis), and space-occupying pituitary and hypothalamic tumors.

The diagnosis of hypoadrenalism is based on the cosyntropin (synthetic ACTH) stimulation test in which 0.25 mg of cosyntropin is given. The cortisol level is obtained at 0, 30, and 60 minutes. Doubling of the baseline level, an absolute rise of 7 mcg/dL, or stimulated levels of 18 mcg/dL are evidence that the adrenal cortical function is intact. In instances when treatment cannot be delayed, dexamethasone can be given and not affect the assay. Although the cosyntropin test does not specifically evaluate function of the hypothalamic-pituitary axis (HPA) in patients who are possibly suppressed with steroids, adrenal responsiveness to ACTH stimulation is presumptive evidence that the entire HPA axis is intact, since adrenocortical atrophy can only follow pituitary hypothalamic hypofunction in this situation. Generally, any patient who has received physiologic doses of steroids (greater than 5 mg/day of prednisone) for 2 to 3 weeks in the past year is at risk for HPA suppression.

The cosyntropin stimulation test cannot distinguish primary from secondary causes of Addison's disease. To do so requires either the 4-day ACTH stimulation test, the hypoglycemic stimulation test, or the metyrapone test.

Hyperaldosteronism

Hyperaldosteronism may be primary—low plasma renin activity (PRA)—or secondary (high PRA). Any flow disturbance to the kidney, decreased blood volume, or diminished sodium load may cause high PRA. Primary hyperaldosteronism is usually due to a functional adrenal adenoma (Conn's syndrome) or bilateral nodular hyperplasia; much more rarely, glucocorticoid-suppressible hyperaldosteronism or aldosterone-secreting adrenocortical carcinoma can cause the syndrome. Clinically, hyperaldosteronism presents as hypertenison and spontaneous hypokalemia. Only 1 per cent of hypertensive patients are found to have primary hyperaldosteronism. The diagnosis of primary hyperaldosteronism is based on the demonstration of elevated, nonsuppressible aldosterone levels in the absence of high PRA. Suppression of aldosterone can be achieved by salt loading (either with a high-sodium diet or a saline load). If aldosterone remains elevated, then a PRA is checked to confirm primary hyperaldosteronism. Distinguishing between an adrenal adenoma and bilateral hyperplasia is essential since surgery is curative in the first case and not beneficial in the second. The distinction between the two causes is frequently aided by radiographic studies—CT, MRI, and ^{131}I-19 iodocholesterol radionuclide scans.

Congenital Adrenal Hyperplasia

Congenital adrenal hyperplasia (CAH) is a family of virilizing syndromes that arise from inherited, inborn errors in adrenal hormone synthesis that prevent normal cortisol production. Patients present with combinations of virilization, hypertension, and salt wasting, depending on the particular enzymatic defect and the subsequent overproduction of cortisol metabolites caused by uninhibited ACTH production. The most common types are salt-losing and non-salt-losing 21-hydroxylase deficiency, 11-beta-hydroxylase, and 3-betahydroxylase deficiencies. The diagnosis is predicated on the clinical presentation and demonstration of increased urinary 17-ketosteroids, which are suppressible with dexamethasone, a virtually pathognomonic finding. In comparison, virilizing adrenal tumors demonstrate elevated urinary 17-ketosteroids, but no response to dexamethasone suppression.

ADRENAL MEDULLA

Embryology and Histology

The adrenal medulla is derived from the embryonic neural crest and shares neuroendocrine properties with other chromaffin tissue of the so-called amine precursor and uptake decarboxylation system (APUD). Ectodermal cells from the neurocrest migrate and infiltrate the mesodermal coalescence destined to become the adrenal cortex at week seven. Another important potential locus of neurogenic cells formed at this time is the Organ of Zuckerkandl, situated at the aortic bifurcation. This alternate nest of cells becomes important, especially as a common site of extra adrenal pheochromocytoma. The fetal adrenal medulla completes development in utero and is fully functional by birth.

Histologically the adrenal medulla is composed of chromaffin staining cells that are vesiculated due to deposits of epinephrine and norepinephrine. Because it is surrounded by cortex, the microcirculatory environment of the medulla is enriched with high concentrations of steroids. Glucocorticoids have been shown to have a strong stimulatory effect on phenylethanolamine-N-methyltransferase (PNMT), the enzyme catalyzing the last reaction in epinephrine synthesis. Thus, the cortex influences production of catecholamines by the medulla and amplifies the organism's response to stress.

Hormone Biochemistry. The adrenal medulla normally secretes the catecholamines, epinephrine and norepinephrine, although tumors may secrete additional substances, such as dopamine. Epinephrine constitutes the largest proportion of output, usually five times the amount of norepinephrine. Catecholamines are synthesized by the pathway depicted in Figure 19–3. The rate-controlling reaction in catecholamine synthesis is catalyzed by tyramine hydroxylase. Epinephrine and norephinephrine are stored in intracellular vesicles that are secreted by exocytosis in response to membrane depolarization and calcium influx.

The half-life of epinephrine and norepinephrine is short, approximately 2 minutes, with degradation taking place throughout the body via two predominant enzyme systems, catechol-O-methyltransferase (COMT) and monoamine oxidase (MAO). Approximately 70 per cent of epinephrine secreted by adrenal medulla is methylated by COMT, and 25 per cent is oxidized by MAO. Figure 19–4 shows the pathways of catecholamine degradation.

Secretory Control Mechanisms

As part of the sympathetic nervous system, the adrenal medulla is under the control of the central nervous system. Almost any stress, including anxiety, fear, or rage, will produce sympathetic discharge. Physiologic stresses, such as hypothermia, hypovolemia, and hypoglycemia, are well-known stimulants of catechol release from the medulla. The adrenal response to hypoglycemia correlates directly with serum glucose levels, and diabetic patients frequently can judge the degree of hypoglycemia from the intensity of symptoms produced by counter-

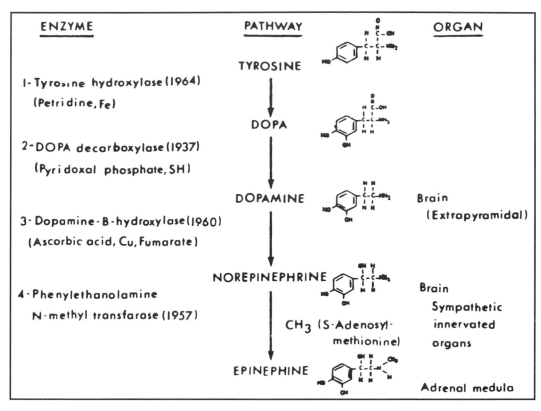

FIGURE 19–3. Pathway of catecholamine biosynthesis. (Reprinted from DeQuattro, V., Myers, M., and Campese, V.M.: Anatomy and biochemistry of the sympathetic nervous system. *In* DeGroot, L.J. (ed.): Endocrinology, 2nd ed. Philadelphia, W.B. Saunders Co., 1989. Chapter 103, p. 1719.)

regulatory sympathetic discharge. Pain is a potent stimulant for catecholamine release, and anesthetic blockade of pain afferents, either by epidural, spinal, or narcotic analgesia, can attenuate the subsequent adrenal medullary response. There is no evidence for feedback inhibition between medulla and catecholamine secretion.

Physiologic Hormone Effects

The effects of epinephrine and norepinephrine are mediated by adrenegenic receptors. There are two classes of receptors, alpha and beta, and each is subdivided into classes I and II. The effects of catecholamines are numerous and depend upon the relative affinity of each hormone for available receptor types. Individual tissues exhibit different receptor density and catecholamine sensitivity. Heart tissue, for instance, is dominated by beta I and beta II receptors, whereas arteriolar cells display both alpha and beta receptors. Thus, vasoconstriction or dilation can be elicited by alpha or beta adrenergic agents, respectively. At the subcellular level, catecholamines bind to adrenegenic receptors and stimulate production of second messengers, such as cyclic AMP in the case of beta stimulation and inositol

1,4,5 triphosphate as proposed for alpha stimulation. In general, the hormones of the adrenal medulla are excitatory and prepare the organism for "fight or flight."

Catecholomines also cause hyperglycemia and are prominent catabolic and counter-regulatory hormones. Epinephrine increases glucose by several mechanisms, including increased hepatic glycogenolysis and gluconeogenesis, inhibition of insulin secretion and stimulation of glucagon secretion, inhibition of glucose uptake by muscle, and finally by increased ACTH secretion and glucocorticoid stimulation.

Diagnostic Assessment of Pathologic Conditions

Pheochromocytoma. Pheochromocytoma is an uncommon tumor of chromaffin cells of neuroendocrine origin that presents with hypertension and episodes of tachycardia, diaphoresis, headache, and palpitations. Although a rare cause of hypertension in screening studies, pheochromocytomas are associated with multiple endocrine neoplasms types IIA and IIB, von Recklinghausen's disease (neurofibromatosis), and von Hippel-Lindau's disease and should be sought in these conditions. Pheochromo-

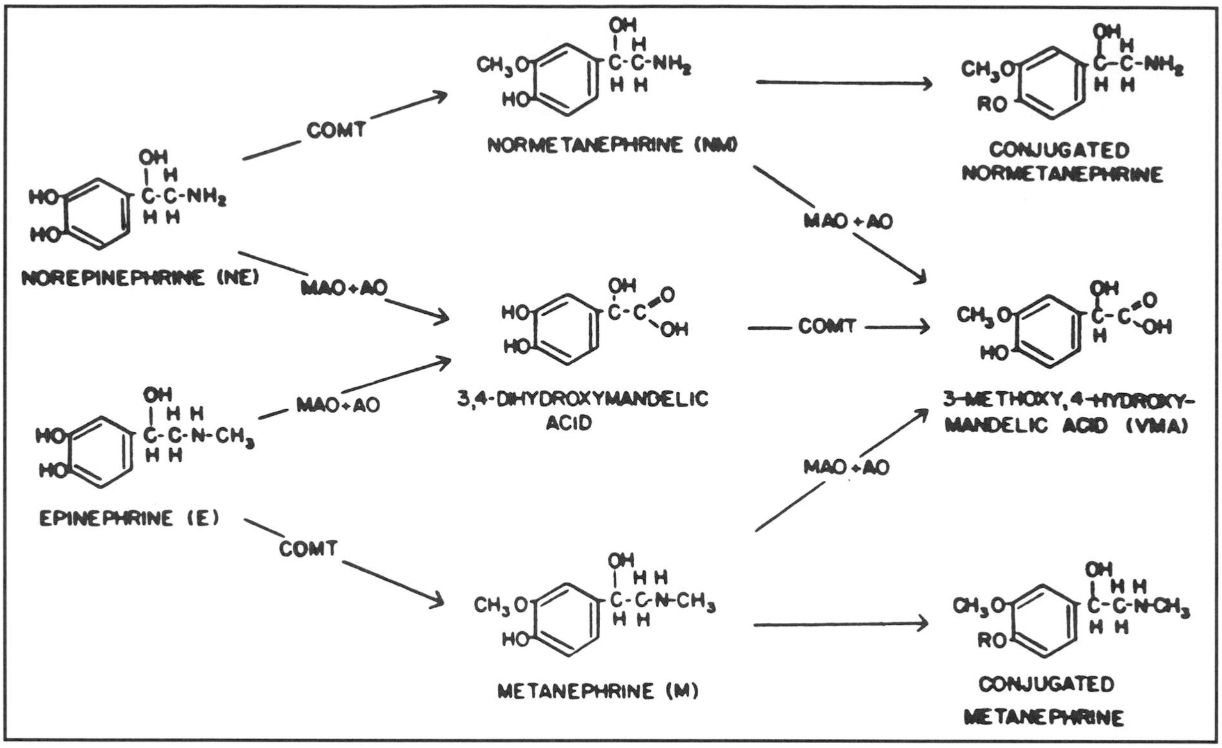

FIGURE 19–4. Pathways of catecholamine degradation. (Reprinted from Dequattro, V., Myers, M., and Campese, V.M.: Anatomy and biochemistry of the sympathetic nervous system. *In* DeGroot, L.J. (ed.): Endocrinology, 2nd ed. Philadelphia, W.B. Saunders Co., 1989. Chapter 103, p. 1719.)

cytomas are nearly all metabolically active, but not always clinically apparent. In contrast to the normal adrenal medulla, norepinephrine secretion predominates in patients with pheochromocytoma, and elevated levels of urinary metabolites of norepinephrine and epinephrine are found in those patients. In general, three classes of metabolites are assayed: (1) free catecholamines, (2) metanephrines (normetanephrine and metanephrine), and (3) vanillylmandelic acid (VMA). Metanephrines are generally considered to be the most sensitive and provide the most reliable screening test, whereas the VMA assay is least reliable. Usually a 24-hour urine collection is performed, but occasionally in cases of a particularly episodic nature, timed collections during an episode are sufficient to make the diagnosis. Serum catecholamines are used in an adjunctive role in making the diagnosis and are very specific. Increased dopamine levels have been found with malignant pheochromocytomas. Only rarely do patients require provocative testing utilizing histamine, glucagon, or tyramine to confirm the diagnosis, and suppression tests may also be used.

Several imaging methods are used to localize pheochromocytoma. Pathologically, 98 per cent of pheochromocytomas are found below the diaphragm, 90 per cent of which arise from the adrenal medulla. However, localization can be quite difficult, especially when one considers that 15 per cent of pheochromocytomas are multiple (particularly true in familial syndromes). CT scanning has been very useful in demonstrating pheochromocytomas, with up to 90 per cent accuracy in multiple series. MRI will undoubtedly evolve into an accurate localization technique, with the additional advantage of differentiating adrenal medullary from cortical neoplasms. Scintigraphic imaging based on tumor uptake of 131 iodine meta-iodobenzylguanidine (131 I-MIBG) provides both functional and localization information.

Neuroblastoma. Neuroblastoma is a tumor usually seen in infants and young children that arises from nonchromaffin cells of neural crest origin. The majority of neuroblastomas are localized to the adrenal medulla (40 per cent) or paraspinal ganglia (25 percent), but 15 per cent are mediastinal in location and 5 per cent are pelvic. Usually presenting as an abdominal mass, neuroblastomas lack the dramatic vasomotor symptoms of pheochromocytoma. Nevertheless, 90 per cent of patients demonstrate elevations of VMA and homovanillic acid (HVA) in urine. Elevations of HVA have been correlated with a poor prognosis, whereas high ratios of VMA to HVA are relatively good prognostic signs. Levels can also be monitored during therapy to provide prognostic information.

BIBLIOGRAPHY

1. Bateman, A., Singh, A., Kral, T., and Saloman, S.: The immuno-hypothalamus-pituitary-adrenal axis. Endocrine Rev., *10*:92, 1989.
2. DeGroot, L.J. (ed.): Endocrinology, 2nd ed. Philadelphia, W.B. Saunders Co., 1989.
3. Mulrow, P.J. (ed.): The Adrenal Gland. New York, Elsevier, 1986.
4. Wilson, D., and Foster, D.W. (cds.): William's Textbook of Endocrinology, 7th ed. Philadelphia, W.B. Saunders Co., 1985.
5. Young, W.F., and Klee, G.G.: Primary aldosteronism: Diagnostic evaluation. Endocrinol. Metab. Clin. North Am., *17*:367, 1988.

20

BONE PHYSIOLOGY

HARRY E. RUBASH

BONE STRUCTURE

The skeletal system serves as a mineral reserve and as a support system to provide protection for the viscera and locomotion of the being. Bone, as is all connective tissue, is composed of cells and an extracellular ground substance. In contrast with other connective tissues, bone has an extensive blood supply that keeps the bone cells in intimate contact with the extracellular fluid. The ground substance of bone is a composite material consisting of collagen fibers (providing tensile strength) and proteoglycans, especially chrondroiton sulfate and hyaluronic acid. The crystalline salts deposited in this organic matrix are composed primarily of calcium and phosphate. These calcium salts have great compressive strength. The degree of bonding between the collagen and the calcium salts provides an extremely strong bony structure that is similar to reinforced concrete. Despite its external appearance, bone is a dynamic tissue that is constantly being renewed (bone accretion) and removed (bone absorption).

The gross structure of a growing long bone is shown in Figure 20–1. The rounded ends of the bond form joints that are covered with hyaline cartilage. Beneath the hyaline cartilage is a subchondral plate of cortical bone that is supported by cancellous bone. The cancellous bone of the metaphysis of a long bone blends with the cortex of the diaphysis of bone. The diaphysis consists of a thick tubular cortical bone and a central medullary cavity containing bone marrow.

The cartilaginous end of a growing long bone is referred to as the epiphysis. The physis or growth plate is a cartilaginous disc with a fibrous periphery where cartilage growth takes place. The cartilage is arranged in a zonal pattern, with the growing cells being closest to the epiphysis and the dying cells, which are being replaced by bone, directed toward the metaphysis (middle) of the bone. One zone in the physis, referred to as a proliferating zone, is the area where longitudinal growth occurs. Cartilage cells rapidly proliferate in this zone and are stacked in long columns separated by cartilage matrix. The

zone closest to the metaphysis of the bone is the hypertrophic zone, which is a relatively avascular, hypoxemic area. The cartilage cells in this zone die and release calcium into the extracellular matrix. Blood vessels grow in from the metaphyseal bone, and bone-forming cells (osteoblasts) lay down fibrous bone (primary spongiosum) on the calcified cartilagi-

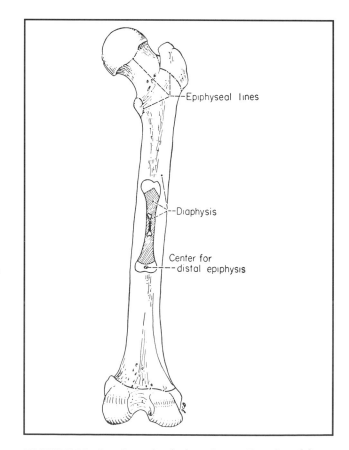

FIGURE 20–1. Growth of a long bone. (Reprinted from Woodburne, R.T.: General concepts in anatomy: The skeletal system. *In* Essentials of Human Anatomy, 5th ed. New York, Oxford Press, 1973, p. 41)

nous bars. The primary spongiosum bone (that which is first made) is remodeled gradually into secondary spongiosum or mature lamellar bone. Thus, the principal events of bone formation are cartilage death, vascular invasion, bone formation, and remodeling of bone.

Bones are surrounded by a layer of connective tissue, the periosteum, which is circumferential except at the articular surface of the bone. The periosteum contributes to formation of new bone when bone exceeds its elastic limit and fractures. It plays an integral part in the healing and the subsequent remodeling of bone that occurs during growth. A dense perichondral ring of fibrous tissue encircles the growing bone at the level of the epiphysial plate. The perichondral ring fosters lateral growth of bone, supplies mechanical support to the growth plate, and is continuous with the periosteum.

The complex process of mineralization (calcification) of bone that occurs during bone growth also occurs in many other tissues and involves the formation of an analogue of the mineral compound of the hydroxyapatite. The chemical composition is $Ca_{10}(PO4)_6(OH)_2$. The mineral is deficient in both calcium and hydroxide ions with respect to true hydroxyapatite. Other ions may either associate with the crystals of apatite or be substituted for ions within the molecule of hydroxyapatite. These include carbonate, citrate, fluoride, and, in addition, many radioactive isotopes. The chondrocytes from the growth plate and the osteoblasts from the metaphysis are the cells that directly control the process of calcification during bone growth. Collagen may also control the orientation of the newly formed bone crystals. Several enzymes, such as alkaline phosphatase and phospholipase, may also play a role in calcification.

Bone is composed of two types of tissue, cortical or "compact bone" and cancellous or "spongy bone." Cancellous bone is composed of bone spicules or trabecula enclosing gaps in the bone matrix that contain bone marrow. Compact or cortical bone is constructed in lamellae or layers that are arranged in concentric rings to form cylindrical structures known as haversian systems or osteons. The lamellae are 3 to 7 μm thick, and each haversian system is made up of 10 to 20 lamellae. The central cavity in each haversian system contains a blood vessel that supplies it. The haversian canals are interconnected by channels called Volkmann's channels. This lamellar bone organization is unique to cortical bone. The bone cells or osteocytes lie in cavities (lacunae) in the bone matrix. The osteocytes can communicate chemically with one another through extensions of the osteocytes called canaliculi. Between the haversian systems lies interstitial bone, which basically fills the gaps between the cylinders.

Cancellous bone has the same lamellar structure as cortical bone. It does not, however, have the haversian canals containing a central blood vessel; instead, the cells are connected by canaliculi to blood vessels on the endosteal side of bone. (Fig. 20–2).

BONE CELLS

Bone cells are composed of osteoblasts, osteocytes, and osteoclasts. The three major physiologic functions of bone cells are calcium transport, maintenance of biophysical or bioelectrical properties, and hormonal responses. Osteoblasts lay down the extracellular matrix including collagen and play a role in mineralization. Osteocytes contribute to mineral matrix homeostasis, and osteoclasts resorb bone. It is currently believed that all cancellous and cortical bone surfaces are covered with either osteoblasts, osteocytes, or thin fibroblastic cells, which together make up the cellular envelope responsible for the control of the flow of ions between the bone matrix and the extracellular fluid compartment. These cells are responsive to calcitonin and parathormone.

Osteoblasts are bone-forming cells that synthesize the collagen and ground substance of the matrix and preside over the poorly understood process of mineralization. The cellular process of collagen synthesis begins with precursor amino acids that are assembled into the three-stranded procollagen molecule extruded by the osteoblast into the soluble extracellular collagen pool. This collagen contributes to the unmineralized osteoid seam of new bone that is laid down upon the calcified cartilaginous bars of the growth plate during fracture healing and during pathologic states in bone, i.e., osteomalacia. The process of mineralization of this seam takes approximately 10 to 20 days, during which time the extrafibular cross-linking of collagen fibers and distribution of glycoaminoglycans help prepare the matrix for mineralization. The concentration of calcium and phosphate in the extracellular fluid is considerably greater than that necessary to cause propagation of the hydroxyapatite crystal. However, inhibitors, such as pyrophosphate and others, prevent the formation of crystals in normal tissues. Most of the mineral is deposited within the first few days, and it is still unknown what causes calcium salts to be deposited in osteoid and how the exact sequence begins and ends.

Osteoclasts are multinucleated giant cells responsible for the resorption of bone. These cells are often seen in shallow depressions on the surface of bone called Howship's lacunae. Unlike osteoblasts and osteocytes, which are intrinsic bone mesenchyme cells, osteoclasts originate from the monocyte/macrophage linage of hematopoietic tissue, but they do not have Fc receptors as does the mature macrophage. When osteoclasts are stimulated by parathormone, the cell membrane close to the matrix becomes ruffled, and a space appears between the bone matrix and the osteoclast itself. It is here where extracellular digestion of the bone matrix by hydrolytic enzymes from the osteoclasts takes place. The min-

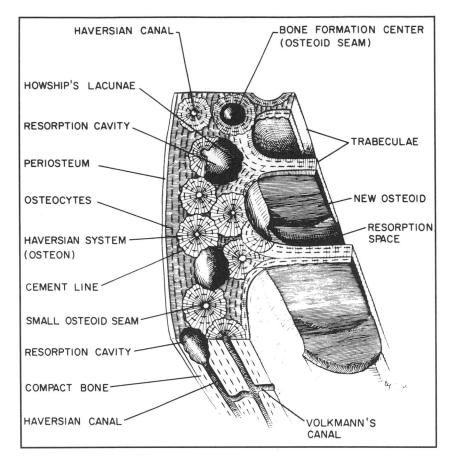

HAVERSIAN CANAL
BONE FORMATION CENTER
(OSTEOID SEAM)
HOWSHIP'S LACUNAE
RESORPTION CAVITY
PERIOSTEUM
OSTEOCYTES
HAVERSIAN SYSTEM
(OSTEON)
CEMENT LINE
SMALL OSTEOID SEAM
RESORPTION CAVITY
COMPACT BONE
HAVERSIAN CANAL
TRABECULAE
NEW OSTEOID
RESORPTION
SPACE
VOLKMANN'S
CANAL

FIGURE 20–2. The configuration of cortical and endosteal bone showing bone remodeling units. (Reprinted from Parfitt, A.M., and Duncan, H.: Metabolic bone disease affecting the spine. *In* Rothman, R.H., and Simeone, F.A. (eds.): The Spine, 2nd ed, vol. II. Philadelphia, W.B. Saunders Co., 1982, p. 777.)

eral crystals are dislodged and the collagen fibers uncovered for resorption.

BONE FORMATION

In the embryo, bone is produced by osteoblasts by either intramembranous or endochondral ossification. Most of the skull bones and the clavicle are formed by the process of intramembranous ossification, which does not involve cartilage formation. During this process, primitive connective tissue (mesenchymal tissue) undergoes changes, including vascularization and the development of osteoblasts. This first bone to be formed is referred to as woven bone (primary spongiosum); it has randomly oriented collagen fibers and appears rather disorganized. Woven bone is only made in postnatal life in response to injury. Lamellar bone (secondary spongiosum), which is laid down subsequent to primary spongiosum, is organized in haversian systems and responds to the mechanical environment of the bone.

Most bones are formed by endochondral ossification. In this process an embryologic template of cartilage is first seen (Fig. 20–1). After vascular invasion, the cartilage is replaced by bone. The process begins at the primary center of ossification in the diaphysis of the bone during the third month of embryonic life. As the primary center of ossification increases in length, two secondary centers of ossification occur on either end of the bone in response to vascular invasion of the cartilage. At the same time, osteoblasts begin to produce circumferential bone around the periphery of the cartilage. The blood vessels that invade the cartilage carry with them primitive connective tissue cells that subsequently develop into hematopoietic cells and osteoclasts. Ossification progresses from the center of the shaft toward the epiphyses with cartilage being replaced by bone. After birth, secondary ossification occurs in the epiphysis. At the epiphysial region the ossification gradually replaces all but the articular cartilage, and the cartilage between the epiphysis and the diaphysis becomes thinned, forming the epiphysial plate. The epiphysial plates are responsible for increasing the length of the bone during childhood and adolescence. Eventually, the cartilage in the epiphysis is completely replaced by bone, and closure of the growth plate occurs.

BONE REMODELING

Bone remodeling is a continuing process throughout life and is necessary to maintain mechanical strength. Since bone mass is relatively constant in adult life, bone resorption is balanced by bone formation. Most evidence suggests that resorption is a primary event in bone, with formation following resorption within the same microenvironment.

Bone remodeling appears to be partly under hormonal control. It is increased by parathyroid hormone and decreased by calcitonin and estrogens. When induced, osteoclasts advance longitudinally in the cortex, producing a resorption channel that usually runs parallel to an existing osteon. Behind the advancing resorption front, refilling of the hole occurs as osteoblasts lay down new bone in a circumferential manner in the cone of bone that had been removed. In trabecular bone, the osteoclasts are spread out over the surface and gouge out a shallow grove, which corresponds to Howship's lacunae. These osteoclasts are followed by osteoblasts forming new bone into the resorption area. Thus, the dynamics of remodeling may differ on different types of osseous surfaces (periosteal, endosteal, or trabecular), even though the basic process appears to be the same.

The mechanical properties of bone are governed by the density of the material, with its weakest point being the area of least density. Bone geometry also plays a role in determining bone strength. Bone is tubular, and thus it is significantly stronger than a solid tube. As one grows older and bone mass diminishes, the periosteal diameter (outside diameter) of long bones increases, as does the endosteal diameter (inside diameter). These increases shift bone mass further from the center of the bone and maximize the skeletal strength of any given bone mass.

Two concepts govern changes in structural properties of bone: modeling and remodeling. In modeling, appositional growth occurs on the surface of a bone that is loading in an unusual or excessive way. Modeling is visible when external callus formation occurs after there is a fracture on one side of a bone or when new bone formation occurs unilaterally on a bone that is subjected to new bending stresses. This latter process is often seen in stress fractures of the metatarsals or femoral neck.

Remodeling is a process whereby bone can alter its shape. It involves the removal of bone by osteoclasts from within, which temporarily weakens the bone, before it is restrengthened by new bone formation. The body recognizes the skeletal stresses, perhaps by electrical feedback within the bending and compressive structures of bone, and thus will only remodel the least stressed bone. Bone cells respond by depositing bone in an effort to increase the structural strength of loaded areas of the bone (Wolff's law).

A steady-state equilibrium between total formation and total resorption of bone exists in normal adults over an extended period of time. The total volume of bone temporarily missing as a result of the normal remodeling process is only about 0.5 to 1.0 per cent of total bone volume. More rapid turnover would impair the mechanical integrity of the skeleton. Bone that is undergoing significant remodeling has a markedly weakened microstructure and may fracture. Such pathologic fractures and microfractures may be seen in osteoporosis and other hypermetabolic states, including hyperparathyroidism, hyperthyroidism, and even Paget's disease. Thus, the term "osteoporosis" refers to a group of disorders with decreased bone mass that are the result of an imbalance between bone absorption and deposition.

BONE REPAIR

Bone can be strained 0.75 per cent before irreversible deformation occurs (plastic deformation). When it is deformed 2 to 4 per cent, it breaks, and the complex process of fracture healing begins. The initial phase of all fracture healing is localized hematoma formation followed by an inflammatory repair. Within the first 8 hours, polymorphonuclear leukocytes and macrophages migrate into the area and begin removing damaged tissue and debris. As the fracture enters the reparative stage, increased cell division begins both on the endosteal and periosteal surfaces of bone. The cells involved directly in the repair of bone are mesenchymal in origin and are pluripotential. This cellular response takes place within 2 weeks of injury and involves formation of a callus of collagen, cartilage, and immature bone in the initial area of hematoma next to the opposed fractured surfaces of bone. The callus quickly envelops the bone ends, gradually increasing the stability of the bone fragments. Compression of the bone ends, or the avoidance of tension, encourages callus formation and the healing response. The cartilage that is formed in the callus is eventually resorbed by the process of enchondral bone formation. Bone, however, is formed without intermediate cartilage formation in some areas. Early in this repair process, cartilage formation predominates, and mucopolysaccharides (glycosaminoglycans) are found in high concentrations. This phase is followed by a gradual increase in the concentration of collagen and eventually the accumulation of calcium hydroxyapatite crystals and bone. Thus, as this next phase of repair takes place, the bone ends gradually become enveloped in a fusiform-like mass of callus that contains increasing amounts of bone. Clinical union occurs when the fracture no longer moves, and it is not painful.

If the bony ends are not in continuity, an external bridging callus forms. This bridging callus is able to span large gaps between the bone ends. It depends upon the availability of viable external soft tissue to bridge the gap and form the callus necessary for healing. Medullary callus formation occurs directly from the ends of the bone fragments along with the external bridging callus. A final type of bone healing, primary cortical healing, occurs only when mechanical immobilization and apposition of the bone ends are almost perfect. When an extremely rigid system is obtained (i.e., open reduction and internal fixation with plates and screws), the formation of external bridging callus is suppressed severely, and the fracture heals mainly by late medullary callus formation and by primary cortical healing of the opposing ends.

Wolff's Law

In 1892, Wolff recognized that the architecture of our skeletal system reflected the system's mechanical requirements. The final phase of fracture healing involves remodeling of bone to meet the stresses of the system. The control mechanism that modulates the cellular behavior is believed to be electrical. When a bone is stressed, electropositivity occurs on the convex surface and electronegativity on the concave surface. These electrical changes may influence bone formation and resorption so that in regions on electropositivity there is osteoclastic activity and in regions of electronegativity there is increased osteoblastic activity. The end result of this remodeling phase is a bone that may not have returned to its original form, but has been altered to meet the functional demands of the new bony architecture.

Normal vitamin D and calcium levels are required for fracture healing. Augmented levels of vitamin D, calcium, or growth hormone do not increase the final fracture healing outcome, but may accelerate the normal process. Many of the anti-inflammatory drugs have been shown to decrease the rate of fractrue healing in laboratory animals.

MINERAL METABOLISM

Calcium and Phosphate Homeostasis

Calcium homeostasis is a complex process that involves multiple organs and hormones. Calcium is critically involved in many different cellular processes (i.e., enzyme control, secretion of hormones, blood coagulation, membrane electrical potential, neurologic function), and its concentration (intracellular and extracellular) is rigidly controlled. Fifty per cent of the calcium in the circulation is bound to plasma proteins and albumin.

All calcium intake is dietary, and significant calcium is lost or reabsorbed via the kidneys. Approximately 900 mg to 1 gm of calcium is required daily. Bone represents a potential reservoir for calcium and phosphate as calcium hydroxyapatite crystals binds large amounts of these minerals. Only 1 per cent of calcium is located outside of the bones. Approximately 1 kg of body weight is made up of calcium. Children, pregnant women, lactating women, adolescents, and postmenopausal women have the greatest calcium requirements, ranging from one to two times the normal requirement.

The normal intestine has a huge reserve capacity available for absorbing calcium. The kidney reabsorbs over 98 per cent of the calcium filtered, and less than 200 mg of calcium usually is present in a 24-hour urine collection (less than 2 mg/kg/day). Calcium resorption occurs throughout the nephron and is closely regulated by parathormone (PTH).

Calcium moves between bone and body fluids by two processes. The first method is the relatively slow process of bone remodeling. The other process for movement of calcium between bone and body fluid is both rapid and reversible and has the ability to control the minute-by-minute calcium level. Osteocytes and osteoblasts respond quite rapidly to hormonal changes, and it appears that the major site of calcium exchange is the perilacunar material surrounding osteocytes. Parathormone appears to increase bone remodeling, osteocyte stimulation, and the release of calcium from the perilacunar material.

Vitamin D and parathyroid hormone are intimately involved in calcium metabolism. Vitamin D is formed in the skin when 7-dehydrocholesterol is exposed to ultraviolet light (Fig. 20–3). One hour of sunlight seems to supply the adequate daily requirement in Caucasians. The endogenous form of vitamin D is cholecalciferol or vitamin D_3. Ergocalciferol or vitamin D_2 is a form of vitamin D found in the diet. The highest concentration of this dietary form of the vitamin is found in muscle and fat. In the liver, vitamin D is converted into 25-OH-cholecalciferol by a vitamin D 25-hydroxylase. The 25-OH-vitamin D is bound to a serum alpha globulin and is the major circulating form of vitamin D. The next and most important step of vitamin D metabolism is that of 1-hydroxylation. The metabolically active form, 1-25-vitamin D, is formed in the mitochondria of kidney cells. The target tissues of this activated steroid hormone are bone, intestine, parathyroid gland, and kidney. In the kidney, it increases resorption of phosphate and perhaps calcium. In the bone, it promotes the mobilization of calcium from bone by an unknown mechanism. In the intestines, its major function is to promote intestinal calcium and phosphate absorption, and in the parathyroid gland, 1-25-OH vitamin D has a negative effect on the production of parathormone. The net effect is to increase the absorption of calcium into the body.

Parathyroid hormone (PTH) regulates the extracellular concentration of calcium. PTH is produced in and secreted exclusively from the parathyroid glands in humans. Secretion of parathyroid hormone is very tightly regulated. Its three major target organs are intestine, kidney, and bone. A very small

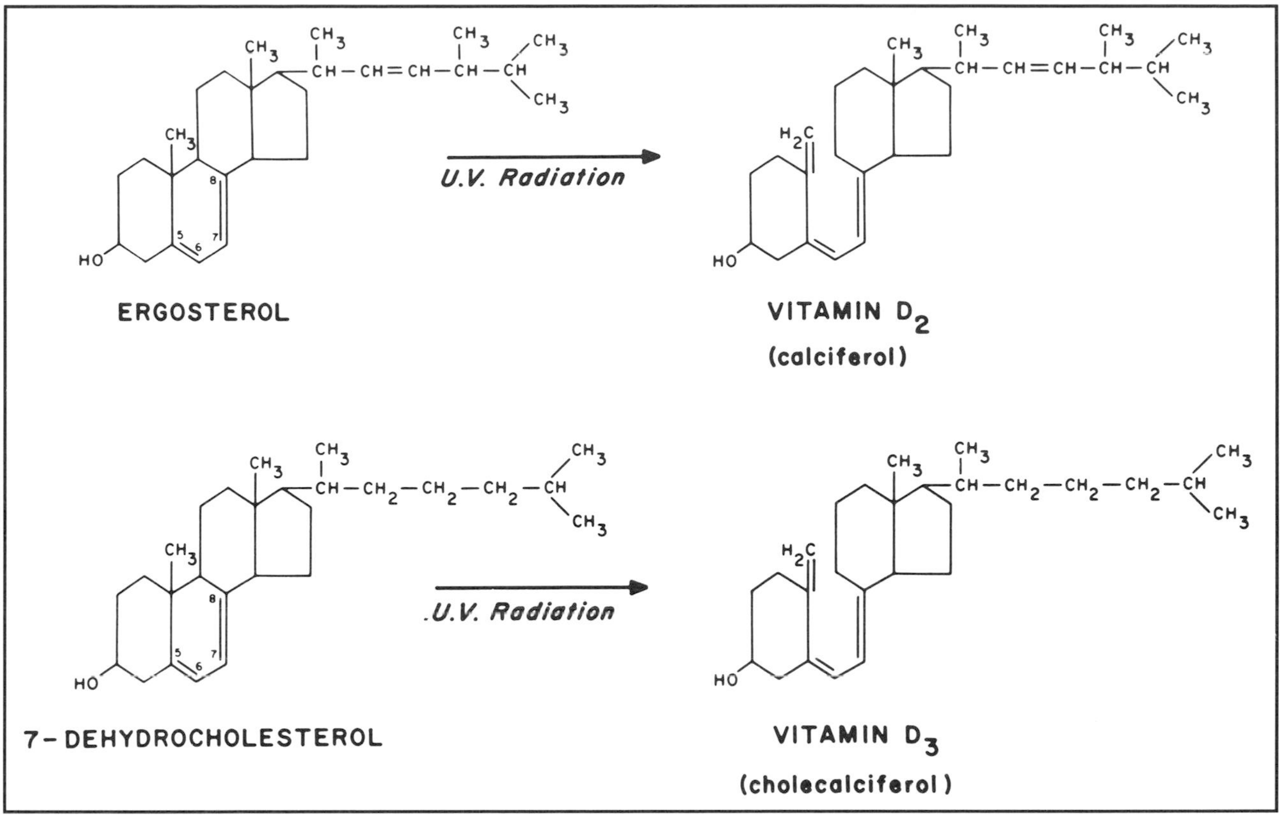

FIGURE 20–3. Activation of provitamins by ultraviolet radiation. (Reprinted from Zaleske, D.J., Doppelt, S.H., and Mankin, H.J.: Metabolic and endocrine abnormalities of the immature skeleton. *In* Lovell, W.W., and Winter, R.B. (eds.): Pediatric Orthopaedics, 2nd ed., vol. 1. Philadelphia, J.B. Lippincott Co., 1986, p. 88.)

change in the ionized calcium concentration will stimulate release of the hormone. In the intestine, PTH works in synergy with vitamin D to increase the absorption of calcium from the diet. PTH increases the level of production of 1-25-OH vitamin D by the kidneys. In addition, it closely controls the amount of calcium excreted by the kidney. Administration of small amounts of PTH significantly increases the amount of calcium reabsorbed by the kidney. It seems to decrease the resorption of calcium in the proximal tubule and increases the resorption in the distal tubule. Phosphate is secreted in the renal tubule, and this process is augmented by increased levels of PTH. In bone, PTH and osteoclast-activating factors stimulate the formation of the osteoclasts' ruffled border and potentiate the activity of osteoclasts, thereby increasing the mineral resorption from bone. This is a relatively slow process, and long-term stimulation by PTH increases both the number and activity of the osteoclasts and, ultimately, the resorption of bone. Osteocytes and osteoblasts respond rapidly (within 5 minutes) to PTH injection by changing their shape and by resorbing materials surrounding the osteocytes as the primary source of calcium on a short-term basis. It is this perilacunar material that is transferred rapidly into the body fluid compartment from the bone surface to increase the calcium concentration in response to PTH.

Calcitonin is a third hormone that may influence calcium metabolism. It is produced and secreted by the C cells (perifollicular cells) in the thyroid gland. It does seem to have a significant calcium- and phosphate-lowering action at physiologic doses in humans. Hypercalcemia stimulates secretion, and low calcium suppresses its release. Calcitonin deficiency causes no known disorder of mineral metabolism in humans. It, however, has several pharmacologic uses, including the treatment of Paget's disease, prevention of disuse osteoporosis, and the rapid lowering of serum calcium in severe hypercalcemic states.

CONDITIONS OF OSTEOPENIA

Osteopenia, or a relative decrease in the amount of bone in the skeleton, is often caused by osteoporosis (Table 20–1) or osteomalacia (Table 20–2). These two entities are quite different.

Approximately 15 per cent of white women over

TABLE 20–1. CAUSES OF OSTEOPOROSIS

Endocrine
Hyperthyroid
Hyperadrenocorticalism
Hyperparathyroidism
Nutritional
Calcium deficiency
Protein deficiency
Intestinal malabsorption
Drugs
Heparin
Anticonvulsants
Others
Disuse
Trauma

age 65 have significant osteoporosis. From the age of 30 until menopause, bone is lost at the rate of approximately 3 per cent per decade. After menopause, cortical bone is lost at a rate of two to three times that level. The rate of loss of cancellous (trabecular bone) does not appear to differ between sexes and progresses at a steady rate of 6 per cent per decade.

The typical patient with osteoporosis is a slender, sedentary woman of northern European descent who smokes and has breast fed children. Her diet is usually deficient in vitamin D and calcium, and she has little exposure to the sun. The cause of postmenopausal osteoporosis has not been clearly delineated. There is clearly an uncoupling of the rate of bone resorption and bone formation. Thus, either increased bone resorption or decreased bone formation can be the causes. The pathologic manifestations of osteoporosis are vertebral and femoral fractures (hip). The cost of the treatment of these conditions is astronomical and is a major impetus for osteoporosis research.

Several different treatment modalities for postmenopausal osteoporosis have been studied. Calcium supplementation decreases the fracture rate by one half, and further supplementation of the diet with fluoride or estrogen may reduce the fracture rate an additional 30 to 50 per cent. Thus, a combination of calcium, fluoride, and estrogen reduces the fracture rate of patients with postmenopausal osteoporosis to 10 per cent of the untreated group. Exer-

TABLE 20–2. CAUSES OF OSTEOMALACIA

Deficiency states
GI disorders
Vitamin d.-resistant rickets
Renal osteodystrophy
Vitamin D deficiency
Phosphorus deficiency
Gastric rickets
Enteric disorders

cise is an important, but poorly understood factor affecting the treatment of osteoporosis. Vigorous training programs have been shown to build bone mass even in elderly osteoporotic patients.

Osteomalacia, as well as its pediatric equivalent, rickets, has a multitude of causes. These causes can be grouped into dietary or endogenous vitamin D deficiency, intestinal malabsorption disorders, acquired or hereditary renal disorders, and a miscellaneous group, which includes anticonvulsant therapy (Dilantin).

The clinical diagnosis of osteomalacia is difficult and requires histologic material. Patients usually have nonspecific complaints, such as muscle weakness or diffuse aches and pains—symptoms that are quite common in elderly patients. Frequently, the diagnosis is not made until the disorder is far advanced with evidence of axial skeletal height decrease or multiple stress fractures. Radiographic evidence of osteomalacia is also nonspecific. The presence of "losers lines" (radiolucent areas in bone that are the result of microstress fractures) is one radiographic sign of osteomalacia. Other radiographic signs are biconcavity of the vertebral bodies and general bowing of the long bones.

As the etiology of the disease implies, the histologic hallmark of osteomalacia is an increase in the width and extent of the osteoid seams that form before mineralization to make bone. The osteoblasts that form the osteoid are not actively stimulated, and calcification of the osteoid is diminished. Over a period of several years, this failure to mineralize newly formed osteoid results in the development of weakened bone. In the immature skeleton, the normal zonal pattern of the epiphysis shows gross distortion, with loss of the ordered columns of chondrocytes and an increased height of the epiphysis. The zone of calcification of the epiphysis is irregular and poorly calcified.

Classic osteomalacia is caused by a decrease in vitamin D content in the diet. Many of these patients often have unusual dietary habits (i.e., strict vegetarianism) or general malabsorption, which is frequently seen in the elderly. Changes in gastrointestinal physiology, such as blind loops, Crohn's disease, and gluten-sensitive enteropathy, may cause steatorrhea and malabsorption of vitamin D and osteomalacia. There are also several known hereditary renal causes of osteomalacia and rickets. Patients with these disorders, such as X-linked dominant hypophosphatemic rickets often develop normally if diagnosis and treatment are made early in life.

The constellation of clinical problems associated with chronic renal failure affect most of the organ systems of the body. The skeletal system shares in this disability to an extraordinary degree. Damage to the glomerulus causes retention of phosphate, producing hyperphosphatemia. In addition, tubular injury leads to a reduction in the production of 1-25 dihydroxyvitamin D. Calcium transport in the gut is inhibited by the increased concentration of phosphate, thus reducing absorption of calcium to minimal levels. The negative feedback system causes an elaboration of parathyroid hormone in response to decreases in serum calcium. A marked secondary hyperparathyroidism develops. Thus, the syndrome that occurs includes not only osteomalacia but also osteitis fibrosa cystica (hyperparathyroidism). Three pathophysiologic entities result: osteomalacia, osteitis fibrosa cystica (secondary hyperparathyroidism), and ectopic calcification. The ectopic calcification occurs when the patient's calcium level rises to near-normal levels. With the pre-existing increased phosphate level, calcium salts precipitate in a variety of ectopic sites. The treatment of renal osteodystrophy remains in the hands of the internists and involves dialysis and phosphate binders.

Increased Osteodensity

The incidence of Paget's disease of bone is approximately 3 per cent of the U.S. population older than 40. No genetic link has been found. Paget's disease is associated with bone resorption in the early phases, which is followed by accelerated bone formation in the later phases of the disease. The bone turnover rate is markedly increased in pagetic bone to as high as 10 to 20 times normal. This hypermetabolic state causes increased alkaline phosphatase to appear in the serum and increased levels of the amino acid hydroxyproline (endogenous to type I collagen) to be excreted in the urine. The alkaline phosphatase activity correlates directly with the osteoblastic activity and therefore with bone production.

Paget's disease is often found as an incidental finding on radiographs and may present with early findings of back pain, usually with some component of osteoarthritis. The treatment of Paget's disease relies upon three important drugs: calcitonin, mithramycin, and diphosphonates. Calcitonin is effective initially in most patients and decreases both osteoclastic activity and the absolute number of osteoclasts. Mithramycin is believed to act by inhibiting the synthesis of specific RNA during rapid bone turnover. Diphosphonates, which function as an analogue of pyrophosphate, interfere with the mineralization of bone.

A second disorder of bone that produces increased bone density is osteopetrosis. The skeletal lesions in osteopetrosis are caused primarily by a markedly decreased rate of cartilage and bone resorption. Thus, the intramedullary canal and hematopoietic system are crowded out by the increased bone presence. Recently, patients with juvenile osteopetrosis have been cured by bone marrow transfer.

BIBLIOGRAPHY

1. Guyton, A.C.: Parathyroid homone, calcitonin, calcium and phosphate metabolism, vitamin D, bone, and teeth. Text book of Medical Physiology, 7th ed. Philadelphia, W.B. Saunders Co., 1986, pp. 937–953.
2. American Academy of Orthopaedic Surgeons.: Orthopaedic Knowledge Update Home Study Syllabus, 1984, Update 1, pp. 15–28.
3. American Academy of Orthopaedic Surgeons.: Orthopaedic Knowledge Update Home Study Syllabus, 1990, Update 3, pp. 29–46.
4. Vass, G.: Cellular biology and biochemical mechanisms of bone resorption: A review of recent developments of formation, activation, mode of action of osteoclasts. Clin. Orthopaedics, 231:239–271, 1988.
5. Carter, D.R., and Spangler, D.M.: Mechanical properties and composition of cortical bone. Clin. Orthopaedics, 135: 192–217, 1978.
6. Parfitt, A.M., and Duncan, H.: Metabolic bone diseases affecting the spine. In Rothman, R.H., and Simeone, F.A. (eds.): The Spine, 2nd ed. Philadelphia, W.B. Saunders Co., 1982, pp. 775–905.
7. Salter, R.B.: Normal structure and function of the musculoskeletal tissues. In Textbook of Disorders and Injuries of the Muscoloskeletal System, 2nd. ed. Baltimore, Williams & Wilkins Co., 1970, pp. 3–16.
8. Lovell, W.W., and Winter, R.B.: Pediatric Orthopaedics, 2nd ed. Philadelphia, J.B. Lippincott Co., 1986.

21

SKELETAL MUSCLE

PAUL D. FADALE

EMBRYOLOGY

Skeletal muscle is also known as voluntary, striated, stripped, or segmental muscle. Limb buds appear during the fourth week of development and consist of a core of mesenchyme covered by the apical ectodermal ridge. As the limb bud grows, the proliferating mesenchyme eventually gives rise to all skeletal rudiments. Myotome cells from the adjacent somites invade the limb buds to give rise to all the skeletal muscles. Distinct muscle formation reaches the level of the hand and foot during the seventh week.

The upper limb bud lies opposite the lower five cervical and first thoracic myotomes. The lower limb bud is positioned opposite the second through fifth lumbar and upper three sacral myotomes. Branches of the spinal nerves that supply these myotomes reach the base of the limb bud. As the bud elongates to form a limb, the nerves grow into it.

Establishment of neurocontacts with developing skeletal muscle fibers (weeks 6 to 10) is critical for muscular development and the complete differentiation and function of muscle fibers. The large somatic motor neurons begin to ramify among developing motor fibers of the muscles and establish formation of the neuromuscular junctions. Voluntary control of skeletal muscle contraction is completed at approximately the end of the first year after birth when myelination of the nerve fibers of the corticospinal tract is complete. At this time, the child has sufficient voluntary control over the skeletal muscles to be able to stand and begin walking.

ORGANIZATION OF SKELETAL MUSCLE
(Figure 21–1)

Approximately 40 to 45 per cent of the body is skeletal muscle. Skeletal muscles are surrounded by well-defined fascial layers. The epimysium is a fascial layer that completely surrounds an individual mus-cle. From it, extensions of the fascia divide the muscle belly itself into fascicles. This dividing fascial layer is called the perimysium. Further division of the muscle is done by the fascial endomysium, which extends into each fascicle and surrounds the individual muscle fibers.

All skeletal muscles are made up of numerous fibers ranging from 10 to 80 μm in diameter. Each of these fibers in turn is made up of successively smaller subunits called myofibrils. These muscle fibers extend the entire length of the muscle and are innervated by only one nerve ending. End muscle fiber cell membrane (sarcolemma) fuses at the end of the muscle fiber with tendinous tissue, which in turn collects into bundles to form muscle tendons.

The muscle fiber exerts its force by contracting (shortening). Each muscle fiber contains several hundred to several thousand myofibrils. Myofibrils are longitudinally oriented bundles of thick and thin filaments. The thick filaments (myosin) and thin filaments (actin) are protein molecules that provide the mechanical force of contraction by sliding past one another. The thin filaments of the myofibrils are anchored at one end by a structure that is made up largely of proteins oriented at right angles to the filaments: the Z-band. These Z-bands occur at regular intervals along the whole length of the myofibrils. They give skeletal and cardiac muscles their striated appearance.

The section of myofibril between two adjacent Z-bands is called the sarcomere (Fig. 21–1), which is the basic unit of contractile action. Thus, myofibrils are constructed of many sarcomeres linked end to end. The sarcomere can further be divided into an A-band, which is a section of the sarcomere containing the interdigitation of actin and myosin filaments. In the middle of the A-band is the M-band, which is created by the middle portion of adjacent thick filaments that line up exactly through the sarcomere. I-bands contain only actin where it does not interdigitate with the myosin molecules. In the relaxed state, the thin filaments of a sarcomere are attached at either end of the Z-band and point toward one another. Normally, they do not touch. Therefore,

316

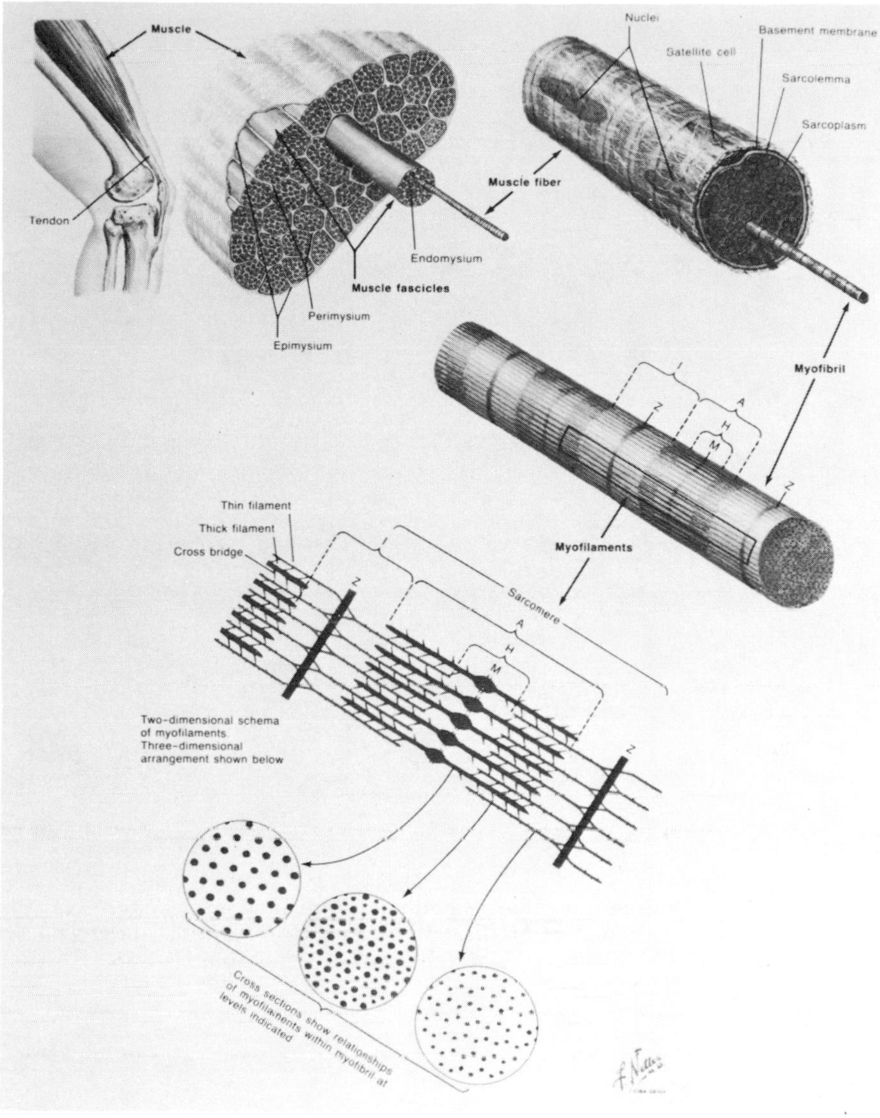

FIGURE 21–1. Structural arrangement of skeletal muscle. (Reprinted from Netter, E.H.: Physiology. *In* The Ciba Collection of Medical Illustrations, vol. 8, Musculoskeletal System, Part 1: Anatomy, Physiology, and Metabolic Disorders. Summit, NJ, CIBA-GEIGY Corp., 1987, p. 150.)

there is a region in the middle of the sarcomere where thick filaments are not overlapped by the thin filaments. This is called the H-zone.

On three-dimensional analysis of the structure of the sarcomere, one can see a recurring and very regular pattern. Each filament is surrounded by six thin filaments, and each thin filament is equidistant to three thick filaments (Fig. 21–1).

Thick filaments are composed primarily of a protein called myosin. This is a large protein with a molecular weight of approximately 500,000. The myosin molecule on electron microscopic exam looks like a long rod with two paddles attached at one end (Fig. 21–2). These paddles form the cross-bridges between the thick and thin filaments. Normally, the paddles in a relaxed muscle state point toward the Z-bands. During muscle contraction, the angle between the cross-bridges and the rod portion of the myosin becomes more acute. This change of angle occurs when the end of the paddle or head group is bound to a nearby thin filament, thereby pulling the thin filament to the center of the sarcomere. This is called the sliding filament mechanism of contraction. By approximating the Z-bands, the sarcomeres shorten. When repeated throughout the length of the myofibril, the result is contraction of the muscle belly.

Thin filaments consist chiefly of a protein called actin. The actin molecule has a molecular weight of approximately 42,000 and is therefore much smaller than myosin. In its normal state, actin resides in the form of a double helix. Along the notches between the two strands of actin are molecules of a globular protein, troponin. Attached to each troponin is a molecule of tropomyosin, which lies along the grooves of the double helix (Fig. 21–2).

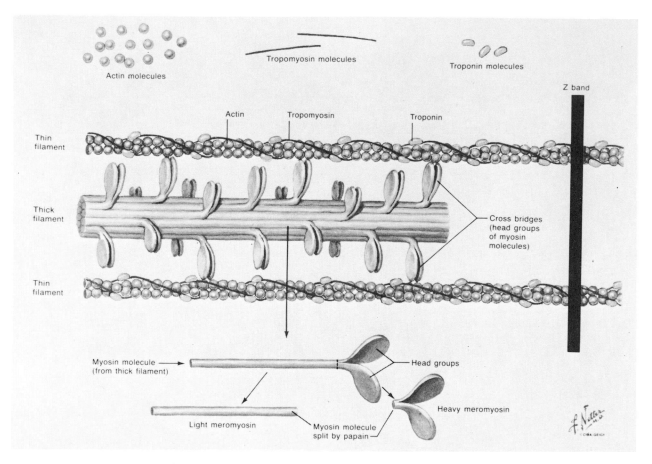

FIGURE 21–2.   Composition of myofilaments. (Reprinted from Netter, F.H.: Physiology. *In* The Ciba Collection of Medical Illustrations, vol. 8. Musculoskeletal System, Part 1: Anatomy, Physiology, and Metabolic Disorders. Summit, NJ, CIBA-GEIGY Corp., 1987, p. 152.)

MUSCLE CONTRACTION

Skeletal muscle fibers are innervated by neurons, the cell bodies of which are located in the anterior horn of the spinal cord. Nerves enter the muscle at a region called the end-plate zone (Fig. 21–3). Each motor neuron branches several times and innervates many muscle fibers. Each muscle fiber is innervated by only one motor neuron. This combination of a single motor neuron and all the muscle fibers it innervates is called the motor unit.

The strength of muscle contractions depends upon the number of muscle fibers active at the same time. The central nervous system is unable to activate single muscle fibers, but must work through an individual motor neuron and its surrounding muscle fibers of the motor unit. Therefore, the degree of control that is exerted on the strength of a contraction depends upon the number of muscle fibers in each motor unit. This organization enables large muscles, such as the gastrocsoleus complex, to exert a great deal of power by containing over a thousand muscle fibers in each motor unit. Conversely, when strength needs are minimal but fine control of the muscle is needed, such as in the extraocular muscles, the motor units contain as few as six muscle fibers each. In general, smaller motor neurons innervate fewer muscle fibers and therefore have smaller units. These neurons are usually activated first. If more power is needed with less fine control, larger motor units are progressively recruited. This is the size principle of motor control. Because the muscle fibers of the smaller motor unit are often activated first, they must be relatively resistant to fatigue and are of a slow twitch nature. When more power is required, larger neurons recruit fast-twitch fibers.

Two separate types of motor units—fast twitch (FT) and slow twitch (ST)—can be identified anatomically and have significant metabolic and functional differences. For a short time, muscles are able to function without oxygen by using the glycolytic pathway to generate adenosine triphosphate (ATP). Muscle fibers that are specialized for high power output over a short time (fast twitch) make extensive use of this pathway. These fibers release energy rapidly from ATP, but energy stores are regenerated

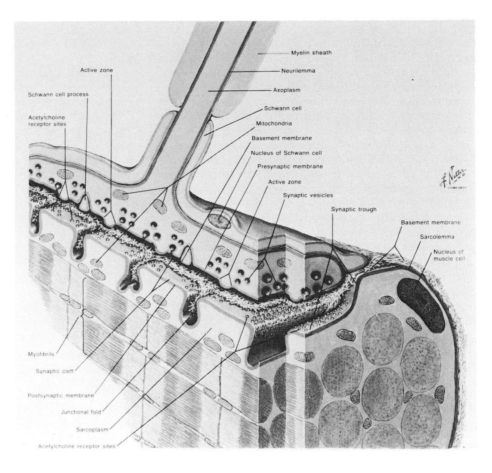

FIGURE 21–3. The neuromuscular junction. (Reprinted from Netter, F.H.: Physiology. *In* The Ciba Collection of Medical Illustrations, vol. 8. Musculoskeletal System, Part 1: Anatomy, Physiology, and Metabolic Disorders. Summit, NJ, CIBA-GEIGY Corp., 1987, p. 158.)

poorly. Therefore, they become fatigued easily. Fast-twitch motor units are larger and can generate more strength than the slow-twitch fibers. The fast-twitch fibers have higher enzymatic activity for phosphagen and glycolytic systems and predominate during activities dependent upon anaerobic energy.

Muscle fibers that are active over a long time period (slow-twitch fibers) are rich in mitochondria. These fibers are stained darkly for enzymes of the oxidative pathway and have a much greater aerobic capacity. They tend to be small and are often used in fine manipulations. In addition, they are the first fibers to be activated when a lower level of power is required.

The distribution of muscle fibers in any one individual is believed to be determined genetically. During physical activity, there is a selective recruitment of the appropriate fibers that are best suited for that specific activity. At this point, it is felt that the ratio of fast twitch and slow twitch fibers in any one individual cannot be altered with specific training. However, such training may selectively improve the abilities of one or the other fiber types. Endurance athletes have a relatively high percentage of slow-twitch fibers, whereas fast-twitch fibers predominate in athletes involved in activities requiring explosive strength.

Motor axons to the motor unit are generally large myelinated fibers. At the end of the neuron, finger-like processes are found between the membranes of the nerve and the muscle. The nerve terminal lies in a trough within the sarcolemma. The nerve terminal itself (Fig. 21–3) is rich in mitochondria and contains numerous synaptic vesicles that contain the neurotransmitter acetylcholine. Acetylcholine is released by exocytosis of the vesicles. The presynaptic and postsynaptic membranes are separated by a space (synaptic cleft) approximately 20 nm wide. In the muscle membranes opposite the site of acetylcholine release are junctional folds containing both acetylcholine receptors that mediate the action of the neurotransmitter and acetylcholinesterase, which destroys the neurotransmitter (Fig. 21–3).

Electrical impulses are propagated along the motor axon toward the neuromuscular junction. When the action potential arrives at the end of the motor nerve, the depolarization opens up calcium channels in the axon terminal. As a result, calcium becomes concentrated in the presynaptic nerve terminal. This sudden increase in the intraterminal concentration of calcium causes the release of acetylcholine. The acetylcholine binds to receptor molecules on the postsynaptic membrane, which results in the opening of channels to permit the influx of sodium ions and the efflux of potassium ions. The net effect is depolarization of the muscle membrane and the triggering of the muscle action potential. The acetylcholine is then rapidly hydrolyzed by acetylcholinesterase into choline and acetate.

Neuromuscular transmission can be blocked by many drugs. A calcium channel blocker, such as verapamil, prevents calcium from entering the nerve terminal and thus blocks the release of acetylcholine. Curare can block the acetylcholine receptors. Succinylcholine can produce muscle relaxation by keeping the acetylcholine channels open for too long a period of time. By keeping the acetylcholine channel open for so long, the depolarizing blockers keep the muscle membrane depolarized and refractory to impulse initiation. Physostigmine and edrophonium chloride inhibit acetylcholinesterase and strengthen transmission by delaying the breakdown of acetylcholine. These agents may be used for the diagnosis or treatment of the neuromuscular disease, myasthenia gravis.

The muscle action potential is propagated along the entire length of the muscle fiber (Fig. 21–4). Between adjacent myofibrils are elements of the conducting pathway called the sarcoplasmic reticulum-transverse tubule system (vertical bars in Fig. 21–4). The T-tubules are internal extensions of the cell membrane. When an action potential propagates along a muscle fiber membrane, it progresses along the T-tubules into the interior of the muscle fiber as well.

The sarcoplasmic reticulum contains calcium ions in a very high concentration. When an adjacent T-tubule is excited, these calcium ions are released and diffuse to the nearby myofibrils where they bind strongly to troponin (Fig. 21–4). This in turn causes conformational changes that allow actin to bind to myosin cross-bridges, thereby eliciting a muscle contraction (Fig. 21–5). A calcium pump is located in the walls of the sarcoplasmic reticulum. This pump resets the muscle for contracting by removing the calcium from the myofibril and concentrating it back into the sarcoplasmic reticulum at the completion of a single contraction. If a second contraction is elicited before the first one has relaxed, a stronger contraction results. This process is the summation of muscle response to increasing frequency of stimulation. If this frequency of activation is high enough, a continuous contraction (tetanus) will result.

The tension that a muscle may generate is also dependent upon the length of the muscle. The muscle length-tension relationship, represented by the Blix curve (Fig. 21–6), is as follows. At the normal resting length of the muscle fiber, there is a maximal overlap of a cross-bridging between the thick and thin filaments. This allows maximum tension to be

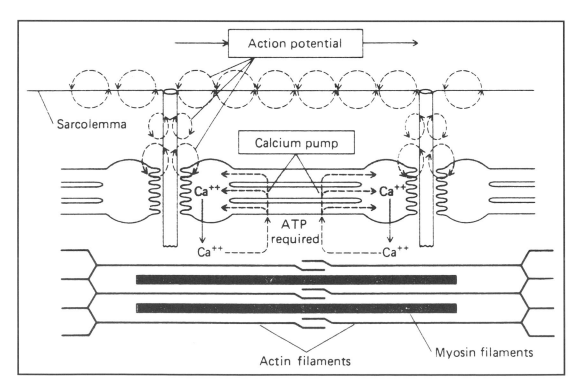

FIGURE 21–4. Excitation-contraction coupling in the muscle, showing an action potential that causes release of calcium ions from the sarcoplasmic reticulum and then reuptake of the calcium ions by a calcium pump. (Reprinted from Guyton, A.C.: Textbook of Medical Physiology, 7th ed. Philadelphia, W.B. Saunders Co., 1986, p. 128.)

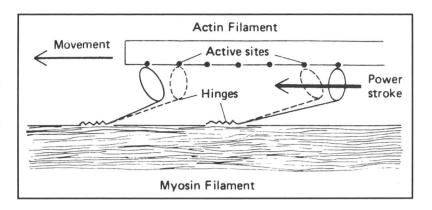

FIGURE 21–5. Muscle contraction by the actin-myosin interaction. (Reprinted from Guyton, A.C.: Textbook of Medical Physiology, 7th ed. Philadelphia, W.B. Saunders Co., 1986, p. 125.)

developed in the resting stage. If a muscle is in a contracted position, the thin actin filaments overlap one another, which interferes with cross-bridging of the thick filaments, thereby reducing the maximal tension possible. Conversely, if the muscle is stretched to the point where thin filaments give minimal cross-bridging to the myosin group, then tension created by cross-bridging is weak. A greatly stretched muscle with almost no overlap at all is able to produce minimal tension in response to stimulation.

ENERGY METABOLISM

Adensosine triphosphate (ATP) is the immediate source of energy needed for muscle activity. Energy is directly released from the high energy phosphate bonds when ATP is broken down into ADP and inorganic phospate. The body must then recreate ATP from one of three available sources. The most readily available source of energy in muscle cells is phosphocreatinine, which is enzymatically broken down, releasing energy to form ATP. It is primarily used in high-intensity, short-duration activities since the amount of energy available utilizing this system is limited. Anaerobic glycolysis utilizing the lactic acid system is the second source of energy available in muscle cells. Partially metabolized glucose releases energy and forms lactic acid as a byproduct. Accumulation of this lactic acid in the muscle causes symptoms of fatigue. Anaerobic glycolysis is also a limited source of energy. Aerobic glycolysis occurs when glycogen is completely broken down to carbon dioxide and water in the presence of oxygen. This process occurs in the mitochondria of muscle cells and is responsible for the release of large amounts of energy for ATP resynthesis. This energy source is utilized primarily in prolonged endurance type of activities. The amount of oxygen available to the cell is the limiting factor in aerobic glycolysis.

The system the body will use depends upon the intensity and duration of the specific activity undertaken. This variation has been described as the energy continuum.

One definition of conditioning is the time that it takes the body to return to its pre-exercise state after vigorous activity. For this to occur, lactic acid must be removed from the muscle, muscle glycogen must be replenished, phosphagen and ATP must be restored, and any remaining oxygen debt must be eliminated. The concept of "warming down" is based on the fact that light exercise hastens the removal of lactic acid from the body. Muscle glycogen can be resynthesized in as short as 1 to 2 hours after moderate exercise or as long as 48 hours after prolonged endurance activities. Muscle phosphagen store replacement is quite active and usually can occur within minutes. Oxygen debt recovery is a two-phase process. Replenishing myoglobin with oxygen and the aerobic recovery of phosphagen stores occur within a few minutes. Recovery from the oxygen debt needed to assist the conversion of lactic acid, however, requires 1 to 2 hours. The recovery

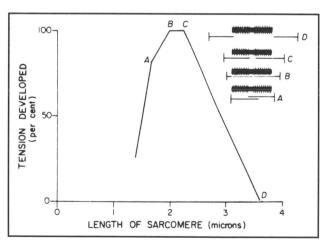

FIGURE 21–6. Length-tension diagram (Blix curve) for a single sarcomere, illustrating maximum strength of contraction when the sarcomere is 2.0 to 2.2 μm in length. At the upper right are shown the relative positions of the actin and myosin filaments at different sarcomere lengths from point A to point D. (Reprinted from Guyton, A.C.: Textbook of Medical Physiology, 7th ed. Philadelphia, W.B. Saunders Co., 1986, p. 128.)

process, like the energy support processes, is dependent upon the particular type of athletic endeavor with its variations and durations in intensity of activity. Conditioning can shorten all recovery times.

MALIGNANT HYPERTHERMIA

Malignant hyperthermia is an autosomal dominant abnormality of muscle that most commonly develops after the administration of general anesthesia, but may be triggered by many stimuli. It is one of the leading causes of anesthetic-related deaths in North America. Halothane and succinylcholine are most commonly implicated as the cause of a hyperthermic reaction. Men and women appear to be equally at risk during childhood, but most postpubescent victims are men. The peak incidence in adults occurs around the age of 30 years.

The pathogenesis of malignant hyperthermia appears to involve an abnormality in the calcium transport system of cell membranes of the sarcoplasmic reticulum and mitochondria. The presence of a trigger agent precipitates a leak of calcium ions from the sarcoplasmic reticulum, resulting in a sustained actin-myosin combination that causes recurrent sarcomeric contraction and muscle rigidity. This process produces heat, metabolic acidosis, and carbon dioxide production with concomitant respiratory acidosis. The end result is a cellular death, which worsens the acidosis. Protein denaturation causes coagulopathy, and the final result is the patient's death.

Patient evaluation for susceptibility to this condition is difficult. An accurate family and personal history is often the best tool. However, it is not reliable. Susceptible patients tend to be healthy and athletic, with large muscle masses. A history of nocturnal leg cramping and exercise intolerance in hot weather may also provide a clue to the disease process. Attacks do not necessarily occur with the first exposure to a general anesthetic; more than 50 percent of reported cases occur during the first, second, or even third experience. Conclusive testing can only be achieved by muscle biopsy with specific in vitro muscle fiber testing.

Careful intraoperative monitoring is important for the management of malignant hyperthermia. Early signs are often nonspecific and include tachycardia, ventricular arrhythmias, and an unstable blood pressure. The most consistent finding is a combined respiratory and a metabolic acidosis. An increase in temperature of 1°C or more requires further investigation.

If malignant hyperthermia is suspected, the surgical procedure is terminated as rapidly as possible. Dantrolene sodium is the treatment of choice. It inhibits calcium release from the sarcoplasmic reticulum. It should be administered intravenously in doses of 5 to 6 mg/kg of body weight. Acidosis is corrected by hyperventilation with 100 percent oxygen and administration of sodium bicarbonate. Procanamide in a 0.2 percent solution (2 mg/cc) is an effective treatment for arrhythmias. Mannitol or Lasix is used to maintain the urine output, which will clear away the products of muscle degradation that could lead to tubular necrosis and renal failure. Glucose may be used to decrease the serum potassium level. Surface cooling by an ice bag and intravenous use of iced fluids may be helpful in reducing core temperature in excess of 39°C. Dantrolene should be administered for at least 48 hours. Since the process of muscle necrosis may continue, it is important to maintain adequate urine output.

COMPARTMENT SYNDROME

A compartment syndrome is a condition in which high pressure within a closed fascial space or muscle compartment results in a reduced capillary blood perfusion level below that necessary for tissue viability. Local ischemia produced by a compartment syndrome must be relieved by decompression of the muscle compartment to prevent muscle and nerve necrosis. Muscle microcirculation is compromised at tissue pressures as low as 30 to 40 mm Hg. Although capillary perfusion is inadequate to meet the metabolic demands of the muscle, central arterial blood flow is typically normal in compartment syndromes.

The first and most important symptom of an impending compartment syndrome is pain that is greater than expected from the primary problem. Pain with passive stretch of the muscles in the involved compartments is a common finding. The first sign of nerve ischemia is the alteration of sensation, which is manifested early on by subjective paresthesia in the distribution of the involved nerve. This sign is followed by hypoesthesia and later by anesthesia of the nerve distribution. Nerve dysfunction of a specific compartment is a reliable but late sign of increased intracompartmental pressure. Paresis, secondary to nerve dysfunction and elevated compartmental pressure, is a relatively late physical finding. Except in the presence of major arterial injury or disease, the peripheral pulses and capillary filling are routinely intact in compartment syndrome patients. Compartment pressure measurements greater than 30 to 40 mm Hg may confirm a clinical suspicion of compartment syndrome. Surgical decompression, which allows the volume of the compartment to increase, is the only means of treatment.

TETANUS

Tetanus is an acute disease caused by an exotoxin produced in a wound by *Clostridium tetani*. It can be a fatal disease. Mortality rates of 25 per cent to 50 per cent have been reported; even in modern facilities. Tetanus is characterized by generalized skeletal muscle rigidity and convulsive spasms. *Clostridium tetani* is an anaerobic, gram-positive rod which readily forms endospores. The production of the exotoxin, tetanus toxin (tetanospasmin) is responsible for the clinical manifestations of the disease. The tetanus bacillus is found as a saprophyte in the intestinal tract of man and certain animals, as well as in the superficial layers of the soil.

Tetanus can only occur after spores or vegetative bacteria gain access to tissue and produce the toxin locally. Because *clostridium tetani* is a noninvasive organism, the usual mode of entry is through a puncture wound or cut of an extremity. Tetanus may also follow elective surgery, burn wounds, dental work, and abortions. Wounds are undoubtedly frequently contaminated with spores of *clostridium tetani,* but the clinical manifestations of tetanus rarely develop because germination of spores occur only when the oxygen tension is much lower than that of normal tissue. Toxin production in wounds is favored by necrotic tissue, foreign bodies, calcium salts, and associated infections which establish a low oxidation-reduction potential. Clinical features of tetanus prone wounds are listed in Table 21-1. Although infection caused by the tetanus bacillus remains localized, the toxin produced is transported to the central nervous system via neuropathways. The tetanus toxin attacks synaptic junctions to produce disinhibition. Generalized muscle rigidity arises from uninhibited afferent stimuli entering the central nervous system from the periphery. When the stimuli become more vigorous, spasms may occur. The tetanus toxin has other effects. It may produce a neuromuscular blockade similar to the botulinum toxin. Direct stimulation of muscle may produce a contraction which is unaccompanied by an action potential in nerves.

The time between injury and the appearance of the clinical manifestations of tetanus will usually occur within 14 days from the time of injury. The most common presenting complaints are pain and stiffness of the jaw, abdomen, or back with difficulty swallowing. Trismus is the most common manifesta-

TABLE 21-1. CLINICAL FEATURES OR WOUNDS PRONE TO DEVELOP TETANUS

CLINICAL FEATURES	NONTETANUS-prone WOUNDS	TETANUS-prone WOUNDS
Age of wound	≤6 hours	>6 hours
Configuration	Linear wound	Stellate wound, avulsion, abrasion
Depth	≤1 cm	>1 cm
Mechanism of injury	Sharp surface (eg, knife, glass)	Missile, crush burn, frostbite
Signs of infection	Absent	Present
Devitalized tissue	Absent	Present
Contaminants (dirt, feces, soil, saliva, etc.)	Absent	Present
Denervated, and/ or ischemic tissue	Absent	Present

tion of tetanus and is responsible for the familiar descriptive name of lock jaw. Sustained contractions of the facial muscles produce a characteristic expression called risus sardonicus. The intensity and sequence of muscle involvement is quite variable. As the disease progresses, minimal stimuli produce more intense or longer lasting spasms with increasing frequency. Respiration maybe impaired by laryngospasm or the tonic contraction of respirator muscles. Low grade fever, profuse sweating, and tachycardia are common.

The diagnosis of tetanus is a clinical one that is not dependent on bacteriologic confirmation. *Clostridium tetani* can be cultured from the wound in only about 30 per cent of cases at best. The patient should be hospitalized in an intensive care unit. Tetanus prophylaxis is administered early as outlined in Table 21-2. All necrotic tissue and foreign bodies should be removed from the infected wound and abscesses should be drained. Skeletal muscle relaxation is important in the management of the patient.

TABLE 21-2. SUMMARY OF TETANUS PROPHYLAXIS FOR THE INJURED PATIENT

HISTORY OF ADSORBED TETANUS TOXOID (DOSES)	NONTETANUS-prone WOUNDS		TETANUS-prone WOUNDS	
	TD[1]	TIG	TD[1]	TIG
Unknown or ≤ three	Yes	No	Yes	Yes
≥ three[2]	No[3]	No	No[4]	No

Key: 1. For children under seven years old: DTP (DT, if pertussis vaccine is contraindicated) is preferred to tetanus toxoid alone. For persons seven years old and older, Td is preferred to tetanus toxoid alone. 2. If only three doses of fluid toxoid have been received, a fourth dose of toxoid, preferably an adsorbed toxoid, should be given. 3. Yes, if more than ten years since last dose. 4. Yes, if more than five years since last dose. (More frequent boosters are not needed and can accentuate side effects.)

Td, Tetanus and diphtheria toxoids adsorbed—for adult use; TIG, Tetanus Immune Globulin—Human.

Barbiturates, phenothiazines, and muscle relaxants are generally used alone or in combination to control muscle spasms and convulsions. In severe tetanus, intubation or a tracheostomy is performed to protect against suffocation and reduce the risk of aspiration. Although surgical debridement remains the cornerstone for the treatment of patients with tetanus, penicillin is also used because it is highly effective against the tetanus bacillus. The recommended dose is one to ten units of penicillin a day for ten days. Because tetanus is a lethal disease, prevention becomes the most efficacious treatment. This carried out through an effective immunization program.

HYPOPARATHYROIDISM

Hypoparathyroidism is a metabolic abnormality characterized by hypocalcemia and hyperphosphatemia, resulting in neuromuscular symptoms of tetani and convulsions. Classically the etiology of hyperparathyroidism can be broken down into Iatrogenic, idiopathic, and functional hypoparathyroidism. Iatrogenic hypoparathyroidism may be the result of excision of the parathyroid glands or damage during surgery for thyroid disorders, hyperparathyroidism and radical neck dissections for cancer. This is a much less frequent disease than it has been in the past. Better medical therapy for thyrotoxicosis and improved surgical awareness have made this disease uncommon. Idiopathic hyperparathyroidism is a relatively rare disease. When occurring at an early age, the disease is transmitted most frequently as a autosomal recessive trait. This type of hypoparathyroidism is called multiple endocrine deficiency-autoimmune-candidiasis (MEDAC) syndrome or juvenile familial endocrinopathy-hypoparathyroidism-Addison's disease-moniliasis (HAM) syndrome. Circulating antibodies are frequently present. Functional hypoparathyroidism occurs in patients with severe and prolonged hypomagnesemia. Magnesium is essential for release of parathyroid hormone from the parathyroid glands. Eucalcemia can be restored by the restoration of normal levels of magnesium.

The signs and symptoms of hypoparathyroidism are those of hypocalcemia. Clinical manifestations reflect the severity and duration, as well as the rate of decrease of serum calcium. Hypocalcemia causes a decrease in the threshold of excitation, resulting in a greatly increased neuromuscular excitability. Tetany is the most striking manifestation. A prodrome of numbness and tingling around the mouth, and in the finger tips may occur. During an attack, the thumb is adducted, the metacarpophalangeal joints are flexed, the fingers extend, and the wrists are flexed (Fig. 21-7). A more generalized form of tetany may be followed by prolonged tonic spasms or a typical epileptiform seizure. Chvostek's sign is elicited by

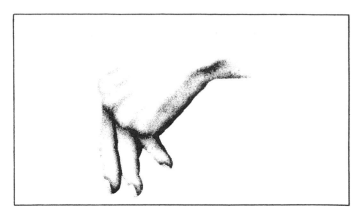

FIGURE 21–7. Attitude of hand during tetany. (Reprinted from Ganong, W.F. (ed.): Review of Medical Physiology, 11th ed. Los Altos, CA, Lange Medical Publications, 1983, p. 319.)

tapping the facial nerve in front of the ear. The response varies from minimal twitching of the lip, to contraction of all the facial muscles on the stimulated side. Trousseau's sign is demonstrated by occluding the circulation of the arm by inflation of a blood pressure cuff to above systolic pressure for 2 to 3 minutes. A positive response is the development of ipsilateral carpal spasm, with relaxation occuring soon after the cuff is deflated.

The diagnosis of hypoparathyroidism is considered in patients who present with symptoms of hypocalcemia and are found to have both hypocalcemia and hyperphospatemia in the presence of normal renal function. Specific laboratory tests include parathyroid hormone radioimmunoassay and measurement of cyclic AMP excretion after the administration of parathyroid hormone. Treatment is geared to restore calcium toward normal by the use of supplementary calcium and vitamin D. It is important also to evaluate the patient for the possibility of hypomagnesemia, which must be corrected before successful treatment with vitamin D and calcium in these patients. These patients should be followed closely for the detection of any complications.

BIBLIOGRAPHY

1. Schwartz, S.I. (ed.): Principles of Surgery, 5th ed. New York, McGraw-Hill, 1989.
2. Walton, Sir John. (ed.): Brian's Diseases of the Nervous System, 9th ed. Oxford, Oxford University Press, 1985.
3. Adelman, G. (ed.): Encyclopedia of Neuroscience. Boston, Birkhauser, 1987.
4. DeGroot, L. (ed.): Endocrinology, 2nd ed. Philadelphia, W.B. Saunders Co., 1989.
5. Wyngaarden, J.B., and Smith, L.H. (ed.): Cecil Textbook of Medicine, 18th ed. Philadelphia, W.B. Saunders Co., 1988.
6. American College of Surgeons Committee on Trauma. Advanced Trauma Life Support Program. American College of Surgeons, 555 Erie Street, Chicago, Illinois, 1989.

7. Guyton, A.C.: Textbook of Medical Physiology, 7th ed. Philadelphia, W.B. Saunders Co., 1986.

8. Netter, F.H.: The Ciba Collection of Medical Illustrations, vol. 8. Musculoskeletal System, Part 1: Anatomy, Physiology, and Metabolic Disorders. Summit, NJ, CIBA-GEIGY Corp., 1987.

9. American Academy of Orthopaedic Surgeons. Orthopaedic Knowledge, Update 1, Home Study Syllabus. American Academy of Orthpaedic Surgeons, 444 North Michigan Ave, Suite 1500, Chicago, Illinois 60611, 1984.

10. Cruess, R. (ed.): The Musculoskeletal System: Embryology, Biochemistry, and Physiology. New York, Churchill Livingstone, 1982.

22

THE SKIN AND ITS CONNECTIVE TISSUE

BRUCE A. BROD *and* J. BLAKE GOSLEN

The skin is the largest organ of the body and the primary site of interface between the human being and the environment. It is a tough yet pliable covering that serves as a highly effective barrier, acts as a sensory receptor, functions in thermoregulation, and is highly involved in immunologic surveillance. Remarkably, the skin has a capacity to regenerate into a nearly perfect, anatomically and functionally diverse organ system even after physical damage.

ANATOMY

The skin is composed of two mutually dependent layers: the outer epidermis, of ectodermal origin, and the inner dermis, of mesodermal origin. These layers rest upon the fat-containing subcutaneous tissue, the panniculus adiposus (Fig. 22–1). In certain areas of the body (i.e., head and neck), fibrous septae from the subcutaneous or superficial fascia (superficial musculoaponeurotic system) insert into the dermis and are responsible for transmitting forces of underlying muscle contraction. On the head and neck, these attachments are instrumental in facial expression and animation.

Epidermis

The epidermis is composed of two types of cells: keratinocytes and dendritic, clear cells. As the keratinocytes differentiate into an outer layer of anucleate cells known as the stratum corneum or horny layer, they are arranged into four layers: (1) the basal cell layer, (2) the squamous cell layer or spinous layer, (3) the granular layer, and (4) the horny layer. The basal layer or stratum germinativum is a single layer of columnar cells attached by hemidesmosomes to the basement membrane zone and named for its property of proliferation. A considerable degree of

heterogeneity exists among the cells of the basal cell layer. Up to 50 per cent of these cells may be noncycling or only slowly proliferative. They may provide a reserve population of cells upon which the epithelium can rely to increase its proliferative rate in response to injury or other extraneous physiologic or pharmacologic stimuli, e.g., epidermal growth factor, vitamin A derivatives, or the hormones progesterone and estrogen. After the basal cells divide, they move upward within the epidermis to replace the cells lost at the surface during normal epidermal turnover.

Above the basal cell layer lies the spinous layer, a zone of cells five to ten layers thick that become more differentiated and flattened as they move outward. These cells are joined by abundant desmosomes, a type of intercellular junction specialized for cell-cell adhesion. Gap junctions, through ionic and electrical coupling, provide an additional pathway for cell-to-cell communication. Glycoproteins on the epidermal cell surface are also important in cell-cell adhesion.

The granular cell layer, which is the most highly differentiated layer of the epidermis, lies beneath the stratum corneum and is the zone where dissolution of the nucleus and other cell organelles is initiated.

Finally, the outermost stratum corneum contains both the greatest number and the largest cells of the epidermis. It ranges from a thin fifteen layers on the face to a hundred or more layers on the plantar surface. A specialized cornified layer of cells comprises the nails situated on the dorsum of the distal end of the fingers and toes. Hair is a similar form of acellular horny material. The stratum corneum limits the passage of water and other molecules into and out of the skin and is our major protection against the outside environment.

Keratins are filament-forming polypeptides, seen initially in the spinous layer, where they attach to desmosomes. They account for up to 80 per cent of the cell mass as keratinocytes differentiate into cor-

326

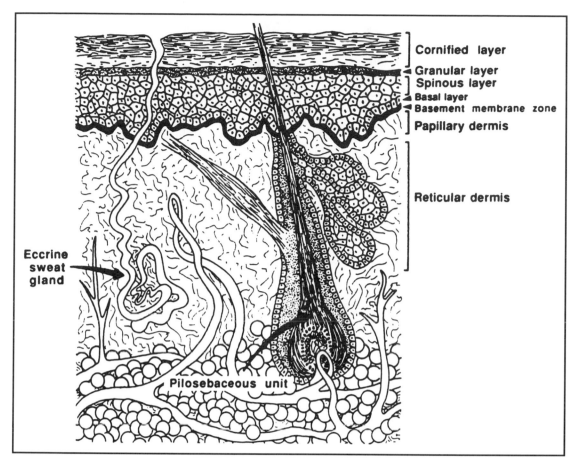

FIGURE 22–1. Normal cutaneous anatomy. (Reprinted from Bauer, E.A., Tabas, M., and Goslen, J.B.: Skin: Cells, matrix, and function. *In* Kelly, W.N. (ed.): Textbook of Internal Medicine. Philadelphia, J.B. Lippincott, 1989. Chapter 153, p. 972.)

nified cells of the horny layer and contribute to this layer's unique barrier properties. In the granular layer, unique keratohyaline granules are present that contain the histidine-rich protein, filaggrin. In the horny layer this protein contributes to the aggregation of keratin filaments. Keratin polypeptides in the spinous layer are largely low molecular weight intermediate filaments, whereas in the horny layer, high molecular weight filaments predominate.

There is constant regeneration of the protective stratum corneum with migration of the cells from the basal layer upward to it. The transit time from the basal layer to the stratum corneum can take 2 weeks, although this can vary greatly with altered hormonal states, as well as proliferating and keratinizing diseases of the skin, e.g., psoriasis and ichthyoses. It usually takes an additional 2 weeks for cells to move to the horny layer and subsequently desquamate.

The epidermis is also a major factor in providing photoprotection. Within the basal layer of the epidermis lie the melanocytes that produce melanin, the pigment that absorbs radiant energy and protects the skin from the harmful effects of ultraviolet light.

Each melanocyte is thought to relate to a specific number of keratinocytes (epidermal melanin units). These neural-crest-derived melanocytes transfer the melanin, packaged in special membrane-bound organelles called melanosomes, to the keratinocytes. The melanocytes possess dendrites that extend to the lower spinous layer and carry the packaged melanin. Variability in pigment among the races is due to differences in the packaging of melanin by melanocytes, rather than to differences in the number of melanocytes. For example, black skin typically contains larger melanosomes than that of more lightly pigmented races.

The skin probably has important immune functions, being the site of foreign antigen presentation. The Langerhans' cell is a bone-marrow-derived dendritic cell present in the basal, spinous, and granular layers of the epidermis, as well as other sites. Langerhans' cells are important antigen-processing accessory cells that can present antigen to lymphocytes in the epidermis or dermis. An example of this complex process is allergic contact hypersensitivity, such as that experienced by many individuals after exposure to rhus antigen (poison ivy). The epidermis also produces important immune-mediating substances. For example, both Langerhans' cells and keratinocytes produce epidermal-cell-derived thymocyte-activating factor (ETAF), an interleukin-1-like molecule. This substance stimulates T lymphocytes to divide and produce interleukin-2; attracts polymorphonuclear leukocytes, mononuclear leukocytes, and T lymphocytes; and stimulates the growth and secretory activity of fibroblasts. Keratinocytes also synthesize or contain thymopoietin, which affects the maturation of T cells in the skin.

Dermal-Epidermal Junction

The dermal-epidermal junction (DEJ) or basement membrane zone (BMZ) of skin lies at the interface between the epidermis and dermis. Although it serves to allow epidermal-dermal adhesion in normal skin, it is also the target of both immunologic and nonimmunologic injury. Disruption of the BMZ at specific anatomic sites accounts for clinically distinct blistering diseases of the skin.

There are two distinct regions of the DEJ. The first, known as the lamina lucida, is the thinner layer parallel to and just beneath the plasma membrane of the basal keratinocytes. The wider lamina densa or basal lamina lies beneath the lamina lucida and is contiguous with the underlying dermis. Within the BMZ are at least 13 distinct antigenic components (Fig. 22–2), many of which are important targets in certain autoimmune and inherited blistering disorders. In bullous pemphigoid, for example, immunoglobulin and complement are deposited in a linear fashion primarily in the lamina lucida, resulting in a blister or split in the skin at this level. Bullous pemphigoid antigen, a 220 to 240 Kd glycoprotein, is thought to be the antigenic target of this immunologic event. In epidermolysis bullosa acquisita (EBA), a disease characterized by tense blisters primarily on the hands and feet, antibodies bind in a linear array to an antigen (EBA antigen) just below the lamina densa. Lastly, in the dystrophic form of epidermolysis bullosa (EB), an inherited but nonimmunologic blistering disease, there is a defect in the expression of some of the basement membrane antigens. For instance, in certain types of dystrophic EB, the anchoring filaments made up of type VII collagen are present in reduced amounts. Their deficiency accounts for the easy fragility of the skin in this disorder.

The DEJ is also thought to play a role in wound healing. A number of animal and in vitro studies suggest a role for bullous pemphigoid antigen in the early phase of wound healing, in which it appears to be the first component of the BMZ that is resynthesized by the newly regenerated epithelium.

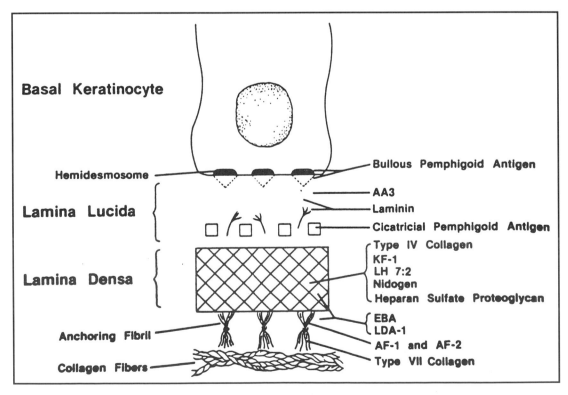

FIGURE 22–2. The basement membrane zone with associated antigens of clinical importance. (Reprinted from Callen, J.P. (ed.): Advances in Dermatology, vol. 2. Chicago, Year Book Medical Publishers, 1987. Figure 2, p. 286.)

Dermis

The biologic functions of the dermis are to provide protection from mechanical injury and to ensure the mobility and elasticity of the skin. It also serves as a reservoir for body water and electrolytes and has a major role in thermoregulation with its rich vascular network.

There are two major layers of the dermis. The more superficial layer or papillary dermis closely abuts the undulating epidermis and contains smaller diameter collagen fibers and a horizontal plexus of capillary-sized vessels and postcapillary venules. Beneath this layer lies the deeper reticular dermis. This layer makes up the bulk of the dermis and consists of larger bundles of collagen and elastin embedded in a ground substance of proteoglycans. Collagen provides the tensile strength of the dermis, whereas the elastic fibers provide elasticity and resiliency. Proteoglycans bind water and contribute to the proper hydration of the skin.

The major cell type of the dermis is the fibroblast, which produces the collagen and other noncellular matrix components. Within the fibroblasts, collagen is produced on membrane-bound ribosomes and compartmentalized on the rough endoplasmic reticulum. Before extracellular secretion, selected proline and lysine residues are hydroxylated. The precursor form of collagen, termed procollagen, is excreted into the extracellular milieu and terminally cleaved by proteolytic enzymes so that the final product spontaneously aggregates into collagen fibrils that further cross-link through disulfide bonds. The final product is a rod-shaped molecule composed of a trimer of alpha chains that aggregate into a right-handed triple helix, leaving only a small nonhelical segment at each end. The phases of collagen synthesis are shown in Figure 22–3.

There are various types of collagen throughout the body. Each type consists of a trimer of alpha chains in varying combinations (Table 22–1). For example, type I collagen, the most abundant collagen in the skin, is a triple helix composed of two different types of polypeptide alpha chains. Type III collagen, a trimer of one alpha polypeptide, is initially more prevalent in fetal skin, granulation tissue, and hypertrophic scars. Lastly, type IV collagen is a major component of the DEJ.

Elastic fibers in the dermis are likewise produced by fibroblasts and consist of two distinct protein components called elastin and elastic fiber microfibrillar protein. Although elastic proteins make up less than 2 to 4 per cent of the dry weight of the dermis, they serve an important role in normal skin function by allowing the skin to return to its original shape after a deforming force. In certain disease states, such as pseudoxanthoma elasticum and cutis laxa, abnormalities in elastin structure occur that produce characteristic skin change and also potentially catastrophic loss of support to the elastin-containing media of larger visceral blood vessels. Elastin is also diminished in scars or keloids, accounting for the poor extensibility of these structures compared to normal skin.

Cutaneous Vasculature

The vascular architecture of the dermis includes both a superficial and deep plexus of horizontally aligned arterioles and venules connected by communicating blood vessels that are oriented perpendicularly to the skin surface. These communicating vessels arise from larger vessels within septae in the subcutaneous fat.

A network of lymphatic vessels parallel the major blood vessel plexuses. They arise from thin-walled lymphatic capillaries that end blindly within the dermal papillae. Collagen fibrils attached at right angles to the walls of these small lymphatics prevent them from collapsing under pressure from interstitial edema fluid that accumulates postoperatively in the skin.

The fact that the blood supply exists as parallel horizontal plexi permits the survival of skin flaps freed from their deeper communicating vessels. Similarly, necrotizing infections can undermine apparently viable skin and subcutaneous tissue as they spread in the facial cleft between subcutaneous tissue and deep fascia.

Cutaneous Appendages

The skin appendages include the pilosebaceous units and the eccrine and apocrine sweat glands. The

TABLE 22–1. SUMMARY OF COLLAGEN TYPES

Type of Collagen	Chain Composition	Tissue Distribution
I	$[\alpha_1 (I)]_2 \alpha_2$	Skin (85%), tendon, bone
II	$[\alpha_2 (II)]_3$	Cartilage
III	$[\alpha_1 (III)]_3$	Skin (15%), blood vessels, GI tract, predominant in fetal skin
IV	$[\alpha_1 (IV)]_2 \alpha_2 (IV)$	Basement membranes, anchoring plaques
V	$[\alpha_1 (V)]_2 \alpha_2 (V)$ or $[\alpha_1 (V)]_3$	Placenta, smooth muscle, vascular tissue
VI	$\alpha_1 (VI) \alpha_2 (VI) \alpha_3 (VI)$	Aortic intima, placenta
VII	$[\alpha_1 (VII)]_3$	Skin (structural components of anchoring fibrils), fetal membranes

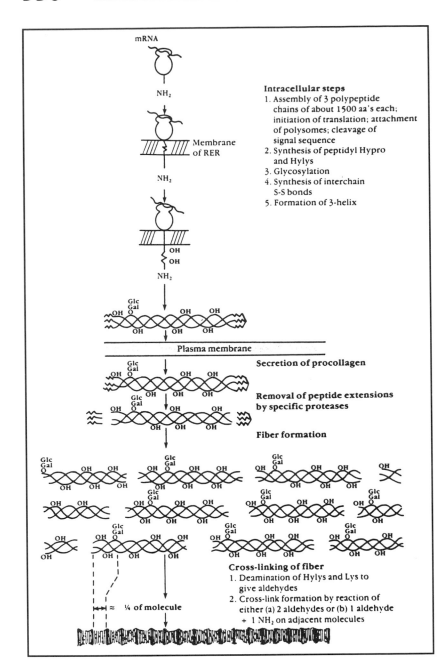

Intracellular steps
1. Assembly of 3 polypeptide chains of about 1500 aa's each; initiation of translation; attachment of polysomes; cleavage of signal sequence
2. Synthesis of peptidyl Hypro and Hylys
3. Glycosylation
4. Synthesis of interchain S-S bonds
5. Formation of 3-helix

Secretion of procollagen

Removal of peptide extensions by specific proteases

Fiber formation

Cross-linking of fiber
1. Deamination of Hylys and Lys to give aldehydes
2. Cross-link formation by reaction of either (a) 2 aldehydes or (b) 1 aldehyde + 1 NH_2 on adjacent molecules

≈ ¼ of molecule

FIGURE 22–3. Normal collagen biosynthesis. (Modified from Thomas, J.R., and Holt, G.R. (eds.): Facial Scars: Incisions, Revision and Camouflage. St. Louis, C.V. Mosby, 1989. Figure 2–2, p. 14.)

principal function of the eccrine gland is to produce sweat, which cools the body by evaporating from the skin's surface. Although these glands are densest in number on the palms and soles, they are distributed over the entire body surface, except for the lips, external ear canal, and labia minora. Each gland consist of a coiled portion in the dermis made up of the secretory coil and proximal duct. This is connected to the epidermis via the relatively straight distal duct that emerges in a spiral fashion through the stratum corneum.

The apocrine glands, although not identical, have a structure similar to the eccrine glands. They are largely found in the axillae and anogenital region and may have a vestigial sexual function, since they are odor producing and do not begin to function until puberty.

The pilosebaceous unit consists of the hair follicle and its associated sebaceous gland. Most of the hair on the body can be elevated by the erector pili muscle that inserts into the hair follicle. Although sebaceous glands are found everywhere on the skin except for the palms, soles, and dorsa of the feet, more glands and larger glands are found on the face and scalp. The sebaceous glands secrete sebum, which is a group of complex oils including triglycerides and the fatty acid breakdown products, wax esters, squalene, cholesterol esters, and cholesterol. Acne, the most common disease seen by dermatologists, develops in sebaceous follicles. The pathogenesis of acne is complex, involving abnormal keratinization within the infundibular portion of the hair follicle, the inflammatory capacity of free fatty acids in the sebum, and possibly the presence of the anaerobic diphtheroid *Propionibacterium acnes* within the hair follicle.

Two types of human hair exist. Terminal hair is the coarse, pigmented hair seen on the scalp, beard area, axillae, eyebrow, eyelids, and pubic area. Vellus hair is the fine, soft, short hair found on the parts of the body thought to be "hairless." Hair grows in a cyclic rather than continuous pattern. The growth phase is termed anagen, and the resting phase is telogen; catagen describes the transition between the two. There is wide variation in the timing of the hair growth cycle in different regions of the body. The length of anagen determines the length of hair so that short hairs are found on the extremities and eyebrows with relatively short anagen periods, whereas long anagen periods occur in scalp hairs. With the exception of the palms, soles, dorsa of the terminal phalanges of the digits, glans penis, and mucocutanous junction, hair follicles populate the entire skin surface.

BARRIER FUNCTION

Skin is uniquely structured to protect against loss of body fluids and external harm from toxins, bacteria, ultraviolet radiation, low-voltage electricity, mechanical forces, and extremes of temperature. For example, because of a deficient skin barrier, the burn victim or a patient with exfoliative erythroderma is prone to dehydration, thermoregulatory disorders, and an increased risk of sepsis. A normal human adult loses about 500 mL of water in 24 hours through the skin by both diffusion and, to a lesser extent, sweating. Such loss is intensified when barrier properties of the skin are abrogated by injury or disease.

The stratum corneum overlying the epidermis is the armor that provides a barrier to water movement. It consists of overlapping thin corneocytes that are each filled with keratin filaments and covered by a tough membrane that is resistant to proteolytic enzymes, organic solvents, and both acidic and basic solutions. Between the corneocytes is a noncharged lipid-rich intercellular material that is analogous to mortar surrounding bricks. It is difficult for water to move through the stratum corneum since it must cross layers of hydrophobic, intercellular lipids and cells that are stacked and tightly packed with keratin filaments. This anatomic arrangement is also effective in protecting against potentially harmful environmental toxins since they must traverse the epithelium by passive diffusion much as does water. The skin loses some of its protective function when the

stratum corneum is traumatically removed or when it is hydrated or rendered free of lipids by certain organic solvents.

The skin protects itself from the damaging effects of ultraviolet (UV) light primarily by the production of melanin. Tanning is the process whereby increased amounts of ultraviolet light induce pigment production in the skin. Upon exposure to UV light, especially longer wave UVA light (320 to 400 nm), immediate pigmentary darkening results from an alteration in melanin that is already present in the dermis. These changes include oxidation of melanin and a redistribution of existing melanosomes. The more clearly photoprotective delayed tanning reaction becomes apparent after 72 hours and is mainly induced by the shorter wave ultraviolet B (UVB) light (290 to 320 nm). This increase in pigment is due to increased production of epidermal melanin. Genetically, darker-skinned individuals are better able to tan than light-skinned people.

The keratin filaments concentrated in the stratum corneum and present throughout the epidermis provide a physical barrier to UV light. This is also inducible, as exposure to UVB light can cause the epidermis to become hyperplastic. Finally, there is also speculation that breakdown products of fillagrin, a protein produced in the granular layer of the epidermis, provides protection by absorbing some of the radiant energy.

The skin provides protection against mechanical forces. Although the stratum corneum is thin, the interdigitation of its cells held together with an intercellular "cement" makes it extremely durable. The epidermis loses much of its resistance to mechanical injury if the stratum corneum is removed. Most of the skin's mechanical protection is provided by the dermis with its strongly cross-linked collagen fibers providing resistance to shearing forces applied to the skin. Additional cushioning is provided by the underlying adipose tissue.

MICROBIOLOGY OF THE SKIN

Although normal skin is colonized by a large variety of organisms, it also functions as a barrier to invasion. Most of this protection comes from the intact stratum corneum and its barrier properties. However, the relative dryness of normal skin also prevents the overgrowth of many pathogenic and nonpathogenic organisms. In addition, the normal microbial nonpathogenic skin flora provide additional protection by competitively inhibiting the overgrowth of potential skin pathogens. This normal flora can be reduced or eliminated by broad-spectrum antibiotics, thereby leading to colonization of skin by more serious, antibiotic-resistant bacterial strains.

This section focuses on the normal resident flora, as listed in Table 22–2, that colonize the outer epidermis and stratum corneum. The two species of *Staphylococci* are the coagulase-negative species and the coagulase positive *Staphylococcus aureus*. Most of the skin surface is not colonized with *S. aureus*, but it can be found occasionally in intertriginous areas, such as the perineum or nasal vestibule. Individuals who are susceptible to recurrent skin infections from *S. aureus* are often persistent nasal carriers. Persistent nasal carriage has been found in 20 to 40 per cent of healthy adults. When there is disruption of the epidermis in certain skin diseases (e.g., psoriasis or eczematous dermatitis), the skin can become heavily colonized with *S. aureus* in both involved and uninvolved sites. Of the many different coagulase-negative species, *S. epidermidis* followed by *S. haemolyticus* are the most common causes of infection, and most of these infections are associated with indwelling foreign devices.

The Gram-negative rods are not commonly found as resident flora. *Acinetobacter* species, nonfermentative aerobic Gram-negative rods, are, however, part of the normal flora in 25 per cent of the population. Most common infections with this species occur in postoperative and burn wounds. *Pseudomonas* and *Proteus* species are common organisms in Gram-negative toe web infections. These infections are characterized by denuded intertriginous toe web spaces with a serous or pustular discharge. They are thought to occur more commonly in patients with tinea pedis, diabetes mellitus, or restricted interdigital spaces or those individuals using germicidal soaps that may deplete protective flora. *Escherichia coli*, *Klebsiella* species, *Enterobacter*, or *Proteus* species are common causes of Gram-negative folliculitis. This condition may present as small pustules or deep nodules on the face or trunk in patients receiving long-term antibiotic therapy, e.g., for therapy of acne vulgaris.

The fungi that are normal resident flora are predominantly the yeast organisms of *Pityrosporum* and *Candida* species. *Pityrosporum* species are lipophilic yeasts that under the proper conditions transform from the resident blastospore stage to the pathogenic hyphal stage. *Pityrosporum orbiculare* is the cause of tinea versicolor, a skin disease characterized by fine, scaly, hyper- and hypopigmented macules found mainly on the chest, back, and proximal extremities. It also causes a folliculitis characterized by red follicular papules or pustules in the same distribution. *Candida* species rarely colonize normal skin, although they are present on 40 per cent of oral mucous membranes. Most limited infections occur in mucous membranes and are facilitated by predisposing factors, such as immunosuppression, broad-spectrum antibiotic therapy, topical or systemic corticosteroids, diabetes mellitus, pregnancy, or debilitating systemic disease. When candidiasis occurs cutaneously, it is more likely to be found on moist, macerated skin or skin that is close to mucous membranes. *Candida albicans* may colonize and infect suture lines that are covered by occlusive dressing material or are treated with broad-spectrum topical antibiotics. Many of these same factors also increase the risk of *Pityrosporum* infection.

Other resident flora include the coryneforms, which are Gram-positive pleomorphic rods found most commonly in intertriginous areas. This group of organisms is thought to play a major role in producing axillary and foot odor by their metabolic interaction with apocrine sweat. *Propionibacteria* are the most prevalent anaerobes of the normal flora and are sometimes referred to as anaerobic coryneforms. *P. acnes*, the most predominant species found in nearly 100 per cent of adults, is largely found in the head and neck region as normal inhabitants of hair follicles and sebaceous glands. It is thought to be a major contributing factor in the inflammatory stage of acne.

Many endogenous and exogenous factors alter the number and ratio of organisms in the normal flora. One such factor is the local skin environment. Most organisms favor increased temperature and humidity and rapidly proliferate under occlusive dressings or body surfaces adjacent to bedding material or other surfaces for prolonged periods. Many bacteria and fungi also proliferate in the moist environment provided by intertriginous areas of the body. Certain medication can dramatically change the normal flora. Both topical and systemic antibiotics can naturally select for the overgrowth of Gram-negative rods and yeasts. Systemic corticosteroids can increase the susceptibility to bacterial, viral, fungal, and parasitic infections by diminishing immunologic defense mechanisms. Hospitalization can rapidly alter the cutaneous flora of patients. These individuals have

TABLE 22–2. COMMON SKIN FLORA

Coagulase-negative staphylococci
  S. epidermidis
  S. hominis
  S. haemolyticus
Staphylococcus aureus (usually intertriginous areas)
Peptococcus
Micrococcus
  M. luteus
Coryneform organisms
  Corynebacteria
  Brevibacterium
Propionibacteria
  P. acnes
  P. granulosum
Gram-Negative Rods
  Acinetobacter (nonfermentive aerobic)
Mycoflora
  Pityrosporum
  Candida (usually mucous membranes)

higher rates of nasal carriage with *S. aureus,* increased colonization with Gram-negative species and yeasts, and an increased number of antibiotic-resistant organisms known as *JK coryneforms.*

THERMOREGULATION

The skin plays a major role in the physiologic regulation of the body's core temperature. Heat is exchanged by the skin's own heat conductivity, convection occurring in cutaneous blood vessels, and by the excretion of sweat. The entire process is regulated by a complex system of negative feedback mechanisms, primarily involving thermosensitive neurons in the anterior hypothalamus.

The skin's vasculature, with its specialized network of interconnecting musculocutaneous arterioles and venules, along with capillaries, arteriovenous shunts, and small venules, is vital in temperature control. Most of the regulative type of blood vessels are located in the distal extremities, ears, and lips with arteriovenous anastomoses regulating temperature by opening and closing. Blood can easily exchange heat through the skin since most of the cutaneous blood is contained in an extensive subcutaneous venous plexus, in which blood can move slowly and relatively closely to the skin surface. In addition, blood returning from the distal extremities can do so by superfical veins near the surface or by deep venae comitantes, allowing for heat loss and conservation, respectively. Large amounts of heat can be exchanged with small changes in the temperature of the blood since blood has a high specific heat and heat conductivity. In addition, the cutaneous flow is very high—10 to 20 times that required for essential metabolites and oxygen. Approximately 8.5 per cent or 450 ml/min of the total blood flow passes through the skin under basal conditions. Much of the blood flow through the skin is controlled by the sympathetic nervous system through the release of epinephrine and norephinephrine.

Response to cold begins when blood colder than normal flows into the preoptic region of the hypothalamus. This results in sympathetic excitation, which causes powerful constriction of the cutaneous blood vessels, thereby shunting blood and thus heat away from the surface. Heat production is also increased both through the sympathetic release of hormones that increase cellular metabolism and from stimuli originating in the preoptic hypothalamus that activate the motor center for shivering. In warmer conditions the blood vessels dilate, allowing blood to accumulate near the skin's surface and heat to be lost by conduction and convection. This occurs through negative feedback on all the heat-conserving mechanisms previously mentioned, as well as reflex vasodilation through direct warming of the skin surface.

Eccrine sweat glands are also important in thermoregulation; however, sweat must be evaporated from the skin surface in order to cool. About 580 cal of heat are lost for every gram of water that is evaporated from the skin. The regulation of sweating is complex and involves both nervous and nonnervous control that allows for increased sweating at or above a certain set core temperature. The firing rate of thermosensitive nerves in the preoptic region increases with both local heating and an elevation of skin temperature. If the skin temperature remains constant, the sweating rate increases linearly with core temperature. The necessary core temperature to be reached to induce sweating becomes lower, however, as skin temperature rises. Through complex pathways, the central sweat center stimulates the nerves that innervate sweat glands. These nerves are sympathetic postganglionic fibers composed of nonmyelinated class C nerve fibers with acetylcholine as the principal terminal neurotransmitter. The importance of sweating in thermoregulation is emphasized by the potential for severe hyperthermia seen in the anhidroses in which there are diminished or absent sweat glands.

DISORDERS OF CONNECTIVE TISSUE

Abnormalities in connective tissue can result in multisystem defects involving skin, joints, bone, blood vessels, and the gastrointestinal tract. Collagen, elastin, and proteoglycans are the major extracellular macromolecules of connective tissue. Therefore, an inherited abnormality in connective tissue may involve any part of the complex biosynthesis and metabolism of these macromolecules or the way these substances are organized. Historically, the connective tissue diseases were thought to include lupus erythematosus, scleroderma, and dermatomyositis; however, except for scerloderma none of these diseases has been shown to have any true abnormality of connective tissue. Instead, the true connective diseases are usually inherited and may be classified as primary or secondary. The primary diseases are caused by gene mutations that interfere with the synthesis or metabolism of collagen and elastin. The secondary disorders result from accumulation of products that damage connective tissue, e.g., homocystinuria.

Some of the inherited connective tissue diseases have great significance for the practicing surgeon. For example, in almost all of the many forms of Ehlers-Danlos syndrome (EDS) the skin is fragile and easily bruised or torn. Suturing can be difficult since the suture material often pulls through the abnormal dermis. Wound healing is slow, and the scar can be paper thin with a characteristic fish-mouth, gaping appearance. The various types of EDS, along with the inheritance and clinical features, can be seen in Table 22–3.

TABLE 22–3. EHLERS-DANLOS SYNDROME

TYPE	INHERITANCE	MAJOR CLINICAL FINDINGS	ULTRASTRUCTURAL FINDINGS	BIOCHEMICAL DEFECT
I: Gravis	AD	Premature rupture of fetal membranes, poor wound healing, fragile skin	Large irregular collagen fibrils	Unknown
II: Mitis	AD	Joint hypermobility of digits	Large irregular collagen fibrils	Unknown
III: Benign hypermobile	AD	Large joint hypermobility, mild skin features	Unknown	Unknown
IV	AD	Marked bruisability, thin fragile skin, arteriolar ruptures	Small collagen fibers, fibrils of variable size	Diminished type III collagen synthesis
	AR	Intestinal perforation		
V	x-Linked recessive	Short stature, hernias, mitral and triscuspid valve prolapse, joint hypermobility, extensible skin	Unknown	Unknown
VI	AR	Marked joint hypermobility, kyphoscoliosis, ocular fragility, hyperextensible and fragile skin	Small collagen bundles, large irregular fibrils	Lysyl hydroxylase deficiency
VII: arthrochalasis multiplex congenity	AD	Marked joint hypermobility, hip dislocation, short stature, moderate skin	Unknown	Defect at amino terminal cleavage site of pro-α2
	AR	Hyperextensibility		
VIII: Periodontitis	AD	Severe generalized periodontitis, marked skin fragility especially over shins	Unknown	Reduced type III collagen
IX: Oxidase cutis laxa	x-Linked recessive	Hyperextensible skin, bony occipital horns	Unknown	Abnormal copper metabolism, x-linked lysyloxidase -deficiency
X: Fibronectin deficient	AR	Easy bruisability, hyperextensible skin and joints	Unknown	Abnormal fibronectin
XI: Familial joint laxity	AD	Marked joint laxity and dislocation	Unknown	Unknown

Aging

The study of skin aging and photoaging is important as many clinical, histologic, and physiologic changes observed in aging skin are implicated in the skin's susceptibility to environmental injury and certain disease states. Dermatologists tend to separate skin aging into two categories: intrinsic aging and actinic aging. There are subtle changes in areas of old but sun-protected skin that consist of laxity, fine wrinkling, and a variety of benign neoplasms. In contrast, strong differences have been demonstrated in the behavior of in vitro cultured skin-derived cells from donors of different chronologic age. For example, there is an inverse relationship between donor age and cumulative population doublings in vitro for keratinocytes, fibroblasts, and melanocytes.

Clinical changes in photoaged skin include coarse wrinkling, sallow color, telangiectasia, irregular pigmentation, and a variety of benign, premalignant, and malignant neoplasms. At the cellular level, both keratinocyte and dermal fibroblast cultures from chronically sun-exposed sites have shorter lifespans. The histologic hallmark of photoaging is dermal elastosis, which is postulated to result from direct UV-mediated damage to the extracellular matrix and to dermal fibroblasts that then produce abnormal elastin.

BIBLIOGRAPHY

1. Dahl, M.V.: Clinical Immunodermatology, 2nd ed. Chicago, Year Book Medical Publishers, Inc., 1988.
2. Fine, J.: The skin basement membrane zone. Adv. Dermatol., *2*:283–304.
3. Fitzpatrick, T.B., et al. (eds.): Dermatology in General Medicine, 3rd ed. New York, McGraw-Hill, 1987.
4. Lever, W.F., and Schaumberg-Lever, G.: Histopathology of the Skin, 6th ed. Philadelphia, J.B. Lippincott Co., 1983.
5. Nordlund, J.J., Abdel-Malek, Z.A., Boissy, R.E., and Rheins, L.A.: Pigment cell biology: An historical review. J. Invest. Dermatol. *92* (suppl.): 53–59, 1989.
6. Rook, A., et al. (eds.): Textbook of Dermatology, 4th ed. Oxford, Blackwell Scientific Publications, 1986.
7. Roth, R.R., and James, W.D.: Microbiology of the skin: Resident flora, ecology, infection. J. Am. Acad. Dermatol., *20:* 367–90, 1989.
8. Sato, K., Kang, W.H., Saga, K., and Sato, K.T.: Biology of sweat glands and their disorders. I. Normal sweat gland function. J. Am. Acad. Dermatol., *20*:537–63, 1989.
9. Soter, N.A., and Baden, H.P.: Pathophysiology of Dermatologic Diseases. New York, McGraw-Hill, 1984.
10. Uitto, J., Olsen, D.R., and Fazio, M.J.: Extracellular matrix of the skin: 50 years of progress. J. Invest. Dermatol., *92* (suppl.) 61–77, 1989.

23

INTRACRANIAL PHYSIOLOGY

JOSEPH M. DARBY

The brain performs a variety of homeostatic and integrative functions, with the neuron serving as the basic functional unit. Neuronal as well as whole brain function and metabolism are critically dependent upon the maintenance of an adequate delivery of glucose and oxygen by the systemic and cerebral circulations. Because the brain functions within a rigid and semiclosed compartment, its function is further dependent on the maintenance and integrity of precise spatial relationships between neurons and specific brain structures within the intracranial compartment. When normal mechanisms fail to maintain homeostasis within the intracranial compartment, neuronal and brain function is impaired or destroyed, resulting in the loss of normal integrative function of the organism as a whole.

ANATOMY

Intracranial Compartments

Enclosing the intracranial compartment is the skull. The major structures contained therein include the brain, meninges, cranial nerves, and blood vessels supplying and draining blood from the brain. The frontal, temporal, parietal, and occipital bones join to form the calvarium and base of the skull. The base of the skull is divided into the anterior, middle, and posterior cranial fossae. The skull is open at the base via the foramen magnum, through which the spinal cord passes. Separating the anterior and middle fossae from the posterior fossa is the tentorium cerebelli, a dural reflection dividing the intracranial compartment into supratentorial and infratentorial compartments (Fig. 23–1). The cerebral hemispheres, basal ganglia, thalamus, and hypothalamus, as well as cranial nerves I and II, are contained in the supratentorial compartment. Within the supratentorial compartment, the hemispheres are further separated by the falx cerebri. Located below the tentorium and above the foramen magnum is the in-fratentorial compartment, which contains the cerebellum, midbrain, pons, medulla, and cranial nerves III to XII.

Meninges

The brain and spinal cord are covered by three protective membranes: the pia mater, arachnoid, and dura mater (Fig. 23–2). The dura is the outermost layer of the meninges; it consists of two tightly adherent, fibrous layers attached firmly to the inner table of the skull and extending onto the spinal cord down to its termination at approximately the second sacral level. The falx cerebri and the tentorium cerebelli are reflections of the dura mater. An opening in the tentorium cerebelli, the tentorial notch or incisura, surrounds the midbrain and associated structures and provides a pathway through which major brain structures may herniate when compartmental pressures are high and compensatory mechanisms have been exhausted. In addition, venous sinuses, the major venous drainage system for the brain, are formed within the two fibrous layers of the dura mater.

The arachnoid and pia mater make up the leptomeninges. The pia is adherent to the surface of the brain and spinal cord, whereas the arachnoid is attached to the pia by the arachnoid trabeculae and is directly adherent to the dura. Between the pia and arachnoid is the subarachnoid space, which contains cerebrospinal fluid (CSF) and through which passes the major arterial vessels supplying blood to the brain. Projections of the arachnoid, called arachnoid villi, evaginate into the dural sinuses and provide a major pathway for CSF drainage into the venous system. The subarachnoid space is enlarged into cisterns in several regions around the brain and named according to anatomic relationships. In addition to the subarachnoid space, the epidural and subdural spaces are spaces in which blood or purulent material may potentially accumulate under pathologic conditions, thereby creating a mass effect on the brain or impairing the normal CSF drainage

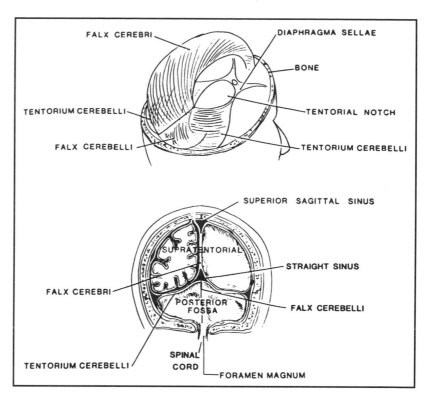

FIGURE 23–1. Cutaway view of the intracranial compartments. The tentorium cerebelli divides the skull into supratentorial and infratentorial compartments, whereas the hemispheres are divided by the falx cerebri. Openings in the falx and tentorium and the foramen magnum provide pathways by which brain tissue may herniate when compartmental pressures are increased. (Reprinted from Daube, J.R., Reagan, T.J., Sandok, B.A., and Westmoreland, B.F. (eds.): Medical Neurosciences: An Approach to Anatomy, Pathology, and Physiology by Systems and Levels, 2nd ed. Boston, Little, Brown and Co., 1986. Figure 3–3, p. 27.)

mechanisms and resulting in either hydrocephalus or increased intracranial pressure (ICP).

Ventricular System

The ventricular system is a series of spaces within the brain that communicate with the subarachnoid space and contain CSF (Fig. 23–3). Two lateral ventricles located within the hemispheres open by way of the foramen of Monro into the third ventricle in the midline between the diencephalon. The third ventricle communicates via the aqueduct of Sylvius with the fourth ventricle, whereas the foramen of Luschka and Magendie provide connections from the fourth ventricle to the subarachnoid space into the basal cisterns (pontine cistern and cisterna magna). The ventricular system is lined with an epithelium, referred to as ependyma, from which arises the choroid plexus, a highly vascularized structure that produces CSF. A choroid plexus is found in each lateral ventricle, as well as the third and fourth ventricles.

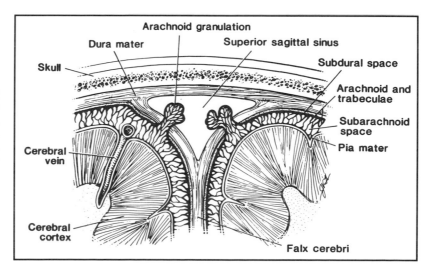

FIGURE 23–2. Coronal section showing meninges, meningeal spaces, and their relationship to the surface of the brain and dural venous sinuses. (Reprinted from Lyons, M.K., and Meyer, F.B.: Cerebrospinal fluid physiology and the management of increased intracranial pressure. Mayo Clin. Proc., 65: 684–707, 1990. Figure 2, p. 687.)

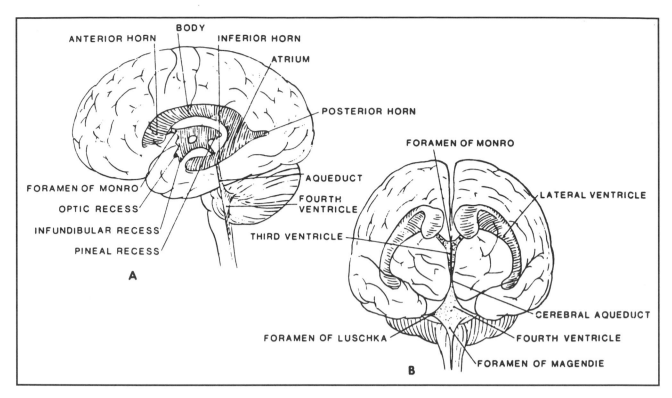

FIGURE 23–3. Lateral and anterior views of the cerebral ventricular system. (Reprinted from Daube, J.R., Reagan, T.J., Sandok, B.A., Westmoreland, B.F. (eds.): Medical Neurosciences: An Approach to Anatomy, Pathology, and Physiology by systems and Levels, 2nd ed. Boston, Little, Brown and Co., 1986. Figure 6–6, p. 97.)

Arterial Blood Supply

The arterial blood supply to the brain is provided anteriorly by the internal carotid arteries and posteriorly by the vertebrobasilar system (Fig. 23–4). These two systems communicate at the base of the brain via a series of anastomoses known as the Circle of Willis. The main branches of the internal carotid artery include the anterior and middle cerebral arteries, which supply blood to the majority of the supratentorial structures. The two vertebral arteries join at the pons to form the basilar artery. This verte-

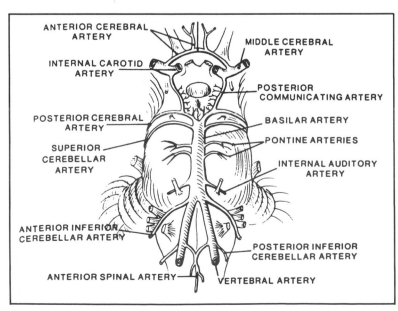

FIGURE 23–4. Arterial blood supply to the brain. (Reprinted from Daube, J.R., Reagan, T.J., Sandok, B.A., and Westmoreland, B.F. (eds.): Medical Neurosciences: An Approach to Anatomy, Pathology, and Physiology by Systems and Levels, 2nd ed. Boston, Little, Brown and Co., 1986. Figure 3–10, p. 31.)

brobasilar system supplies blood to structures in the posterior fossa, as well as the occipital lobe of the hemispheres, by the posterior cerebral artery. A complete and intact circle of Willis is present in only 15 to 40 per cent of the population.

Venous Drainage

The venous drainage of the brain can be divided into cerebral and dural sinus systems. The cerebral component includes a superficial system that drains superficial cortical structures and a deep system that drains the deeper structures of the brain. Anastomotic veins connect the superficial and deep cerebral venous systems.

The dural venous sinuses drain blood mainly from cerebral venous system and the meninges (Fig. 23–5). The posterosuperior group of sinuses includes the superior and inferior sagittal, straight, transverse, sigmoid, and occipital sinuses. The anterointerior group includes the cavernous and posterior petrosal sinuses, as well as the basilar plexus. Venous spaces called lateral lacunae provide connections from superficial hemispheric veins to the superior sagittal sinus. Venous blood generally courses posteriorly to empty into the sigmoid sinuses and finally drains into the systemic circulation via the internal jugular veins or into the cavernous sinuses, orbital veins, or basilar plexus.

Extracranial venous connections with the dural sinuses are made possible by way of emissary veins draining blood from the scalp and by diploic veins draining blood from the skull. Under conditions in which normal venous drainage may be impaired, these extracranial connections can provide alternate routes for venous drainage of the brain.

BRAIN METABOLISM AND BLOOD FLOW

Metabolism

Although the brain represents only 2 per cent of the total body weight, it uses 20 per cent of the systemic oxygen consumption for the oxidation of glucose, its exclusive metabolic substrate under normal conditions. Brain and neuronal function there-

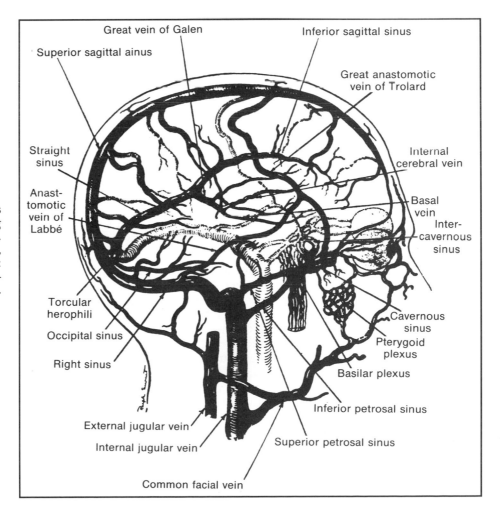

FIGURE 23–5. The venous drainage of the brain, including the major dural venous sinuses. (Reprinted from Shenkin, H.A., Harmel, M.H., and Kety, S.S.: Dynamic anatomy of the cerebral circulation. Arch. Neurol. Psychiatr. 60: 245, 1948.)

Great vein of Galen

Inferior sagittal sinus

Superior sagittal ainus

Great anastomotic vein of Trolard

Straight sinus

Internal cerebral vein

Anasttomotic vein of Labbé

Basal vein

Intercavernous sinus

Torcular herophili

Cavernous sinus

Occipital sinus

Pterygoid plexus

Right sinus

Basilar plexus

External jugular vein

Inferior petrosal sinus

Internal jugular vein

Superior petrosal sinus

Common facial vein

fore is fundamentally dependent upon an adequate supply of oxygen and glucose. Interruption of cerebral blood supply for only 10 seconds will result in loss of consciousness. Although almost half of the volume of the brain is composed of nonneuronal glial cells, the neuronal pool has a much higher metabolic rate, accounting for its extreme functional and structural sensitivity to oxygen and glucose deprivation.

The continual electrical activities of the brain require a high rate of neuronal oxidative metabolism, mainly for active ionic transport processes that are involved in the restoration of neuronal membrane potentials. In addition, energy is required for protein synthesis; the production, release, degradation, and uptake of neurotransmitters; and the maintenance of structural integrity of neuronal membranes. Although carbohydrate is the preferred substrate for brain metabolism, ketone bodies (hydroxybutyrate and acetoacetate) can be metabolized for energy in such conditions as starvation or alcohol ingestion or in the neonatal period. Ketone bodies, however, cannot be used as an exclusive substrate to maintain or restore normal function.

Neuronal activity and metabolism are normally tightly coupled events. A general scheme of energy metabolism is shown below. Oxidative metabolism of glucose results in the production of ATP, which is utilized for energy-requiring neuronal processes, yielding ADP and inorganic phosphate (A). When neuronal metabolic activity is high or there is a relative lack of oxygen, excess glycolytic activity may ensue, resulting in the production of lactate and hydrogen ion (B) or a shift in the adenylate kinase equilibrium toward the production of AMP (C). The accumulation of AMP can, through removal of phosphate, result in the accumulation of adenosine (D).

A. $ATP + H_2O \longrightarrow ADP + P_i + energy$
B. $Glucose \longrightarrow Lactate + H^+ + ATP$
C. $ADP + ADP \Longleftrightarrow ATP + AMP$
D. $AMP \xrightarrow{5'nucleotidase} Adenosine + P_i$

The importance of H^+ and especially adenosine accumulation is that these metabolic byproducts are important feedback regulators of cerebral blood flow in response to changes in neuronal activity. Both mediators result in vasodilation, increasing oxygen and glucose delivery to meet neuronal metabolic demand. These same metabolic byproducts may be produced under pathologic conditions (e.g., hypoxia, ischemia) and help maintain neuronal homeostasis by enhancing oxygen delivery. The loss of compensatory mechanisms to maintain adequate supplies of oxygen and glucose and the resultant energy failure cause intracellular potassium release, influx of Ca^{+2}, as well as intracellular acidosis. A cascade of events is subsequently set into motion, mediated primarily by Ca^{+2}, which result in cell swelling and ultimately cell death.

The metabolic rate of the brain is expressed in terms of its rate of oxygen or glucose consumption ($CMRO_2$ or CMR_{glu}). The cerebral metabolic rate (CMR) for oxygen or glucose can be determined using the Fick principle, which states that brain uptake is equal to the cerebral blood flow times the arteriovenous concentration difference across the brain.

$$CMR = CBF \times (Art - Ven) \qquad (Eq.\ 1)$$

Normal $CMRO_2$ is approximately 3.5 mL/100 gm brain/min, whereas normal CMR_{glu} is 5.5 mg/100 gm brain/min. For the normal adult brain, these values translate into a whole brain oxygen consumption of approximately 49 mL/min and glucose consumption of approximately 77 mg/min. Brain oxygen consumption, glucose consumption, and cerebral blood flow can be measured simultaneously in humans using positron emission tomography.

Cerebral Blood Flow

Approximately 15 per cent of the total cardiac output is distributed to the brain, which amounts to approximately 750 ml/min. Since brain metabolism and neuronal function are tightly coupled to cerebral blood flow (CBF), increases or decreases in brain metabolism are associated with parallel changes in CBF to meet metabolic demand. Changes in blood flow may be generalized when overall brain metabolism and neuronal function are affected (e.g., by fever or coma), or they can be localized to specific brain regions associated with localized neuronal activity, such as seizures or hand movements. When flow is inadequate to meet metabolic demand, ischemia and tissue injury ensue. Flow in excess of metabolic demand can occur in a variety of pathologic conditions, such as head injury or reperfusion after ischemia and is referred to as luxury perfusion. Diaschisis is the phenomenon of a localized cerebral lesion, such as a stroke, that has the effect of decreasing blood flow and metabolism at a site removed from the area of injury. the mechanisms of diaschisis remain unknown.

CBF can be measured using a modification of the Fick principle. The amount of tracer uptake within the brain (Q_x) is equal to the amount delivered to the brain (flow $\times$ arterial concentration) minus the amount removed from the brain (flow $\times$ venous concentration) over time. Thus,

$$Q_x = Flow\ (A_x - V_x) \qquad (Eq.\ 2)$$

Using a metabolically inert, freely diffusible tracer with a known partition coeffcient between blood and brain, the concentration in the brain can be estimated from measurements of the cerebral venous concentration at tissue saturation and CBF can be calculated according to the Kety-Schmidt relationship.

$$CBF = \frac{V_x \times S}{\int(A_x - V_x)dt} \qquad (Eq.\ 3)$$

where V_x is the cerebral venous concentration, S is the tissue partition coefficient, and A_x is the arterial concentration. CBF is expressed as flow per unit weight of brain tissue (cc/100 gm/min). Normal mean cerebral blood flow in the adult ranges from 45 to 55 cc/100 gm/min. CBF is higher in children and tends to decline with age. CBF values are significantly higher in the gray matter (75 to 80 cc/100 gm/min) than in the white matter (20 to 25 cc/100 gm/min) because the capillary density in the gray matter is approximately five times higher than in the white matter. Highly localized measurements of CBF can be made clinically using either positron emission tomography (PET) or xenon-enhanced computed tomography. PET uses short-lived radioisotopes as blood flow tracers, whereas xenon-enhanced CT uses stable xenon, a radiopaque diffusible tracer. In addition to measurement of cerebral blood flow, PET can also measure cerebral blood volume and local brain metabolism, i.e., brain oxygen and glucose consumption.

Flow Thresholds and Selective Vulnerability

Neuronal functions are critically dependent upon an adequate delivery of oxygen. When oxygen delivery is reduced, cerebral oxygen consumption can only be maintained by an increase in tissue oxygen extraction or by regulatory mechanisms that augment CBF. When these two mechanisms fail, neuronal dysfunction or even infarction will ensue.

Threshold values of cerebral blood flow for neuronal function and ischemic injury exist and vary from one neuronal pool to another—the so-called selective neuronal vulnerability. The threshold for neuronal failure is that level of CBF that results in *reversible* disturbances in neuronal function; the threshold for membrane failure is that level of flow that results in disturbances in neuronal energy metabolism and irreversible functional disturbances. In between these two thresholds is the so-called ischemic penumbra in which neurons with impaired function are still potentially viable (Fig. 23–6). Tissue infarction occurs below the threshold for membrane failure, but is time dependent. To illustrate, a decrease in EEG amplitude occurs at approximately 20 cc/100 gm/min, flattening of the EEG occurs at approximately 15 to 16 cc/100 gm/min, and membrane failure becomes evident at approximately 10 cc/100 gm/min. Under ischemic conditions, tissue infarction is determined by the amount of residual flow present and the duration of the ischemic insult. Tissue viability can be maintained as long as CBF remains above a threshold of 18 cc/100 gm/min. When flow drops below this threshold, tissue infarction will occur var-

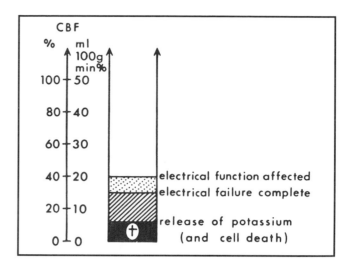

FIGURE 23–6. Flow thresholds for functional and morphologic integrity of neuronal tissue. Between the threshold for impaired electrical function and cell death is the ischemic penumbra in which neuronal function is severely impaired yet potentially viable. (Reprinted from Jafar, J.J., and Crowell, R.M.: Focal ischemic thresholds. *In* Wood, J.H. (ed.): Cerebral Blood Flow. Physiologic and Clinical Aspects. New York, McGraw-Hill, 1987. Figure 28–1, p. 451.)

iably, depending upon the degree and duration of the ischemic insult, as well as the selective vulnerability of the neuron pool involved. The neurons most susceptible to ischemia include those in the cortex, hippocampus, and cerebellum.

Regulation of Cerebral Blood Flow

CBF is very tightly regulated in order to maintain oxygen supply in balance with oxygen demand and to protect brain tissue from the adverse effects of extremes in perfusion pressure, e.g., brain edema, hemorrhage. Although it is likely that the cerebral circulation is modulated by a variety of factors under both normal and pathologic conditions (Fig. 23–7), several theories have been advanced in an attempt to explain the regulation of CBF. The Roy-Sherrington or metabolic hypothesis proposes that local changes in functional neuronal activity cause the release of metabolic byproducts that feed back to the cerebral circulation, thereby adjusting local blood flow to meet changes in metabolic demand. The myogenic theory states that the degree of stretch (perfusion pressure) in the walls of cerebral vessels is sensed and results in an adjustment in the vascular diameter that then maintains a constant flow (autoregulation). Lastly, evidence has accumulated that: (1) there is cerebrovascular innervation by the sympathetic and parasympathetic nervous system, (2) a multitude of vasoactive neurotransmitters, and that (3) there are

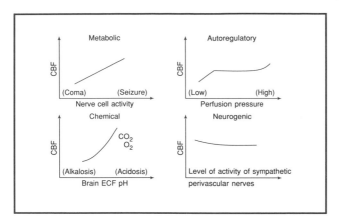

FIGURE 23–7. Regulatory mechanisms for control of cerebral blood flow. (Reprinted from Lassen, N.A.: Cerebral and spinal cord blood flow. *In* Cottrell, J.E., and Turndorf, H. (eds.): Anesthesia and Neurosurgery. St. Louis, C.V. Mosby Co., 1986, Figure 1–1 p. 3.)

specific brain regions that directly influence CBF. This evidence forms the basis for the neural hypothesis. Accordingly, neural influences could act as a generalized coupling mechanism between CBF and metabolism by direct connections between both neurons and cerebral vasculature. A considerable degree of controversy exists as to the relative importance of one mechanism or another in the regulation of CBF.

The understanding of CBF regulation is further confounded by the fact that the intracranial circulation can be divided into extraparenchymal and intraparenchymal circuits, each with separate regulatory control mechanisms. The predominant site of CBF regulation, however, almost certainly occurs in the intraparenchymal circuit at the level of the precapillary sphincter. The data suggest that CBF is tightly regulated at this level by vasoactive metabolites. These metabolites are either produced or washed out, depending on the balance of oxygen supply and demand, and feed back either to augment or reduce CBF. A number of metabolites have been suggested as being involved in metabolic regulation and include hydrogen ion, potassium, calcium, the end products of arachidonic acid metabolism and adenosine. The weight of evidence favors adenosine, a byproduct of cellular energy metabolism, as the primary metabolic regulator of CBF. Adenosine concentrations can increase both with high metabolic activity and under conditions of limited oxygen supply. Since changes in adenosine concentration are dependent on the balance of oxygen supply and demand of the tissue, it is likely that it is also the fundamental mechanism underlying the maintenance of CBF with variations in perfusion pressure. Although adenosine is considered to be the primary metabolic regulator of CBF, other vasoac-

tive mediators (e.g., H^+, K^+), may be released under normal and pathologic conditions and also act to modulate CBF.

Neurogenic regulation is likely the most important mechanism influencing the cerebral venous system. Metabolic factors appear only to influence the venous circulation passively by their effect on the arterial circuit. Sympathetic stimuli can cause an adrenergically mediated venoconstriction and a reduction in the cerebral blood volume. Although 70 to 80 per cent of the cerebral blood volume is in the venous system, sympathetically mediated reductions in cerebral blood volume are relatively small and probably of little clinical significance under pathologic conditions, such as increased ICP and arterial hypercarbia.

Autoregulation

Cerebral autoregulation refers to the capacity of the cerebral vasculature to maintain constant CBF in response to changes in perfusion pressure. Generally, it is operative between a mean arterial pressure of 50 to 150 mm Hg. Reductions in arterial pressure below the limits of autoregulation result in ischemia, whereas a "breakthrough" of autoregulation occurs when the upper limit is exceeded, resulting in capillary injury and edema formation.

The relationship between pressure and flow within the cerebral circulation is such that the cerebral perfusion pressure (CPP) is the primary determinant of CBF across the cerebral resistance vessels. This relationship can generally be described as the perfusion pressure divided by the cerebrovascular vascular resistance (CVR).

$$CBF = \frac{CPP}{CVR} \qquad (Eq. 4)$$

The CPP is generally considered to be the mean arterial pressure (MAP) minus the intracranial pressure (ICP).

$$CPP = MAP - ICP \qquad (Eq. 5)$$

If resistance is assumed to be constant, flow is then directly proportional to the perfusion pressure. In the normal brain, when the CPP is reduced to the range of 40 mm Hg, CBF falls and neurologic dysfunction becomes evident. Although ICP is generally thought to be a major determinant of CPP, flow is largely independent of ICP unless it becomes pathologically elevated. Furthermore, cerebral venous pressure only influences arterial flow to the extent that it increases ICP to a significant degree.

Adjustments in vessel diameter have been thought to be the primary mechanism by which CBF is maintained constant over a wide range of perfusion pressures (autoregulation). Although this may be true for the larger, preresistance conduit vessels, alterations in arteriolar vasomotor tone, rather than changes in vessel diameter, may be the main mechanism by which adjustments in brain tissue flow occur. For example, decreases in arterial pressure are accompanied by a reduction in vasomotor tone, whereas increases in arterial pressure are accompanied by an increase in vasomotor tone, maintaining a constant CPP and CBF. The limits of changes in vasomotor tone define the pressure-flow relationships for CBF autoregulation.

Among factors influencing the range of autoregulation are vessel size and the presence of vascular injury, hypoxemia, hypercarbia, and drugs. The range of autoregulation may be greater for smaller vessels or those with higher vascular tone than for larger vessels or those with reduced vascular tone. When vasomotor tone is impaired, such as in hypoxia, hypercapnia, trauma, and infarction or with the use of certain volatile anesthetic agents, autoregulation may be impaired to the extent that CBF varies directly with blood pressure (vasoparalysis).

Such other conditions as chronic hypertension may alter the autoregulation curve. In this situation, the upper and lower limits of autoregulation are shifted upward, protecting the microcirculation from high systemic pressures. This shift also means, however, that blood flow will decrease at a higher pressure than would normally be expected.

Although the principal site of cerebral autoregulation is believed to be the level of the cerebral arteriole, the larger extraparenchymal conductance vessels, which are influenced mainly by the sympathetic nervous system, can also affect CBF. For example, under conditions of high sympathetic activity and increased systemic blood pressure, constriction of the conductance vessels protects the downstream vasculature from excessive pressure. On the other hand, the same sympathetic response in the presence of hemorrhagic shock results in a decline in CBF at higher pressures than the normal lower limits of autoregulation.

"False autoregulation" is the phenomenon seen after CNS injury in which CBF remains constant under conditions of increased blood pressure but decreases when blood pressure is lowered. It may occur when the increase in mean arterial pressure is accompanied by a parallel rise in intracranial pressure or when there is increased tissue pressure from edema formation, preventing blood flow from increasing passively.

Carbon Dioxide

Carbon dioxide is one of the most potent stimuli affecting CBF. Hypocapnia decreases CBF, whereas hypercapnia increases CBF. Changes in CBF caused by changes in $PaCO_2$ are mediated primarily by changes in interstitial brain pH that occur as a result of the rapid diffusion of CO_2 across the blood-brain barrier (BBB). CBF changes by approximately 2 to 3 per cent per mm Hg change in CO_2 from a $PaCO_2$ of 40 mm Hg. The CBF response to changes in $PaCO_2$ is relatively linear in the CO_2 range of 20 to 80 mm Hg. Below a $PaCO_2$ of 20 mm Hg, further reductions in CBF are limited primarily by the release of vasodilator metabolites resulting from ischemia. Increases in cerebral blood flow above a $PaCO_2$ of 80 mm Hg generally do not occur as the reduction in vasomotor tone has reached its upper limits. Changes in CBF induced by a change in $PaCO_2$ are usually relatively short lived, as regulatory mechanisms restore brain interstitial pH toward normal. As has been noted for cerebral autoregulation, the response of the cerebral vasculature to changes in $PaCO_2$ may also be impaired under pathologic conditions, such as trauma or stroke.

Oxygen and Oxygen Content

CBF remains relatively constant until PaO_2 drops below approximately 50 mm Hg, at which time CBF doubles. However, it is not the PaO_2 that affects CBF, but rather the oxygen content and total oxygen delivery primarily influence the cerebral circulation in hypoxia. This is further supported by the fact that inhalation of carbon monoxide increases CBF in the presence of a normal PaO_2 and that CBF is inversely related to hemoglobin concentration. The changes in blood flow in response to decreases in O_2 content are relatively independent of changes in arterial pCO_2. CBF decreases only slightly with inhalation of 100 per cent oxygen at atmospheric pressure and by approximately 25 per cent at two atmospheres of pressure.

Cardiac Output

In the normal brain, CBF also appears to be autoregulated in response to increases in cardiac output. However, reductions in cardiac output, independent of blood pressure, do result in a decrease in CBF. In contrast, CBF in the ischemic brain with impaired autoregulation appears to be more responsive to increases in cardiac output than the normal condition. Therefore, augmentation of cardiac output may be useful in treating patients with limited perfusion reserve, such as those with vasospasm after subarachnoid hemorrhage or ischemia due to cerebrovascular disease.

Viscosity

CBF may also be regulated in response to changes in blood viscosity. Accordingly, if blood viscosity is reduced (e.g., by acute mannitol administration), vascular resistance decreases, resulting in an increase in flow and oxygen delivery. The increase in delivery is then compensated for by cerebral vasoconstriction to maintain oxygen delivery constant. Similarly, increases in blood viscosity increase vascular resistance, reduce CBF and oxygen delivery, and ultimately result in an autoregulatory increase in CBF. In regions of the vasculature that have impaired autoregulation, there will be no autoregulatory response to changes in viscosity, and flow will change passively in response to the change in blood viscosity.

THE BLOOD-BRAIN BARRIER

Whereas the capillary beds of most tissues permit a wide variety of compounds to traverse the endothelial cells into the interstitium, the CNS possesses a unique capillary bed that is characterized by a high degree of selective permeability, as well as by specialized transport systems. The so-called blood-brain barrier (BBB) is formed by tight endothelial junctions, a thick capillary basement membrane, and astrocytic foot processes that encircle brain capillaries. Several structures, including the choroid plexus, dura mater, the median eminence, neurohypophysis, pineal gland, area postrema, and other regions of the hypothalamus, do not possess a BBB. The BBB functions to maintain and buffer the ionic and solute composition of the brain interstitium, regulate the transport of substrates supporting neuronal metabolism, and control intracranial volume.

The selective permeability of the BBB exists for both organic and inorganic compounds, with the major determinant of permeability being lipid solubility. Highly lipid-soluble compounds, such as alcohol, barbiturates, and antipyrine (a blood flow tracer), are highly permeable, whereas mannitol, urea, and inulin are relatively impermeable. The inorganic electrolytes, such as Na^+, K^+, and Cl^-, are also impermeable, with their transport across the BBB in part dependent upon active transport processes. Another important factor influencing the overall transport of substances across the BBB is the capillary surface area. Brain regions with a high capillary density (gray matter) have a higher rate of transport of a given compound than regions with lower capillary density (white matter). Specialized "carrier-mediated" transported systems have been described for glucose, amino acids, monocarboxylic acids (lactate, pyruvate, fatty acids), nucleic acid precursors (e.g., adenosine), as well as for other nutrients. The transport of glucose and amino acids is linked in part to Na^+ and therefore may be energy requiring.

In addition to the low permeability of the BBB to most solutes, diffusion of water is also low. Because of the low permeability of the BBB to water and most solutes, water flux is driven mainly by osmotic pressure gradients, a major mechanism controlling intracranial volume. The effective osmotic pressure of plasma in brain capillaries is enormous in comparison to the hydrostatic pressure gradient for water filtration (5700 mm Hg versus 36 mm Hg). Therefore, control of bulk water movement across the BBB is mainly achieved by osmotic buffing. Any water traversing the BBB is very dilute, setting up a counteracting osmotic gradient either in brain interstitium or plasma that then tends to minimize either brain swelling or shrinkage. Acute and large changes in plasma osmolarity, such as hyperglycemia or hyponatremia, cause neuronal dysfunction as a result of either brain dehydration or edema formation. In time, these changes in osmolarity can be compensated for by either the generation or inactivation of as yet unidentified osmotically active substances, the so-called idiogenic osmoles. Yet another mechanism permitting osmotic adaptation in the chronic state results from changes in the intracellular binding of sodium and potassium, which buffer alterations in osmolarity and limit further changes in brain water. Breakdown of the BBB under pathologic conditions, such as trauma, abscess, or brain tumor, reduces osmotic buffering capacity, increases bulk transport of water by hydrostatic forces, and results in brain edema and tissue swelling.

THE CEREBROSPINAL FLUID SYSTEM

The components of the CSF system include the meninges and meningeal spaces, the ventricular system, and the CSF itself. The normal adult CSF volume is about 90 to 150 mL, representing approximately 10 per cent of total intracranial volume. CSF is produced primarily by the choroid plexuses at a continual rate of approximately 0.35 mL/min or 500 cc/day. The choroid plexus is a richly vascularized body, the capillary endothelium of which is permeable to both solutes and water. Although a filtrate of plasma is produced through the capillary endothelium, CSF is considered a secretory product of the choroid as both water and electrolyte transport across the epithelium are energy-requiring processes. Although the composition of the CSF differs significantly from that of serum (Table 23–1), it is almost identical in its biochemical composition with brain interstitial fluid.

The secretion of CSF is linked to the active transport of Na^+. Consequently, CSF production generally continues even in the face of high intraventricular pressure (i.e., ICP) and is not significantly affected by osmotic pressure gradients. Such drugs as acetazolamide, furosemide, digoxin, corticosteroids, and alkalosis can all decrease CSF production.

Once produced, the CSF flows unidirectionally from the ventricular system through the foramen of Luschka and Magendie and into the basal cisterns. Once in the basal cisterns, CSF flows into the spinal subarachnoid space or through the tentorium,

TABLE 23–1. COMPARISON OF HUMAN CSF AND SERUM COMPOSITION

	CSF	SERUM
Sodium (mEq/L)	138	140
Potassium (mEq/L)	2.8	4.0
Calcium (mEq/L)	2.4	4.6
Magnesium (mEq/L)	2.7	1.8
Chloride (mEq/L)	124	99
Glucose (mg/dL)	60	99
Protein (gm/dL)	.015-.050	7.0

coursing over the surface of the brain in the subarachnoid space. Finally, from the subarachnoid space, CSF drains into the cerebral venous sinuses via the arachnoid granulations (Fig. 23–8). Drainage of CSF into the venous sinuses via the arachnoid villi is the principal mechanism for CSF removal and is driven primarily by the hydrostatic pressure gradient between the CSF and dural sinus. The circulation of CSF itself is driven by the ciliary action of ependymal cells, as well as by pulsatile changes in intracranial volume that occur with systolic cardiac activity and from fluctuations in venous pressure associated with respiration. Obstruction of CSF drainage may result in hydrocephalus or increased intracranial pressure or both.

The CSF system serves several important functions within the intracranial compartment. First, CSF provides a mechanical fluid cushion for the brain, buffering it from traumatic injury. Second, it helps maintain homeostasis of the perineuronal environment. Because the CSF is in functional continuity with the brain interstitium, it acts as a "sink" for the removal of the products of brain metabolism or other compounds traversing the BBB. Substances gaining entrance to the brain interstitium generally do not reach equilibrium with the plasma; rather, the sink action of the CSF provides a concentration gradient down which they can diffuse from the plasma, to the interstitium, across the ependyma, and into the CSF from where they are eventually returned to the circulation when CSF is absorbed. Finally, the CSF system provides a mechanism by which increases in brain volume (e.g., brain edema) can be accommodated by increasing the rate of CSF absorption.

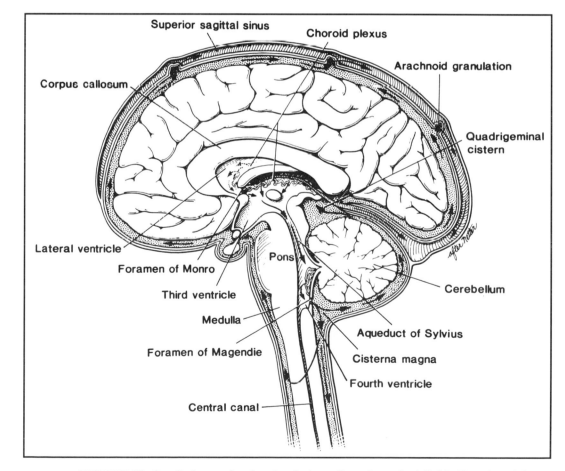

FIGURE 23–8. Pathways for the circulation of cerebrospinal fluid. (Reprinted from Lyons, M.K., and Meyer, F.B. Cerebrospinal fluid physiology and the management of increased intracranial pressure. Mayo Clin. Proc., *65:* 684–707, 1990. Figure 1, p. 687.)

Intracranial Pressure

Intracranial pressure (ICP) is the pressure measured within the intracranial compartment. The ICP waveform itself is a reflection of the arterial pulsations as they are transmitted to the CSF via the cerebral veins. Its configuration may change both under normal physiologic and pathologic conditions. ICP measurements can be obtained from a variety of intracranial locations, including the epidural, subdural, and subarachnoid spaces, as well as within the ventricles. ICP is most reliably measured within the ventricle and is normally less than 10 mm Hg.

The ICP itself is a reflection of the aggregate effects of several forces interacting within the intracranial compartment, including both vascular and nonvascular factors, such as focal pathologic lesions or impaired absorption of the cerebrospinal fluid. Although changes in any of these factors may change ICP acutely, the steady-state ICP is determined by the CSF production rate (I_f), CSF outflow resistance (R_o), and dural sinus pressure (P_d).

$$ICP = (I_f \times R_0) + P_d \qquad \text{(Eq. 6)}$$

The CSF formation rate is normally equal to the rate of CSF absorption and is largely unaffected by changes in ICP. Therefore, the steady-state ICP is determined primarily by the dural sinus pressure and CSF outflow resistance. Although CSF outflow resistance can decrease with increases in ICP, anatomic obstruction of the CSF outflow pathways (e.g., subarachnoid hemorrhage) increases CSF outflow resistance and results in an increase in the steady-state ICP. Increases in dural sinus pressure (e.g., when high intrathoracic pressure increases systemic venous pressures causes a rise in ICP, especially when baseline ICP is low. When baseline ICP is high, however, increased sinus pressure has less of an effect on ICP as the cerebral veins tend to collapse and minimize dural sinus pressure transmission. The level to which the ICP will change when any of these factors are changed is dependent upon the volume-buffering capacity of the intracranial compartment.

The Monro-Kellie hypothesis states that the intracranial contents are incompressible and that changes in the volume of one compartment (blood, brain, CSF) are accompanied by compensatory changes in the volume of one or another compartment. The magnitude of pressure change required to return compartments to their original size is described by the intracranial compliance. Compliance is an index of intracranial distensibility and is the ratio of the change in volume to the change in pressure (delta v/delta p). Intracranial compliance determines the dynamic ICP response to changes in intracranial volume. The lower the compliance, the lower the buffering capacity of the intracranial compartment and the higher the ICP for a given volume change. The intracranial compliance curve is nonlinear so that compliance decreases as ICP increases (Fig. 23–9). On the flat portion of the compliance curve, changes in intracranial volume are compensated for with little if any change in ICP. When, however, the resting ICP is located on the steeper portion of the curve, the same volume increment results in a much greater increase in ICP.

Approximately two thirds of intracranial buffering capacity is provided by the intracranial compartment itself, with the remainder provided by the spinal compartment. The major buffering mechanism in response to an acute increase in intracranial

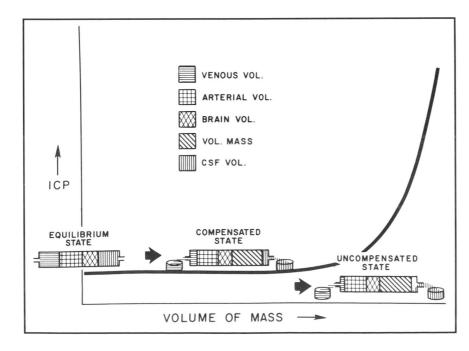

FIGURE 23–9. Intracranial volume-pressure relationship. Compliance is the $\Delta V / \Delta ICP$. Changes in intracranial volume are compensated for by reductions in cerebral blood volume and CSF volume. When compensatory mechanisms are exhausted, ICP increases. (Reprinted from Ward, J.D., Becker, D.P., Mickell, J., and Keenan, R.: Intracranial pressure, head injuries, subarachnoid hemorrhage, nonsurgical coma and brain tumors. *in* Shoemaker, W.C., and Thompson, W.L. (eds.): Critical Care, State of the Art, vol. II (R). Fullerton, CA, Society of Critical Care Medicine, 1981, Figure 1, p. 2.)

volume is a reduction in cerebral venous blood volume. Additional buffering capacity is provided by the displacement of CSF into the spinal subarachnoid space and by an increase in the CSF absorption rate.

An index of the buffering capacity of the CSF system is provided by a linear transformation of the compliance curve and is referred to as the pressure-volume index (PVI). The PVI is the slope of the volume-log pressure curve and is defined as the volume required to raise the resting ICP by a factor of 10.

$$PVI = \frac{\Delta V}{\log_{10} \dfrac{P_p}{P_o}} \qquad \text{(Eq. 7)}$$

where P_p is the peak ICP and P_o is the initial ICP. Unlike compliance, the PVI is not affected by the ICP at which it is measured and thus allows comparison of buffering capacity at various levels of ICP. The normal PVI in an adult is 25 mL. Measurement of the PVI in the clinical setting is performed by injection or withdrawal of small volumes of fluid and then measuring the change in pressure. The PVI allows a better overall evaluation of CSF dynamics and may also permit elevations in ICP to be anticipated.

The ICP is fundamentally important because of its effect on CBF. When intracranial buffering mechanisms have been exhausted, rises in ICP reduce CPP, ultimately causing cerebral ischemia and infarction when CPP becomes critically reduced. Pathologic increases in ICP can occur in a number of clinical conditions, including head injury, stroke, intracerebral hemorrhage, hepatic failure, and hydrocephalus. ICP monitoring is frequently employed in the clinical setting to detect changes in intracranial dynamics (e.g., expanding mass lesions) and for monitoring the progress of treatment in order to avoid secondary ischemic injury to the brain. Local and generalized increases in ICP can also cause mechanical herniation and compression of brain tissue from one intracranial compartment to another (Fig. 23–10).

Under pathologic conditions, sudden periodic increases in ICP may occur (Fig. 23–11). The A or plateau wave is a sudden increase in ICP as high as 50 to 100 mm Hg and lasting anywhere from a few minutes to as long as 30 minutes. B waves are oscillations in ICP usually occurring at a frequency of every 30 seconds to 2 minutes that are of much lower amplitude and of shorter duration than A waves. These periodic increases in ICP are likely due to cerebrovascular dilation resulting in an increase in cerebral blood volume in a cerebrovascular bed that is able to vasodilate in response to decreases in cerebral perfusion pressure.

Acid-Base Homeostasis

Acid-base balance of the CSF and brain is important not only for neuronal function but also in controlling the central respiratory response to changes in systemic acid-base balance. In addition, the pH of interstitial fluid bathing the intraparenchymal cerebral vasculature modulates, in part, cerebral blood flow.

Despite the absence of large qualities of protein for buffering, the pH of the CSF is maintained in a relatively narrow range, even when major changes in systemic arterial pH occur. The importance of pH homeostasis is further emphasized by the fact that the range of CSF pH compatible with life is very narrow (7.19 to 7.38) in comparison to systemic pH (6.9 to 7.8). CSF pH is normally lower than the pH of arterial blood due primarily to a higher CSF pCO_2, whereas CSF bicarbonate levels are only slightly lower than arterial bicarbonate levels (Fig. 23–12).

A number of important mechanisms are involved in CNS pH homeostasis. Carbon dioxide diffuses rapidly across the blood-brain barrier, but both bicarbonate and hydrogen ion are relatively impermeable. Therefore, when pCO_2 is held constant, CSF and brain interstitial pH resist isolated acute changes in systemic acid-base balance that are metabolic in origin. Paradoxic changes in CSF pH in response to acute metabolic acidosis or alkalosis may, however, be seen; they occur as a result of changes in CSF pCO_2 arising from peripherally mediated respiratory compensation for the primary metabolic disturbance. For example, acute metabolic acidosis results in compensatory hyperventilation, a reduction in

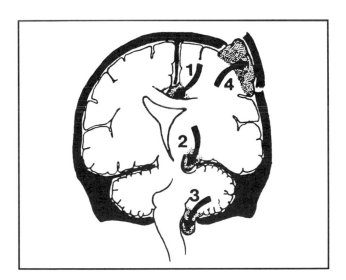

FIGURE 23–10. Examples of brain herniation. (1) Cingulate gyrus herniation across the falx, (2) temporal uncus herniation across the tentorium, (3) cerebellar tonsil herniation through the foramen magnum, (4) herniation of brain tissue through craniotomy defect. (Reprinted from Fishman, R.A.: Brain edema. N. Engl. J. Med., 293(14): 706–741, 1975. Figure 1, p. 706.)

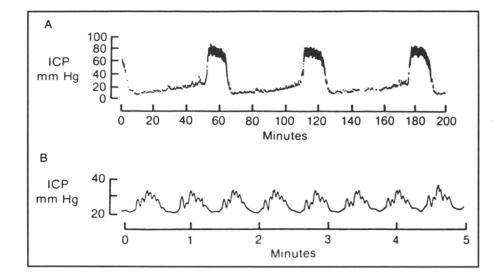

FIGURE 23–11. Pathologic ICP waves. *A,* "plateau" waves; *B,* "B" waves. (Reprinted from Sokoll, M.D.: Monitoring intracranial pressure. *In* Blitt, C.D. (ed.). Monitoring in Anesthesia and Critical Care Medicine, 2nd ed. New York: Churchill Livingstone, 1990, pp 413–425. Figure 19–2, p. 527.)

CSF pCO_2, and a paradoxic CSF alkalosis. Similarly, acute administration of bicarbonate can result in a paradoxic CSF acidosis as hypoventilation, in response to the alkalosis, increases systemic pCO_2, which then diffuses across the BBB and reduces CSF pH. Compensation in the case of paradoxic CSF changes occurs by intracellular buffering, the generation of bicarbonate, or alterations in CBF in response to changes in pCO_2 that result in either washout of CO_2 CSF acidosis or decrease the washout of CO_2 CSF alkalosis. In the example of acute metabolic acidosis and paradoxic CSF alkalosis, perivascular alkalosis results in a decrease in CBF and reduces the washout of carbon dioxide, returning interstitial and CSF pH toward normal. As a consequence of the relative impermeability of the BBB to bicarbonate and hydrogen ion and these homeostatic mecha-

nisms, systemic acid-base disturbances in themselves have little if any direct effect acutely or chronically on cerebral function.

Because of the rapid diffusion of CO_2 across the BBB, the pH of the CSF and brain interstitium is less well buffered in acute respiratory acid-base disorders. In the acute phase of respiratory acidosis or alkalosis, the CSF and brain interstitial pH tracks systemic pH and can result in impaired cerebral function. However, compensatory mechanisms return CSF and brain interstitial pH toward normal in a matter of hours. In acute respiratory acidosis, CSF pH decreases concomitantly with systemic pH. In time, carbonic-anhydrase-catalyzed generation of bicarbonate by the choroid plexus and glial cells returns pH toward normal. Ammonia produced by the deamination of glutamic acid can also buffer hydrogen ion in compensation for respiratory acidosis, resulting in the generation of bicarbonate and ammonium ion. The rise in CBF associated with respiratory acidosis also minimizes the increase is CO_2 in comparison with the systemic CO_2. When hypocapnia is induced, for example, with therapeutic hyperventilation, the CSF alkalosis is buffered by a decline in CSF bicarbonate and rise in CSF lactate. The lactate generation likely occurs in part as a result of anaerobic glycolysis associated with a reduction in CBF that in turn is associated with interstitial alkalosis.

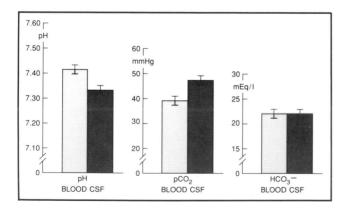

FIGURE 23–12. Relationship between arterial blood and CSF acid-base variables. (Reprinted from Arieff, A.I.: Effects of water, acid-base, and electrolyte disorders on the central nervous system. *In* Arieff, A.I., and DeFronzo, R.A. (eds.): Fluid Electrolyte and Acid-Base Disorders. New York, Churchill Livingstone, 1985, pp. 969–1040. Figure 21–1, p. 971.)

BIBLIOGRAPHY

1. Siesjo, B.K.: Cerebral circulation and metabolism. J. Neurosurg., *60*:883–908, 1984.
2. Davson, H., Welch, K., Segal, M.B.: Physiology and Pathophysiology of the Cerebrospinal Fluid. New York, Churchill Livingstone, 1987.
3. Arieff, A.I.: Effects of water, acid-base, and electrolyte disorders on the central nervous system. *In* Arieff, A.I., and

DeFronzo, R.A. (eds.): Fluid Electrolyte and Acid-Base Disorders. New York, Churchill Livingstone, 1985, pp. 969–1040.

4. Daube, J.R., Reagan, T.J., Sandok, B.A., Westmoreland, B.F. (eds.): Medical Neurosciences: An Approach to Anatomy, Pathology, and Physiology by Systems and Levels, 2nd ed. Boston, Little, Brown and Co., 1986.

5. Lyons, M.K., and Meyer, F.B.: Cerebrospinal fluid physiology and the management of increased intracranial pressure. Mayo Clin. Proc., 65:684–707, 1990.

6. Ward, J.D., Becker, D.P., Mickell, J., and Keenan, R.: Intracranial pressure, head injuries, subarachnoid hemorrhage, nonsurgical coma and brain tumors. In Shoemaker, W.C., and Thompson, W.L. (eds.): Critical Care, State of the Art, vol. II(R). Fullerton,CA, Society of Critical Care Medicine, 1981, pp. 1–31.

7. Fishman, R.A.: Brain edema. N. Engl. J. Med., 293(14):706–741,1975.

8. Lassen, N.A.: Cerebral and spinal cord blood flow. In Cottrell, J.E. and Turndorf, H. (eds.): Anesthesia and Neurosurgery. St. Louis, C.V. Mosby Co., 1986, pp. 1–21.

9. Early, C.B., Dewey, R.C., Pieper, H.P., et al.: Dynamic pressure flow relationship of brain blood flow in the monkey. J. Neurosurg., 41:590–596, 1974.

10. Sokoll, M.D.: Monitoring intracranial pressure. In Blitt, C.D. (cd.): Monitoring in Anesthesia and Critical Care Medicine. New York, Churchill Livingstone, 1985, pp. 413–425.

11. Marmarou, A., Shulman, K., and LaMorgese, J.: Compartmental analysis of compliance and outflow resistance of the cerebrospinal fluid system. J. Neurosurg., 43:523–534, 1974.

12. Astrup, J., Siesjo, B.K., and Syman, L.: Thresholds in cerebral ischemia—The ischemic penumbra. Stroke, 12 (6):723–725, 1981.

13. Berne, R.M., Winn, H.R., and Rubio, R.: The local regulation of cerebral blood flow. Prog. Cardiovasc. Dis., 24(3):243–260, 1981.

14. Keller, T.S., McGillicuddy, J.E., LaBond, V.A., et al.: Modification of focal cerebral ischemia by cardiac output augmentation. J. Surg. Res., 39:420–432, 1985.

15. Davis, D.D., and Sundt, T.M.: Relationship of cerebral blood flow to cardiac output, mean arterial pressure, blood volume, and alpha and beta blockade in cats. J. Neurosurg., 52:745–754, 1980.

16. Muizelaar, J.P., Wei, E.P., Kontos, H.A., et al.: Mannitol causes compensatory cerebral vasoconstriction and vasodilation in response to blood viscosity changes. J. Neurosurg., 59:822–828, 1983.

17. Jafar, J.J., and Crowell, R.M.: Focal ischemic thresholds. In Wood, H.H. (ed.): Cerebral Blood Flow. Physiologic and Clinical Aspects. New York, McGraw-Hill, 1987, pp. 449–457.

18. Shenkin, H.A., Harmel, M.H. and Kety, S.S.: Dynamic anatomy of the cerebral circulation. Arch. Neurol. Psychiatr., 60:240–252, 1948.

24

REPRODUCTIVE PHYSIOLOGY

RONALD R. JOHNSON

MALE REPRODUCTIVE SYSTEM

Characterization of the male reproductive system involves description of the differentiation of the gonad, its effect on the development of male internal and external sex organs, and the function of these organs in the phenotypic expression of maleness, as well as gamete production. These separate functions of the testes, including testosterone production and gametogenesis, are intimately related and controlled by the hypothalamic-anterior pituitary axis.

Fetal Development

The primitive gonad remains indistinct until the sixth or seventh fetal week. Primitive germ cells join with mesenchymal elements of the mesonephric ridge in the midabdomen. In genetic males, the gonad then develops into a testis, a process that seems to be controlled by the influence of an inducer substance, the HY antigen, which is a membrane-bound protein coded for by the Y chromosome. The cortex regresses and the medulla forms cords that later become the seminiferous tubules (Fig. 24–1). Between the developing tubules and the loose connective tissue lie the interstitial cells of Leydig, which are responsible for testosterone production. Human chorionic gonadotropin secreted by the placenta and fetal pituitary gonadotropins stimulate the developing interstitial cells to produce testosterone at an early stage.

The internal and external genital primordia of the developing fetus are identical in both sexes (Fig. 24–2 and 24–3). In genetically determined males, the wolffian ducts develop into seminal vesicles, epididymis, and vas deferens, and the genital tubercle and swelling develop into the penis, scrotum, and prostate gland. Mullerian ducts that give rise to the uterus and fallopian tube normally regress. Differentiation is under the control of the fetal testis. Testosterone is responsible for differentiation of wolffian duct structures and the development of external genitalia. Mullerian regression factor, a protein hormone produced by the Sertoli cells of the developing seminiferous tubules, is responsible for regression of mullerian duct structures.

In the absence of normal testosterone production in genetically determined males, internal and external genital development fails to proceed, and the phenotypic expression is that of a normal female. This condition is termed *male pseudohermaphroditism.* It results from lack of testosterone, absence of androgen receptor, or resistance to the function of testosterone in the presence of normal receptors.

The primitive gonad normally descends in the seventh fetal month through the abdominal wall and into the scrotum. This descent is under the influence of testosterone. Failure of the testis to descend is known as *cryptorchidism.* Failure of descent results in deficient gametogenesis, as the cooler environment of the scrotum is necessary for normal gamete production. The function of the fetal testis in androgen production ceases abruptly after birth, concomitant with withdrawal of gonadotropins. Leydig cells regress and remain quiescent until puberty.

Testis

Eighty per cent of the mass of the adult testis results from the convoluted seminiferous tubules that empty into the rete testis, epididymis, vas deferens, and prostatic urethra.

Spermatogenesis. The seminiferous tubules are lined by primitive germ cells known as spermatogonia, with the formation of sperm occurring throughout the length of the tubule. Spermatogenesis is complex and is divided into three phases: *spermatocytogenesis,* in which the spermatogonia undergo mitotic division to replenish the germ cells; *meiosis,* in which two cell divisions result in a decrease in chromosome number by one half to produce a cluster of spermatids; and finally, *spermiogenesis,* in which the developing spermatids mature into sperm before being shed into the lumen of the tubules. The entire process takes 64 days. Sperm production proceeds throughout life from the time of puberty with no

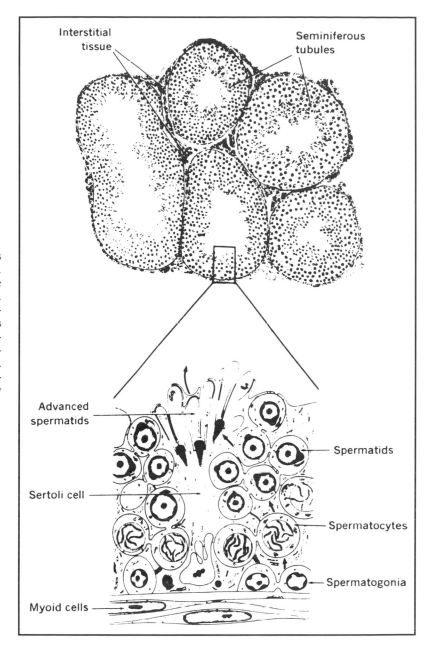

FIGURE 24–1. Histologic section of testis showing the relation of various cell types. Upper figure shows cords of interstitial tissue interspersed between seminiferous tubules. Lower portion shows a high-power magnification of seminiferous epithelium. Arrows indicate migration of germ cells through Sertoli cells as spermatogenesis progresses. (Reprinted from Goodman, M: Reproduction. *In* Mountcastle, V.B. (ed.): Medical Physiology, 14th ed. vol. II. St. Louis, C.V. Mosby Co., 1980, p. 1625.)

equivalent of the female climacteric recognized in males.

The second cell type recognized in the seminiferous tubule is the Sertoli cell, and it too is intimately related to spermatogenesis. Sertoli cells extend the entire distance from the basement membrane to the lumen of the tubule and are connected to one another at the level of the basement membrane by tight junctions (Fig. 24–4). These tight junctions form the so-called blood-testis barrier, which is a semipermeable barrier protecting developing spermatogonia from the constituents of the blood. The progression from spermatogonia to spermatozoa takes place in the intercellular spaces between Sertoli cells, to which the dividing and maturing sperm are attached during their 2 month long period of development into mature sperm (Fig. 24–4). The Sertoli cells also function in phagocytosis of dying spermatids, the conversion of testosterone to estrogen, and the production of mullerian regression factor. The Sertoli cells secrete a clear fluid into the seminiferous tubules, which serves as nourishment for the spermatids in their journey to the epididymis. Androgen-binding hormone produced by Sertoli cells concentrates testosterone in the vicinity of the developing sperm.

Testosterone. Androgens, which are any substance that results in the development of male primary and secondary sexual characteristics, are produced in interstitial cells (Leydig cells) of the testis,

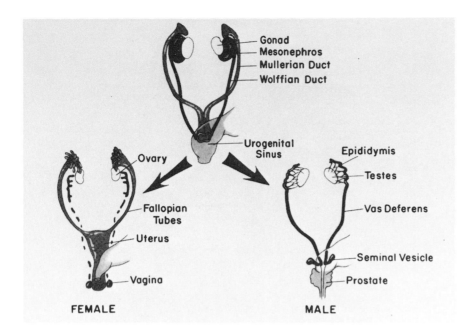

FIGURE 24–2. Internal genitalia development in the male and female. (Reprinted from Jaffe, R.B.: Disorders of sexual development. *In* Yen, S., and Jaffe, R.B. (eds.): Reproductive Endocrinology, 2nd ed. Philadelphia, W.B. Saunders Co., 1986, p. 285.)

with lesser contributions by the adrenal gland. Production of testosterone remains fairly constant from puberty throughout adult life, with only minimal decreases in measured serum testosterone levels. Production of testosterone, as with other sex steroid hormones, occurs through cholesterol precursors under the direction of gonadotropins (Fig. 24–5).

Most secreted testosterone circulates bound to plasma proteins, either albumin (40 per cent) or testosterone-binding globulin (58 per cent). This latter substance is the same sex hormone-binding globulin found in females, but has a much higher affinity for testosterone than estrogens. Free testosterone is degraded in the liver by conjugation with either sulfate or glucuronide and is excreted in the urine.

The mechanism of action of testosterone is similar to that of other sex-steroids. Being lipid soluble, testosterone penetrates the cell membrane and is converted by a 5-alpha-reductase cytoplasmic enzyme system to its active form, dihydrotestosterone (DHT). DHT binds to a cytosolic androgen receptor protein and is transported to the nucleus, where it acts to initiate production of mRNA and resultant protein synthesis. DHT is responsible for the development of the phenotypic characteristics of the male. In the syndrome of testicular feminization,

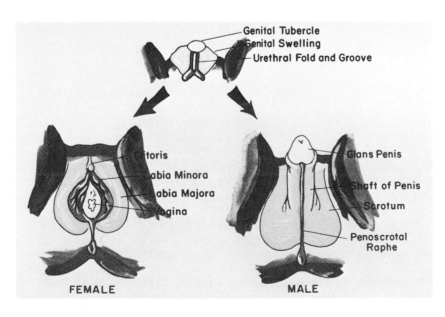

FIGURE 24–3. External genital development, demonstrating homologies and common anlage in the male and female. (Reprinted from Jaffe, R.B.: Disorders of sexual development. *In* Yen, S., and Jaffe, R.B. (eds.): Reproductive Endocrinology, 2nd ed. Philadelphia, W.B. Saunders Co., 1986, p. 285.)

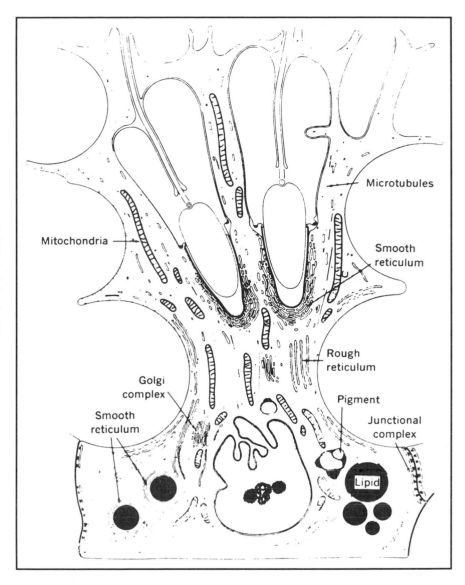

FIGURE 24–4. A typical Sertoli cell. Two advanced spermatids are embedded in cytoplasm near the apical surface. Irregular indentations on lateral borders indicate location of maturing spermatids. Various intracellular organelles are indicated. (Reprinted from Goodman, H.M.: Reproduction. *In* Mountcastle, V.B. (ed.): Medical Physiology, 14th ed. St. Louis, C.V. Mosby Co., 1980, p. 1626.)

genetically determined males with normal testosterone levels develop the external genitalia of a female because of the congenital lack of the cytosolic reductase system responsible for conversion of testosterone to DHT.

The functions of testosterone (Table 24–1) are directed at promoting the growth, differentiation, and function of the accessory organs of reproduction. At the time of puberty, gonadotropin stimulation of dormant interstitial cells results in a dramatic increase in testosterone production. Primary sexual characteristics—growth of the penis, scrotum, and prostate—occur, as well as development of the typical male pattern of secondary sexual characteristics: the male pattern of body hair, expression of the gene controlling male pattern baldness, thickening of the vocal cords resulting in deepening of the voice, and dramatic nitrogen retention with addition of muscle mass. Testosterone also targets the brain to affect the male libido. Estrogens are produced by the testis, as well as by Sertoli cells and peripheral conversion of testosterone in amounts similar to the early proliferative phase of the female cycle. The roles of estrogens in the male are unclear, but they may be involved in feedback inhibition of testicular function.

Pituitary Control of Testicular Function. Control of testicular function occurs at the level of the hypothalamic-pituitary axis. Gonadotropin-releasing hormone (GRH) produced in the hypothalamus is carried to the anterior pituitary by the hypothalamic-pituitary portal venous system and stimulates production and release of the gonadotropic hormones, luteinizing hormone (LH) and follicular-stimulating hormone (FSH).

LH and FSH are protein hormones produced by PAS-positive basophilic cells of the anterior pituitary, which consist of alpha and beta subunits. The alpha subunits are identical for both hormones, and specific function is conferred by differences on the beta chain.

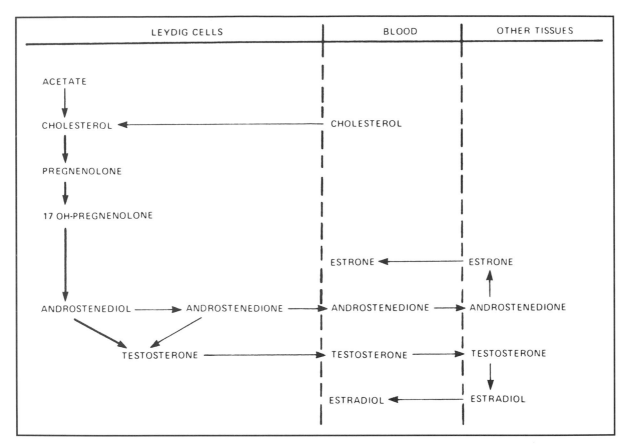

FIGURE 24–5. Androgen biosynthesis in the testis of the human. Testosterone is the major secretory product of the testis. Androgens can be converted to estrogens in peripheral tissues. (Adapted from Bardin, C.W.: Pituitary-testicular axis. *In* Yen, S., and Jaffe, R.B. (eds.): Reproductive Endocrinology, 2nd ed. Philadelphia, W.B. Saunders Co., 1986, p. 182.)

Lutenizing hormone (LH) was named for its role in women, causing formation of the corpus luteum. This trophic hormone is found in males and controls production of testosterone by a classic negative feedback inhibition (Fig. 24–6).

Castration in the males causes a dramatic rise in LH concentrations, whereas the exogenous administration of testosterone results in low levels of LH. LH works by binding to specific LH receptors on the Leydig cell membrane, thereby stimulating the production of cytosolic cAMP, which is actually the trigger for Leydig cell function (Fig. 24–7). Testoster-one, but not dihydrotestosterone, acts at the level of the pituitary and hypothalamus to decrease LH production. It is thought that testosterone conversion to estrogen within the hypothalamus acts as the mediator for decreased GRH production. DHT cannot be converted to estrogen and hence is not involved in the feedback system. Follicular-stimulating hormone (FSH) has a synergistic role with LH in stimulating Leydig cell function, but the mechanism for this remains obscure. No FSH receptors are present on Leydig cell membranes.

The relationship between FSH and sperm production is also not clear. FSH receptors exist within the seminiferous tubules, and FSH is essential for initiating spermatogenesis at the time of puberty. However, once established, spermatogenesis can proceed indefinitely in the absence of FSH, providing that adequate amounts of LH and testosterone are present. The role of LH is probably to serve as a stimulus of testosterone production. The blood-testis barrier is permeable to testosterone, and very high local concentrations of testosterone are reached within the seminiferous tubules. Testosterone functions in the maturation of spermatogonia to mature

TABLE 24–1. EFFECTS OF TESTOSTERONE

Development of primary sexual characteristics: growth of penis, testes, scrotum, prostate, and seminal vesicles
Increased growth at puberty
Development of secondary sexual characteristics: hair growth, deepening voice, muscle mass, male pattern baldness, and facial hair
Maintenance of spermatogenesis
Increased libido and potency

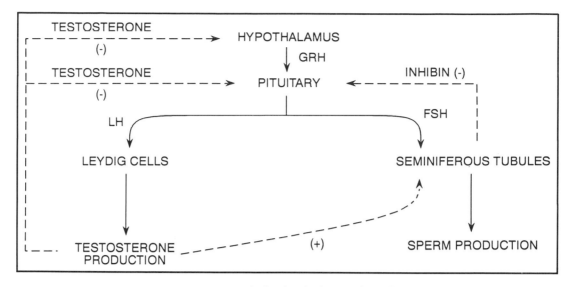

FIGURE 24–6. Hypothalamic-pituitary axis and control of testicular function.

FIGURE 24–7. The mechanism of action of pituitary hormones and testosterone on the seminiferous tubule. *Upper panel,* LH acts by way of its Leydig cell membrane receptor to stimulate cyclic AMP formation, which facilitates the conversion of cholesterol (C) to testosterone (T). Both testosterone and FSH directly on Sertoli cells to stimulate the transport of various substances into the seminiferous tubular lumen. *Bottom panel,* two Sertoli cells are shown. *Left,* germ cells (*stippled circles*) develop, surrounded by Sertoli cell plasma membrane. *Right,* testosterone and FSH stimulate Sertoli cell protein synthesis and androgen-binding protein (ABP). In addition, FSH stimulates the conversion of testosterone to estradiol (E₂). (Reprinted from Bardin, C.W.: Pituitary testicular axis. *In* Yen, S., and Jaffe, R.B. (eds.): Reproductive Endocrinology, 2nd ed. Philadelphia, W.B. Saunders Co., 1986, p. 192.)

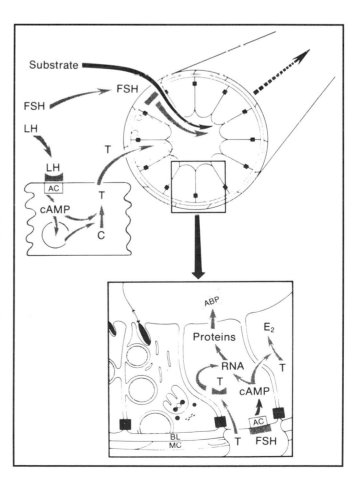

spermatids, probably through an influence on the Sertoli cells that contain testosterone-binding protein.

Castrated animals develop very high serum levels of FSH, as do animals that suffer acquired injuries of the seminiferous tubules. The negative feedback system responsible for this action is controlled by inhibin, a protein substance produced by Sertoli cells that acts at the level of the anterior pituitary to decrease the sensitivity of basophilic cells to GRH (Fig. 24–6).

FEMALE REPRODUCTIVE SYSTEM

Growth and differentiation of the female reproductive system occur under the influence of hypothalamic-pituitary control for the purpose of procreation of the species. Unlike the male, the dual functions of the ovary in gametogenesis and hormone production are intimately related and influence the female in a cyclical rather than constant fashion.

Embryology and Female Reproductive System

As in the male, the female reproductive organs develop from genetically indistinct genital primordia. The embryologic genital ridge in the midabdomen becomes suffused with primitive germ cells. The lack of androgen production during the period from the 6th to 13th week results in the phenotypic expression of the female. The primitive gonad, consisting of cortex and medulla, differentiates with regression of the medulla and development of the cortex (Fig. 24–8). The germ cells, primordial oogonia, are surrounded by the stroma of the developing cortex. The number of germ cells is greatest in midgestation at 6 to 7 million and decreases steadily from this point on, with only 100,000 to 300,000 active gametes at the time of puberty and, at most, 400 developing to maturity during the reproductive years of the adult female.

The internal and external genitalia develop in the female pattern as shown in Figures 24–9 and 24–10. As described in the section on male reproduction, the chief determinants of genital differentiation are testosterone and mullerian regression factor, which

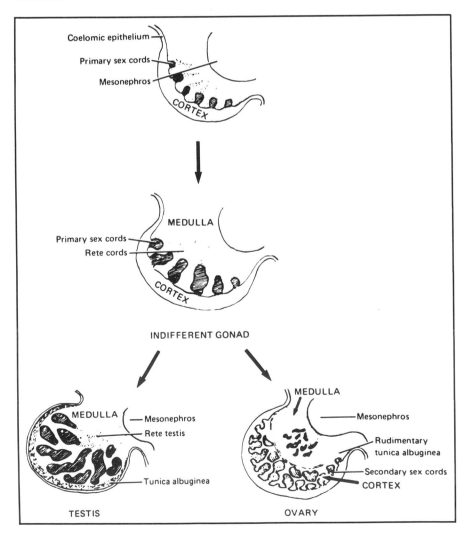

FIGURE 24–8. Development of an ovary from the cortex or a testis from the medulla of a bipotential primordial human gonad. (Reprinted with permission from Grumbach, M.: *In* Astwood, E.B. (ed.): Clinical Endocrinology. New York, Grune & Stratton, 1960.)

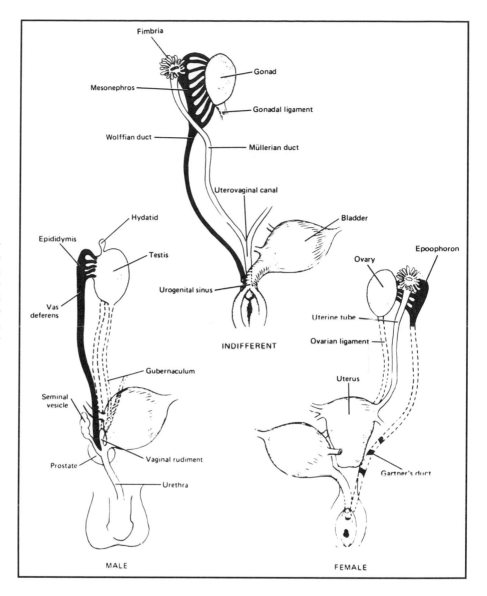

FIGURE 24–9. Embyronic differentiation of male and female internal genitalia (genital ducts) from wolffian (male) and mullerian (female) primordia. (Reprinted from Ganong, W.F. (ed.): *Review of Medical Physiology,* 13th ed. Norwalk, CT, Appleton & Lange, 1987. Figure 23–6, p. 350.)

are both produced by the testis. In the absence of these substances, wolffian duct structures atrophy, and the mullerian ducts fuse to form the fallopian tubes, uterus, and upper portion of the vagina.

Obviously, exposure of the indifferent genital primordia to androgen during the early part of gestation can result in the phenotypic expression of maleness in a genetically determined female. This condition, known as *female pseudohermaphroditism,* results from exogenous administration of androgens to the mother or congenital virilizing adrenal hyperplasia in the embryo.

Unlike the male, the female gonad does not function during gestation despite exposure to trophic hormones secreted by the placenta and fetal pituitary. The gland remains quiescent until puberty.

Puberty

Puberty, by strict definition, refers to the time when gonadal functions of gametogenesis and sex-steroid production have matured to the point where reproduction is possible. It has, by convention, come to mean the beginning of the menstrual cycle, the first of which is known as menarche, but given that the first few cycles are anovulatory, fertilization is not possible.

The average American woman experiences puberty between the ages of 8 to 13 years, the age varying greatly from person to person. Delayed puberty is defined as the lack of normal menstrual cycles by the age of 17 years. The complex factors that control puberty are poorly understood. The ca-

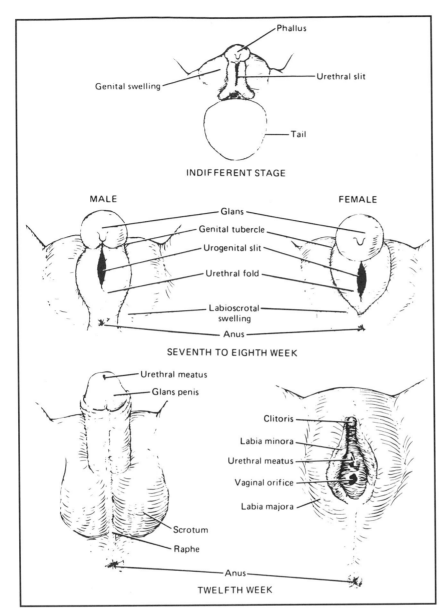

FIGURE 24–10. Differentiation of male and female external genitalia from indifferent primordial structures in the embryo. (Reprinted from Ganong, W.F. (ed.): Review of Medical Physiology, 13th ed. Norwalk, CT, Appleton & Lange, 1987. Figure 23–7, p. 351.)

pability of successful menstrual cycles is in place shortly after birth. Gonadotropin-releasing hormone (GRH) can be identified within the hypothalamus, gonadotropins are present in the anterior pituitary, and sex-steroid production by the ovary is possible, yet some poorly understood neural inhibition prevents the normal cyclical nature of ovarian function until the hypothalamus "matures" at puberty.

Lesions within the ventral hypothalamus have been demonstrated to result in precocious puberty —normal physiologic function of the pituitary ovarian axis at age less than 8 years—but this is very variable. At the time of puberty, GRH is released from the hypothalamus in a pulsatile fashion and is carried to the anterior pituitary by the hypophyseal-portal system. Release of pituitary gonadotropins re-

sults in stimulation of gametogenesis and hormone production, with the consequent development of secondary sexual characteristics and menstrual cycles that are used to identify the onset of puberty.

The Menstrual Cycle

In contrast to the male, the female reproductive physiology undergoes cyclical changes marked by periodic vaginal bleeding known as menstruation. The purpose of the cycle is to provide a mature ovum the proper environment in which fertilization, implantation, and embryogenesis may occur and, failing that, to shed, the "wasted" endometrium to prepare for another cycle.

The average menstrual cycle lasts 28 days, although its length is quite variable. By convention, the first day of bleeding marks the start of a new cycle. Each of the primary sex organs experiences cyclical changes that, for the sake of clarity, are described separately in this chapter.

The Ovarian Cycle

The mature ovaries are 5 cm paired organs floating free in the abdominal cavity, except for attachments at the hilum. The cortex contains many primordial follicles, and the medulla contains blood vessels and autonomic nervous innervation.

Follicular Phase. Many of the primordial follicles beneath the cortex, each containing a single ovum, begin to mature at the beginning of a new cycle. The developing follicle is surrounded by a theca, or container, the outer layer of which is connective tissue, the theca externa, and the inner layer of which contains secretory cells, the theca interna. A basement membrane separates the theca interna from the ovum and its surrounding secretory cells, the granulosa cells.

By the sixth day of the cycle, a combination of factors results in continued development of a single follicle and regression of all others. The single developing follicle is known to have the highest concentration of estrogens within the follicle and the highest estrogen-to-androgen ratio. Development of primordial follicles occurs independent of gonadotropins, as no membrane receptors for FSH have been identified.

As shown in Figure 24–11, the primordial follicle differentiates into a primary follicle with proliferation of granulosa cells, and the development of a fluid-filled cavity, the antrum, and of membrane-bound FSH receptors. Estrogen production increases dramatically because of a complex interaction between the theca interna and granulosa cells as depicted in Figure 24–12. The dramatic midcycle increase in estrogen concentration results in the LH surge responsible for rupture of the mature graafian follicle and extrusion of the mature ovum and liquor folliculi into the abdominal cavity, known as ovulation.

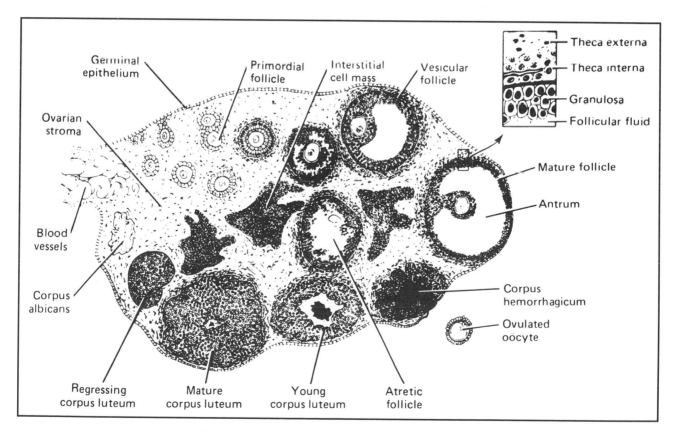

FIGURE 24–11. A mammalian ovary, showing the sequential development of a follicle, formation of a corpus luteum, and, in the center, follicular atresia. A section of the wall of a mature follicle is enlarged at the upper right. The interstitial cell mass is not prominent in primates. (Reprinted from Patten, B., and Eakin, R.M. *In* Gorbman, A., and Bern, H. (eds.): Textbook of Comparative Endocrinology. New York, Wiley, 1962.) Garong, W.F. (ed.): Review of Medical Physiology. Norwalk, CT, Appleton & Lange, 1987. Figure 23–21, p. 365.)

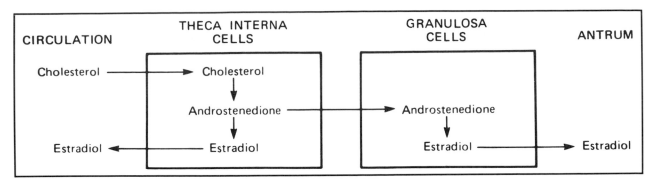

FIGURE 24–12. Interactions between theca and granulosa cells in estradiol synthesis and secretion. (Reprinted from Ganong, W.F. (ed.): Review of Medical Physiology, 13th ed. Norwalk, CT, Appleton & Lange, 1987. Figure 23–28, p. 370.)

Luteal Phase. After ovulation, the ruptured follicle fills with blood, forming the corpus hemorrhagium. "Mittelschmerz," or intermenstrual pain, results from irritation of the parietes secondary to follicle rupture. The granulosa cells and cells of the theca interna rapidly proliferate, and the blood-filled follicle is replaced by lipid-rich luteal cells, which secrete estrogens and progesterones (Fig. 24–11).

If successful implantation of the ovum occurs, the corpus luteum persists and continues to secrete sex hormones throughout most of the pregnancy. Failing implantation, the rate of steroid sex hormone production falls, and the corpus luteum regresses to be replaced by a fibrous white scar, the corpus albicans.

Ovarian Hormone Production

Production of steroid sex hormones by the ovary follows the pattern of steroidogenesis seen in the male, with androgen precursors derived from cholesterol being converted to estrogens by the action of cytosolic aromatases (see Fig. 24–13). Active estrogens include estrone, 17B estradiol, and estriol, with estradiol being by far the most potent and most important physiologically. Estrogen production within

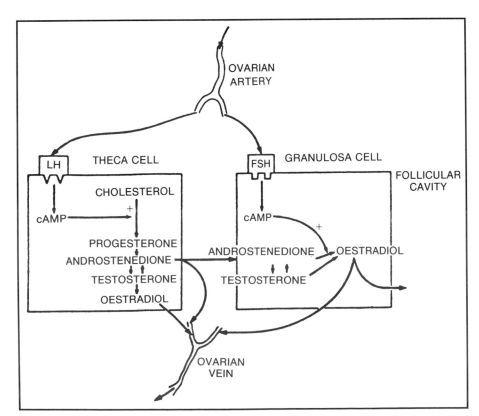

FIGURE 24–13. Action of FSH and LH on the ovarian follicle. (Reprinted from MacDonald, R.R. (ed.): Scientific Basis of Obstetrics and Gynaecology, 3rd ed. New York, Churchill Livingstone, 1985. Figure 2.5, p. 40.)

the graafian follicle requires an intimate relationship between the cells of the theca interna, which present androgen precursors, and granulosa cells responsible for aromatization to estrogen. The plasma levels of estrogens vary throughout the menstrual cycle, with the majority bound to plasma constituents. Binding between sex-steroids and albumin is less secure than in the male, and the same sex hormone-binding globulin (SHBG) is present in the female. About 3 per cent of estrogens circulate freely and represent the active hormone. Estrogens are degraded by a single pass through the liver where they are conjugated to glucuronide or sulfate metabolites. They enter the enterohepatic circulation, but little estrogen is lost in the GI tract, with most being reabsorbed in the gut and excreted in the urine.

The mechanism of action of estrogens is similar to other steroid sex hormones. They cross membrane barriers and, in cells containing cytosolic estrogen receptors, are transported to the nucleus where they stimulate synthesis of mRNA.

Effects of Estrogens

Like testosterone in the male, the foremost effect of estrogens in the female is to promote growth and differentiation of the primary organs of reproduction, fallopian tubes, uterus, vagina, and external genitalia (Table 24–2). There is also a sustaining quality of this hormone in that castration results in atrophy of the above organs in adult life. Estrogens have an anti-atretic effect on the ovary itself and may contribute to deciding which follicle will persist to maturation and which become atretic. Within the granulosa cells, estrogen is responsible for regulation of FSH receptors, production of aromatase enzyme systems, and a general upregulation of steroid production. The effects of estrogens on the fallopian tube and uterus are described in detail later, but act to promote implantation of the ovum in a safe and nourishing environment in the uterus. Secondary sexual characteristics, such as deposition of body fat, female patterns of body hair, and early epiphyseal closure, occur under the direction of estrogens.

Progesterone

The other sex-steroid, progesterone, is a C_{21}-steroid derived from cholesterol. It is formed principally by the cells of the corpus luteum postovulation, although the adrenal cortex and granulosa cells may contribute in much smaller amounts. Similar to estrogens, the progesterone circulates bound to plasma proteins, is degraded by the liver, and is excreted in the urine. Its mechanism of action is similar to testosterone and estrogens producing an increase in mRNA production.

TABLE 24–2. EFFECTS OF ESTROGENS

Growth and differentiation of primary sex organs
Upregulation of steroid production from the ovary
Promotion of fallopian tube contraction and ciliary action
Development of uterine endometrium
Development of secondary sexual characteristics
Development of duct system in breasts
Increase in libido

Progesterone is the "hormone of pregnancy." Its action is to promote and foster an environment in which implantation, development, and growth of the embryo can occur. Specific effects on the primary organs of reproduction are described below.

Relaxin

Relaxin is a polypeptide hormone with an amino acid sequence that resembles insulin. Secreted by both the corpus luteum and the placenta, this hormone acts to relax the pubic symphysis and pelvic joints. Important in parturition, relaxin also softens and dilates the cervix during pregnancy and decreases the excitability of the uterine musculature.

Hypothalamic-Pituitary-Gonadal Control Mechanisms

Control mechanisms governing the female reproductive cycle are quite complex. At puberty, maturation of the hypothalamus occurs, allowing for the production of gonadotropin-releasing hormone (GRH) or luteinizing-hormone-releasing hormone (LHRH), which is then secreted into the hypophyseal-portal system in a pulsatile fashion throughout the day and is responsible for cyclical ovarian activity. GRH is a decapeptide with a very short half-life. Concentrations within the hypophyseal-portal system vary widely, depending on when in the episodic rhythm the levels are measured. Specific receptors for GRH exist on the plasma membranes of gonadotropic cells in the anterior pituitary. High levels of GRH stimulate gonadotropic activity with increased production and release of LH and FSH. Low levels of circulating sex-steroids are the stimulus of increased GRH release, whereas high levels inhibit GRH production in a classic negative feedback pattern (Fig. 24–14).

The pituitary gonadotropins, LH and FSH, are identical to the glycoprotein hormones described in the section on the male reproductive system. In broad terms, FSH is responsible for maturation of the graafian follicle, whereas LH is responsible for ovulation and corpus luteum formation. The gonadotropes are glycoproteins produced by PAS-positive

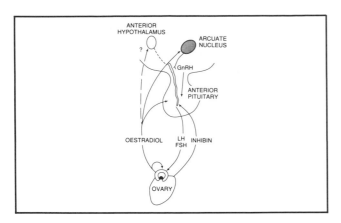

FIGURE 24–14. Estradiol secreted by the graafian follicle feeds back at the anterior pituitary and the hypothalamus to regulate the secretion of gonadotrophins. A nonsteroidal product of the ovary (inhibin) suppresses FSH secretion by its inhibitory action at the anterior pituitary. GnRH is released by the axons of neurones that project into the median eminence to enter the long portal vessels. (Reprinted from MacDonald, R.R. (ed.): Scientific Basis of Obstetrics and Gynaecology, 3rd ed. New York, Churchill Livingstone, 1985. Figure 2.1, p. 30.)

basophilic cells of the anterior pituitary. Each consists of an identical alpha subunit and variable beta subunit, which confers its specific function. Each acts at the level of the plasma membrane to promote cytosolic cAMP as a secondary messenger.

FSH acts at the level of the granulosa cells to promote estrogen production, increase the number of estrogen receptors, and increase the number of LH receptors. LH activates steroidogenesis to increase estrogen/progesterone production via the complex interaction between theca cells and granulosa cells previously described.

The feedback mechanisms for pituitary gonadotropes are more complex than in the male. Generally, low levels of sex-steroids act at the level of the pituitary to stimulate LH/FSH production, and vice versa, in a classic negative feedback loop. However, estrogen also acts in a positive feedback mechanism during the immediate preovulatory period. Increased plasma concentrations of estrogen occurring at midcycle result in a surge of LH responsible for ovulation, which occurs approximately 9 hours later.

Postovulation, gradually increasing levels of estrogen and progesterone inhibit gonadotrope production. If implantation does not occur, luteolysis or degeneration of the corpus luteum follows, and the fall in sex-steroids allows for gradually increasing gonadotrope levels. The stimulus for luteolysis, which actually confers the cyclical nature to the female cycle, is unknown.

Uteral Cycle

The clinically obvious indication of the cyclical nature of the female reproduction process is the periodic shedding of blood and debris from the uterus known as menstruation. Similar to the ovary, the uterus undergoes predictable changes in response to variable hormone levels.

Proliferative Phase. The proliferative phase of the uterine cycle occurs concomitant to the follicular phase of the ovarian cycle. The duration of this phase is generally 14 days, but is quite variable. Increasing estrogen levels from the maturing follicle result in rapid growth of the uterine endometrium with elongation of the uterine glands (Fig. 24–15).

Secretory Phase. The secretory phase of the cycle equates with the luteal phase of ovarian function. It is quite constant in length at 14 days. Progesterone produced by the functioning corpus luteum results in continuous development of the endometrium. The glands become highly convoluted (Fig. 19–15) and secrete a clear fluid. The blood supply to the endometrium is divided into stratum basale and stratum functionale. The stratum basale consists of short, straight arteries, whereas the functionale becomes longer and coiled with progression of the secretory phase. The coiling is thought to contribute to the ischemic necrosis that results in menstruation.

Menstruation

Luteolysis after failure of implantation results in dramatically diminishing sex-steroid levels, which in turn result in menstruation. The local stimulus is thought to be prostaglandin PGF$_2$ alpha, which results in vasoconstriction of the long spiraled arteries and ischemic necrosis of the stratum functionale. Menstruation generally lasts 3 to 5 days and consists of both arterial and venous blood and debris. Average blood loss ranges from 35 to 50 cc. No clots are formed secondary to fibrinolysis present within the endometrium. At the conclusion of menstruation, a new endometrium is formed from cells of the stratim basale.

Cervical Cycle

The cervix of the uterus does not experience the endometrial changes of the uterine corpus, but cyclical changes of the cervical mucus are produced. During the follicular phase of the cycle, estrogens result in a thinner, more alkaline cervical mucus, which is thought to promote sperm motility and survival. The luteal phase of the cycle sees a change in the cervical mucus to a more cellular thick form, secondary to progesterone. The elasticity of cervical mucus, or spinnbarkheit, is greatest at the time of ovulation

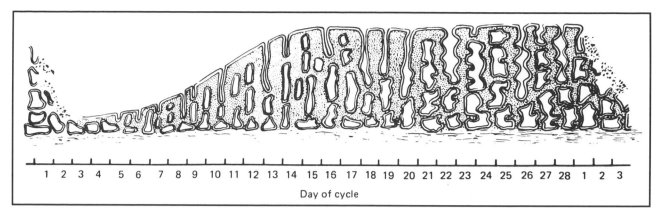

FIGURE 24–15. Changes in the endometrium during the menstrual cycle. (Reprinted from Ganong, W.F. (ed): Review of Medical Physiology, 13th ed. Norwalk, CT, Appleton & Lange, 1987. Figure 23–22, p. 366.)

when mucus dries on a slide in a characteristic fern-like pattern. After ovulation the mucus is thick, and the fern-like pattern disappears. The usefulness of this simple test is obvious in assessing fertility problems, allowing one to determine if a cycle was ovulatory or not.

Pregnancy

A successful cycle is marked by conception and implantation of the embryo within the uterus. Cyclical activity of the uterus, ovary, and cervix ceases. Fertilization generally occurs within the fallopian tube. The ovum spends 3 days within the tube and, immediately after fertilization, undergoes cell division. The developing embryo spends 3 days within the uterine cavity and develops to the blastocyst stage, with an inner cellular layer, the cytotrophoblast, and an outer multinucleate mass, the syncytiotrophoblast. Implantation generally occurs in the dorsal wall of the uterus, with the blastocyst burrowing into the wall and the outer layer developing into the placenta.

The corpus luteum fails to regress and actually enlarges secondary to placental gonadotropins. The corpus luteum of pregnancy continues to secrete estrogen, progesterone, and relaxin, which result in a nourishing stable environment for the developing embryo. Castration before 6 weeks of pregnancy results in abortion. After this period, the placenta produces adequate quantities of sex-steroids such that castration is not harmful. The contribution of the corpus luteum diminishes throughout pregnancy, but persists in some fashion.

The placenta becomes the major endocrine organ of pregnancy. Along with sex-steroids, the placenta is responsible for the production of trophic hormones. Human chorionic gonadotropin (HCG) is a glycoprotein hormone similar to LH with very little

FSH activity and is produced by the syncytiotrophoblast. It can be recognized within the blood and urine of the mother at very early time periods and is the basis for pregnancy testing. This "luteinizing" hormone is responsible for sustaining the corpus luteum of pregnancy until the placenta can take over production of progesterone. It peaks at the end of the first trimester and gradually diminishes during the remainder of pregnancy.

Human chorionic somatomammotropin (HCS) is a protein hormone similar in structural characteristics to growth hormone. It results in development of the body and particularly the breasts during pregnancy. Levels of HCS and prolactin rise steadily through pregnancy and contribute to breast development. The amount produced is proportional to placental size, and hence assays for this hormone can be used as a marker for placental insufficiency.

Parturition

It remains uncertain what triggers the expulsion of the products of conception. The length of pregnancy is generally 270 days from conception or 284 days from the last menstrual period, but is quite variable. The fetoplacental unit may in fact trigger the onset of labor, but the mechanisms for this remain obscure.

With the onset of labor, the cervix becomes softer and dilates, and the myometrium undergoes rhythmic contractions. In early labor, the plasma oxytocin levels are normal, but uterine contraction and cervical dilation cause dramatic rises in the oxytocin concentration in plasma via afferent nervous pathways. A positive feedback loop is established whereby oxytocin increases the force and rate of contractions.

Oxytocin also increases uterine contractions by stimulating prostaglandin synthesis in the endometrium. Prostaglandin inhibitors prolong labor, and both mechanisms appear to be important in successful labor.

Menopause

Unlike the male, the female reproductive term is limited by the availability of viable ova. The average age of the female climacteric is about 50 years, but most women experience irregular menstrual cycles for 1 to 2 years before becoming amenorrheic.

The symptoms commonly associated with the "change of life" are those of estrogen deficiency. The loss of the sustaining qualities of estrogens results in atrophy of the vagina and breast tissue. "Hot flashes," which occur in 80 per cent of women, may be related to the loss of negative feedback inhibition of pituitary gonadotropes. Measurement of serum FSH levels are useful in recognizing ovarian failure as FSH levels rise dramatically before the onset of amenorrhea. Symptoms respond to estrogen therapy, which may also have some role in preventing the medical complications of menopause; namely, accelerated atherogenesis and osteoporosis.

BIBLIOGRAPHY

1. Patton, Fuchs, Hille, Scher, Steiner (eds). Textbook of Physiology, 21st ed. Philadelphia, W.B. Saunders Co., 1989.
2. McDonald, R.R. (ed.): Scientific Basis of Obstetrics and Gynaecology, 3rd ed. New York, Churchill Livingstone, 1985.
3. Yen, S., and Jaffe, R.B. (eds.): Reproductive Endocrinology, 2nd ed. Philadelphia, W.B. Saunders Co, 1986.
4. Goodman, H.M.: Reproduction. *In* Mountcastle, V.B. (ed.): Medical Physiology, 14th ed. St. Louis, C.V. Mosby Co., 1980, pp. 1602–1637.
5. Ganong, W.F.: Review of Medical Physiology, 13th ed. Norwalk, CT, Appleton & Lange, 1987.
6. Bardin, C.W.: Hormonal regulation of growth and development. *In* West, J.B.: Best and Taylor's Physiological Basis of Medical Practice, 11th ed. Baltimore, Williams & Wilkins, 1985, pp. 902–969.

25

THE BREAST

RONALD R. JOHNSON

Breasts are skin appendages arising from ectodermally derived mammary ridges in the embryo. Normally, a single pair of breasts develops, but supernumerary breast tissue may be found anywhere along the mammary ridge. Accessory nipples are most common in the axillae, but can frequently be found beneath the breast and as low as the groin.

PHYSIOLOGIC DEVELOPMENT

At all periods of female life, the breast is under hormonal control. Estrogen generally leads to ductal elongation and branching and fat deposition; progesterone governs alveoli formation and prepares for lactation; prolactin, with estrogen and progesterone, develops the alveoli for secretion during pregnancy and, after parturition, along with cortisone, it triggers milk production (Fig. 25–1).

Fetus

Development of the breasts proceeds identically in both sexes during fetal life and is uninfluenced by sex-steroids until the seventh month. Epithelial and mesenchymal elements combine to form the duct system and supporting structures, respectively. Epithelially derived precursor tissue resembling sweat glands proceed through a branching stage to form 15 to 25 epithelial strips that later canalize to form ducts. The primitive duct system begins peripherally and proceeds toward the eventual nipple/areola complex.

After the seventh month, the developing duct systems become arranged into lobuli, with end-vesicle formation resembling secretory alveoli under the influence of maternal progesterone and, to a lesser extent, estrogen.

Neonate

The abrupt withdrawal of female sex-steroids allows prolactin to act directly on the alveolar epithelium. Consequently, colostrum ("witches' milk") can be expressed from the breast bud of newborns of both sexes in 80 to 90 per cent of cases. Lack of steroid production by the newborn results in regressional changes. End-vesicles disappear, and the breasts remain dormant until puberty.

Puberty

Mammary glands are once again exposed to increasing levels of sex-steroids at puberty. Because the initial menstrual cycles are generally anovulatory, estrogens, predominantly estradiol, are produced without progesterone. Breast development under the influence of estrogens includes branching and elongation of existing duct structures and the obvious increases in the supporting mesenchymal elements and fat deposition. The addition of progesterone, produced by the corpus luteum in ovulatory cycles, allows for the development of lobular-alveolar structure, and the breast gradually assumes the mature size and shape.

Menstruation

The period from menarche to menopause is marked by monthly cyclical changes in hormone production by the ovary in preparation for pregnancy. During the proliferative phase of the cycle, estrogens secreted by the maturing graafian follicle produce increased development of the breast by enhancing duct proliferation and budding. With the addition of progesterone secreted by the corpus luteum, the breast size increases by 15 to 30 cubic centimeters as the result of increased mammary blood flow, lobular edema, thickening of the base-

365

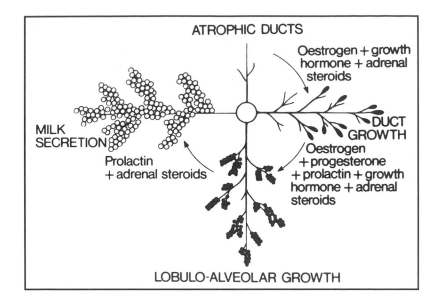

FIGURE 25–1. The multihormonal interaction in the growth of the mammary gland and the initiation of lactogenesis and lactation, delineated in the hypophysectomized-ovariectomized-adrenalectomized rat. (Reprinted from Yen, S.: Prolactin in human reproduction. *In* Yen, S., and Jaffe, R.B. (eds.): Reproductive Endocrinology, 2nd ed. Philadelphia, W.B. Saunders Co., 1986, p. 250.)

ment membrane, and especially enlargement of the alveolar diameter with the appearance of secretory material. Failure of implantation results in an unsuccessful cycle, marked by rapidly failing levels of sex-steroid production from the corpus luteum. This releases the hormonal inhibition of prolactin, allowing for mild milk secretion in the premenstrual period, but the production of milk in this situation is rarely recognized. At the end of menstruation, regressive changes that resemble those occurring shortly after birth again occur, with the lobular-alveolar units becoming smaller. Tissue edema decreases, and hyalinization of the basement membranes occurs. These regressive changes are quickly reversed by the appearance of sex-steroids during the next cycle. The overall result is a net increase in mammary size with each successive cycle.

Pregnancy

The capability of the breast to develop into an essential organ for milk production is realized during pregnancy. The intense stimulation of both development and differentiation occurs under the influence of sex-steroids (luteal and placental), prolactin, placental lactogen, and human chorionic gonadotropin.

First Trimester. During the first weeks of pregnancy, an intense ductular sprouting and elongation occur that far surpasses any changes seen during the menstrual cycle. Noticeable enlargement of the breasts is evident by 5 to 8 weeks of pregnancy, with superficial venous hypertension and the sensation of breast heaviness. The nipple and areola become more heavily pigmented, and the areola enlarges.

Second Trimester. A relatively greater inhibition by progesterone results in less activity of ductular sprouting and greater development of the lobular units. Secretory epithelium of the lobular-alveolar units becomes single layered in anticipation of increasing function, and colostrum, containing little fat, is secreted into the alveoli, resulting in dilation. Progressive enlargement of the breast also results from progesterone-induced changes in the mesenchymal elements of the breasts with dramatic increases in mammary blood flow. From midpregnancy on, the proliferative phase of mammary development decreases, with differentiation of existing structures in anticipation of function.

Third Trimester. The dramatic increase in breast size toward the conclusion of pregnancy is the result of dilation of existing alveoli with colostrum. The average increase in weight approximates 350 grams.

Lactation

The production of milk is a complex process under the hormonal control of the hypothalamus, anterior pituitary, gonad, placenta, and adrenals. Lactation refers not only to the production of milk but also to the periodic release of milk from the breast, which is controlled from the posterior pituitary.

Milk Production. Prolactin or lactogen is the most powerful hormone responsible for milk production, but the secondary action of adrenocorticoids, insulin, and growth hormone is also required. Prolactin is produced in the anterior pituitary and has a similar chemical composition to growth hormone. Serum levels of prolactin rise steadily during pregnancy and, together with placental sex-steroids, contribute to the development of the breast. Milk production before birth, however, is inconsequential in comparison with the amount produced postpartum. High estrogen levels in the blood exhibit inhibitory activity in preventing development

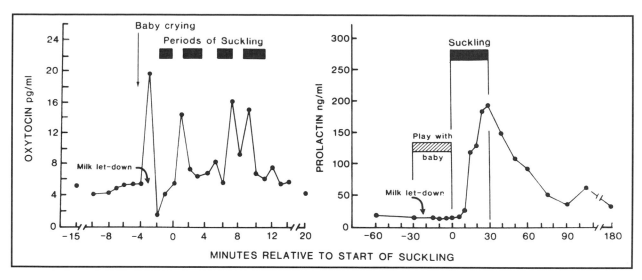

FIGURE 25–2. Plasma oxytocin (*left*) and prolactin (*right*) concentrations in response to the anticipation of nursing and suckling in lactating women. Milk "let down" occurred in association with acute release of oxytocin but not prolactin. (Reprinted from Yen, S.: Prolactin in human reproduction. *In* Yen, S., and Jaffe, R.B.: Reproductive Endocrinology, 2nd ed. Philadelphia, W.B. Saunders Co., 1986, p. 251.)

of prolactin receptors by mammary alveoli. After birth, the concentration of sex-steroids declines rapidly, allowing the full expression of prolactin activity.

Prolactin levels return to near-normal levels postpartum, but periodic surges of prolactin from the pituitary are stimulated by suckling (Fig. 25–2). The act of suckling presumably blocks the release of prolactin-inhibitory factor (PIF) from the hypothalamus. This periodic burst of prolactin activity can maintain lactogenesis indefinitely.

For the first few days postpartum, colostrum is secreted, later to be replaced by mature human milk. Colostrum is a thick, yellow substance that differs from mature milk in that it contains a high protein content in the form of lactoglobulin. IgG is secreted into the colostrum and is absorbed intact by the newborn gastrointestinal tract, although its role in conferring specific immunity is unclear. Within 1 to 2 weeks, colostrum is replaced by mature milk with its high content of lactose and fat.

Milk Letdown. No amount of negative pressure exerted upon the nipple will result in the movement of milk from its site of production in the alveoli to the ducts. A complex neurohumoral reflex exists whereby the act of suckling or tactile stimulation of the nipple is transmitted to the hypothalamus via spinal reflexes and results in the release of oxytocin from the posterior pituitary. Oxytocin produces the contraction of myoepithelial cells surrounding the alveoli. Positive pressure within the alveoli is generated and results in movement of milk from the lobuli into the major ducts—a process known as "milk letdown" (Fig. 25–3). Emotional factors, such as pain or anxiety, can interfere with this reflex and result in a failure to eject milk.

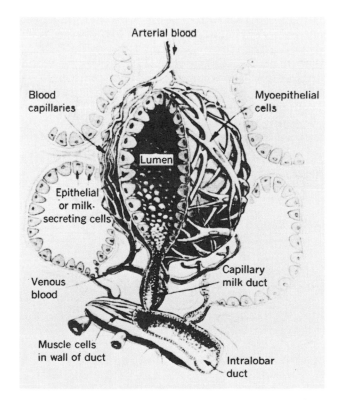

FIGURE 25–3. A mammary alveolus encased in myoepithelial cells. (Reprinted from Goodman, H.M.: The pituitary gland. *In* Mountcastle, V.B. (ed.): Medical Physiology, 14th ed. St. Louis, C.V. Mosby Co., 1980, p. 1489.)

Cessation of lactation occurs when the mother makes a conscious decision to allow it. When suckling stops, milk letdown does not occur. Local factors, such as the distension of alveoli with milk, result in involutional changes responsible for decreased secretory activity of the breast. Prolactin levels remain low, and the duct system returns to the prepartum state. The connective tissue and fat remain with the result that postpartum breasts are enlarged.

Menopause

At the time of menopause, ovarian regression results in dramatic decreases in the serum levels of sex-steroids. Involution of the mammary glandular tissue follows rapidly, with preservation of the connective tissue elements. The breasts decrease in size or remain fairly constant with replacement of ductal tissue by fat.

PATHOPHYSIOLOGY OF BREAST DISEASE

Fibrocystic Disease

Fibrocystic disease or mammary dysplasia actually represents a spectrum of benign breast disease ranging from replacement of breast by fibrous tissue through glandular hypertrophy up to the development of gross cystic disease. The etiology is uncertain, but the overwhelming evidence points to a disturbance in the response of the breast to existing hormonal conditions. Fibrocystic disease is unheard of in young women before menarche and only rarely observed in the years immediately after menarche.

Seven per cent of middle-aged women have symptoms or histologic evidence of fibrocystic disease. Symptoms are generally greatest in the premenstrual period when estrogen and progesterone levels are high. Relief of symptoms occurs after menopause, although the exogenous administration of estrogen-containing compounds to prevent "hot flashes" can result in continuing breast symptoms.

Breast Cancer

No single etiologic agent has to date been identified, but an association exists between the development of breast cancer and the length of time that the mammary epithelium is exposed to unopposed estrogens. Women who have undergone early menarche, remain nulliparous or have a late first pregnancy, or experience late menopause are all at higher risk of developing mammary cancer. The harmful effects of estrogen or the protective effects of progesterone have yet to be identified.

BIBLIOGRAPHY

1. Mountcastle, V.B. (ed.): Medical Physiology. St. Louis, C.V. Mosby Co., 1980.
2. Turner, C.W.: Harvesting Your Milk Crop. Oak Brook, IL, Babson Bros. Co., 1969.
3. Vorherr, H.: The Breast: Morphology, Physiology, and Lactation. New York, Academic Press, 1974.
4. Yen, S.S.C.: Neuroendocrine regulation of gonadotropin and prolactin secretion in women: Disorders in reproduction. *In* Vaitukaitus, J.L. (ed.): Current Endocrinology: Clinical Reproductive Neuroendocrinology Section. New York, Elsevier Biomedical, 1982, p. 137.
5. Yen, S., and Jaffe, R.B. (eds.): Reproductive Endocrinology: Physiology, Pathophysiology, and Clinical Management, 2nd ed. Philadelphia, W.B. Saunders Co., 1986.
6. West, G.B.: Best and Taylor's Physiological Basis of Medical Practice, 11th ed. Baltimore, Williams & Wilkins Co., 1985.

26

PHYSIOLOGY OF THE PEDIATRIC PATIENT

SAMUEL D. SMITH

Infants and children have unique physiologic characteristics created by differences in maturity and growth. These unique physiologic factors affect the surgical care of the pediatric patient.

WEIGHT AND GESTATIONAL AGE

The normal full-term infant has a gestational age of over 38 weeks with a body weight of over 2.5 kg. Infants weighing less than 2.5 kg are classified as low birthweight infants, and most are born prematurely. Infants weighing less than 2.5 kg who are born before 38 weeks gestation are classified as preterm infants, whereas those weighing less than 2.5 kg but born after 38 weeks gestation are classified as small for gestational age (SGA). SGA babies are thought to suffer from intrauterine growth retardation. Intrauterine growth retardation may result from placental and maternal abnormalities, as well as abnormalities in the fetus. Infants born 42 weeks or later are considered postterm.

Small for Gestational Age Infants (SGA)

SGA infants can usually be recognized by their physical characteristics of low body weight, normal body length, and normal head circumference. To classify an infant as SGA the gestational age must be estimated from physical examination. These physical findings are summarized in Table 26–1.

Although an SGA baby may weigh the same as a premature infant, they have different physiologic problems. Because of the longer gestational period and resultant well-developed organ systems, the metabolic rate in the SGA infant is much higher in proportion to body weight. Fluid and caloric needs of the SGA patient are increased. Thermal regulation is frequently difficult in SGA infants because of their larger body surface area, lack of body fat, and higher metabolic demands. Hypoglycemia, hypocalcemia, and marked polycythemia are also commonly noted in SGA infants.

The Preterm Infant

Infants born before 38 weeks gestation, regardless of birth weight, are considered premature. The differentiation of prematurity from SGA requires careful physical examination as outlined in Table 26–1. In general, on physical examination, premature infants have head circumferences below the 50th percentile. The skin is thin and transparent with an absence of plantar creases. The ears are soft and malleable with poorly developed cartilage. Breast tissue is not palpable, and the areolae are not visible. In males, the testicles are usually undescended with an undeveloped scrotum. In females the labia minora appear enlarged, but the labia majora are small.

Special problems of the preterm infant include

- nutritional deficiency due to a weak suck reflex
- inadequate gastrointestinal absorption
- high incidence of hyaline membrane disease (35 per cent in the moderately premature infant at 31 to 36 weeks gestational age)
- increased incidence of hypoglycemia, hypocalcemia, anemia, intraventricular hemorrhage, and hypothermia
- persistence or reopening of the ductus arteriosus with bidirectional shunting and subsequent congestive heart failure

THERMOREGULATION

A homeotherm is a mammal who can maintain a constant deep body temperature. The newborn human homeotherm has difficulty maintaining con-

369

TABLE 26–1.   CLINICAL CRITERIA FOR CLASSIFICATION OF LOW BIRTHWEIGHT INFANTS

CRITERIA	36 WEEKS (PREMATURE)	37–38 WEEKS (BORDERLINE PREMATURE])	39 WEEKS (FULL-TERM)
Plantar creases	Rare, shallow	Heel remains smooth	
Size of breast nodule	Not palpable to < 3 mm	Palpable—creases	Visible—7 mm
Head hair	Cotton wool quality		Silky; each strand can be distinguished
Earlobe	Shapeless, pliable with little cartilage		Rigid with cartilage
Testicular descent and scrotal changes	Small scrotum with rugal patch; testes not completely descended	Gradual descent	Enlarged scrotum creased with rugae; fully descended testes

Adapted from Avery, M.E., Villee, D., Baker, S., and Wharton, R.: Neonatology. *In* Avery, M.E., and First, R.L. (eds.): Pediatric Medicine. Baltimore, Williams & Wilkins Co., 1989, p. 148. Table 4.13.

stant deep body temperature due to its relatively large surface area, poor thermal insulation, and small amount of mass to act as a heat sink. Infants therefore produce heat by increasing metabolic activity either by shivering or by nonshivering thermogenesis. Catecholamine-mediated nonshivering thermogenesis in brown fat is important in maintaining temperature in the human newborn, as well as in cold-adapted animals and hibernating animals. This dependency has practical consequences since brown fat may be rendered inactive by blockage induced by certain drugs, such as anesthetic agents, or by nutritional depletion. The optimal thermal environment for the newborn—*thermoneutrality*—is defined as the range of ambient temperatures in which a baby with normal body temperature has a minimal metabolic rate and can maintain a constant body temperature by vasomotor control. *Critical temperature* is defined as the temperature below which a metabolic response to cold is necessary to replace lost heat.

No single temperature range is appropriate for all sizes and conditions of babies. The appropriate neutral thermal temperature is determined by the patient's weight and postnatal age as seen in Figures 26–1 and 26–2. Thermoneutrality is approximately 34° to 35°C for low birthweight infants up to 6 weeks in age and 31° to 32°C at 12 weeks of age. Larger or term infants weighing 2 to 3 kg have a thermoneutrality zone of 31° to 34°C on the first day of life and 29° to 31°C at 12 days.

Heat loss can occur from radiation, convection, evaporation, and conduction. Evaporation heat loss is increased with increasing prematurity. The ambient humidity is also important in regulating this source of heat loss. Placing a clear plastic drape or a radiant heat shield over a baby facilitates thermoregulation by decreasing air movement and increasing the humidity of the microenvironment around the baby. Measuring the temperature gradient between skin and rectal temperatures is an effective method of determining whether an infant has increased its metabolic output in order to maintain a normal core temperature. A decreasing skin temperature in the face of a constant rectal temperature suggests that there is increased metabolic activity. The optimal gradient between the rectal and skin temperature should be approximately 1.5°C.

GLUCOSE AND CALCIUM METABOLISM IN THE NEWBORN INFANT

The abrupt termination of the placental supply of glucose, calcium, and magnesium results in profound changes in energy and mineral metabolism. Rapid changes in plasma, glucose, and calcium occur

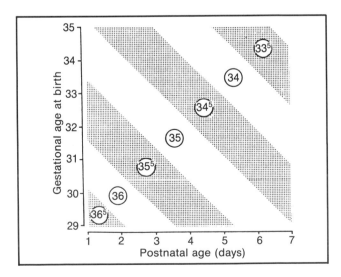

FIGURE 26–1. Neutral thermal environment during the first week of life, calculated from the measurements. Dewpoint of the air 18°C, flow 10 L/min. (Reprinted from Sauer, P.J.J., Dane, H.J., and Visser, H.K.A.: New standards for neutral thermal environment of healthy very low birthweight infants in week one of life. Arch. Dis. Child. *59:* 18–22, 1984. Figure 1, p. 19.)

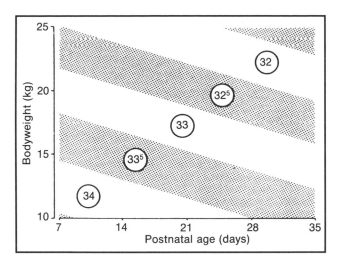

FIGURE 26–2. Neutral thermal environment (°C) from days 7 to 35. Dewpoint of the air 18°C, flow 10 L/min. Body weight is current weight. Values for body weight over 2.0 kg are calculated by extrapolation. (Reprinted from Sauer, P.J.J., Dane, H.J., and Visser, H.K.A.: New standards for neutral thermal environment of healthy very low birthweight infants in week one of life. Arch. Dis. Child., 59:18–22, 1984. Figure 2, p. 19.)

during the first days of life. The fetus receives glucose by facilitated diffusion across the placenta, maintaining fetal blood glucose at approximately 70 to 80 per cent of maternal levels. During the later stages of fetal development, there is a build-up of glycogen stores in liver, skeletal, and cardiac muscle, but very little gluconeogenesis. After delivery, the infant depletes its hepatic glycogen stores within 2 to 3 hours and becomes dependent on gluconeogenesis to maintain its blood glucose levels. Fat metabolism does occur, but the availability of fat substrate in SGA infants for synthesizing glucose is severely limited and serum glucose can fall progressively. The rate of fall of the serum glucose level depends upon the adequacy of the substrate stores, which are related to the gestational age and the energy demands placed on the infant. The infants at greatest risk for development of hypoglycemia are SGA infants. The symptoms of hypoglycemia are nonspecific and include a weak or high-pitched cry, cyanosis, apnea, apathy, or seizures. Once symptoms have developed, permanent brain damage is common; thus, symptomatic hypoglycemia should be avoided by careful monitoring of blood sugars. Neonatal hypoglycemia is defined as a serum glucose level less than 35 mg/dL in a full-term infant and less than 25 mg/dL in the low birthweight infant. After 72 hours, plasma glucose should be 45 mg/dL or higher. Although the newborn infant is at the highest risk for developing hypoglycemia, it must be of concern in older infants and children as well.

In contrast, hyperglycemia is a common problem of the very immature infant on intravenous support.

The cause appears to be a lesser insulin response to glucose. Hyperglycemia can be anticipated in infants below 30 weeks gestation and 1.1 kg birthweight who are usually less than 3 days of age and are receiving 10 per cent glucose at 100 mL/kg/24 h. Problems related to hyperglycemia include osmotic changes that can cause intraventricular hemorrhage, as well as renal water and electrolyte losses from glucosuria. The treatment is to adjust the glucose infusion rate by giving more fluids with lower glucose concentration.

The placenta actively transports calcium to the fetus and maintains fetal total and ionized calcium levels about 1 mg above respective maternal levels. Seventy-five per cent of the total amount of calcium is transferred after the 28th week of gestation. At birth, the neonate has a natural tendency toward hypocalcemia due to decreased calcium stores, renal immaturity, and relative hypoparathyroidism secondary to suppression by high fetal calcium.

Calcium levels usually reach their nadir between 24 to 48 hours after delivery. Hypocalcemia is defined as an ionized calcium level less than 1 mg%. The majority of babies who experience hypocalcemia are either preterm low birthweight infants, the products of complicated pregnancies, or those receiving bicarbonate infusions.

BLOOD VOLUME

Total red blood cell volume is at its highest point at delivery. Six hours after delivery, plasma shifts out of the circulation, but total blood volume continues to remain high, primarily because of a relatively elevated red cell volume. Estimation of blood volume for prematures, term newborns, and infants over 1 month of age is summarized in Table 26–2. At about 3 months of age, total blood volume per kilogram is nearly equal to adult levels of 70 mL/kg.

During the newborn period, total blood volume varies according to the maturation of the infant, the infant's size in relation to maturation, and the presence or absence of a placental transfusion. At birth, blood is normally transferred from the placenta to the infant, with one fourth of the placenta

TABLE 26–2. BLOOD COMPONENT REPLACEMENT GUIDELINES

Estimation of Blood Volume	
Premature infants	85–100 mL/kg
Term newborns	85 mL/kg
> 1 month	75 mL/kg
3 months—adult	70 mL/kg

Adapted from Rowe, P.C. (ed.): The Harriet Lane Handbook, 11th ed. Chicago, Year Book Medical Publishers, Inc., 1987, p. 25.

transfusion occurring within 15 seconds of birth and one half by the end of the first minute. Because the placenta contains 75 to 125 cc of blood at birth, infants delivered after delayed cord clamping have higher hemoglobin values. Placental transfusion may be prevented or anemia created by holding the newborn above the level of the placenta before cord clamping. The neonate's hematocrit can be used as a rough guide to the presence or absence as well as the volume of placental transfusion. Hematocrits over 50 per cent suggest that placental transfusion has occurred. Cord hemoglobin values of less than 13 gm/dL are abnormally low.

Anemia present at birth or appearing in the first weeks of life can be broadly characterized into three groups based on its etiology: blood loss, underproduction of erythrocytes, or hemolysis. Erythroblastosis fetalis (hemolytic disease of the newborn) can result in severe chronic anemia and occasionally death. It is caused by the passage of maternal antibodies to the Rh+ cells of the fetus from the sensitized Rh-negative mother. The common signs of hemolytic disease in the newborn are jaundice, pallor, and enlargement of the spleen and liver. The most severely affected infants manifest hydrops fetalis, with massive edema, pleural effusions, and ascites. Erythroblastosis is best prevented by the administration of anti-Rh immunoglobulin to an Rh-negative mother after either delivery or abortion of an Rh-positive infant. In affected infants with a positive-reacting Coombs' test—a cord hemoglobin less than 10.5 g/dl or a cord bilirubin of over 4.5 mg/dL—immediate exchange transfusion is indicated. For less severely affected infants, exchange transfusion is indicated when the total indirect bilirubin is over 20 mg/dL.

Neonatal polycythemia occurs in infants of diabetic mothers or of mothers with toxemia of pregnancy and infants who are SGA. A hemoglobin over 22 g/dL or a hematocrit over 65 during the first week of life is defined as polycythemia. The manifestations of polycythemia appear to be a primary consequence of the associated increase in blood viscosity. After the central venous hematocrit reaches 60 to 65, any further increase in hematocrit results in an exponential increase in blood viscosity. The treatment of polycythemia is a partial exchange of the infant's blood with fresh whole blood.

In the normal adult, when oxygen tension has fallen to 27 mm Hg at a pH of 7.4 and temperature of 37°C, 50 per cent of the oxygen bound to hemoglobin has been released. The P_{50} is thus stated to be 27 torr. When the affinity of hemoglobin for oxygen is reduced, more oxygen is released in the tissues at a given oxygen tension. The hemoglobin equilibrium curve is shifted to the right of normal.

Fetal hemoglobin has a p_{50} value of some 6–8 mm Hg lower than that of a normal adult. The lower P_{50} of fetal hemoglobin allows more efficient O_2 delivery from the placenta in utero. The low P_{50} is due to the failure of fetal hemoglobin to bind 2,3 diphosphoglycerate to the same degree as adult hemoglobin. In the term infant, the hemoglobin equilibrium curve gradually shifts to the right, and the P_{50} value is approximately that of a normal adult by 4 to 6 months of age.

NEONATAL JAUNDICE

The liver and spleen can convert the tetrapyrrol of hemoglobin to bilirubin. Bilirubin is a lipid-soluble substance that is transported into the hepatocytes for clearance. After birth, lipid-soluble bilirubin or indirect bilirubin is transported into the hepatocytes where it is conjugated with glucuronic acid and rendered water soluble (conjugated or direct bilirubin) for elimination in bile. Without this mechanism, the unconjugated bilirubin accumulates and acts as a neural cell poison interfering with cellular respiration (Levine), especially in the face of anoxia. This clinical condition of bilirubin neural damage is known as kernicterus or chronic bilirubin encephalopathy. In its severest form, infants develop athetoid cerebral palsy and sensorineural hearing loss.

After birth, the infant's liver has a metabolic excretory capacity for bilirubin that is not equal to its load. Thus, even healthy full-term babies can experience a rise of unconjugated bilirubin (physiologic jaundice), which peaks around the fourth day of life at about 10 mg/100 mL and returns to normal near the sixth day of life. A total bilirubin level over 12 mg/100 mL in a full-term newborn warrants investigation. The causes of prolonged indirect hyperbilirubinemia are noted in Table 26–3.

BODY COMPOSITION IN THE NEONATE

At 12 weeks gestation, the fetus has a total body water content of 94 per cent of body weight. This figure decreases to 80 per cent by 32 weeks gestation and 78 per cent by term (Fig. 26–3). A reduction of 3 to 5 per cent occurs in the first 3 to 5 days of postnatal

---

TABLE 26–3.   CAUSES OF PROLONGED INDIRECT HYPERBILIRUBINEMIA

Breast milk jaundice
Hemolytic disease
Hypothyroidism
Pyloric stenosis
Crigler-Najjar syndrome
Extravascular blood

Adapted from Maisels, M.J.: Neonatal jaundice. *In* Avery, G.B. (ed.): neonatology: Pathophysiology and Management of the Newborn. Philadelphia, J.B. Lippincott Co., 1987, p. 566.

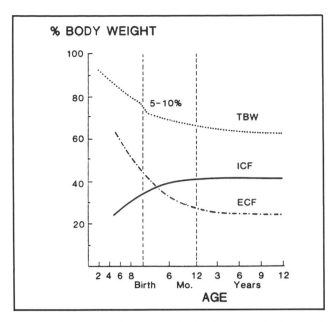

FIGURE 26–3. Friss-Hansen's classic chart relating total body, extracellular, and intracellular water to percentage of body weight, from early gestation to adolescence. (Adapted from Rowe, M.I.: Fluid and electrolyte management. *In* Welch, K.J., Randolph, J.G., Ravitch, M.M., O'Neill, J.A., and Rowe, M.I. (eds.): Pediatric Surgery, 4th ed. Chicago, Year Book Medical Publishers, Inc., 1986. Figure 4–2, p. 24.)

life. Body water continues to decrease and reaches near adult levels by 1 ½ years of age. Extracellular water falls in parallel with total body water content and reaches adult levels by 1 to 3 years of age (Fig. 26–3). In contrast, intracellular water increases with fetal maturation from 25 per cent of body weight to 44 per cent or adult levels by 3 months of age.

These compartment changes progress in an orderly fashion in utero, but premature delivery requires the neonate to complete both fetal and term water-unloading tasks. Amazingly, the premature infant can complete fetal water unloading by 1 week after birth. This postnatal reduction in extracellular fluid volume has such a high physiologic priority that it is achieved even in the face of relatively large variations in fluid intake. Immature infants occasionally receive such large volumes of parenteral fluid to "replace urine volume" that it counteracts their water unloading. Thus, excess parenteral fluid therapy may unfavorably alter clinical outcome by increasing the incidence of patent ductus arteriosus, left ventricular failure, respiratory distress syndrome, or bronchopulmonary dysplasia.

RENAL FUNCTION

The glomerular filtration rate (GFR) of all newborn infants is less than that of adults. From 21 mL/min/1.73 square meters at birth in a term infant, GFR quickly rises to 60 mL/min/1.73 square meters by 2 weeks of age. GFR reaches adult levels by 1 ½ to 2 years of age. In premature infants less than 30 weeks gestation, GFR is only slightly lower (16 mL/min/1.73 square meters) than that of the full-term infant. The discrepancy in GFR between the term and preterm baby persists for approximately 1 month. In addition to differences in GFR, the concentrating capacity of the preterm and full-term infant's kidney is well below adult levels. A term infant responding to water deprivation can increase urine osmolality to a maximum of only 500 to 600 mosm/kg. The adult, in contrast, can concentrate to 1200 mosm/kg. the regulation of extracellular osmolality is principally achieved by variations in antidiuretic hormone (ADH) levels. The capacity to produce antidiuretic hormone is fully developed in both the term and preterm infant. It appears that the difference in concentrating capacity is due to insensitivity of the collecting tubules to ADH in the newborn. Although the newborn cannot concentrate urine as efficiently after a water load, the infant can excrete a very dilute urine of 30 to 50 mosm/kg, in contrast to adult levels of 70 to 100 mosm/kg.

Compared with the adult, the full-term newborn infant has a diminished capacity to excrete excess sodium when in positive balance. The principal defect again is thought to be tubular. The preterm infant has a similar difficulty in handling excess sodium, yet is considered a "salt waster" unless excess sodium is administered.

INSENSIBLE WATER LOSS

Insensible water loss is the invisible loss of water from the lungs and skin. In the adult, insensible loss is between 9 to 14 mL/kg/day. Insensible water loss can reach enormous levels in the premature infant.

Transepithelial water loss (TEWL) is the major component of insensible water loss in newborns of all ages. The greatest losses occur in the first postnatal day in infants 25 to 27 weeks gestation (129 gm/kg/24 h; (Table 26–4). TEWL then decreases steadily as postnatal age increases. A major environmental condition that produces profound changes in TEWL is exposure to radiation by infant warmers and phototherapy. The associated increase in TEWL varies from 38 to 80 per cent depending on the infant's size.

NEONATAL AND FLUID REQUIREMENTS

Classic systems for estimating fluid requirements in the newborn are based on body weight, surface area, or caloric requirements. They are founded on unproven assumptions and do not account for multi-

TABLE 26–4. TRANSEPITHELIAL WATER LOSS IN NEWBORNS*

	GESTATIONAL AGE (MEAN BIRTHWEIGHT)			
POSTNATAL AGE (DAYS)	*25–27 Weeks* *(0.869 ± 0.100 kg)*	*28–30 Weeks* *(1.340 ± 0.240 kg)*	*31–36 Weeks* *(2.110 ± 0.300 kg)*	*37–41 Weeks* *(3.600 ± 0.390 kg)*
1	110 ± 27	39 ± 11	11 ± 5	6 ± 1
3	71 ± 9	32 ± 9	12 ± 4	6 ± 1
7	43 ± 9	24 ± 7	12 ± 4	6 ± 1
14	32 ± 10	18 ± 6	9 ± 3	6 ± 1
28	24 ± 11	15 ± 6	7 ± 1	7 ± 1

* Expressed in gm/kg/24 h.

Adapted from Rowe, M.I.: Fluid and electrolyte management. *In* Welch, K.J., Randolph, J.G., Ravitch, M.M., O'Neill, J.A., and Rowe, M.I. (eds.): Pediatric Surgery, 1986. Chicago, Year Book Medical Publishers, Inc., 1986, p. 27. Table 4–1.

ple variables that affect fluid balance. Newer systems utilize multiple physiologic factors that include (1) renal water needs, (2) evaporative water losses, (3) metabolic demands, (4) third-space losses, (5) external losses, and (6) pre-existing deficits.

Renal water can only be calculated in retrospect. Metabolic needs and evaporative water losses can only be measured as a research tool. Currently, third-space losses and deficits cannot be determined accurately, and external losses can only be measured in ideal circumstances. Therefore, the most effective approach to fluid management of the critically ill infant is to approach the fluid needs dynamically. The dynamic approach has two components: (1) choosing and giving a starting volume that is safe for the patient's status, termed a *bogey volume,* and (2) utilizing a monitoring system so that the effects of the bogey volume are assessed constantly and appropriate adjustments are made depending on the infant's response.

A table of bogey volumes expressed in rates of mL/kg/24 h for various surgical conditions has been developed (Table 26–5). These patients were divided into three groups:

1. Moderate conditions—colostomies, laparotomies for repair of intestinal atresias
2. Severe conditions—midgut volvulus, operations for meconium peritonitis, gastroschisis
3. Necrotizing colitis with perforation or bowel necrosis

After administering the bogey volume for a period of 4 to 8 hours, the patient is reassessed by monitoring urine output and urine concentration. Using these two measures it is possible to determine the state of hydration of most neonates and their responses to the bogey volume.

Urine output and concentration are determined by multiple factors: osmolar load, available renal water, excess body water, and renal concentrating and diluting capacities. Osmolar load is the material that the kidney must excrete to maintain homeostasis. The osmolar load is made up of intrinsic components, which are waste products and electrolytes, and extrinsic components, which are measured from the osmolar intake. Renal water is the amount of water that is available to allow the kidneys to clear the osmolar load presented to them within their concentration capacity. Excess water is the volume of water above the amount needed for metabolic functions and osmolar excretion.

Renal capacity is the range of renal tubule function resulting in excretion or reabsorption of water to produce an isotonic urine. There is no normal urine output. Ideal urine volume per unit of time can be estimated by measuring the osmolar load presented to the kidneys for excretion and then calculating the amount of urine necessary to clear this load at an isotonic urine level of 280. In three surgical groups studied, the mean ideal urine output varied between 2 mL/kg/h to 3.5 mL/kg/h (Table 26–6). This large variation was due to the variability of

TABLE 26–5. NEWBORN "BOGEY" VOLUME REQUIREMENTS FOR VARIOUS SURGICAL CONDITIONS*

GROUP	DAY 1	DAY 2	DAY 3
Moderate surgical conditions—colostomies, laparotomies for intestinal atresia, Hirschsprung's, disease, etc.	80 ± 25	80 ± 30	80 ± 30
Severe surgical conditions—gastroschisis, midgut volvulus, meconium peritonitis, etc.	140 ± 45	90 ± 20	80 ± 15
Necrotizing enterocolitis with perforation	145 ± 70	135 ± 50	130 ± 40

* Expressed in mL/kg/24 h.

TABLE 26–6. NEWBORN IDEAL URINE OUTPUT FOR VARIOUS SURGICAL CONDITIONS*

GROUP	DAY 1	DAY 2	DAY 3
Moderate surgical conditions—colostomies, laparotomies for intestinal atresia, Hirschsprung's, disease, etc.	2 ± 0.96	2.63 ± 1.71	2.38 ± 0.92
Severe surgical conditions—gastroschisis, midgut volvulus, meconium peritonitis, etc.	2.67 ± 0.92	2.96 ± 0.54	2.96 ± 1.0
Necrotizing enterocolitis with perforation	2.58 ± 1.04	3.17 ± 1.67	3.46 ± 1.46

* Expressed in mL/kg/24 h.

the excreted osmolar load (13 mosm/kg/day to 21 mosm/kg/day). The maximum measured urine output for a newborn surgical patient was 8.3 mL/kg/h or 197 mL/kg/day. The infant has a striking ability to clear water, and most urine output values should be at least 2 mL/kg/h. A level below 1 mL/kg/h should be considered abnormal.

GASTROINTESTINAL PHYSIOLOGY

The intestinal tract of a full-term newborn is approximately 240 to 300 cm in length, which is only one third the length of the adult tract. The musculature and elastic fibers of the bowel are not well developed at birth, in contrast to the digestive and absorptive surfaces. At term, the human infant's stomach holds 10 to 20 mL and empties more slowly than at any other age. Gastric emptying in the neonate is dependent on the osmolarity and caloric density. Air swallowing begins almost immediately after birth so that air should reach the jejunum in 15 minutes and be in the cecum by 2 hours. The rate of intestinal air transport is an important aid in diagnosing congenital GI malformations. Initially sterile, the gut acquires a characteristic polymicrobial flora in the first few days after birth. With the exception of pancreatic amylase, the characteristic digestive enzymes are present even in small premature infants.

Carbohydrate digestion in infants begins with salivary amylase. Breakdown is continued by the brush border mucosal cells of the small intestine, which contain the four disaccharidases: lactase, sucrase, maltase, and isomaltase. These disaccharides liberate the monosaccharides: glucose, galactose, and fructose. Glucose and galactose are actively transported into the mucosal cell. Fructose, however, is absorbed by facilitated diffusion. The gradient for fructose is generated by the rapid conversion of fructose to galactose. In normal circumstances, most carbohydrate absorption is completed in the midjejunum.

The newborn is deficient in pancreatic amylase. This enzyme remains low during the first few months of life. However, amylase activity is present in fresh or nonpasteurized human milk. There is also a glycoamylase present among the small bowel brush border enzymes. Lactose is the principal dietary carbohydrate present in the milk-fed infant. Lactose is normally well absorbed, although the enzyme lactase is particularly sensitive to any disease damaging the small bowel mucosa, so that lactose intolerance is the first disaccharidase deficiency that is usually noted after any inflammatory disease of the bowel, such as infectious diarrhea.

Carbohydrate malabsorption can be detected by one of three techniques: (1) fecal pH, (pH less than 6 is abnormal and strongly suggests carbohydrate intolerance), (2) fecal-reducing substances or fecal glucose (Clinitest Tablets; reduction greater than 1.4% or glucose greater than 1+ is considered abnormal), (3) disaccharide tolerance test, in which lactose is given orally in a dose of 2 gm/kg, serum glucose levels are measured, and failure to note a rise of serum glucose over 20 mg/100 mL within 2 hours is considered abnormal.

Protein digestive mechanisms are well developed even in the low birthweight infant. Protein malabsorption, even in pathologic states, is virtually unknown. The most active site of amino acid absorption is in the jejunum.

Fat digestion normally begins in the stomach under the influence of lingual lipase, an enzyme secreted by salivary glands. This enzyme may be particularly important in the newborn because it does not depend on bile salts. Absorption of lipids in low birthweight infants is poor partly because the bile salt pool is only 50 per cent that of the adult patient and partly because pancreatic lipase is quantitatively less in premature compared with term infants. Human milk fat is better absorbed than butter fat (cow milk fat). Other vegetable fats, notably corn, coconut, or soy oil, are better absorbed than butter fat. As a consequence, most commercial formulas are now made with vegetable fats. Medium chain triglycerides (MCT) composed of fatty acids of 8 to 10 carbon atoms are absorbed directly into the circulation and require neither lipase nor bile salts for digestion. For this reason, MCT are useful as a dietary supplement for pediatric patients with fat absorption problems.

It is difficult to settle on an ideal caloric balance for newborns because of the many variables involved. Term infants appear to require about 110 to 120 kcal/kg/day. The full-term infant has a basal metabolic rate of 32 cal/kg/day, which rises to a peak of 48 cal/kg/day by 2 weeks of age. The greatest caloric expenditures for growth and development approximate 33 cal/kg/day in infancy, which falls to 18 cal/kg/day by 3 months of age. Surgical operations increase caloric demands in all patients by approximately 10 to 25 per cent. Basal calories must be exceeded by 60 to 85 cal/day to achieve catch-up growth in the cachexic infant, and caloric requirement may range as high as 160 to 185 cal/day.

Kwashiorkor is the state of malnutrition with predominantly protein deficiency. It is characterized by edema, growth failure, listlessness, abdominal distension, hypoproteinemia, and diarrhea. Marasmus is the state in which both proteins and calories are proportionally reduced. It is characterized by generalized wasting and growth failure.

The body has considerable ability to interconvert amino acids, but nine are considered essential: arginine, lysine, leucine, isoleucine, valine, methionine, phenylalanine, threonine, and tryptophan. In addition, the newborn has a temporary specific requirement for histidine and cystine and may also, for a time, be unable to convert phenylalanine to tyrosine or methionine to cystine. Currently, 3 gm/kg/day of protein are recommended at birth. This requirement decreases to 2.2 gm/kg/day by 6 months and to 1.6 gm/kg/day at 1 year. Protein should equal approximately 9 per cent of the total caloric intake.

Unique biologic and anti-infective properties make human milk more than just a food. Its high fat, high lactose, and low casein composition makes it easily digestible by most infants and provides an environment for the development of nonpathogenic flora in the intestine. A comparison of breast milk to other formulas is provided in Table 26–7. The chemical composition of human milk varies with individual mothers, as well as during different stages of lactation. Colostrum contains a higher concentration of protein but less fat and carbohydrates than mature human milk. It is higher in sodium, potassium, and chloride and is a rich source of vitamin A, vitamin E, and immunoglobulins, especially secretory IgA. It has been estimated that a breast-fed infant receives on an average about 1 gram of IgA each day and approximately 10 mg of IgM and IgG. These immunoglobulins help provide protection against gastrointestinal infections. The same immunoglobulins in colostrum are found in mature human milk, but in lower concentrations. Mature human milk provides 65 to 75 calories/mL and is composed of 85 to 95 per cent water, 0.9 per cent protein, 2.7 to 4.5 per cent fat, and 6.0 to 7.6 per cent carbohydrate. The major portion of protein in human milk is alpha-lactalbumin (whey), whereas in cow's milk it is beta-lactoglobulin (casein). Casein is more likely to coagulate in the acidic environment of the stomach and form curds.

Commercial infant formulas approximate the composition of human milk as closely as possible. However, they do not provide the immunoglobulins of human milk. Most formulas consist of nonfat cow's milk with the following modifications:

• Protein is heat modified to produce a more digestible curd and may contain added whey to resemble more closely the protein composition of human milk.

TABLE 26–7. COMPARISON OF COMPOSITION OF HUMAN MILK AND SELECTED FORMULAS*

	MATURE† HUMAN MILK	ENFAMIL® AND ENFAMIL® WITH IRON 20 (STD MILK-TYPE FORMULA)	ENFAMIL® PREMATURE FORMULA®20	ISOMIL® 20	PREGESTIMIL® 20	NUTRAMIGEN® 20
Energy, Cal	730	670	670	676	670	670
Protein, gm	11	15	20	18.0	19	22
Percentage of total calories	6	9	12	11	11	13
Source	Mature human milk	Reduced minerals, whey, and nonfat milk	Demineralized whey and nonfat milk solids	Soy protein isolate	Casein hydrolysate, cystine, tyrosine, and tryptophan	Casein hydrolysate
Fat, gm	45	38	34	36.9	27	22
Percentage of total calories	55	50	44	49	35	35
Source	Mature human milk	Coconut and soy Oils	Medium chain triglycerides, soy and coconut oils	Soy and coconut oils	Corn oil and medium chain triglycerides	Corn oil
Carbohydrate, gm	71	69	74	68.3	91	88
Percentage of total calories	39	41	44	40	54	35
Source	Lactose	Lactose	Corn syrup solids, lactose	Corn syrup and sucrose	Corn syrup solids and modified tapioca starch	Sucrose and modified tapioca starch

* Approximate analyses per liter: Values calculated from nutrient values per 100 cal.

† Composition of human milk varies with the stage of lactation and from mother to mother.

Adapted from Avery, M.E., Masland, R., Ferber, R., Ware, J., and First, L.R.: Section 1, Chapter 2, Well Child Care. *In* Avery, M.E., and First, L.R. (eds.): Pediatric Medicine. Baltimore, Williams & Wilkins Co., 1989, pp. 30–31. Table 1.4.

- Polyunsaturated vegetable fats are added to provide essential fatty acids.
- The calcium content is decreased by dilution.
- Vitamins and minerals are added to approach the concentration of human milk.
- In some formulas the sodium content is reduced by dialysis.

The standard caloric density is .67 kcal/oz. There are three categories of commercial formulas. Breast milk substitutes are used for the normal term infant. Soy protein-based lactose-free formula are used for infants who are sensitive to lactose. Protein-modified formulas are used for infants with allergies to milk protein, such as cow's milk or soy protein or those who have severe chronic malabsorption, such as short gut syndrome. Fat-modified formulas facilitate the absorption of fat when intestinal malabsorption is present. Portogen contains medium chain triglycerides as its major fat component. It is useful in children with liver disease, such as biliary atresia.

Total parenteral nutrition (TPN) has reversed the previous high mortality associated with congenital surgical anomalies such as gastroschisis, necrotizing enterocolitis, and the like. Table 26–8 summarizes the indications for parenteral nutrition, whereas the daily requirements for total parenteral nutrition are presented in Table 26–9.

PULMONARY AND CARDIOVASCULAR SYSTEM OF THE NEWBORN

At around 18 to 20 weeks gestation the lungs have a solid glandular appearance. At around 24 to 26 weeks gestation, most of the epithelial lung tissue is made up of glycogen-rich cuboidal cells with only a few type 1 epithelial cells present. The air-blood sur-

TABLE 26–8.   INDICATIONS FOR PARENTERAL NUTRITION IN NEWBORNS

Surgical lesions
  Omphalocele
  Gastroschisis
  Complicated anastomoses
  Short gut $\geq$ 18 cm with ileocecal value
           $\geq$ cm without ileocecal value
Necrotizing enterocolitis
Intractable nonspecific diarrhea
Premature infants—feedings not tolerated or in conjunction with increasing oral calories
Chronically ill infants of any size—feedings not tolerated.

Adapted from Avery, G.B., and Fletcher, A.B.: Nutrition. *In* Avery, G.B. (ed.): Neonatology: Pathophysiology and Management of the Newborn. Philadelphia, J.B. Lippincott Co., 1987, p. 1206.

TABLE 26–9.   DAILY REQUIREMENTS OF TOTAL PARENTERAL NUTRITION FOR NEWBORNS

Protein	2.5–3.5 gm/kg
Fat emulsion	2–4 gm/kg
Calories	90–110 mL/kg or
H_2O	125–150 mL/kg
Na	3–4 mEq/kg
K	2–3 mEq/kg
Ca	50–100 mg/kg, depending on size of infant
P	1–1.5 mM/kg
Mg	0.5–1 mEq/kg
Multivitamins*	10 mL (65% of dosage to infants less than 3 kg; 33% to infants less than 1 kg)

* Multivitamin preparations are undergoing scrutiny because of the preservatives in them. Practitioners must keep abreast of current recommentations.

Adapted from Avery, G.B., and Fletcher, A.B. Nutrition. *In* Avery, G.B. (ed.): Neonatology: Pathophysiology and Management of the Newborn. Philadelphia, J.B. Lippincott Co., 1987, p. 1206. Table 47–16.

face area for gas effusion is therefore very limited, and should the fetus be delivered at this gestational age, survival would be difficult. Between 26 and 32 weeks gestation, small terminal air sacs give way to air spaces. From 32 to 36 weeks further budding occurs from these alveolar ducts, and alveoli become more numerous.

At the time that these anatomic events are occurring, biochemical changes are also necessary for fetal lung development. A combination of surface active phospholipids or pulmonary surfactant lines the mature lung terminal air spaces and is extremely important in maintaining alveolar stability, especially at low transmural pressures. The two principal components of sufactant are phosphatidylcholine (PC) and phosphatidylglycerol (PG). The acyl component of both is an esterified palmitic acid. These components are produced by type 2 alveolar cells.

Material discharged from cells lining potential air sacs finds its way into the amniotic contents. Therefore, the changing pattern in amniotic fluid phospholipids can be used to assess the maturation of surfactant production. Thus, phosphatidylcholine (lecithin) concentration increases as gestation progresses, whereas sphingomyelin is fairly stable in concentration with a small peak at 28 to 30 weeks. The ratio of lecithin to sphingomyelin (L/S ratio) in amniotic fluid has been widely used as index of fetal lung maturity. A ratio over 2 is considered compatible with relatively mature lung function. In order to prevent the problems related to the immaturity of the newborn lung, glucocorticoids have been used to induce lung maturation. However, glucocorticoids are only effective in (1) fetuses treated between 27 to 34 weeks, (2) when the infant is delivered no more than 7 days after treatment, and (3) when treatment is begun at least 48 hours before delivery.

The presence of adequate amounts of surfactant to line the air spaces is critical for postnatal pulmonary adaptation. In normally growing infants, abundant numbers of type 2 cells are well differentiated and capable of supplying sufficient surfactant at 35 weeks. The absence of adequate surfactant results in hyaline membrane disease (HMD), which is responsible for 30 per cent of all neonatal deaths in the United States. Clinical trials are currently underway to evaluate the use of exogenous surfactant to treat HMD. Other conditions associated with pulmonary distress in the newborn include delayed fetal lung absorption or wet lung syndrome, intrauterine aspiration pneumonia (meconium aspiration), and intrapartum pneumonia. In all these conditions, mechanical assistance to ventilation may be required for hypoxia, CO_2 retention, or apnea. The premature newborn infant frequently requires an artificial airway or intratracheal intubation.

The length of the trachea from the vocal cords to the carina varies from 2.6 cm in the smaller premature infants to 6 cm in term infants. A formula of "7-8-9" for oral tracheal and "8-10-12" ("7-8-9 + weight") for nasotracheal tube depth corresponding to body weights of 1, 2, and 3 kg is simple to remember.

The use of mechanical ventilation has been one of the most striking advances in the treatment of neonatal respiratory disorders. Most commercially available neonatal ventilators are pressure-cycled respirators, which regulate the volume of gas delivered by setting a limit on the peak inspiratory pressure (PIP). Most of these ventilators operate by timed cycling, with constant flow as the generating force. These types of respirators prevent excess peak pressure by a pop-off valve while delivering a constant flow. The flow rate, inspiratory time, and inspiratory : expiratory (I : E) ratio may all be adjusted. This type of respirator permits several types of respiratory patterns and will display positive inspiratory pressure (PIP), mean airway pressure, positive end-expiratory pressure (PEEP), I : E ratio, frequency, and inspiratory time (T_I).

To understand the effects of mechanical ventilation on the neonatal lung, some knowledge of respiratory mechanics are necessary. Lung compliance is defined as a change in lung volume per unit pressure change (mL/cm H_2O). Compliance depends on the elastic properties of the lung, which are influenced by lung volume, as well as tissue inflammation or pulmonary edema. Compliance is low if there has been alveolar collapse or if the alveoli are overdistended. The lungs of infants with hyaline membrane disease have areas of collapse and overexpansion, resulting in nonuniform compliance. Other conditions, such as pulmonary consolidation, pulmonary edema, or pneumothorax, also decrease compliance.

Airway resistance is inversely related to the fourth power of the airway radius. Airway resistance in the infant is high due to the small airway size. Airway resistance and compliance affect the rate at which lung areas will inflate. The product of resistance and compliance and how they affect the inflation of the lung is known as the pulmonary time constant. Changes in either airway resistance or pulmonary compliance alter this time constant. Hyaline membrane disease, with its associated atelectasis, increases airway resistance and decreases compliance. This results in a fast time constant, and, therefore, rapid inspiratory and expiratory times are possible on the ventilator. An increased mean airway pressure is needed to improve ventilation. If the expiratory time is shorter than the time constant of the lung for expiration, overdistension may result, known as inadvertent PEEP. If the time constant for the lung is longer than the ventilator inspiratory time, inadequate ventilation can result. Hand ventilation with a pressure monitor and bag at various pressures and flow rates can be helpful in many cases in estimating the optimal settings for the ventilator. Adjustments of the peak inspiratory pressure, inspiratory time, the positive-end expiratory pressure, and the frequency of ventilation all affect mean airway pressure. Appropriate ventilator adjustments require balancing these interrelated settings to avoid the potential hazards of each of these factors. With appropriate ventilator settings, the tidal volume in the average infant is approximately 8 mL/kg, with one third of this volume consisting of dead space.

The assessment of adequate oxygenation has been greatly improved by use of pulse oximetry. Measurement of pulse oximetry depends on changes in light transmittance that occur with each arterial pulse of blood through the tissues. At a given wavelength, oxyhemoglobin (HbO_2) and reduced hemoglobin (Hb) have different absorptions. These changes are detected by a transducer that contains a photodiode and two light-emitting diodes (LEDs) in the visible red spectrum (660 nm) and in the infrared spectrum (940 nm). Transillumination of the tissue by the LEDs allows the photodiode to receive a combination of transmitted and scattered light from the vascular bed. O_2 saturation is directly related to the amplitude of these waveforms and is calculated using the ratio of the two wave amplitudes. Pulse oximetry has a rapid (5 to 7 seconds) response time, requires no calibration, and may be left in place for hours. The limitations of pulse oximetry are noted when there is loss of adequate arterial pulsations, inadequate hemoglobin, extraneous movement, or pulsating venous blood. Fetal hemoglobin results in a lower saturation reading. To obtain an accurate measurement, a correction formula is required.

The other method of monitoring adequate oxygenation noninvasively is the use of transcutaneous PO_2 measurement. With this method, the skin is warmed to 43° to 45°C, and a miniature polarographic electrode is utilized to measure gas tension across the skin and the dilated capillaries. Correlation between transcutaneous O_2 and PO_2 has been remarkably good over a wide range of infant sizes. However, the frequent need for calibration and the poor correlation in infants with poor perfusion must be kept in mind when utilizing this device.

The principal characteristic of the circulatory pattern of the fetus is two ventricles working in parallel, rather than in series as in the adult. Newborn circulation must accommodate the transition from the parallel pattern of the fetus to the series pattern of the adult in order to adapt successfully to extrauterine life. During fetal life, pulmonary vascular resistance is high compared with total systemic vascular resistance. It is maintained by the low PO_2 (around 24 mm Hg) of the blood perfusing the fetal lung. This level of PO_2 causes marked pulmonary artery vasoconstriction. Lower total systemic resistance is maintained by the available run-off into the low-resistance placenta, which functions as the fetal lung. Due to the presence of fetal hemoglobin, which shifts the oxygen dissociation curve to the left, blood returning to the fetus from the placenta is well saturated, despite a low PO_2.

After placental separation with assumption of gas exchange by the neonatal lung, the fetal circulatory pattern undergoes profound adjustments. Pulmonary blood flow is increased as a consequence of mechanical lung expansion and the progressively better oxygenation of the blood perfusing it. Simultaneously there is a rise in systemic vascular resistance with the removal of the low-resistance placenta. The overall effect of these changes is to reverse the pressure gradient across the ductus arteriosus. As these changes progress, blood flow through the ductus arteriosus becomes directionally left to right. This further increases the pulmonary venous return to the left atrium. With increasing oxygenation associated with better pulmonary perfusion, the ductus begins to constrict and closes within approximately 24 hours after birth. This vasoconstrictive mechanism of the ductus arteriosus may not be completely operative in the immature infant, which helps explain the frequent persistence of the ductus in the immature infant. Prostaglandin E2 has been shown to maintain ductal patency when perfused in the pulmonary artery. This property has led to the hypothesis that the intraductal production of prostaglandins plays a role in normal duct closure. Blockers of prostaglandin production, such as indomethacin, are used to induce pharmacologic closure of the ductus in small preterm infants.

Persistent pulmonary hypertension of the newborn (PPHN) develops when right-to-left shunting occurs through the foramen ovale and ductus arteriosus due to persistence of high pulmonary vascular resistance. Conditions that result in persistent pulmonary hypertension include cardiac defects that are associated with pulmonary venous hypertension and with large increases in pulmonary blood flow. Other causes of PPHN include primary pulmonary vascular bed secondary to pulmonary hypoplasia or functional obstruction of the pulmonary vascular bed, as is associated with hyperviscosity syndrome. With PPHN, in only those patients without parenchymal pulmonary disease or structural pulmonary vascular or cardiac defects and without evidence of neurologic or hematologic disease should the classification of persistence of the fetal transitional circulation be made. The management of infants with hypoxemia associated with PPHN depends on its origin. When the problem is secondary to pulmonary diseases, such as hyaline membrane disease, treatment is directed toward the underlying cause. The treatment of idiopathic PPHN consists of hyperventilation to lower PCO_2 (20 to 25 mm Hg) to decrease pulmonary vascular resistance. If hypovolemia or systemic hypotension is present these conditions should be corrected. Although vasodilators have been utilized, their effects are variable and unpredictable. When all other treatment fails, extracorporeal membrane oxygenation has become more frequently utilized for this and other reversible pulmonary conditions in the newborn period.

BIBLIOGRAPHY

1. Karlberg, P., Moore, R. E., and Oliver, T.K.: The thermogenic response of the newborn infant to noradrenaline. Acta Paediatr. Scand., 51:284, 1962.
2. Landsberg, L., and Young, J.B.: Fasting, feeding, and regulation of the sympathetic nervous system. N. Engl. J. Med., 198:1295, 1978.
3. Ziegler, E.E., O'Donnell, A.M., Nelson, S.E., et al.: Body composition of reference fetus. Growth, 40:329, 1976.
4. Stone, H.O., Thompson, H.K., and Schmidt-Nielsen, K.: Influence of erythrocytes on blood viscosity. Am. J. Physiol., 214:913, 1968.
5. Blanchett, V., and Zipursky, A.: Neonatal hematology. In Avery, G.B. (ed.): Neonatology: Pathophysiology & Management of the Newborn. Philadelphia, J.P. Lippincott Co., 1987, pp.638–686.
6. Koldovsky, O.: Digestion and absorption during development. In Stave, U. (ed.): Physiology of the Perinatal Period. New York, Appleton-Century-Crofts, 1970, pp. 379–416.
7. Rowe, M.I.: Fluid and electrolyte management. In Welch, K.J., et al. (eds.): Pediatric Surgery. Chicago: Year Book Medical Publishers, Inc., 1986, pp. 22–30.
8. Stahlman, M.T.: Acute respiratory disorders in the newborn. In Avery, G.B. (ed.): Neonatology: Pathophysiology and Management of the Newborn. Philadelphia, J.B. Lippincott Co., 1987, pp. 418–445.
9. Farrell, P.M., and Hamush, M.: The biochemistry of fetal lung development. Clin. Perinatol., 5:197–229, 1978.
10. Toomasian, J.M., Snedecov, S.M., Cornell, R.G., et al.: National experience with extracorporeal membrane oxygenation for newborn respiratory failure. Trans. Am. Soc. Artif. Intern. Organs., 34:140, 1988.

Part IV

BIOLOGY OF SURGICAL TREATMENTS

27

PRINCIPLES OF SURGICAL NUTRITION

JAMES J. REILLY, JR.

Adequate nutrition is essential for function, growth, and healing. Many patients cannot maintain optimal nutrient intake because of anorexia, depression, GI tract obstruction, or dysmotility. Additionally, catabolic stress and metabolic disorders alter nutrient requirements or utilization or both.

Many surveys of surgical patients document a significant incidence (25 to 54 per cent) or protein-calorie malnutrition, hypoalbuminemia, and hypovitaminosis. Patients may be malnourished on admission; they often become more depleted during hospitalization.

Poor nutritional status results in organ dysfunction, including skeletal muscle weakness, cardiomyopathy, gastrointestinal atrophy, neurologic abnormalities, delayed wound healing, and depressed immune function. In concert, these changes result in significant morbidity, mortality, and prolongation of the hospital stay. Mortality risk increases by approximately 37 per cent for each gram deficit of serum albumin if malnutrition is untreated.

In starving patients oxygen consumption and metabolic rate are typically reduced, and caloric requirements decline over several weeks to months. The reduced energy requirements are met by the mobilization of fat, and a certain level of obligatory skeletal muscle breakdown occurs to support gluconeogenesis. Hepatic ketogenesis provides an alternate substrate for the central nervous system and other tissues that in health preferentially oxidize glucose. This metabolic adaptation to chronic starvation allows patients to conserve their most precious metabolic reserve, skeletal and visceral protein, and expend their generally abundant caloric reserves, fat. The loss of skeletal muscle mass results in generalized weakness, including loss of diaphragmatic muscle, which may result in death from respiratory infection and insufficiency. These characteristic steps in the pathogenesis of malnutrition take weeks to months to evolve, and, in practice, should be aborted by the initiation of adequate nutritional support.

NUTRITIONAL ASSESSMENT AND CLASSIFICATION

Nutritional treatment begins with nutritional assessment to detect patient who are sufficiently malnourished to increase morbidity. The assessment also enables the nutritionist to establish reasonable goals. Finally, assessment repeated at intervals permits one to determine the efficacy of the nutritional regimen. In general, the techniques employed in such an assessment can be categorized as "static" or "functional." Static measurements describe nutritional parameters at a single point in time and are used to categorize patients into nutritional groups. Examples include weight, height, serum albumin, etc. Functional nutritional parameters describe the impact upon physiologic processes. For example, in children, the most important functional determinant of good nutrition is growth. In adults, weight loss over time and urinary nitrogen determinations, collected over 24-hour periods, are particularly useful tests.

The first step in assessing nutritional adequacy is the physical examination, with special attention paid to signs of fat and muscle wasting and manifestations of vitamin, mineral, and essential fatty acid (EFA) deficiency. These include skin rash, pallor, cheilosis, glossitis, gingival lesions, hepatomegaly, edema, Trousseau's sign, neuropathy, and dementia.

Body weight is expressed as a percentage of ideal body weight (IBW) for age, sex, and height, obtained from the newly revised Metropolitan Life weight tables. "Ideal" weights are, of course, only an estimate; the relevance of an ideal weight in the surgical patient is questionable. In fact, comparison to a subjects's usual body weight might be a more accurate assessment of current nutritional status. Anthropometric parameters, such as triceps skinfold thickness (TSF) and midarm muscle circumference (MAC), are proportional to body fat stores and skeletal muscle mass, respectively. Values are reported as

383

a percentage of the reference standard for sex and height. Other measures of lean body mass—urinary creatinine and 3-methylhistidine excretion—are proportional to muscle mass because muscle creatine hydrolysis to creatinine is relatively constant and 3-methylhistidine release occurs only with muscle protein breakdown.

"Visceral" protein comprises the visceral organs, hematopoietic system, plasma, and transport proteins. Thus, serum albumin, transferrin, retinol-binding protein, lymphocyte count, and delayed hypersensitivity (DH) skin tests, when not influenced by other disease processes, reflect the adequacy of the visceral protein compartment. Because nonnutritional factors may affect each measurement, none by itself possesses sufficient sensitivity and specificity to diagnose malnutrition.

Knowing an individual's exact body composition would greatly facilitate nutritional assessment. Numerous methods to determine body composition have been devised, including anthropometry, body densitometry, calculation of lean body mass from total body water (TBW) with or without measurement of total body potassium (TBK), neutron activation analysis of nitrogen and other elements, and total body electrical conductivity. Each suffers from technical disadvantages, including invasiveness, lack of reliability, required specialized equipment, or the need for technically skilled operators. For practical purposes, a high degree of clinical suspicion, plus a dietary history, physical examination, and the constellation of anthropometric and laboratory data allow a reasonably accurate evaluation of nutritional status.

Various tests of immune function are simply too nonspecific to be reliable. Nonetheless, because of its simplicity, delayed hypersensitivity skin testing is often part of the nutritional assessment.

One important goal of the nutritional assessment is to evaluate the risks due to malnutrition. The prognostic nutritional index (PNI) relates risk to four nutrition parameters: serum albumin, serum transferrin, the triceps skinfold thickness, and the results of delayed hypersensitivity skin testing.

$$\text{PNI} = 158 - 16.6 \text{ (Alb)} - 0.78 \text{ (TSF)} -$$
$$0.20 \text{ (TFN} - 5.8 \text{ (DH)} \qquad \text{(Eq. 1)}$$

Where Alb = serum albumin level (gm/100 mL) TSF = triceps skinfold (mm), TFN = serum transferrin (mg/100 mL) and DH = reactivity to any of three recall antigens:

0 = nonreactive, 1 = >5 mm induration, and 2 = >7.5mm induration).

Such a quantitative analysis of the relationship between malnutrition and risk is important because it may identify patients in whom nutritional morbidity is sufficiently high to warrant the expense and risk of aggressive nutritional support.

Malnourished patients may be grouped into three often overlapping categories (Fig. 27–1). *Marasmus*

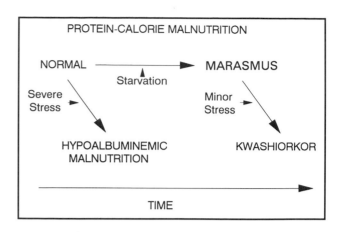

FIGURE 27–1.   Three types of malnutrition.

patients become malnourished due to a prolonged period of semistarvation; weight loss is prominent, and anthropomorphic measurements are depressed. Typically, however, serum protein levels remain at low normal levels, and skin tests are reactive. *Hypoalbuminemic malnutrition* develops rapidly in victims of trauma or sepsis as a consequence of severe metabolic stress. Weight changes and anthropomorphic measurements are unreliable because of salt and water retention; the serum albumin level is typically less than 2.5 gm/dL, and skin tests demonstrate anergy. The *adult kwashiorkor* patients are usually marasmus patients who are subjected to stress. The normal or low normal serum albumin typical of the marasmus patient falls dramatically in response to increased metabolic demands, and anergy becomes evident. Marasmus patients lack the nutritional reserves necessary to cope with planned or accidental metabolic stress; when they decline into the kwashiorkor category, they suffer the highest nutrition-related morbidity and mortality of all malnourished patients.

COMPONENTS OF THERAPY

Estimated Energy Requirements

Estimating energy requirements is generally simple for the simple starvation patient without extraordinary needs, but is more complex and difficult for the critically ill, hypermetabolic patient. Three techniques are commonly used.

The simplest technique estimates energy expenditure on the basis of weight. The starving patient expends approximately 30 kcal/kg/day. When mild to moderate stress is present, caloric expenditure is adjusted upward to 35 kcal/kg/day and, when stress is more severe, to 40 to 50 kcal/kg/day. This method is obviously limited in the edematous patient and in those with significant obesity (over 30 per cent above IBW).

The second technique calculates the patient's basal energy expenditure (BEE) and multiplies it by a factor related to estimated expenditures above a basal level due either to muscular work or stress. BEE may be calculated from the Harris-Benedict equations:

$$BEE\ (women) = 655 + (9.6\ W) + (1.8\ H) - (4.7\ A)$$
$$(Eq.\ 2)$$

$$BEE\ (men) = 66 + (13.7\ W) + (5\ H) - (6.8\ A)$$
$$(Eq.\ 3)$$

where W = weight in kg, H = height in cm, and A = age in years.

Finally, one may calculate energy requirement from measured oxygen consumption and carbon dioxide production, a technique known as indirect calorimetry (Fig. 27–2). Oxygen consumption and CO_2 production are directly measured during breathing into a spirometer with immediate gas analysis (the "metabolic cart"). Total nitrogen excretion is measured in a timed, usually 24-hour urine specimen. Energy expenditure can be calculated according to this equation:

$$Metabolic\ rate\ (kcal/m^2/h) =$$
$$\frac{[(3.9 \times VO_2(L/min)] + 1.1 \times VCO_2(L/min) \times 60(min/h)}{Body\ Surface\ Area\ (M^2)}$$
$$(Eq.\ 4)$$

This technique is often limited by the inherent difficulties in gas collection and analysis. Metabolic carts produce widely varying values in patients breathing high inspired oxygen fractions. If accurate, however, this technique permits one to calculate not only the total energy expenditure but also to define the substrate utilization patterns through the respiratory quotient (RQ). The RQ is the ratio of carbon dioxide production to oxygen consumption. The RQ of glucose oxidation is 1.0, that of fat is 0.7, and that of protein is 0.8. Mixed fuel utilization generally results in a total body RQ of 0.7 to 0.8 (Table 27–1).

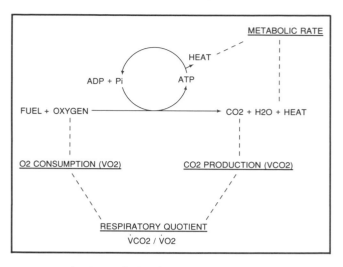

FIGURE 27–2. Relation between oxygen consumption, metabolic rate, and generation of high energy intermediates. (Reprinted from Schlichtig, R., and Ayers, M.: Nutritional Support of the Critically Ill. Chicago, Year Book Medical Publishers, Inc., 1988, p. 50.)

Carbohydrate Requirements

The minimum amount of carbohydrate necessary for the brain and red blood cells, both of which prefer glucose as oxidative substrate, is 100 to 150 gm/day. Larger quantities serve as an energy source for the remainder of the body. Carbohydrate reserves in normal humans consist of glycogen stored in both skeletal muscle and the liver. These stores are relatively small, comprising about 300 gm or about 1200 kcal. These stores are depleted in 48 to 72 hours in the starving individual and in as little as 12 to 24 hours in the stressed individual.

Fasting healthy humans normally produce glucose via glycogenolysis and gluconeogenesis (from amino acids) at the rate of 2.53 +/− 0.58 mg/kg/min and utilize it at the same rate. Gluconeogenesis is sup-

TABLE 27–1. QUANTITY OF HEAT AND ATP PRODUCED DURING COMBUSTION OF CARBOHYDRATE (CHO), LIPID, AND PROTEIN*

	KILOCALORIES PRODUCED/L OF O_2	MOLES OF ATP/L OF O_2	KCAL/GM SUBSTRATE	RQ†
CHO	5.047	3.15	4.1	1.0
Lipid	4.735	2.85	9.3	0.718
Protein	4.463	Variable, depending on amino acid composition	5.3	0.802

* Per mole of oxygen consumed, production of heat and of ATP is similar for all three substrates; however, more potential energy is contained within an equal weight of liquid.

† Respiratory quotient.

Reprinted from Schlichtig, P., and Ayers, M. Nutritional Support of the Critically Ill. Chicago, Year Book Medical Publishers, Inc, 1988, p. 51.

pressed by as little as 2 mg/kg/min of exogenous glucose, but the rate of utilization is not linearly related to the rate of glucose infusion. When glucose intake exceeds the maximal oxidative rate, the excess is converted to fat, even though total caloric intake may not meet caloric needs.

Stressed patients exhibit a maximum glucose oxidation rate of 3 to 5 mg/kg/min, regardless of how much is infused. Hyperglycemia is more common in this setting, reflecting the impact of stress hormones —cortisol, catecholamines, and glucagon—that inhibit glycogenolysis and gluconeogenesis. This conversion of excess exogenous carbohydrate into fat is deleterious for two reasons. First, fat synthesis is an energy-requiring process (Table 27–2). To the extent that available ATP must be consumed during fat synthesis, less is available for protein synthesis and for other energy-dependent cellular processes.

Second, converting glucose to long chain fatty acids releases large amounts of CO_2. This augmented CO_2 production is reflected in a rise in the respiratory quotient, and the patient must increase minute ventilation to sustain a normal arterial pCO_2, thus increasing the work of breathing. Although this compensation is relatively easy for normal individuals, patients with impaired respiratory function, particularly those requiring mechanical ventilation, may experience obvious difficulties. For these reasons, it is wise to limit carbohydrate intake to approximate the maximal rate of glucose oxidation, generally less than 5 mg/kg/min.

Fat Requirements

Fats serve as metabolic fuel, both as a source of glycerol and from the direct oxidation of long chain fatty acids. Fatty acids are a major fuel of the heart, liver, and skeletal muscle. Ketone bodies (autoacetate and beta-hydroxybutyrate), derived from the partial oxidation of fatty acids by the liver, are preferred by the heart, skeletal muscle, and the starvation-adapted brain. In the fed state, insulin promotes fat synthesis and storage and inhibits the hormone-sensitive lipase of the adipocyte. Fasting stimulates this lipase, effecting lipolysis and the release of fatty acids and glycerol. Hormone-sensitive lipase is also stimulated by catecholamines; thus, lipolysis and fatty acid oxidation are augmented during stress.

Fat is a high-density energy source (9 kcal/gm dry weight). Dietary triglycerides may be composed of medium chain length fatty acids (6 to 12 carbons) or long chain fatty acids (more than 12 carbons). Medium chain triglycerides (MCT) are absorbed throughout the small intestine directly into the portal venous system. Long chain triglycerides must be emulsified by bile salts in the proximal bowel to form micelles and then undergo hydrolysis by pancreatic lipase. Longer fatty acids are absorbed, re-esterified to triglycerides, and enter the bloodstream as chylomicrons via the intestinal lymphatics and the thoracic duct. Peripheral hydrolysis via endothelial lipoprotein lipase produces fatty acids and glycerol, which may be oxidized by all tissues.

The metabolism of parenterally administered fat proceeds similarly; the chylomicron-like particles infused into the blood are initially hydrolyzed by peripheral lipoprotein lipase. The liver further metabolizes the resultant remnant particles and synthesizes lipoproteins, triglycerides, and ketones.

Essential fatty acid (linoleic acid) deficiency is manifested by a dry skin rash, ecchymoses, alopecia, anemia, edema, thrombocytopenia, and respiratory distress; fat-free total parenteral nutrition will produce this clinical syndrome in 4 to 6 weeks. The diagnosis can be confirmed by measuring the serum triene and tetraenoic acids, the metabolic products of oleic and linoleic acids, respectively. A triene : tetraene ratio greater than 0.4 is diagnostic and ap-

TABLE 27–2.   METABOLIC "COST" OF SYNTHESIZING LIPID FROM EXOGENOUSLY ADMINISTERED FUELS

Precursor	Converted to	Moles of ATP required per Mole of Precursor Converted	O_2 Used per Kilocalories of Precursor* (mL of O_2/kal)	Moles of CO_2 Produced per Mole of Precursor†
Glucose	Fat	4	1.43	2.6
Medium chain triglyceride (average chain length, C_8)	Triglyceride in adipose tissue	7	0.325	1.0
Long chain triglyceride (average chain length, C_{18})	Triglyceride in adipose tissue	7	0.154	1.0

* Assumes 1 mole of O_2 is required to make 6 moles of ATP.

† Includes CO_2 produced by synthesis of ATP, assuming approximately 1 mole of CO_2 per 7 moles of ATP.

Reprinted from Schlichtig R., and Ayers, M.: Nutritional Support of the Critically Ill. Chicago: Year Book Medical Publishers, Inc., 1988, p. 68.

pears within 10 days of fat-free intravenous alimentation. As little as 3.2 per cent of total caloric intake in the form of an intravenous fat emulsion (containing approximately 54 per cent linoleic acid), or 15 per cent of the caloric intake as oral fat (assuming a 6.5 per cent linoleic acid content) prevents EFA deficiency.

Intravenous lipid emulsions at high doses have attendant side effects. Pyrogenic reactions occur in 3 per cent of patients. Fat administration in excess of 3 gm/kg/day in infants and 4 gm/kg/day in adults produces a fat overload syndrome, consisting of hyperlipidemia, coagulopathy, fever, cholestatic jaundice, and gastrointestinal distress. Lipid microaggregates may deposit in the liver. In the lung, impaired diffusion capacity may produce a respiratory distress syndrome. This syndrome probably occurs when the rate of infusion exceeds peripheral clearance; lipid particle coalescence results in aggregation and deposition in reticuloendothelial cells, thereby releasing cellular inflammatory and vasoactive mediators.

Fat should be provided in any enteral or parenteral nutritional program, not only to prevent essential fatty acid deficiency but also as a caloric source. Stressed patients are often relatively glucose intolerant, and caloric goals are more difficult to achieve with glucose alone. Furthermore, excessive glucose in the stressed patient may contribute to the fatty liver and abnormal liver function tests commonly seen in TPN patients. Persistent catabolic states are often resistant to reversal with glucose alone. Twenty to 40 per cent of calories should be supplied by fat (up to 2.5 gm/kg/day).

Protein

The protein "stores" of the body comprise about 14 kg in a 70-kg adult, and, if oxidized, will provide about 54,000 kcal. However, there are no true protein stores; all body protein is functional, i.e., a component of the cellular structure or matrix, a component of an enzymatic system, or a transport protein, such as hemoglobin. When catabolism reduces total body protein stores, organ dysfunction and failure inevitably follow.

Twenty common amino acids comprise most dietary proteins. The eight essential amino acids (isoleucine, leucine, valine, lysine, methionine, phenylalanine, threonine, and tryptophan), must be supplied from exogenous sources since the body cannot synthesize them. Other amino acids are synthesized from these essential amino acids or keto acid precursors.

Ingested protein is hydrolyzed by the digestive enzymes of the gut and absorbed from the proximal small intestine, primarily in the form of small peptides. Gut mucosal cells metabolize some amino acids, particularly glutamine, and completely hydrolyze the peptides. Amino acids then pass via the portal vein to the liver. There, amino acids may be incorporated into intact protein, oxidized, or incorporated into other nitrogenous compounds, such as purines, pyrimidines, uric acid, and urea. The liver regulates the flux of amino acids from the gut to peripheral sites, maintaining plasma amino acid levels within relatively narrow ranges.

During normal protein turnover, protein synthesis balances degradation and catabolism. Amino acid nitrogen recycles within the total body pool. Amino acids may also be oxidized to CO_2 as an energy source or converted to carbohydrate or fat; in either instance, nitrogen is eliminated, usually as urea.

Much amino acid metabolism occurs in the liver, which is the exclusive catabolic site of all the essential amino acids, except the branch chain amino acids—isoleucine, leucine, and valine.

Skeletal muscle is the largest protein reservoir in the body, undergoes considerable protein turnover, and is the primary site of branch chain amino acid metabolism. In the fed state, insulin regulates amino acid disposition and anabolism by facilitating amino acid transport, especially of the branch chain amino acids, into muscle. During fasting, muscle cells catabolize protein and convert most amino acids to alanine or glutamine. These "transport" amino acids are released into the circulation and provide the liver with precursors for gluconeogenesis. Skeletal muscle branch chain amino acids are catabolized locally to provide energy. Protein degradation can be monitored by urinary 3-methylhistidine excretion because this methylated amino acid is not recycled. Steroids, thyroxine, and catecholamines all increase skeletal muscle protein catabolism.

Intact proteins are lost from the skin surface, in secretions, and from the turnover of gut mucosa. Monomeric nitrogenous compounds, such as urea, creatinine, ammonia, uric acid, and some amino acids, are excreted in urine. Most amino acids are reabsorbed after glomerular filtration, whereas other nitrogenous wastes undergo active tubular secretion. The kidney synthesizes ammonia from glutamine. Nitrogen excretion is thus coupled to renal gluconeogenesis.

Recognizing that proteins and amino acids are in dynamic equilibrium, global nitrogen balance can be calculated from total input and output.

$$\text{Nitrogen balance in grams} = \frac{\text{Dietary protein}}{6.25} - (\text{UNN} + 4 \text{ gm}) \quad \text{(Eq. 5)}$$

Additional extraordinary losses from diarrhea, excessive desquamation of the skin, bleeding, or surgical tubes and drains can be measured and added to the output side of the equation.

The daily oral protein requirement of unstressed healthy adults is approximately 0.8 gm/kg/actual body weight. Children require more, up to 1.5 gm/kg, since growth, rather than simple maintenance, is desired. Older adults have slower rates of protein turnover, but chronic illness and less efficient absorption affect their requirements.

The patient's metabolic state also alters protein utilization and requirements. Starvation and immobilization retard protein synthesis. Further stress augments protein catabolism and induces negative nitrogen balance. Accelerated skeletal muscle and visceral protein breakdown occurs during stress to meet energy needs and persists without the adaptive protein conservation and augmented lipolysis that occur in starvation.

Nitrogen balance depends not only upon the quantity of nitrogen intake but also upon potassium, magnesium, phosphate, and vitamin intake. Of greatest importance, however, is the intake of adequate nonprotein calories (Fig. 27–3). Nitrogen retention to increase body cell mass will not occur if the protein supplied is diverted to meet energy needs via oxidation or gluconeogenesis. A desirable calorie : nitrogen ratio in unstressed states approximates 150 : 1 (kcal : gm of nitrogen). During stress, more nitrogen is required, and the calorie : nitrogen ratio is reduced to 100 : 1. Glucose utilization is impaired, and more amino acids are required—at the same time that the total caloric intake is increased.

The qualitative nature of administered protein also affects the quantitative requirement. For example, enteral formulas containing crystalline amino acids produce less nitrogen retention than do those comprised of hydrolyzed casein. Digested protein is probably the most physiologic source. Plasma amino acid patterns are more physiologic in enterally fed subjects, demonstrating the importance of gut and liver function. Intravenously administered amino acids are less well utilized. Urinary excretion of free or conjugated amino acids during TPN may be fivefold greater than in the physiologic postprandial state. Certain amino acids appear in the urine in proportion to their concentration in TPN; others, with low renal reabsorption, appear in higher levels, suggesting inefficient utilization.

Essential amino acid requirements vary widely, but adults probably require 20 per cent of their protein intake as essential amino acids. Depleted patients may need proportionately more essential amino acids (up to 40 per cent) for lean body mass replacement.

Vitamins

Vitamins are essential to many metabolic processes. Most function as enzyme co-factors (Table 27–3). The recommended dietary allowances (RDAs) established for the four fat-soluble and the nine water-soluble vitamins exceed the biologic requirements of most normal individuals. In stressed surgical patients, however, the RDAs frequently un-

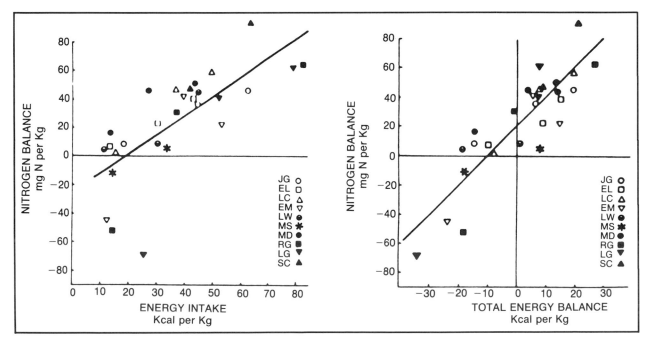

FIGURE 27–3. Relationship between total energy intake (kcal/kg) and nitrogen balance at fixed nitrogen intake in ten malnourished patients. Slope = 1.4 mg of N/kal (*left*). When energy intake was recalculated as a function of measured calorie expenditure, it appeared that nitrogen equilibrium was attained at near-energy equilibrium (*right*). (Reprinted from Elwyn, D.H., Gump, F.E., Munro, H.N., et al.: Changes in nitrogen balance of depleted patients with increasing infusions of glucose. Am. J. Clin. Nutr., 32: 1604, 1979.)

TABLE 27–3. VITAMINS IN HUMAN NUTRITION

Vitamin	Co-Enzyme or Active Form	Function	Deficiency	Toxicity	Requirements	
					RDA	Parenteral
Vitamin A	Retinol (in rhodopsin)	Active site of rhodopsin glycoprotein synthesis	Xerophthalmia, keratomalacia, impaired epithelial integrity, hypogonadism	Altered mental status, hepatic fibrosis, portal hypertension Elevated CSF pressure, bone changed, hypercalcemia	4000–5000 IU	3300 IU
Vitamin D	1,25-dihydroxy-cholecalciferol	Intestinal absorption, bone remodeling	Rickets, osteomalacia	Hypercalcemia	400 IU	200 IU
Vitamin E	α-Tocopherol	Antioxidant	Hemolytic anemia, ataxia nystagmus, loss of DTRs, myopathy, edema	Weakness, fatigue, hypertension, antagonist of vitamin K, GI complaints	12–15 IU	10 IU
Vitamin K	Menaquinones	δ-Carboxylation of glutamic acid in clotting factors and osteocalcin	Coagulopathy	Hemolysis	0.5–1.0 mgm/kg	5–10 mg/wk
Thiamin	Thiamin pyrophosphate	Decarboxylation of α-keto acids, transketolase reaction	Wernicke's encephalopathy, peripheral neuropathy (dry beriberi) ± heart failure (web beriberi)	Rare anaphylaxis, neurologic abnormalities	1.0–1.5 mg	3.0 mg
Riboflavin	Flavin monomucleotide Flavin adenine dinucleotide	Oxidation-reduction reactions	Dermatitis, glossitis, mucositis, anemia, neuropathy, photophobia, lipid abnormalities	Unknown	1.1–1.8 mg	3.6 mg
Niacin	Nicotinamide adenine	Oxidation-reduction reactions	Pellegra (dermatitis, diarrhea, dementia, and death)	Induction of histamine-mediated reactions; elevated serum glucose, uric acid, and hepatic enzymes; GI complaints; hypotension	12–20 mg	40 mg
Pantothenic acid	Co-enzyme A	Acyl transfer	Erythromelalgia, altered mental status, GI complaints	Occasional diarrhea	5–10 mg	15 mg
Vitamin B$_6$	Pyridoxal phosphate	Amine transfer synthesis of niacin from tryptophane, DOPA decarboxylase	Sideroblastic anemia, pellegra, mucositis, peripheral neuropathy	Ataxia, neuropathy, seizure, acceleration of drug metabolism	1.6–2.0 mg	4.0 mg
Folate	Tetrahydrofolate	Methyl transfer, purine and thymidine synthesis	Megaloblastic anemia	Antagonist of seizure medications, seizures		400 mg

Table continued on following page

TABLE 27–3. VITAMINS IN HUMAN NUTRITION *Continued*

| | | | | | REQUIREMENTS | |
VITAMIN	CO-ENZYME OR ACTIVE FORM	FUNCTION	DEFICIENCY	TOXICITY	*RDA*	*Parenteral*
Vitamin B$_{12}$	Cobalamine	1-->2 carbon shift	Megaloblastic anemia, mental changes, peripheral neuropathy	Unknown	3.0 mgm	5.0 mg
Vitamin C		Antioxidant, proline hydroxylation in collagen carnitine synthesis	Scurvy, Sjögren's syndrome	Osmotic diarrhea, bone mineral resorption, impaired B$_{12}$ and Cu absorption, false urine glucose and stool guaiac tests	45 mg	100 mg
Biotin	Biotinyl-lys-enzyme	Carboxyl transfer	Dermatitis, mucositis, GI complaints, altered mental status, paresthesia	Unknown	0.50–300 mg	60 mg

Modified from Reilly J.J., and Gerhardt, A.L.: Modern surgical nutrition. Curr. Prob. Surg., 22:18–19, 1985.

derestimate requirements. Specifically, vitamins A, B$_1$, B$_2$, and C and folate are necessary in greater amounts postoperatively, but how much more is needed is not known. The bioavailability of parenteral vitamins or oral vitamins taken alone, administered with elemental enteral formulas, or in various enteric disorders will vary.

The recommended parenteral vitamin dosages therefore differ slightly from the RDA. Intravenous vitamins are subject to adsorption (fat-soluble vitamins) onto the administration apparatus, inactivation by light (vitamins A, E, B$_2$, B$_6$, B$_{12}$, folic acid), and incompatibility with TPN components. Nevertheless, the doses recommended in Table 27–3, with the exception of that of vitamin A, which may be insufficient, are adequate and safe for daily use.

During deprivation or stress, water-soluble vitamins are more prone to depletion because body stores are small, except for the large stores of B$_{12}$. Serum levels of water-soluble vitamins B$_{12}$, C, and erythrocyte folate content are inaccurate indicators of vitamin status, so that a diagnosis of deficiency must be made clinically, and treatment is empiric.

Fat-soluble vitamins are stored in body fat and excreted in the bile. Serum levels, which are usually normal even when only minimal body stores are present, are relatively insensitive to acute changes in nutrition. However, low serum levels are diagnostic of deficiency and are treatable by a single or a few large parenteral doses. Overadministration of vitamin A, however, is toxic.

Minerals

Minerals are necessary to prevent deficiency states that interfere with nitrogen retention and anabolism. Malabsorption syndromes, the consequences of diverse diseases, and drug side effects alter mineral balances.

Calcium, the most abundant cation in the body, plays a vital role in muscular and cardiac contractility, neuromuscular excitability, coagulation, membrane permeability and adhesiveness, and hormone secretion. Bone is the vast storehouse for the homeostatic control of plasma calcium levels. Parathyroid hormone, calcitonin, thyroxin, sex-steroids, and 1,25-dihydroxyvitamin D regulate bone resorption, intestinal absorption, and renal tubular reabsorption of calcium. The RDA for calcium is 800 mg/day. The recommended intake for adolescents and postmenopausal women, because of bone growth and poor calcium balance, respectively, increases to 1.2 to 1.5 mg/day. Normal adults consuming the RDA absorb 30 to 50 per cent of dietary calcium. The recommended parenteral calcium intake is 12–20 mEq/day. A calcium:phosphorus (mg:mg) dietary ratio of 1.0 is optimal for maintenance of skeletal integrity.

Hypervitaminosis A or D and milk-alkali syndrome are nutritional causes of hypercalcemia and hypercalciuria that persist regardless of calcium intake until weight-bearing activity is resumed. Hypocalcemia is often associated with other nutritional defects, such as hypoalbuminemia, hypomagnesemia, hyperphosphatemia, and vitamin D deficiency states.

Magnesium is the second most abundant intracellular cation; it serves as a co-factor for innumerable enzymes and as a regulator of membrane permeability and neuromuscular excitability. Normal serum levels of 1.5 to 2.5 mEq/L (55 per cent is ionized) are maintained by sensitive renal homeostatic mechanisms. Intestinal absorption is depressed by rapid intestinal transit time and high dietary intake of calcium, phosphate, and fiber and is augmented by vitamin D, protein, and lactose. In subjects consuming the magnesium RDA (300 to 350 mg/day), about 40 per cent of an oral dose is absorbed. The recommended daily parenteral dose during TPN is approximately 1000 mEq (120 to 290 mg), usually as the sulfate or chloride salt.

Magnesium deficiency is identified by a low serum level or by daily urinary excretion less than 80 per cent of an intravenous magnesium load. Although dietary insufficiency will produce hypomagnesemia in any subject, low serum levels are common in patients with pancreatitis, fat malabsorption, short bowel syndrome, and severe diarrheal disease. Augmented renal loss due to nephritis, renal tubular acidosis, thiazide or loop diuretics, ethanol, aminoglycosides, cis-platinum, hyperparathyroidism, and hyperaldosteronism also predispose to deficiency. Magnesium salts ingested as laxatives and antacids may cause toxicity, especially in patients with renal failure. Deficiency responds acutely to doses of 1 to 2 gm $MgSO_4$ IM or IV as a slow infusion. Maintenance oral therapy with magnesium oxide (1 to 2 gm/day in divided doses) then sustains normal serum levels. Diarrhea may limit the maximum tolerable oral dose, necessitating intermittent parenteral therapy.

Phosphorus plays important roles in intermediary metabolism and cellular and skeletal structure. Most body phosphorus exists as hydroxyapatite in bone. Inorganic phosphates are major intracellular anions. Phospholipids contribute to membrane stability, clotting factor activity, and lipoprotein structure. Metabolic intermediates (such as ATP, cyclic AMP, 2,3-DPG glycolytic intermediates), vitamins (including niacin, thiamin, pyridoxine), nucleic acids, and multiple enzymes require phosphorylation.

The clinically important inorganic portion of plasma phosphorus consists of the mono- and dibasic orthophosphates. Because the valence varies, the most accurate means of expressing serum phosphate concentration is in milligrams or millimoles (rather than mEq) of phosphorus. The normal serum inorganic phosphorus is 2.5 to 4.5 mg/dL.

The RDA for phosphorus is 800 mg/day. In total body depletion, shifts of intracellular phosphate to the extracellular compartment maintain near-normal serum phosphate levels. Acute intracellular phosphate shifts may produce severe hypophosphatemia. Phosphorus deficiency impairs glycolysis, oxy-gen transport, and phagocyte function. Hemolysis, bleeding, rhabdomyolysis, congestive cardiomyopathy, respiratory failure, altered sensorium, neuropathy, seizures, and coma may also occur. Therapy with 0.08 to 0.24 mmol/kg phosphate IV over 6 hours should be monitored with frequent serum phosphorus and calcium determinations.

The parenteral requirement for phosphorus is 0.5 to 1 mmol/kg/day in stable patients without renal failure. Starved patients who are refed may require more; the best method of determining requirements is to follow serum levels.

Trace Elements

Trace elements are those components of the diet present in small quantity, generally less than 0.1 per cent of the diet. The essential trace elements include the minerals—iron, zinc, manganese, cobalt, chromium, copper, molybdenum, and selenium—and the halogens, iodine, and fluorine. Requirements for tin, nickel, vanadium, and silicon are inferred from animal studies. Their importance in human nutrition is unknown.

Trace elements function as necessary components of the metalloenzymes, which are crucial to most metabolic pathways. Although trace elements function at a molecular level, deficiency states present as multiple organ dysfunction and a variety of skin abnormalities. Table 27–4 describes the biochemical functions of most trace elements, the metabolic consequences of deficiency, and recommended intravenous allowances.

Iron additives are unnecessary in the short-term TPN patient with sufficient iron stores. However, pre-existing iron deficiency, anticipated blood loss, or long-term TPN necessitate daily (0.5 to 1 mg/day) or weekly (10 mg/week) supplementation. Routine vitamin B_{12} supplementation supplies cobalt.

The consequences of iodine and fluorine deficiencies are well recognized, and intravenous additives exist. Yet, reports of TPN-related deficiency are rare, and routine supplementation is probably unnecessary. Reports of selenium deficiency within 4 weeks of unsupplemented TPN make routine daily selenium supplementation advisable. Selenous acid, 80 to 100 gm/day, prevents deficiency and 200 to 400 g/day treats depleted patients. Because molybdenum deficiency only occurs after more than 1 year of TPN, molybdenum additives (0.02 to 0.03 mg/day) should only be used in long-term TPN patients. On the basis of available information about vanadium, nickel, silicon, and tin requirements, these trace elements are not generally provided.

Altered requirements in specific disease states or in stressed patients are poorly defined. In some, excessive losses (e.g., over 0.5 mg iron/mL blood loss, or zinc lost from the bowel in Crohn's disease) may

TABLE 27–4.   BIOCHEMICAL FUNCTIONS AND MANIFESTATIONS OF DEFICIENCY OF ESSENTIAL TRACE ELEMENTS

ELEMENT	SITES OF ACTION	KEY BIOCHEMICAL FUNCTIONS	SIGNS OF DEFICIENCY	REQUIREMENTS RDA	REQUIREMENTS Parenteral
Zinc	Metalloenzymes, e.g., alcohol dehydrogenase carboxypeptidase, and DNA polymerase	Metabolism of lipids, protein, carbohydrates, and nucleic acids	Parakeratosis (swine), acrodermatitis enteropathica (humans), (?) hypogonadism	.5 mg	2.5–4.0 mg
Chromium	"Glucose tolerance factor"	Glucose metabolism— (?) mediates insulin effects on membranes	Impaired glucose clearance (many species); impaired growth, reproduction, and life-span (rats and mice)	0.05–0.2 mg	1.0–1.5 mgm
Cobalt	Co-enzyme B_{12}	Biologic methylation, e.g., methionine synthesis	Pernicious anemia (humans) methylmalonic aciduria (humans)	See Vitamin B_{12}	
Copper	Metalloenzymes (e.g., cytochrome oxidase)	Mitochondrial function, collagen metabolism, melanin formation	Menkes' syndrome (humans); anemia, leukopenia, neuropenia (animals and humans)	2–3 mg	0.5–1.5 mg
Fluorine	Unknown	(?) Iron absorption	Anemia (mice), impaired growth and reproduction (rats)	1.5–4 mg	0.9–4.0 mg
Iodine	Thyroglobulin, thyroxine, triiodothyronine	Cellular oxidation processes	Thyroid diseases (animals and humans)	150 mgm	70–140 mgm
Mn*	Pyruvate carboxylase	Oxidative phosphorylation; fatty acid metabolism; synthesis of proteins, mucopolysaccharides, and cholesterol	Defective growth, bony anomalies, reproductive dysfunction, and central nervous system abnormalities in many species	2.5–5.0 mg	0.15–0.8 mg
Mo⁺	Flavoenzymes	Xanthine, hypoxanthine metabolism	Growth retardation, impaired urate clearance (chicks)		

Table continued on following page

TABLE 27–4. BIOCHEMICAL FUNCTIONS AND MANIFESTATIONS OF DEFICIENCY OF ESSENTIAL TRACE ELEMENTS
Continued

ELEMENT	SITES OF ACTION	KEY BIOCHEMICAL FUNCTIONS	SIGNS OF DEFICIENCY	REQUIREMENTS	
				RDA	*Parenteral*
Selenium	Glutathione perioxidase, (erythrocytes), "cytochrome" (muscle)	Degradation of intracellular peroxides, oxidation of glutathione	Liver necrosis (rats), "white-muscle disease," exudative diathesis (chicks)	0.15–4 mg	0.02–0.03 mg
Nickel	Ribonucleic acid	(?) Nucleic acid stabilization, (?) membrane structure and function	Impaired reproduction, deranged liver, lipid, and phospholipid metabolism (chicks)	?	?
Silicon	Mucopolysaccharides	(?) Connective tissue structure	Impaired growth and connective tissue formation (chicks)	?	?
Tin	Fatty tissue	(?) Redox catalyst	Growth and dentition (rats)	?	?
Vanadium	Hemovanadin	Oxygen transport, (?) redox catalyst	Impaired growth, reproduction, bone, and lipid metabolism (chickens, rats)	?	?

* Mn = manganese

† mo = molybdenum

Modified from Reilly J.J., and Gerhardt, A.L.: Modern surgical nutrition. Curr. Prob. Surg. *22*:26–27, 1985.

necessitate additional supplementation. Diseases affecting the liver or kidney might reduce exogenous requirements for copper and manganese (primarily biliary excretion) and for chromium, selenium, and molybdenum (excreted via the kidneys). Although serial serum trace element determinations are recommended to monitor therapy in TPN patients, serum levels are poor indicators of target tissue levels, e.g., of iodine in the thyroid and zinc in the liver. Intravenous requirements become ever less firm when the patient can eat and absorb some food.

Patients fed only enteral formulas, especially elemental diets, have the same predisposition to trace element deficiency as TPN patients. Trace elements have been added to some, but not all, formulas. Trace element content should be considered in the choice of formula for patients on long-term (greater than 4 weeks) tube feedings.

DELIVERY SYSTEMS: ENTERAL AND PARENTERAL

The choice between enteral and parenteral hyperalumentation depends primarily on the patient's GI function and the rapidity with which the desired nutrients must be delivered. When enteral formulas or parenteral nutrition are required, not only the special requirements of the stressed patient but also variations necessitated by the purified nutrient form and the route of administration must be considered.

Enteral Alimentation

When there are no serious contraindications, enteral alimentation is preferable to parenteral feeding. Advantages of enteral alimentation include maintenance of intestinal structure and function by the trophic effects of intraluminal nutrients, the augmented physiologic insulin response to enterally administered carbohydrate, provision of more nutritionally complete feeding solutions, economy, and safety. Small-bore nasogastric, nasoduodenal, gastrostomy, gastroduodenostomy, or jejunostomy tubes have made intubation at any level of the gut possible.

Numerous commercial enteral feeding mixtures are available, so that an appropriate choice can be made to satisfy any given patient's specialized needs. Enteral products fall into three broad categories based on composition: polymeric, chemically defined, and modular formulas. Products differ in nutrient complexity, nutrient concentration, osmolarity, viscosity, and caloric density.

Polymeric formulas may be food-based or contain combinations of intact macronutrients. Blenderized feedings contain intact protein and lactose and are typically high in residue, osmolarity, and viscosity. Such preparations are nutritionally complete, cause few gastrointestinal side effects if delivered into the stomach, promote normal gut function, and are inexpensive. However, due to their high viscosity, such feedings may require a large-bore feeding tube or gastrostomy.

Other polymeric products contain mixtures of variably intact macromolecular components. They may be milk-based or lactose-free and contain whole milk, egg, or soy protein; fat with or without medium chain triglycerides; and carbohydrate polymers. They are nutritionally complete, low in residue, and of low to moderate osmolarity and moderate viscosity. Some are isosmolar, permitting initial use at full strength. Most flavored supplements are palatable, and, with high-caloric density formulas, fluid restriction is possible.

Chemically defined formulas are intended for patients with impaired digestive capabilities; they contain monomeric or short chain hydrolysis products of protein and carbohydrate macronutrients. Fats are generally intact; some products add medium chain triglycerides. All are lactose-free. The chemical simplicity (monosaccharides, amino acids, and short peptides) creates hypersomolar, low residue, nutritionally complete, defined formulas. The fat content, although low, is usually sufficient to prevent EFA deficiency. However, energy needs may not be met efficiently with the predominantly carbohydrate calorie source, especially in stressed patients. Other disadvantages include relative unpalatability and high cost.

Special formulas have been designed to nourish patients with liver and or renal diseases. A branch chain amino acid (BCAA) enriched formula with MCT and low electrolytes attempts to improve the presumed metabolic deficiencies of hepatic failure. Other formulas are designed to stabilize elevated blood urea nitrogen, phosphate, and potassium while improving the nutritional status of patients in renal failure. More recently, high BCAA mixtures (15 to 25 per cent) have been designed for use in stressed surgical patients.

Variations in electrolyte, mineral, and vitamin content may also influence the choice of product; for example, sodium content for the cardiac failure patient or vitamin K content for the anticoagulated patient. This information is available with each product and in some product comparison charts.

Gastrointestinal side effects, including bloating, distension, nausea, and diarrhea, occur in 10 to 20 per cent of tube-fed patients. Such symptoms often subside after reduction of the infusion rate. Hyperosmolar solutions introduced beyond the pylorus may produce a "dumping syndrome." Isosmolar solutions at lower infusion rates typically correct this problem. Diarrhea results from excess volume, hyperosmolarity of the diet, and, in the chronically starved patient, malabsorption due to functional atrophy of the intestine. This is the most common and vexing gastrointestinal side effect of tube feeding. Diarrhea usually responds to lowering the infusion rate and reducing the osmolality of the solution or pharmacologic manipulation (paregoric or dilute tincture of opium).

Diarrhea is often associated with significant hypoalbuminemia (less than 2.5 gm/dL). Presumably, the resultant lowered plasma oncotic pressure impairs nutrient absorption. Correcting hypoalbuminemia with a parenteral salt-poor albumin infusion may improve diarrhea, and when adequate intake is achieved, the serum level will remain elevated. When diarrhea persists or is particularly massive, the prudent course is often to discontinue feeding for a few days and then change the enteral formula or consider parenteral nutrition. Serum hyperosmolarity and associated electrolyte disturbances may occur when diarrhea volume is excessive or underestimated. Liver function test abnormalities are less frequent than in parenteral nutrition.

Parenteral Nutrition

Parenteral nutrition solutions are formulated from a "base" solution of amino acids, to which are added variable amounts of glucose, electrolytes, vitamins, etc. Synthetic amino acid solutions, compared to natural protein sources, are generally enriched in essential amino acids, as well as alanine, arginine, histidine, and proline. Glutamine is unstable in solution and is notably absent from parenteral formulas. Amino acid concentrations range from 2.75 to 5 per cent. Special formulas are available with increased content of essential amino acids or branch chain amino acids.

Dextrose may be added to the amino acid solutions to achieve a final concentration of from 10 to 35 per cent. Dilute solutions (5 to 10 per cent) must be used for peripheral intravenous regimens, but higher concentrations are permissible in central TPN. Dextrose supplies 3.4 kcal per gram wet weight; therefore, a 5 per cent solution supplies 170 kcal/L, and the 25 per cent solution most commonly used in central TPN supplies 850 kcal/L.

Intravenous fat emulsions should be used to provide from 15 to 40 per cent of the desired calories. Intravenous lipid emulsions are available in 10 per cent or 20 per cent solutions and are rendered isotonic with 2.5 per cent glycerol. The fat and glycerol contribute to a caloric density of 1.1 kcal/mL in the 10 per cent solution.

Electrolytes, vitamins, and trace elements may be added individually or as premixed solutions. The quantities necessary to maintain normal serum levels vary widely. During anabolism, large requirements for potassium, phosphate, and magnesium are often apparent. Serum levels should be monitored frequently, particularly in the face of extraordinary initial deficiencies or ongoing losses. The recommended maintenance quantities may be insufficient to correct deficiencies.

Carbohydrate infusion during TPN stimulates a subphysiologic insulin response compared to that associated with enteral feeding. Resultant hyperglycemia may progress to dehydration, hyperosmolarity, and coma unless corrected by insulin added directly to the solution. In the patient with respiratory insufficiency, and excessive glucose load can cause hypercapnia due to increased CO_2 production. Conversely, reactive hypoglycemia may occur within 1 to 2 hours after abrupt cessation of a glucose-rich TPN solution, since the physiologic half-life of insulin (1 to 2 hours) exceeds that of the infused glucose.

Reversible hepatic fatty infiltration and mild hepatocellular enzyme elevation may be caused by glucose administration in excess of oxidative capacity, phosphate deficiency, or protein excess. Cholestasis and cholelithiasis may develop in as many as one third of long-term home TPN patients.

Metabolic bone disease, typically osteomalacia, also complicates the course of long-term TPN patients. Vitamin D levels are usually normal. Hypercalciuria accompanying amino acid infusions may be the cause.

BIBLIOGRAPHY

1. Alpers, D.H., Clouse, R.E., and Stenson, W.F.: Manual of Nutritional Therapeutics. Boston, Little, Brown and Co., 1988.
2. Reilly, J.J., and Gerhardt, A.L.: Modern surgical nutrition. Curr. Prob. Surg., 22:18–19, 1985.
3. Schlichtig, R., and Ayrea, S.M. Nutritional Support of the Critically Ill. Chicago, Year Book Medical Publishers, Inc., 1988.
4. Kinney, J.M., Jeejeebhoy, K.N., Hill, G.L., and Owen, O.E.: Nutrition and Metabolism in Patient Care. Philadelphia, W.B. Saunders Co., 1988.

28

RADIOLOGY

CARL R. FUHRMAN

RADIATION: GENERAL CONCEPTS AND BASIC CONSIDERATIONS

X-rays are a form of electromagnetic radiation first discovered by Wilhelm Conrad Roentgen in 1895. As with any type of electromagnetic radiation, there are observed properties that necessitate consideration of this form of energy as both waves and particles.

Electromagnetic radiation travels in a vacuum as a wave, maintaining a constant velocity, which is the speed of light. A wave is always characterized by its frequency and wavelength. This is expressed in the equation:

$$c \text{ (velocity of light)} = \text{wavelength (meters)} \times \text{frequency (per seconds)} \quad \text{(Eq. 1)}$$

X-rays differ from ordinary visible light only by differences in frequency and wavelength. The wavelengths of x-rays are very much smaller than visible light, which permits x-rays to pass through a patient and to be recorded by an imaging device.

Electromagnetic waves that have very short wavelengths, such as x-rays, have certain features that are best explained if the electromagnetic radiation is considered as a beam of separate particles of energy, rather than as waves. This is a very complex topic that is the basis of quantum physics. These discrete particles of energy are known as photons, and they also travel at the speed of light. The energy of each of these photons is directly proportional to the frequency of the electromagnetic radiation as defined by the equation:

$$E = \text{(Planck's constant)} \times \text{frequency} \quad \text{(Eq. 2)}$$

X-rays are considered a form of ionizing radiation since the photons of high frequency x-rays have enough energy to eject electrons from atoms with which they interact.

The original unit of measurement for dose was the *roentgen* (R), which was defined as the quantity of x-rays or gamma rays necessary to produce 2.58×10^{-4} coulombs/kg of air at standard conditions. This unit of measurement was limited to x- and gamma rays and could not be used for high-energy radiation. The *rad* was later introduced as a measurement of absorbed dose. It could be used for all forms of radiation and did not depend on measurement in air as did the roentgen. It was particularly useful for measurements in biologic tissues. For practical purposes in diagnostic radiology, 1 (R) ≈ 1 rem in soft tissues for x-rays used in routine diagnostic procedures. Such a simplification is not applicable for the high-energy x-rays used in radiation therapy. By international agreement, the Système Internationale (SI) has been adopted in which the unit of radiation is measured by the *Gray* (Gy) with 1 Gy = 100 rads. Although the SI units are currently used in most scientific publications, rad units are still more commonly used in daily practice in most radiology departments in the United States. The term *rem* is used as a dose-equivalent unit of measurement since the biologic effect of the same dose of radiation may differ when different forms of radiation are used. This is expressed by the equation;

$$\text{rem} = \text{rads} \times \text{quality factor} \quad \text{(Eq. 3)}$$

The quality factor for x-rays is 1. The quality factor for protons, for example, is approximately 5. Therefore, the biologic absorbed dose for irradiation with a proton source is on the order of five times the absorbed dose with standard x-rays for the exact same dose in rads. Since relatively low-energy X-rays are used in diagnostic procedures, the following equation can be used as a practical guide to the often confusing measurements of radiation dose.

$$1 \text{ (R)} \approx 1 \text{ rad} = 1 \text{ rem} = 0.01 \text{ Gy} \quad \text{(Eq. 4)}$$

Patient doses from various radiographic procedures differ greatly. The mean skin dose/film (in rads) for various diagnostic exams are listed in Table 28–1. As there are considerable variations dependent upon equipment used, film speed, patient size, beam collimation, fluoroscopic time, and beam filtration these values are only meant to represent estimated typical doses. Gonadal doses are of special consideration in patients of reproductive age and can be considerably higher in women because of the intrapelvic position of the ovaries.

TABLE 28–1. MEAN SKIN DOSE/FILM FOR DIAGNOSTIC EXAMINATIONS

EXAMINATION	MEAN SKIN DOSE/FILM (RADS)	GONADAL DOSE/EXAM Male (rads)	GONADAL DOSE/EXAM Female
Chest	0.05–0.10		
Abdomen KUB	0.5–1.0	0.1	0.2
Mammography	0.6–1.0		
Lumbar spine	1.0–2.5	0.2	0.7
Barium enema	0.6–1.0	0.3	1.7

There are strict recommendations on the maximum permissible doses for medical personnel exposed to radiation. Radiation detectors (film badges or other devices) should always be worn by occupationally exposed individuals. Monthly readings are obtained to ensure that maximum permissible doses are not exceeded.

PRINCIPLES OF IMAGING TECHNIQUES

Conventional Radiography

Despite the many impressive advancements in diagnostic imaging technologies in the last several decades, conventional radiography remains the most commonly used imaging procedure. It is almost universally available, generally reliable, and relatively inexpensive. It is well suited for most common diagnostic problems and is adaptable for portable use at the bedside or in the operating room.

X-rays are produced in a vacuum tube. A beam of electrons is generated in a filament at the cathode end of the x-ray tube and is rapidly accelerated to a tungsten target at the anode end of the tube. The rapid deceleration of the electrons as they hit the target causes the emission of low wavelength electromagnetic waves known as x-rays. Since the wavelength of light is inversely proportional to its frequency (frequency × wavelength = speed of light) and as the energy of an electromagnetic wave is directly proportional to its frequency, these high frequency x-rays have much more energy than visible or ultraviolet light and are therefore capable of penetrating body tissues.

The high energies necessary for x-ray production are provided by generators. One inherent limitation of portable x-ray machines is their inability to produce the high energies that are obtainable with the standard generators available in the radiology department.

The x-rays that leave the tube are collimated by lead restrictors to limit excessive patient radiation and to decrease scatter radiation, which degrades image quality by blackening the x-ray film without providing anatomic information. The x-ray beam that leaves the tube is also filtered to remove its low-energy portion. Patient dose is decreased by beam filtration since the low-energy photons that are excluded are unlikely to exit the patient (and thus expose the film) and would only be deposited in the skin and subcutaneous tissues, resulting in a higher absorbed patient dose without providing any diagnostic information.

The x-ray photons used in diagnostic radiology can react with matter in the patient in two important ways: the photoelectric effect and Compton scattering. In the photoelectric effect an incident x-ray photon is energetic enough to eject an electron from the inner-shell electrons (K shell) of an atom. The x-ray photon disappears, giving all of its energy to the ejected electron, which is now known as a photoelectron. This photoelectron will travel only a very short distance since atomic particles have little penetrating power, and it will deposit all of its energy in adjacent tissue, which will result in a major contribution to patient dose. An electron from one of the outer electron shells of the atom will immediately fall to the lower-energy K shell to replace the ejected electron. As it falls to the lower-energy K shell, this electron will lose some of its energy, which will be emitted as characteristic radiation. Atoms with high atomic numbers are more likely to undergo a photoelectric interaction with an x-ray photon. This is the most common interaction of x-ray photons with contrast agents, such as barium and iodine.

The other major interaction of x-rays with matter in clinical radiology is Compton scattering. In this interaction the x-ray photon strikes an outer-shell electron and ejects it from the atom. The x-ray photon does not disintegrate as in the photoelectric interaction, but rather gives up some of its energy to provide kinetic energy for the ejected electron. The remainder of its energy is retained by the incident x-ray photon, which is now deflected in a different direction as scatter radiation. It will carry no diagnostic information if it leaves the patient and strikes the x-ray film. Compton scatter not only degrades film quality because of scatter but it can also be a major safety hazard to operating room personnel during fluoroscopic examinations using a C-arm intensifier. The scatter radiation that results from Compton interactions can be almost as energetic as the primary beam and can be a significant source of radiation exposure to the operator and other exposed personnel. Caution must always be used during fluoroscopy to ensure that adequate collimation is used that allows only the minimal field size necessary for diagnostic information and that appropriate shielding is used by all exposed personnel.

The x-ray photons that exit the patient contain anatomic information, as well as the randomly directed scatter photons. A grid device containing thin lead strips is often placed between the patient and the film to absorb the scattered x-rays. The perpendicularly directed diagnostic photons pass between the lead strips to carry anatomic information to the x-ray film cassette. This grid can move to prevent the annoying lead lines that would otherwise be present on the film. A grid improves radiographic contrast and image resolution by removing scatter radiation, but does require a higher initial dose of x-ray photons and thus results in a higher patient dose. This increased patient dose is usually justified by the resultant improvement in the x-ray images. Most portable examinations cannot be done with moving grids, which results in poorer image quality that is particularly noticeable in larger patients. Portable abdominal examinations suffer from relatively long exposure times necessitated by the portable equipment, as well as the large amounts of scatter radiation. They are never of the same diagnostic quality as those obtained in the department with stationary equipment. This is less of a problem with portable chests unless the patient is very large.

The actual x-ray film is enclosed in a cassette between two light-emitting screens. The x-ray photons that passed through the grid are absorbed by the material in the screens, which in turn emit multiple photons of lower-energy visible light for each x-ray photon that strikes the screen. It is this visible light emitted from the intensifying screens, and not the actual x-ray photons, that actually exposes the x-ray film. The silver emulsion of the x-ray film chemically interacts with these light photons to produce a latent image on the film. The film is chemically developed, fixed, washed, and dried and is then ready for viewing. Many different film-screen combinations are commercially available to satisfy the requirements of any particular examination. Faster film-screen combinations result in a decreased patient dose, although there is always some loss of image sharpness related to the larger silver halide grains used in the manufacture of these faster films.

Xeroradiography

Xeroradiography differs from conventional radiography in the design of the x-ray detector. Instead of using a film-screen combination, an electrically charged material known as a photoconductor is used. Photoconductors can only conduct an electrical current when they are exposed to x-rays. After the charged cassette is exposed to x-rays, an electrostatic latent image is retained on the plate. Tiny electrically charged blue particles known as toner are used during the development process, which accounts for the standard appearance of xeroradiographs. A unique advantage of the xeroradiographic system is the intrinsic edge enhancement that results from the application of the electrically charged toner to the exposed plate. This resultant edge enhancement is particularly advantageous for tissues with low intrinsic tissue contrast, such as breasts, and can also be used in the detection of foreign bodies in soft tissues. Microcalcifications that occur in breast diseases are particularly well seen because of this edge enhancement effect. Xeromammography usually requires a higher patient dose than most modern film-screen mammographic techniques, and many institutions have switched to film-screen systems in recent years.

Tomography

During tomography an x-ray tube moves in one direction while the film moves in an opposite direction at the same speed as the tube. This results in a plane of tissue being left in focus while the tissues above and below it are blurred. Tomography is frequently necessary in examination such as intravenous pyelography in which overlying bowel can obscure optimal visualization of the kidneys. Tomography can involve either a linear or complex motion (trispiral or hypocycloidal), depending on the brand of equipment and the requirements necessitated by the examination being performed. Tomography does not really improve radiographic resolution. It only allows the intrinsic detail of the area of interest to be better seen by obscuring the tissues in front of and below the section plane.

Ultrasonography

Ultrasonography has some unique advantages over other imaging modalities and does not involve the use of ionizing radiation. An ultrasound beam is produced in a piezoelectric crystal located in the head of an ultrasound transducer. The beam is then directed into the patient's body where it interacts with tissue interfaces. Some of the sound waves are reflected back to the transducer where they transmit their energy back to the same crystal from which they originated. In this way the ultrasound transducer functions as both the source of the ultrasound beam and the receiver for echoes that are reflected from tissue interactions in the patient's body. The energy from the returning echoes is converted to an electrical signal that can be corrected for the time and depth of the reflective tissue source. This information is then processed electronically to produce a two-dimensional image for display.

The ultrasound beam can be focused to allow sharper resolution at various depths within the body. The intensity of the ultrasound beam must be strong enough to allow adequate depth penetration, but the original beam does not itself contribute to image production. The image is produced only by that portion of the beam that is reflected back to the transducer. Some of the initial beam will be absorbed and converted to heat within the patient, and some will also be refracted, which results in a bending of the sound wave as it passes from one medium to another. When the primary beam meets a soft tissue-air interface, almost the entire beam is reflected back to the transducer so that none of the original beam is left to penetrate beyond the air interface. This is the reason that bowel gas interferes with the evaluation of the soft tissues beyond it. A similar process will occur with bone, metal, and other very dense interfaces. This principle also explains the common appearance of gallstones in which the strongly reflective echogenic interfaces essentially stop the ultrasound beam, with the reflected sound waves making the gallstones appear as strongly echogenic foci. No echoes are seen beyond the gallstones, and this is referred to as acoustical shadowing. Interaction with highly reflective structures, such as the diaphragm, results in a bright curvilinear echogenic focus appearing on the final image, but it does not reflect the entire beam back to the transducer and will allow for the visualization of a pleural effusion above the diaphragm if one is present. The homogeneous nature and lack of interfaces in liquids, such as are encountered in the urine-filled bladder, cysts, and the gallbladder, allow most of the beam to be transmitted through them with very little of the beam being reflected back to the transducer. This makes these structures appear as echo-free areas on the final image. This appearance can totally change depending on the nature of the fluid. An abscess can be completely liquid, but its inhomogeneous consistency may produce many echogenic interfaces that can make the collection appear solid on the final image. Conversely, the homogeneous cellular arrangements in some lymphomas can allow near-complete transmission of the beam because of lack of echogenic interfaces. Thus, they produce a nearly hypo-echoic image that can look similar to a cyst on the final image.

Many newer ultrasound machines are now equipped with Doppler capabilities that allow the determination of flow and direction of flow within vessels. Doppler technology is based on the physical principle that there will be a shift in the perceived frequency of sound when it is emitted by a moving source, such as blood within a vessel. The difference in frequency shift will allow the determination of the direction of blood flow. Continuous-wave Doppler is particularly well suited for superficial vessels, such as the carotid arteries or arteries of the feet. The frequency shift can be audibly detected by the examiner after appropriate amplification. Pulsed Doppler is better suited for evaluation of deep vessels, but is considerably more expensive than the equipment for continuous-wave Doppler. Pulsed Doppler allows the determination of the depth of the Doppler shift signal, as well as flow. This capability is very useful in determining vascular patency in transplant patients and can be crucial in the distinction between a simple cyst and a pseudoaneurysm, which can have identical appearances on conventional ultrasound images.

Color-flow Doppler allows detection of both flow and depth simultaneously and displays the image in shades of red and blue. The choice of colors is not meant to necessarily represent arterial or venous flow, but merely to indicate the direction of flow with respect to the ultrasound transducer.

Extracorporeal shock-wave lithotripsy (ESWL) is currently being used for biliary and renal calculus disease. High-pressure shock waves are created and are acoustically focused and directed to the area of interest. Considerable care must be taken to ensure the accurate localization of the stones to be disintegrated since these high-power shock waves can injure adjacent tissues. Delayed renal hypertension has been reported in up to 8 per cent of patients treated with renal lithotripsy. These high-pressure ultrasound waves are created by one of three methods in currently available equipment: (1) spark-gap discharge, (2) electromagnetic shock wave, or (3) piezoelectric crystal. Some units require the patient to be submerged in a water bath during the procedure, although most gallstone lithotripsers do not. Oral cholecystography is now often used before the procedure to better document the number and size of the stones, as well as the ability of the gallbladder to function. The early results from gallstone lithotripsy suggest that 90 per cent of patients with one or two nonopaque gallstones and a functioning gallbladder will be successfully treated with few complications. The role of ESWL in gallstone disease compared to surgical or medical therapeutic alternatives is presently under active investigation.

Computed Tomography

Computed tomography has revolutionized the field of radiology and has significantly changed the practice of medicine in the last decade. The theoretical basis for computed tomography is the premise that the internal composition and structure of any object can be determined by measuring the amount of x-rays absorbed by the object when it is radiographed in multiple projections. Most scanners now use a ring of x-ray detectors to surround the patient within a doughnut-shaped structure known as the gantry. An x-ray tube rotates around the patient, and the transmitted x-rays that leave the patient are detected by each detector in the ring. The x-ray detectors usually contain compressed xenon gas, which functions as a type of ionization chamber that can measure radiation. These detectors are connected to photomultiplier tubes that allow the detected x-ray energies to be proportionally converted into electrical signals that are then transmitted to a computer. Using very complicated mathematics the computer allows the image to be reconstructed using a series of complex computer algorithms. Such complicated calculations would be impossible without high-speed computers. Each CT slice is divided into multiple tiny squares known as pixels. A separate linear attenuation number (a measurement of x-ray absorption in the patient) is calculated by the computer for each pixel. The attenuation number for water is arbitrarily assigned a value of zero, and the attenuation numbers can range from -2000 to $+2000$ on most scanners. These CT numbers are also referred to as Hounsfield units in honor of the developer of CT. On this scale bone usually measures around $+500$ and air around -500. Since fat is less dense than water it measures around -50, and most soft tissue structures measure in the range between $+25$ and $+80$.

CT allows excellent anatomic resolution, which is directly related to its ability to detect very small density differences between contiguous anatomic structures. Within the brain the CT attenuation of gray and white matter differs by only about 5 Hounsfield numbers, but this small difference is readily perceptible on modern scanners. CT also provides potential insight into the composition of a structure by its CT number. For example, the detection of fat density within a solid renal mass will allow a confident diagnosis of angiomyolipoma to be made. Oral and intravenous contrast agents are frequently used during CT examinations to enhance intrinsic contrast differences and allow accurate identification of vessels and bowel.

Magnetic Resonance Imaging

Magnetic resonance imaging uses no ionizing radiation. The patient is placed in a strong magnetic field within the scanner. A basic principle of nuclear physics is that atomic nuclei that have an odd number of protons, neutrons, or combined protons and neutrons have a property known as nuclear spin (or angular momentum) and behave like small magnets when placed in a strong magnetic field. This nuclear spin is a vector with both direction and magnitude. Outside of a strong magnetic field the direction of these vectors is random, resulting in no net magnetization. When placed in a strong magnetic field, almost all of these dipole vectors align with the magnetic field and precess (rotate about an axis like a spinning top) with a frequency that is directly proportional to the external magnetic field. It is the hydrogen nucleus that is clinically used for imaging during MRI since it yields a strong MRI signal and is the most abundant paramagnetic substance in the human body. Cortical bone, which has few paramagnetic hydrogen nuclei, are not influenced by the magnetic field and thus do not produce an MRI signal but appear as a black signal void on the final images.

A radiofrequency pulse (a radio wave) is then applied to the patient, and this transfers energy into the patient and causes perturbations in the precessions of the hydrogen nuclei dipoles within the magnetic field. When the pulse is terminated, the dipoles lose energy as they return to their original lower energy state (a process known as relaxation). This release of energy is detected as the MRI signal, which is used to construct an image. The relaxation rates differ depending on the hydrogen nuclei concentration and thus the composition of the tissue. Two components of relaxation known as T1 and T2 can be measured and vary for different body tissues. Numerous pulsing sequences are possible and differ for various examinations. An image that is "T1 weighted" uses image parameters to produce an image in which contrast between tissues is mainly related to the T1 relaxation differences of the tissues, whereas a "T2 weighted" image produces an image dependent on the intrinsic differences of the T2 relaxation properties of the tissues. For example, CSF appears black on a T1 image and white on a T2 image. Flowing blood is usually devoid of signal since the radiofrequency-pulsed blood quickly passes out of the scan slice and is thus unavailable for measurement of relaxation parameters that produce the MRI signal. The ability to detect flowing blood without the use of contrast or ionizing radiation is a distinct advantage of MRI. This modality has been proven to be excellent for evaluation of brain, spine, and spinal cord. MRI provides superb soft tissue and bone information in evaluation of tumors, marrow disorders, and musculoskeletal disease. Applications in the thorax and upper abdomen usually necessitate the use of cardiac and respiratory gating to decrease the motion artifacts associated with the long scan times necessary to acquire an image. MRI imanges can be directly obtained in any anatomic plane, and this imaging advantage may be particularly useful in such areas as the pelvis where direct coronal sections offer a perspective that is not possible with typical axial CT images. Gadolinium, which is a paramagnetic agent, can be injected intravenously as a contrast agent for MRI and results in improved detection and characterization of many lesions.

CONTRAST MATERIALS FOR RADIOLOGY

Contrast agents are used in diagnostic radiology to facilitate the differentiation of normal and abnormal anatomic structures from surrounding tissues with similar intrinsic radiographic densities. This differentiation is usually achieved by the administration of compounds with high atomic numbers since these elements will more likely undergo photoelectric interactions with the incident x-ray photons. This use of such compounds results in an improvement in tissue contrast and a superior quality radiograph because of the decrease in scatter radiation. The elements, iodine (atomic number 53) and barium (atomic number 56), are the usual contrast agents used in diagnostic radiology. Use of these contrast agents significantly increases the absorbed patient dose. Patient doses from barium enemas and excretory urograms are among the highest in diagnostic radiology; a abdominal radiograph with barium in the bowel results in a higher patient dose than one without barium in the bowel.

Barium sulfate is a biologically inert substance that has been used for gastrointestinal studies since the earliest days of radiology. Numerous additives are present in commercial preparations to ensure an adequately uniform suspension. High-density preparations are used to provide adequate mucosal coating for air-contrast studies of the esophagus, stomach, small bowel, and colon. Dilute barium sulfate suspensions are generally used for routine single-contrast gastrointestinal studies. The use of barium is contraindicated in the presence of a suspected visceral perforation. Oral barium has the potential to form concretions in the colon because of water absorption proximal to a segment of complete colonic obstruction. Barium aspiration is generally well tolerated and clears in several days with adequate pulmonary toilet. Rarely a patient may have an idiosyncratic allergy to an additive or flavoring compound used in the preparation of the commercially available barium products.

Oral cholecystography has largely been replaced by biliary ultrasound, but has regained some importance with the development of biliary lithotripsy. Iopanoic acid (Telepaque) contains three iodine atoms substituted on a phenolphthalein ring. Minor other substitutions are the basis for the other commercially available compounds. The contrast agent must be absorbed across the gastrointestinal mucosa, transported by the portal circulation to the liver, conjugated by the liver, excreted in the bile, and finally concentrated in the gallbladder. Vicarious excretion by the kidneys may occur, especially in the presence of hepatic dysfunction. Failure of visualization of the gallbladder may be related to any of the above biologic steps. Nausea, vomiting, and diarrhea are common minor side effects. A rare serious complication is nephrotoxicity of uncertain etiology. Intravenous cholangiography using iodipamide (Cholograffin) for the post cholecystectomy patient carries a significant risk of serious allergic reaction and has generally been replaced by other imaging procedures.

Water-soluble contrast agents for the gastrointestinal tract are indicated whenever there is suspicion of perforation or closed-loop small bowel obstruction, for upper intestinal studies in the presence of large bowel obstruction, for the demonstration of fistulas and sinus tracts, and for the evaluation of anastomotic leaks in the postoperative period. Sodium diatrizoate (Hypaque) is generally used for enema studies since it is considerably cheaper, whereas flavored diatrizoate methylglucamine (Gastrograffin) is usually used for the esophagus and upper intestinal studies. These agents are strongly hypertonic and draw fluid from the circulation into the bowel lumen.

This can result in circulatory collapse, particularly in dehydrated elderly patients and infants, and careful evaluation of the fluid and electrolyte status of the patient must be done before the examination is started. For this reason, some institutions are beginning to use the newer and more expensive low-osmolality intravenous contrast agents for gastrointestinal studies in critically ill infants and children. Diagnostic-quality Hypaque enemas are usually possible, but because of the dilutional effect of the hypertonic contrast, adequate visualization of the small bowel beyond the jejunum is often not achieved with Gastrograffin and the mucosal detail is never as good as with barium. Considerable caution must be used in the evaluation of esophageal perforations if communication to the tracheobronchial tree is suspected since Gastrograffin aspirated into the lung can result in fulminant pulmonary edema and death. Allergic reactions to oral contrast agents are rare.

Diagnostic bronchography is rarely performed since the development of flexible fiberoptic bronchoscopy and computed tomography. Various iodized oils are commercially available, and the most commonly used agents are aqueous or oily suspensions of Dionisil. They are usually well tolerated and safe and are rapidly cleared from the lung by mucociliary function and absorption.

There are numerous intravascular contrast agents that are commercially available. They are used for arteriography, venography, excretory urography, arthrography, sialography, percutaneous cholangiography, endoscopic retrograde cholangiopancreatography, hysterosalpingography, and seminal vesiculography. They are extensively used in computed tomography for evaluation of vascular anatomy and abnormalities, as well as for enhancement of both normal and abnormal tissues.

Intravascular contrast media can be divided into two broad categories: ionic and non-ionic compounds. Common commercial varieties of ionic contrast use a cation of either sodium or meglumine or a combination of both and anions of either diatrizoate or iothalamate. Osmolality is hypertonic for most ionic contrast agents, which can have osmolalities as high as 2938 mosm/kg (Hypaque-M, 90 per cent). There are nearly 40 different commercial products currently available, and the iodine percentage in solution can vary from 24 to 90 depending on the intended use of the product. The higher iodine concentration products are generally needed for arteriography. A new ionic contrast agent known as ioxaglate (Hexabrix), which has low osmolality, has been shown to decrease the pain and heat associated with the intra-arterial injections of the usual ionic compounds.

Metrizamide (Amnipaque) was the first non-ionic compound introduced in the 1970s for myelography. It has been largely replaced by two newer non-ionic compounds, iohexol (Omnipaque) and iopamidol (Isovue). These non-ionic contrast agents have the added advantage of low osmolality and are associated with a significant decrease in adverse reactions and patient discomfort. However, they are considerably more expensive (by a factor of 10 to 20 times) than standard ionic agents. Most radiology departments have developed some guidelines for the use of these more expensive non-ionic compounds. Generally accepted indications include a history of prior allergic reaction or allergies, asthma, renal impairment, multiple myeloma, diabetes, young infants and elderly patients, pre-existing cardiopulmonary disease, and cerebral disease associated with disruption of the blood-brain barrier.

Contrast reactions occur more frequently from intravenous injections than from intra-arterial administration. Mild reactions—nausea and vomiting, injection pain, urticaria, and mild dyspnea—can occur in up to 5 per cent of patients and are probably related at least in part to the hyperosmolality of most ionic compounds. More severe reactions—urticaria, bronchospasm, and transient hypotension—occur in up to 2 per cent of patients and generally require treatment with epinephrine, antihistamines, or even steroids. Life-threatening reactions—cardiopulmonary arrest, laryngospasm, angina, prolonged hypotension, myocardial infarction, or seizure—occur in less than 1 per cent of patients with the use of standard ionic contrast agents, and death rates as high as 1 in 40,000 administrations have been reported. The risk of death after use of non-ionic compounds has been reported to be three times lower than with ionics and may be even ten times lower in some high-risk groups.

Intravascular contrast should never be administered unless appropriate medical personnel and equipment are readily available for immediate resuscitation. Patients with a prior history of allergic reaction are usually premedicated before the procedure and are generally given non-ionic contrast. The renal dysfunction associated with contrast is dose-related, and typically an examination should generally not exceed a limit of 40 gm of iodine in an adult. This upper limit may need to be adjusted because of age, impaired renal function, or patient size.

The use of lymphangiography has declined markedly since the development of newer cross-sectional imaging modalities. An intradermal injection of blue dye is made between the toes (or fingers for upper extremity studies) to allow visualization of the tiny lymphatic channels. A lymph vessel is cannulated with a tiny needle, and an iodized oil (Ethiodol) is injected into the peripheral lymphatic channel. This results in the accumulation of the contrast in the lymphatics and nodal chains. Excess contrast is drained into the systemic venous system by the thoracic duct. Minor oil embolization often occurs and is usually well tolerated, but can cause morbidity and even death, particularly in patients with underlying lung disease. Central nervous system embolization is very rare, but can result in serious CNS dysfunction

and death. To prevent these complications, most radiographers use intermittent filming or fluoroscopy to terminate the injection of contrast after it has reached the upper lumbar lymph nodes. A low-grade fever is common after the procedure, which may be related to embolized oil in the lungs.

Several contrast agents are available for myelography. Pantopaque (iophendylate), an iodized oil made from poppy seeds, has been used for many years. It is very dense, and the contrast column can be manipulated to the appropriate position in the spinal canal by tilting the table. Its high contrast density generally obscures the spinal nerves and makes it unacceptable as an intrathecal contrast agent for computed tomography. It is generally removed at the end of the examination because of the possible later complication of arachnoiditis. Its use as a contrast agent has generally been discarded in favor of the newer non-ionic compounds that do not need to be removed at the end of the examination. In addition, postmyelography CT has become an important addition to the routine myelogram and can be satisfactorily performed with the non-ionic contrast agents. Iohexol is the agent generally used for myelographic studies at this time. It is usually well tolerated and generally considered safe. Special caution must be used in patients who are taking medications that can lower seizure threshold. Headache, nausea, and vomiting can occur after the study, but are generally self-limited. Seizures and other serious complications are rare.

Magnevist (gadopentetate dimeglumine) has been introduced as an intravenous contrast agent for magnetic resonance imaging. It is a paramagnetic agent that allows excellent visualization of intracranial lesions and can be helpful in the differentiation of recurrent herniated disc from scar. It is considered safe, and the most significant adverse reaction is transient headache.

RADIOISOTOPES IN IMAGING

A nuclide refers to any atomic nucleus characterized by its atomic number (number of protons), atomic mass (number of protons and neutrons), and its energy state. Almost all radionuclides used in nuclear medicine are artificially produced in either cyclotrons or nuclear reactors. Isotopes are groups of radionuclides that have the same atomic number (i.e., number of protons), but differ in the number of neutrons within the nucleus. An isotope may be either stable or unstable. If there is an imbalance between the numbers of protons and neutrons within the nucleus, the isotope is likely to decay to a more stable energy state. Nuclear decay results in either an energetically more stable isomeric state of the parent compound or a totally new element. The rate of decay determines the half-life of an isotope, which is the amount of time necessary for one half of any isotope to decay to a lower energy state. Detection of the energy released during decay is the basis for clinical nuclear medicine. During decay an isotope may emit high-energy particles, such as alpha particles (helium nuclei), electrons, or positrons (positively charged electrons), which travel very short distances and deposit their energy in the patient. These emitted particles provide no diagnostic information and contribute in a large degree to the radiation dose received by the patient during the procedure. Most of clinical nuclear medicine depends on the detection of the gamma rays (high-energy photons of light) that are emitted during isotope decay. These gamma rays must be of sufficiently high energy to exit the patient's body and be detected by a collimated camera detection device.

Nuclear medicine differs from conventional radiology in that the patient acts as the radiation source after injection or ingestion of an appropriate isotope. The distribution of the isotope within the patient can be directly related to the physiology of the element itself (e.g., radioactive iodine accumulates within the thyroid) or to the distribution of a pharmaceutical compound to which an isotope has been attached as a tracer, e.g., a radioactive isotope of technetium attached to albumin that will accumulate in the precapillary arterioles of the lungs after injection into the peripheral venous system. Nuclear medicine images provide both anatomic and physiologic information. Only minute amounts of the radiopharmaceuticals are needed, and allergic reactions are virtually nonexistent. Patient dose is related to the site of accumulation of the isotope (the "target organ"), the half-life of the isotope, and the mechanism of physiologic clearance. As an example, the usual dose of ingested I-131 for a thyroid scan is 50 to 80 μCi. The isotope has a half-life of 8.1 days, and the whole body dose to the patient is approximately 0.04 rads, with an absorbed dose to the thyroid ranging from 25 to 150 rads depending on the actual uptake by the gland. Larger doses can be given for therapeutic ablation of the gland, and in those cases considerable care must be taken to ensure the safe disposal of body wastes and to avoid possible contamination of hospital personnel and family members. Such therapy is usually monitored under the close supervision of the nuclear medicine physician and radiation safety officer.

Usual caution must be taken to ensure that an examination is not accidentally performed on a pregnant patient; that employees are not exposed to the patients' readioactive excrement, blood, and body fluids; and that any areas of possible contamination be reported immediately to the radiation safety officer. Appropriate lead shielding is necessary for the preparation and storage of the radioactive compounds within the department.

The most commonly used isotope in daily practice is the metastable isotope of technetium (Tc-99m). It is readily available since it can be eluted from a generator within the department on a daily basis. The generator is usually replaced on a weekly or biweekly basis. This isotope decays by isomeric transition to Tc-99, a more stable energy state of the same isotope, and emits a single gamma ray that has a photon energy peak that is ideal for imaging. Its half-life is only 6 hours, which considerably decreases the absorbed dose to the patient. It can be injected as free technetium (99mTc-sodium pertechnetate) and will accumulate in the salivary glands, thyroid, and gastric mucosa. This agent can be used clinically for thyroid scans; its localization in the thyroid is dependent only on the trapping of the isotope and not on the organification necessary with iodine isotopes. It is also used for the localization of ectopic gastric mucosa in Meckel's diverticulum and for vascular perfusion studies in cases of suspected testicular torsion.

The technetium isotope is frequently tagged to other pharmaceutical preparations for organ-specific types of scans. It can be attached to sulfur colloid for liver-spleen and bone marrow scans, DTPA for glomerular clearance renal function studies, macroaggregated albumin for lung perfusion, various phosphate compounds for bone scans, iminodiacetic acid derivatives for biliary scans, and glucoheptonate for brain and kidney imaging. It may also be reduced with tin compounds and attached to red blood cells. This blood pool labeling is the basis for cardiac wall motion and ejection fraction studies, as well as for gastrointestinal bleeding studies. Technetium can also be combined with pyrophosphate for use in myocardial infarct scanning.

Two isotopes of iodine are commonly used. I-131 is inexpensive and readily available. It has a half-life of 8.1 days and emits a beta particle (electron) during its decay, which increases the absorbed patient dose. I-123 is considerably more expensive, has a half-life of 13.3 hours, and emits no particles during decay. It may not always be readily available since it is not produced in the department and cannot be stored for long periods because of its short half-life. It delivers a significantly decreased dose to the patient and is the preferred isotope for younger patients. Visualization of radioactive iodine isotopes in the thyroid is dependent on both the uptake and organification in the gland. Clinical applications include the evaluation of thyroid function, nodules, thyroiditis, and malignancies. High doses of I-131 are also used in the treatment of hyperthyroidism and some thyroid malignancies. Radioactive iodine can also be attached to hippuran for renal plasma flow studies and to fibrinogen for thrombus detection.

Nuclear medicine applications in the central nervous system have been largely replaced by CT and MRI. However, isotope cerebral angiography is still used at some institutions in the evaluation of brain death. Cysternography using 131-I HSA or 169-Yb-DTPA is occasionally still performed in the evaluation of normal pressure hydrocephalus, CSF rhinorrhea, and ventriculoperitoneal shunt function.

Radioactive xenon gas is used for ventilation studies and is usually done in combination with a lung perfusion scan for the detection of pulmonary embolus. Care must be taken to provide proper ventilation when using this agent since 133-Xe has a half-life of 5.3 days and can be a source of significant radiation exposure to department employees.

Gallium citrate is used for the detection of abscess, some tumors (notably melanoma and lymphomas), and the evaluation of some inflammatory processes in the lungs and kidneys, e.g., staging the activity of sarcoid lung disease. The mechanism of gallium localization in inflammatory and neoplastic cells is unclear. Gallium accumulates in the colon normally, which can detract from its usefulness in the search for abdominal abscesses. Leukocytes obtained from a patient can be selectively labeled in vitro with radioactive Indium and then re-injected into the same patient for evaluation of abscess and other inflammatory lesions.

Radioactive thallium behaves as a potassium analogue and is particularly useful for the evaluation of myocardial ischemia, but can also be used for parathyroid gland imaging. The adrenal can be imaged with various labeled cholesterol precursors (131 I-MIBG); this test can be very helpful for evaluation of pheochromocytomas not identified by CT or in patients with syndromes associated with multiple endocrine abnormalities that have a high incidence of pheochromocytomas. Isotopes have been increasingly used for the evaluation of gastrointestinal motility and esophageal reflux. Isotopes can also be instilled into the urinary bladder for evaluation of ureteral reflux, and these studies have a significantly decreased patient dose than conventional fluoroscopic studies. Radioactive phosphorus (P-32) is used only for the treatment of polycythemia vera. During its decay it emits electrons, but since it emits no gamma rays it cannot be used for conventional imaging.

The development of isotope-labeled monoclonal antibodies to various tumor markers, such as CEA, is an exciting new development for tumor detection and possible future therapy. Antibodies to purified tumor markers are produced in animals, labeled with a radioactive tracer, and then injected into patients. The localization of the tracer can be useful for staging of a malignancy, as well as for detection of metastases. It is particularly helpful in patients in whom the metastatic lesions may be too small to be detected by conventional imaging modalities, such as CT.

BIBLIOGRAPHY

Diagnostic Radiology

1. Curry, T.S., Dowdey, J.E., and Murry, R.C.: Christensen's Introduction to the Physics of Diagnostic Radiology, 4th ed. Philadelphia, Lea & Febiger, 1990.
2. Sprawls, P.: The Physical Principles of Diagnostic Radiology. Rockville, MD, Aspen Publications, 1987.
3. Pizzarello, D.J., and Witcofsky, R.L.: Medical Radiation Biology. Philadelphia, Lea & Febiger, 1982.
4. Hendee, W.R.: Medical Radiation Physics: Roentgenology, Nuclear Medicine & Ultrasound. Chicago, Year Book Medical Publishers, Inc., 1979.

Contrast Agents

1. Fischer, Harry W.: Catalog of intravascular contrast media. Radiology, 159:561–563, 1986.
2. Miller, Roscoe E., and Skucas, Jovitas.: Radiographic Contrast Agents. Baltimore, University Park Press, 1977.
3. Latchaw, Richard E.: Intravascular contrast agents: Guidelines for use. In Straub, W.E. (ed.): Manual of Diagnostic Imaging, 2nd ed. Boston, Little, Brown and Co., 1989, pp. 17–22.

Nuclear Medicine

1. Chandra, R.: Introductory Physics of Nuclear Medicine, 2nd ed. Philadelphia, Lea & Febiger, 1982.
2. Fogelman, I., and Maisey, M.: An Atlas of Clinical Nuclear Medicine. St. Louis, C.V. Mosby Co., 1988.
3. Iturralde, M.P.: Dictionary and Handbook of Nuclear Medicine and Clinical Imaging. Boca Raton, FL: CRC Press, 1990.

29

PRINCIPLES OF ANESTHESIOLOGY

CHARLES H. RICHARDS

In its 1990 *Booklet of Information,* the American Board of Anesthesiology defines the range of activities of anesthesiologists as (1) the assessment of, consultation for, and preparation of patients for anesthesia; (2) the provision of insensibility to pain during surgical, obstetric, therapeutic, and diagnostic procedures, and the management of patients so affected; (3) the monitoring and restoration of homeostasis during the perioperative period, as well as homeostasis in the critically ill, injured, or otherwise seriously ill patient; (4) the diagnosis and treatment of painful syndromes; (5) the clinical management and teaching of cardiac and pulmonary resuscitation; (6) the evaluation of respiratory function and application of respiratory therapy in all its forms; (7) the supervision, teaching, and evaluation of performance of both medical and paramedical personnel involved in anesthesia, respiratory, and critical care; (8) the conduct of research at the clinical and basic science levels to explain and improve the care of patients insofar as physiologic and the response to drugs are concerned; and (9) the administrative involvement in hospitals, medical schools, and outpatient facilities necessary to implement these responsibilities.

This chapter is a limited survey of principles pertinent to the practice of anesthesiology. The era of insufflation of volatile organic solvents with haphazard effects has now been supplanted by the metered and monitored administration of diverse agents. Astounding developments in monitoring and therapeutics enhance the precision of care, but do not supplant clinical acumen.

PHARMACOLOGY OF ANESTHETIC AGENTS

An enlightened practice of anesthesiology is founded upon an understanding of clinical pharmacology. Pharmacologic concepts and models enable the practitioner to design a rational anesthetic plan and to anticipate its effects. Pharmacodynamics and pharmacokinetics describe the effect and course of a drug.

Pharmacodynamics

Pharmacodynamics is the analysis of the relationship between the concentration of a drug and its effect. Simply stated, it is the effect of a drug on the body. Concentration-response relationships require measurement of the concentration of the drug at its site of action. These relationships are frequently described in terms of the concentration of the drug in the blood, which may not be equal to its concentration at its site of action. The effect of a drug is described in terms of its efficacy, potency, and selectivity. Efficacy is the maximum effect of a drug. Potency is the amount of a drug required to produce an effect. Selectivity is the relationship between a dose of a drug and the number of its effects. Dose-response curves graphically represent the efficacy and potency of a drug, with the slope of the curve depicting the increment in dose required to increase the effect (Fig. 29–1).

Receptor. A drug's pharmacodynamic properties are determined by its interaction with its site of action. For anesthetics, this site is often, but not always, a cell-membrane-bound protein or lipoprotein referred to as a receptor. The drug-receptor interaction is the first in a series of cellular events culminating in a physiologic response. Both the drug's concentration and physicochemical properties and the receptor's quantity and functional status contribute to the drug-receptor interaction. The development of new anesthetic drugs is facilitated by exploitation of the relationship between a drug's structure and its receptor-mediated effect.

Receptors cannot be invoked to explain all actions of drugs. Small molecule interactions (e.g., the che-

405

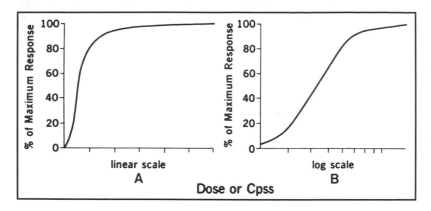

FIGURE 29–1. *A,* The relationship of drug dose or steady-state plasma concentration to percentage of maximal response plotted on a linear scale. *B,* The same relationship plotted on a logarithm scale. (Reprinted from Stanski, D.R., and Watkins, W.D.: Drug Disposition in Anesthesia. Orlando, FL, Grune and Stratton, Inc., 1982. Figure 1–12, p. 39.)

lation of Ca++ by citrate) and physicochemical mechanisms (e.g., osmotic effects of mannitol, membrane effects of volatile anesthetics) are examples of non-receptor-mediated effects observed during the course of an anesthetic.

Drug. A drug is any chemical agent that affects living processes. An agonist is a drug that activates a receptor. An antagonist binds to a receptor without activating it and thus prevents activation of the receptor by an agonist. Competitive antagonism is the activation or inhibition of a receptor by varying concentrations of the agonist and antagonist drugs. Noncompetitive antagonism is receptor inhibition by an antagonist drug that cannot be overcome by high concentrations of an agonist drug. This interplay of drugs at the receptor is the basis of several routine anesthetic techniques, e.g., reversal of both narcotic effects and neuromuscular blockade.

Pharmacokinetics

Pharmacokinetics is the analysis of the relationship between the dose of a drug and its concentration. The concentration of a drug is influenced by its absorption, biotransformation, distribution, and excretion.

Absorption. Absorption is influenced both by the drug's concentration and solubility and the absorption site's area and blood flow. Drug administration may be achieved by either enteral or parenteral administration. Parenteral administration encompasses intracompartmental injection, pulmonary absorption, and topical application. Compartments accessible to injection include the epidural, intrathecal, muscular, peritoneal, pleural, subcutaneous, and vascular spaces. Considerations involved in the selection of a route of administration include accuracy in achieving the desired concentration, availability of a suitable drug preparation, bioavailability, convenience, cost, patient cooperation, reliability in achieving and maintaining the desired effect, safety, and the urgency of the situation.

Distribution. Distribution is the movement of a drug between body compartments. The volume of distribution (Vd) has no direct anatomic or physiologic correlate, yet it is influenced by alterations in both anatomy and physiology. It is based on two assumptions. First, the body is considered to be a single compartment. Second, the drug is uniformly distributed within that compartment. Thus, Vd equals the total amount of drug in the body divided by the concentration of the drug in the plasma. Vd is used to compare the distribution of drugs, anticipate their dosing requirements, and predict the influence of disease processes. It is also useful in predicting drug clearance (see below).

The one-compartment model is the simplest model of drug distribution. It assumes the rapid and uniform distribution of an administered drug that is eliminated as modeled by exponential kinetics. In exponential kinetics, a rate constant (k) describes a proportional change per unit time. In pharmacokinetics, a commonly used k is the elimination half-life ($t_{1/2}$). It is the time elapsed for a 50 per cent reduction of the plasma concentration of a drug. This rate is independent of the drug's concentration and dose.

Clearance is the volume of a compartment that is cleared of drug per unit time. Total body clearance is the product of the Vd and the elimination rate constant.

The distribution of many anesthetic drugs is better represented by the two-compartment model. The plasma drug concentration has an initial rapid decline followed by a subsequent slower decline. The initial decrease in blood drug concentration is explained by the distribution of a drug from the plasma to the tissues. The subsequent slower decline in blood drug concentration is attributed to the more gradual elimination of the drug from the body (Fig. 29–2).

Elimination. Elimination is the irreversible loss of active drug. It is the sum of both drug excretion and metabolism. Anesthetic drug metabolism predominates in the liver and plasma, whereas anesthetic drug excretion occurs via the biliary tract, kidneys, and lungs. Disease processes affect elimination via altering clearance within the affected system and also by altering Vd.

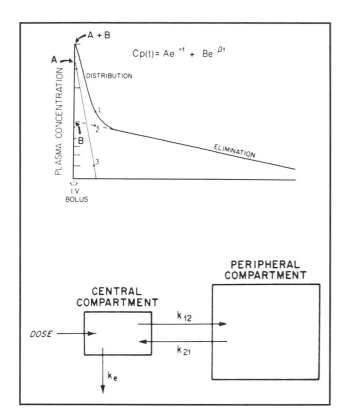

FIGURE 29–2. *Top,* The plasma concentration versus time curve for a drug with distribution and elimination phases. *Bottom,* A two-compartment pharmacokinetic model. (Reprinted from Stanski, D.R., and Watkins, W.D.: Drug Disposition in Anesthesia. Orlando, FL, Grune and Stratton, Inc., 1982. Figures 1–5 and 1–6, p. 13.)

ANESTHETIC AGENTS

General anesthesia is a controlled, drug-induced, reversible coma during which a patient is insensible to pain. A complete general anesthetic blocks mental, motor, sensory, and reflex activity. It is usually produced by a combination of drugs with variably selective effects (Fig. 29–3). This polypharmacy tends to limit both the dose-related side effects and the potential for toxicity of each drug. The effect of general anesthesia upon the central nervous system (CNS) is a depression of autonomic outflow, consciousness, and motor responses. Peripheral input to the CNS is also modulated. General anesthetic agents include both inhaled (gases and volatile liquids) and injected (barbiturates, benzodiazepines, etomidate, ketamine, opioids, and propofol) drugs. The selection of an anesthetic drug or technique is based on its utility in controlling certain aspects of a patient's physiology. This serves the frequently concomitant goals of making the surgeon's task easier and increasing the patient's tolerance for the simultaneous trespasses of illness and surgery.

Inhaled Anesthetics

Inhaled anesthetics (gases and volatile liquids) interact with hydrophobic lipids and proteins (Table 29–1). Their desired effects include sedation, analgesia, amnesia, and muscle relaxation (Fig. 29–4).

Nitrous oxide (N_2O), introduced early in the history of anesthesiology, is the only gas still in common use as a component of many general anesthetics. N_2O lacks potency, and it is associated with increased intracranial pressure; inhibition of methionine synthetase, polymorphonuclear leukocyte migration, and phagocytosis; myocardial depression; and expansion of gas-filled cavities. Nevertheless, it has retained its popularity because of its convenience and reliability in producing amnesic and analgesic effects. It is used to supplement other anesthetic agents and reduce their dose requirements.

The presently popular volatile liquid anesthetics are halothane (an alkane derivative) and enflurane and isoflurane (derivatives of methyl ethyl ether). The potency of volatile liquid anesthetics is expressed in terms of the minimum alveolar concentration (MAC). MAC is the partial pressure (at 1 atmosphere) of an inhaled anesthetic that prevents movement of skeletal muscle in response to skin incision in 50 per cent of subjects. MAC is a pharmacodynamic term used to compare the effects of volatile liquid anesthetics relative to their inspired concentrations. The range of potencies of enflurane (1

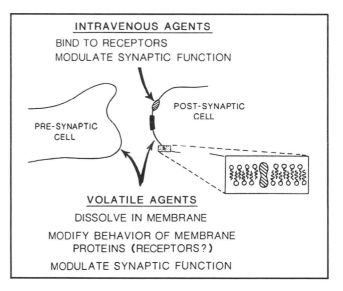

FIGURE 29–3. Anesthesia results from the reversible modulation of synaptic communication between neurons. Most intravenous agents bind to receptors and influence the effects of neurotransmitters. Volatile agents influence membrane function by causing physiocochemical changes within membrane lipids and proteins. (Reprinted from Barash, P.G., Cullen, B.F., and Stoelting, R.K. (eds.): Clinical Anesthesia. Philadelphia, J.B. Lippincott Co., 1989. Figure 10–6, p. 289.)

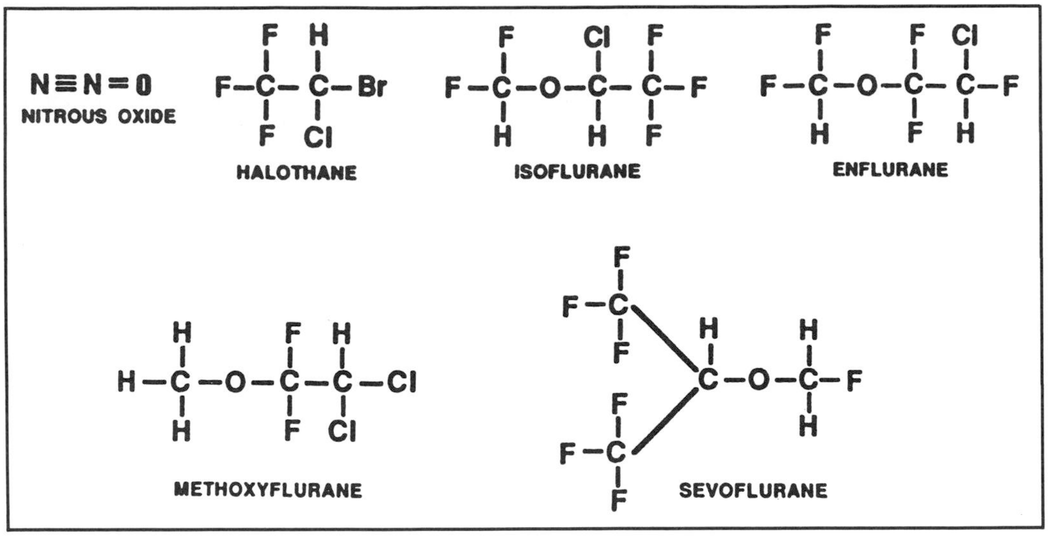

FIGURE 29–4. Molecular structures of inhaled anesthetics. (Reprinted from Barash, P.G., Cullen, B.F., and Stoelting, R.K. (eds.): Clinical Anesthesia. Philadelphia, J.B. Lippincott Co., 1989. Figure 11–1, p. 294.)

MAC = 1.68 per cent), halothane (1 MAC = 0.75 per cent), and isoflurane (1 MAC = 1.15 per cent) is relatively small, particularly when compared with nitrous oxide (1 MAC = 105 to 110 per cent). The volatile liquid anesthetics are chosen on the basis of their selectivity of effects, side-effects, and relative toxicities.

The volatile liquid anesthetics induce a disordering of lipid membranes and their protein content. Synaptic function is disturbed, and cell excitability is depressed. At the organism level, general anesthesia is divided into four stages (Table 29–2). These effects occur with progressive increases in the inspired concentration of volatile liquid anesthetic (FI_{VLA}), which effects an increase in the alveolar partial pressure (PA_{VLA}) and a proportional increase in the partial pressure of the volatile liquid anesthetic in the brain (Pb_{VLA}) and other tissues. This creates a dose-response curve. A unifying theory incorporating a precise delineation of the sundry molecular mechanisms of anesthesia remains to be written. It might include some enduring hypotheses explaining the effects of anesthetics. The Meyer-Overton hypothesis relates the lipid solubility of an anesthetic to its potency. Potency is thus defined as the amount of anesthetic dissolved in a membrane to achieve a defined effect. Additional hypotheses propose the existence of membrane-bound receptors for the volatile liquid anesthetics and alterations of neurotransmitter availability secondary to the presence of a volatile liquid anesthetic.

The uptake and elimination of inhaled anesthetics

TABLE 29–1. PHYSICAL CHARACTERISTICS OF ANESTHETICS

Agent	Molecular Weight	Boiling Point (760 mm Hg°C)	Vapor Pressure (mm Hg @ 20°C)	Liquid Density	Vapor/ Liquid (mL)	Chemical Stabilizer Necessary	Flammability Limits
Enflurane	184.5	56.5	175	1.517(25°C)	198	No	None
Halothane	197.4	50.2	241	1.86 (20°C)	227	Yes	None
Isoflurane	184.5	48.5	238	1.496(25°C)	196	No	None
Methoxyflurane	165	104.7	22.5	1.43 (20°C)	208	Yes	7% in air 5.4% in O$_2$
Nitrous oxide	44	−88.0	39,000	—	—	—	
Sevoflurane	200	58.5	160	1.505(20°C)	181	—	None in air 11% in O$_2$ 10%in N$_2$O

Physical data are from manufacturer's literature; Wallin W.F., Regan B.M., Napoli, M.D. et al.: Sevoflurane: A new inhalational anesthetic agent. Anesth. Analg. *54:*758, 1975; Vitcha, J.E.: A history of Forane. Anesthesiology, 35:4, 1971; Halsey, J.M.: Physiochemical properties of inhalational anesthetics. *In* Gray, T.C. Nunn, J.E., and Utting, J.E. (eds.): General Anaesthesia. London, Butterworths, 1980, p. 45.

TABLE 29–2. STAGES OF GENERAL ANESTHESIA

STAGE	CHARACTERISTICS
1	Analgesia: decreased dorsal horn activity and reduced spinothalamic tract transmission
2	Excitation: enhanced excitatory and depressed inhibitory transmission
3	Unconsciousness: depression of the ascending pathways of the reticular activating system
	Skeletal muscle relaxation: inhibition of spinal reflex activity
4	Severe cardiorespiratory depression: depression of medullary control centers

are described in terms of their distribution of partial pressures across various compartments. The effect of a volatile liquid anesthetic is considered to be directly proportional to its arterial partial pressure (Pa_{VLA}). Pa_{VLA} measurements are cumbersome; therefore PA_{VLA} is accepted as a reliable approximation of Pa_{VLA}. Pa_{VLA} and PA_{VLA} correlate best in the steady state. Variations in the inspired concentration of an inhaled anesthetic necessarily create disparities of Pa_{VLA} and PA_{VLA}. Other reasons for poor correlation include physiologic dead space and intrapulmonary shunting of blood.

The biotransformation of volatile liquid anesthetics is variable, with a tendency to increased metabolism of volatile liquid anesthetics with greater solubility in blood and tissue lipids. They are primarily excreted unchanged via the lung when the partial pressure of the volatile liquid anesthetic in the pulmonary capillary (Pc_{VLA}) exceeds the PA_{VLA}. The amount and duration of exposure, expressed as MAC-hours, determine the extent of metabolism of a volatile liquid anesthetic. Fluoride ion is produced via metabolism of enflurane and methoxyflurane. Oxidative metabolism of halothane produces trifluoroacetic acid, bromide, and chloride. Reductive metabolism of halothane produces reactive intermediary metabolites and fluoride.

Organ Effects of Volatile Liquid Anesthetics

Cardiac. Depression of contractility and of stroke volume are dose-related effects of the volatile liquid anesthetics. Halothane has little effect on heart rate, but it is associated with junctional rhythm and re-entrant ventricular arrhythmias. Increases in heart rate are associated with both isoflurane and enflurane, the latter being dose-dependent. Isoflurane is associated with coronary artery dilation and the potential for "steal" of blood flow and related myocardial ischemia.

Cerebral. Enflurane lowers the seizure threshold. Although the volatile liquid anesthetics decrease cerebral metabolism, they can elevate intracranial pressure (ICP) via cerebral vasodilation.

Hepatic. Splanchnic blood flow is decreased during general anesthesia. Liver function is not clinically impaired unless injury due to hypoxia and hepatotoxic halothane intermediary metabolites occurs. Halothane hepatotoxicity is rare and is a diagnosis of exclusion. Risk factors include atopy, female sex, middle age, obesity, and repeated exposure to halothane.

Pulmonary. Volatile liquid anesthetics decrease tidal volume (V_T), increase respiratory rate, dilate bronchioles, diminish responsiveness to hypercarbia and hypoxia, diminish minute volume, and impair hypoxic pulmonary vasoconstriction. The last effect is not significant at the usual FI_{VLA}.

Renal. Dose-dependent reductions in the glomerular filtration rate and urine output follow changes in cardiac output. Fluoride ion nephrotoxicity occurs when the fluoride ion concentration exceeds 50 μML^{-1} and results in polyuria with an inability to concentrate the urine. This occasional consequence of the administration of methoxyflurane explains its replacement by less extensively metabolized inhalation anesthetic agents.

Intravenous Anesthetics

Intravenous anesthetics effect general anesthesia by interfering with membrane receptor proteins. The profusion of intravenous anesthetics with short elimination half-lives affords increased flexibility and control in the design and management of an anesthetic. The disadvantages of inhaled anesthetics may be decreased or eliminated by the partial or complete substitution of intravenous anesthetic agents. Predicting the duration and extent of a response to a dose of an intravenous anesthetic is complicated by interindividual variability in pharmacokinetics. This variability demands the presence of a responsive anesthesiologist.

Nonopioids

Nonopioid anesthetic drugs are effective at producing amnesia and unconsciousness. Their inability to provide total blockade of sensory, reflex, and motor function means they must be administered with other drugs to achieve a complete anesthetic. The most commonly used drugs are discussed below, and Table 29–3 lists their pharmacokinetic properties.

Barbiturates (Thiopental). Barbiturates depress synaptic function, perhaps both by decreasing excitatory neurotransmitter release and by inhibiting the dissociation of inhibitory neurotransmitter from ion channels. Barbiturates have a selective depressant effect on the reticular activating system. Cerebral blood flow (CBF) is decreased due to both reduced cerebral metabolism ($CMRO_2$) and cerebral vasocon-

TABLE 29–3. PHARMACOKINETIC PROPERTIES OF COMMONLY USED NONOPIOIDS

DRUG	CLEARANCE (mL/kg/min)	ELIMINATION $T_{1/2}$ (h)	VOLUME OF DISTRIBUTION (V_d) (L/kg)
Thiopental	3	12	3
Propofol	59	1	5
Ketamine	19	3	5
Etomidate	18	3	5
Midazolam	6-8	1-4	1-1.5

striction. Consequently, intracranial pressure (ICP) may be decreased.

Barbiturates are negative inotropes and decrease vascular tone via diminishment of central sympathetic outflow. Baroreceptor-mediated increases in heart rate offset the potential for hypotension and decreased cardiac output. Barbiturate-induced depression of the medullary respiratory center causes both diminished CO_2 responsiveness and apnea.

The uses of barbiturates in anesthesiology include premedication for anesthesia, the induction and occasional maintenance of anesthesia, treatment of seizures, and cerebral protection. The last includes protection both from injury due to increases of ICP and transient focal ischemia.

Benzodiazepines (Midazolam, Diazepam). Benzodiazepines selectively enhance the inhibitory effect of gamma aminobutyric acid (GABA) in the CNS. Unlike the barbiturates, the effects of benzodiazepines may be offset by physostigmine, an anticholinesterase, or the specific antagonist flumazenil. Used alone, benzodiazepines cause minimal circulatory depression. They also decrease CBF and $CMRO_2$.

Clinical effects of the benzodiazepines include amnesia, sedation, and anticonvulsant activity. They are suitable for the premedication, induction, and maintenance of anesthesia. Diazepam is associated with pain on injection, phlebitis, and prolonged effect because of a long elimination half-life and active metabolites. Midazolam has gained popularity because it lacks these disadvantages.

Ketamine. Ketamine is an arylcyclohexylamine that increases CNS sympathetic outflow and has dose-dependent effects on the sensorium varying from catalepsy to unconsciousness. It produces amnesia, analgesia, cerebral vasodilation, bronchodilation, cardiovascular stimulation, and sialism. Ketamine is empolyed as an analgesic for brief repetitive painful procedures and as an induction agent in patients with hypovolemia or reactive airways disease.

Etomidate. Etomidate is a corboxylated imidazole derivative. It is characterized by a rapid onset and offset of unconsciousness. Etomidate decreases CBF, $CMRO_2$ and ICP. Its cardiovascular effects are minimal. Decreased seizure threshold, myoclonus, transient adrenal suppression, pain with intravenous

injection, and postoperative nausea and vomiting are observed with its use. Etomidate is an attractive choice in situations where rapid emergence or cardiovascular stability is at a premium.

Propofol. Propofol, an alkyl phenol, is a unique new agent suitable for both the induction and maintenance of anesthesia. Its short elimination half-life and lack of accumulation with prolonged administration allow for a rapid emergence from anesthesia. Its recognized side effects are respiratory depression, hypotension, bradycardia, pain on injection, phlebitis, and thrombosis. The emulsion preparation is not associated with anaphylactoid reactions or histamine release. Exaggerated hypotension may be expected in the presence of hypovolemia or impaired cardiac function.

Opioids

An opioid is an exogenous substance that binds to an opioid receptor (see Chapter 30). The effects of opioids are mediated by distinct receptors at numerous locations, including the CNS and the bowel. A comprehensive classification system for the opioids does not exist. Opioids may be classified by their relative efficacies (e.g., weak or strong) or by their receptor effects, e.g., agonist, antagonist, partial agonist, and mixed agonist-antagonist. Therapeutic effects of opioids include analgesia, suppression of the cough reflex, and depression of bowel hypermotility. Opioid side effects include biliary spasm, convulsions, delirium, dysphoria, emesis, euphoria, miosis, nausea, pruritus, respiratory depression, sedation, thoracoabdominal muscle spasm, and urinary retention. In anesthesiology, opioids are used alone to provide analgesia and in combination with other drugs to produce anesthesia. Extending the dose of an opioid beyond that sufficient for analgesia alone, past the point of mental clouding to unconsciousness, cannot be relied upon to provide adequate surgical anesthesia. Awareness and sensomobility are not reliably ablated even by high doses of potent opioids.

Local Anesthetics

Local anesthetics are used in a broad variety of clinical situations. They are administered systemically as components of general anesthetics and to treat cardiac arrhythmias. They are administered regionally to aid in the diagnosis and treatment of painful conditions and to allow a patient to tolerate a diagnostic or therapeutic procedure. The concentration, point of administration, type, and volume of local anesthetic may be exploited to achieve a specific effect. The extent, duration, and intensity of motor, sensory, and sympathetic neural blockade are all subject to control.

Local anesthetics are small molecules composed of an aromatic lipophilic group and amine hydrophilic group linked by either an amide or an ester group. Categorization of the local anesthetics is based on the type of linkage. The ester local anesthetics have higher pKas than the amides. The ester local anesthetics are metabolized by plasma pseudocholinesterase, and the amides are metabolized in the liver. Local anesthetics are weak bases with pKas above 7.4 and are dispensed as acidic salts to enhance their water solubility. Local anesthetics exist in an equilibrium between ionized (water-soluble) and non-ionized (lipid-soluble) forms.

The site of action of local anesthetics is the nerve membrane's sodium channel. The local anesthetic, in its lipophilic form, diffuses through to the interior of the membrane and, in its hydrophilic form, interferes with sodium channel function. The clinical effect of a local anesthetic is the sum of its physicochemical properties, the chemical milieu, and tissue composition of the site of deposition and the nerve fiber's diameter, myelination, and position within a nerve bundle.

Local anesthetics are associated with general, category-specific, and agent-specific complications. General effects include cardiovascular and CNS toxicity and skeletal muscle irritation. The manifestations of toxicity are characterized by a concentration-response curve. Local anesthetic toxicity (both CNS and cardiovascular) correlates with its anesthetic potency. At lower concentrations, mild effects on the sensorium predominate. As the concentration increases, the CNS excitation progresses to convulsions. Cardiovascular compromise, with inhibition of pacemaker activity, conduction, and contractility, eventually supervenes. Prompt treatment is mandatory because the development of acidosis in the affected organ tends to trap the local anesthetic and perpetuate its toxic effects.

Allergic reactions are relatively uncommon. Mild systemic local anesthetic toxicity or effects of added epinephrine are occasionally mistaken for true allergy. The higher incidence of allergy to the esters is attributed to their derivation from para-aminobenzoic acid. Prilocaine is associated with methemoglobinemia.

Neuromuscular Blocking Drugs

The interaction of acetylcholine (Ach) with the nicotinic receptor in the neuromuscular synapse results in end-plate depolarization and muscular contraction. Neuromuscular blocking drugs (NMBs) impair muscle function through their actions at the neuromuscular synapse. The effects are both pre- and postjunctional and involve the impairment of delivery of substrate for Ach formation, impairment of Ach release, and Ach receptor antagonism.

Depolarizing NMBs

Depolarizing NMBs are Ach receptor agonists. The only depolarizing NMB in clinical use is succinylcholine. Succinylcholine causes sustained depolarization (and fasciculations) via the Ach receptor, resulting in decreased muscle excitability. Succinylcholine is metabolized by pseudocholinesterase (plasma), rather than by acetylcholinesterase (synaptic cleft), and its effect is terminated by dissociation from the receptor and diffusion from the cleft to the plasma. It is categorized as a short-acting drug because of its fast onset and brief duration of action.

Succinylcholine's side effects include cardiac arrhythmias; hyperkalemia; increased pressure within the cranial, gastric, and ocular spaces; myalgia, trismus; and the triggering of malignant hyperthermia.

Nondepolarizing NMBs

Nondepolarizing NMBs are Ach receptor antagonists (Table 29–4). They are categorized according to their duration of action, which is either intermediate or long acting. They are ionized at physiologic pH, and their volume of distribution is considered to be equivalent to the distribution of the extracellular fluid. The long-acting nondepolarizing NMBs are excreted by the kidneys and have variable cardiovascular effects. The intermediate-acting nondepolarizing NMBs are not dependent on renal function for their elimination and have minimal circulatory effects.

The effects of the nondepolarizing NMBs may be reversed by the use of anticholinesterase drugs. Anticholinesterases increase the concentration of Ach within the synapse and thus effect displacement of the nondepolarizing NMB from the nicotinic receptor. Anticholinesterase drugs also increase the concentration of Ach available to muscarinic receptors and have pronounced muscarinic effects, e.g., bradycardia.

Many antibiotics enhance the effects of neuromuscular blocking drugs. Increased potency and duration of action are usually observed, particularly with the nondepolarizing agents. Carbemazepine and phenytoin are associated with a decrease in the duration of action of nondepolarizing NMBs because they induce hepatic enzymes.

RISK OF ANESTHESIA

Anesthesia carries an inherent risk of morbidity and mortality. Without meaning to diminish the multiplicity of sources of risk and the complexity of their interactions, the major factors of risk are from the anesthetic, the patient, and the operation. Additional factors include the operating room environ-

TABLE 29–4. SUGGESTED MUSCLE RELAXANT DOSES (mg · KG⁻¹) FOR CLINICAL USE

DRUG	ED$_{95}$	INTUBATING DOSE	SUPPLEMENTAL DOSES	
			N$_2$O/OPIOID	INHALATIONAL
d-Tubocurarine	0.51	0.60	0.10	0.05
Metocurine	0.28	0.40	0.07	0.04
Pancuronium	0.07	0.10	0.015	0.007
Vecuronium	0.05	0.08–0.10	0.02	0.015
Atracurium	0.20	0.40–0.50	0.10	0.07
Gallamine	2.8	3.5	0.60	0.30
Pancuronium-metocurine combination	0.018 + 0.072	0.025 + 0.10	0.004 + 0.016	0.003 + 0.012
Pancuronium-d-tubocurarine combination	0.024 + 0.144	0.03 + 0.18	0.005 + 0.03	0.004 + 0.025

Reprinted from Barash, P.G., Cullen, B.F., and Stoelting, R.K. (eds.): Clinical Anesthesia. Philadelphia, J.B. Lippincott Co. 1989. Table 13–2, p, 347.

ment and equipment. With the exceptions of eye, hip, and prostate surgery, the safety of general and regional anesthesia is equivalent. The choice of a particular anesthetic technique depends on the site, nature, and duration of the proposed operation and the condition of the patient.

The physical status (PS) assignment system of the American Society of Anesthesiologists (ASA) allows a statement of general risk (Table 29–5), but does not determine precisely the risk of the anesthetic alone. It is generally agreed that mortality tends to increase with ASA PS. Any pre-anesthetic evaluation ought to include a statement of the patient's ASA PS, which may be regarded as a summary statement of the patient's general medical condition.

General Anesthesia

The risk of a general anesthetic is the sum of the dynamic interaction of drugs, environment, equipment, patient condition, and position, and the trespasses of the operation. Special techniques, such as

controlled hypotension, cooling, EEG burst suppression, extracorporeal circulation, hyperventilation, and normovolemic hemodilution, impose unique risks and are thus selectively applied.

Regional Anesthesia

In addition to the risks described for general anesthesia, the risk of a regional anesthetic is the sum of the potential for injuries specific to the area of the procedure and the nontherapeutic effects of the local anesthetic. The procedure may cause direct tissue trauma with the potential for systemic consequences. The local anesthetic may produce systemic toxicity or induce complications consequent to its expected impairment of neural function. Technique-related risk is primarily determined by the site of the block and the experience of the operator. Superficial infiltration nerve blocks are less prone to complication than deeper blocks performed on the thorax, spinal column, or major peripheral nerves.

The likelihood of developing systemic toxicity from a local anesthetic is determined by its dose and site of deposition. Highly vascular areas tend to absorb local anesthetic solutions rapidly. Abnormalities of CNS and cardiovascular function are anticipated in the presence of high serum levels of local anesthetics.

Environmental Factors

The operating room or anesthetizing area poses the greatest risk to the occupant totally unable to protect him- or herself. Uncontrolled environmental factors may either injure the patient directly or contribute to a cascade of events culminating in a complication.

TABLE 29–5. ASA PHYSICAL STATUS

CATEGORY	DESCRIPTION
I	Healthy with localized pathologic process
II	Mild surgical or systemic disease without functional limitation
III	Severe systemic disease with definite functional limitation
IV	Severe systemic disease that is a constant threat to life
V	Moribund

For example, any operation disrupts defenses against *infection*. Furthermore, anesthesia may mask the early signs of sepsis. Although anesthesia has not been shown to increase infection rates due to the rather mild and transient effects of anesthetic agents on immune defenses, instrumentation associated with the delivery of an anesthetic carries an irreducible risk of contamination and infection. Colonization of the airway inevitably occurs with nasotracheal and orotracheal intubation. Percutaneous intravascular epidural or intrathecal instrumentation may serve as both a nidus and portal of infection. Contaminated intravenous solutions and blood products have induced infection.

Alterations of the patient's body temperature may be either deliberate or unintentional. Deliberate manipulation of temperature-sensitive homeostatic processes may optimize the patient's outcome. However, drift of a patient's body temperature may have an unfavorable effect. Hypothermia may impair cardiovascular function, and thermogenesis (shivering) and hyperthermia may impose excessive metabolic demands.

A change in temperature may be a sign of illness developing during an anesthetic. Such illnesses are usually mediated either by failure of homeostatic processes (central or end-organ), increases in metabolic rate, infections, or pyrogens. Transfusion reaction, infection, thyrotoxicosis, myxedema, adrenal insufficiency, and malignant hyperthermia are examples of such processes.

The position required for optimal operating conditions may amplify, aggravate, or counteract the pharmacologic perturbations of the anesthetic on cardiovascular and respiratory function. Injuries related to position are usually consequences of either compression or traction. Protection is more effective than treatment of hand, breast, and genital injury; corneal abrasion; peripheral nerve injury, and retinal ischemia.

Equipment Factors

The equipment that delivers the anesthetic to the patient and other devices attached to the patient all have the potential for harm.

Modern anesthesia machines control and measure gas flows and pressures. Alarms are intended to notify the operator of potentially hazardous conditions. However, it remains the duty of the operator, not the machine, to prevent the delivery of hypoxic gas mixtures, inadequate ventilation, excessive airway pressures, and inappropriate concentrations of inhaled anesthetics.

Protection of the airway is a constant concern of the anesthesiologist. It is achieved with the use of a wide variety of instruments for inspecting and maintaining the airway. Injury of the dentition, larynx, lips, mucosa, trachea, and turbinates is more effectively prevented than treated. The undeclared displacement of an airway device, resulting in hypercarbia and hypoxia, is potentially more devastating than the injuries listed above. Airway equipment is most dangerous when its presence permits a false sense of security.

Intravenous cannulation is a component of all but the briefest anesthetic. Cannulation of a peripheral vein is usually innocuous. Infection and local tissue trauma are possible, but are of greater concern with central venous cannulation. Air embolism, brachial plexus injury, cardiac arrythmias, carotid artery puncture, hemorrhage, hemothorax, penetrating cardiac trauma, pneumothorax, and vessel laceration are potential complications of central venous cannulation.

Arterial cannulation poses the additional risks of anterograde and retrograde embolism, pseudoaneursym formation, and thrombosis and ischemia in an area with inadequate collateral blood flow.

Electrical Factors

The administration of flammable volatile liquid anesthetics, such as cyclopropane and ether, necessitated grounding objects and people to prevent the accumulation and discharge of static electricity. Otherwise, static electrical discharge would ignite flammable volatile liquid anesthetics with disastrous consequences. The introduction of the nonflammable volatile liquid anesthetics eliminated the risk of fire and explosion. Furthermore, the absence of flammable anesthetics permitted the design of operating room electrical circuits that do not conduct electricity through the operating room personnel. This design may include isolation transformers, line isolation monitors, ground-fault circuit interrupters, nonconductive floors and operating tables, and nongrounded equipment cases.

Macroshock is ventricular fibrillation arising as a result of external application of current to a person. The usually stated threshold for this injury is 100 milliamps. This threshold is well above the lower limits of detectable (by the line isolation monitor) current leakage and would probably not occur because of prior generation of an alarm signal or automatic circuit interruption.

Microshock is ventricular fibrillation arising as a result of internal application of current to a person. The current is usually delivered via a device in direct contact with the heart. The usually stated threshold for microshock is 100 microamps, below the limits of detection of the line isolation monitor. Microshock can thus occur in the absence of an alarm condition or automatic circuit interruption.

Electrosurgical units (ESUs) present several hazards to the patient. Explosive gases in distended bowel in contact with the cautery are now the most common cause of surgical explosions. Electrical burns are usually caused by an improperly placed ESU current dispersion pad ("grounding" pad). The large surface area of the dispersion pad lowers the current density below that required to produce a burn. If the pad is incompletely applied or its gel is partially dried, the patient may experience a burn both at the intended site (the cautery knife) and at the contact point of the dispersion pad.

Use of the cautery knife in proximity to a pacemaker or locating the pacemaker generator between the entry and exit points of the ESU current will either inhibit its function or damage its circuitry. In either event, cardiac function is jeopardized.

ANESTHESIA AND PRESERVATION OF OXYGEN DELIVERY

A patient's illness does not stop at the door when he or she enters the operating room. The anesthetic must therefore accommodate the illness. The provision of insensibility to pain is a shallow achievement if tissue oxygenation is impaired. The following discussion of some conditions directly affecting tissue oxygenation is meant to exemplify the impact of illness upon planning and managing an anesthetic.

Airway Abnormalities

Anoxic brain damage, cardiac arrest, and death are inexorable and swift consequences of inadequate oxygenation and ventilation. The multiplicity of anticipated and emergent reasons for assisting or controlling a patient's respiration during the course of any anesthetic necessitates preparation for control of respiration. Preparation includes assessment of the patient's airway and readying drugs and equipment. The airway must be analyzed in the context of the anesthetic plan and the proposed surgery.

A difficult intubation exists when the trachea cannot be intubated as planned. Assuming thorough preoperative evaluation by an experienced intubationist, it is usually the result of an upper airway configuration that prevents visualization of the glottis and intubation of the trachea by conventional means. When a difficult intubation is encountered, one must resist the temptation to adhere rigidly to the initial approach. Implementation of alternative approaches is determined by the urgency of the surgery and the patency of the airway.

It is imperative to verify tracheal tube position immediately after placement. Endobronchial intubation prevents gas exchange in the contralateral lung and predisposes to hypoxia and pulmonary barotrauma. Unrecognized esophageal intubation with the tracheal tube is usually suspected only at the onset of its calamitous consequences. Only two methods reliably establish the intratracheal position of a tracheal tube. The first method is direct observation of the passage of the tracheal tube through the vocal cords. The limitation of this method is that is a single observation that would not detect subsequent displacement. The second method is the observation of a characteristic capnographic waveform. This method permits continuous observation and confirmation of the tube's patency and position.

Cardiovascular Disease

Organ function depends on the availability of oxygen. Oxygen uptake and delivery are the conjoined functions of the blood, heart, and lungs. Oxygen delivery is the product of cardiac output and arterial oxygen content. Thus, during the perioperative period, cardiac output is assessed continuously, and if necessary, it is supported. The significance of cardiovascular disease lies in the diminished reserves of the heart and its increased tendency to arrhythmia, failure, ischemia, and arrest.

Arrhythmias. Arrhythmias compromise myocardial function and all that depends on it. Abnormalities of heart rate and rhythm may increase myocardial oxygen consumption and decrease cardiac output. Continuous monitoring of the electrocardiogram during surgery is routine both because of its low cost and risk and the importance of the monitored variable.

Coronary Artery Disease. Coronary artery disease (CAD) is a process characterized by both broad prevalence and abrupt and irregular progression. The balance of myocardial oxygen supply and demand is subject to more variables than the anesthesiologist can monitor or control. Myocardial ischemia and its consequences can occur despite impeccable management of afterload, contractility, preload, and heart rate and rhythm. These hemodynamic variables may influence the relationship between the constituents of the blood and the walls of the coronary arteries. Coronary artery thrombosis probably underlies the majority of episodes of acute coronary artery compromise. Its predictability and treatment remain incomplete.

Knowledge of the presence and extent of CAD is essential to the design of an anesthetic. The patient's exercise tolerance, history (e.g., myocardial infarction), medication regimen, and symptoms, such as angina, exertional dyspnea, or orthopnea, are investigated to determine whether additional evaluation and treatment are required before the planned surgery. The anesthetic monitoring and technique are proportional to the condition of the patient and the stress of the proposed surgery.

Myocardial infarction (MI) in the perioperative period is associated with a high mortality rate. The presence of congestive heart failure, recent MI, unstable angina, critical aortic stenosis, and prolonged operation within a major body cavity is associated with an increased risk of perioperative MI.

Valvular Heart Disease. Valvular heart disease (VHD) compromises cardiac function via either valvular incompetence or stenosis or both. Cardiac output is compromised either by the valvular heart disease itself or its consequences of arryhthmias and impaired myocardial function. In addition, valvular heart disease predisposes to cardiac and systemic infection and systemic embolism.

Perioperative anesthetic management of valvular heart disease strives to keep myocardial function at its most efficient. Anesthetic drugs are selected according to their side effects on the cardiovascular system. The anesthetic technique frequently entails the use of cardioactive and vasoactive drugs to control afterload, contractility, heart rate, and preload.

Cardiomyopathy. Cardiomyopathy occurs as a primary or secondary process, and its presence modifies the degree of cardiovascular support provided to the patient. The type of support provided is tailored to the hemodynamic characteristics of the cardiomyopathy. Cardiomyopathy is commonly a consequence of both coronary artery disease and valvular heart disease and is also associated with other diseases (e.g., endocrine, infiltrative, and infectious) and their treatment, such as chemotherapy and radiation. Cardiomyopathy is occasionally discovered to be the cause of perioperative mortality, which might otherwise have been attributed to the anesthetic, emphasizing the importance of postmortem examination.

Hypertension. Hypertension is occasionally a presenting sign of disorders of CNS, endocrine, or renal function. It is more commonly a primary process affecting the function of the arterial side of the circulation and the brain, heart, and kidneys. Altered cerebral and renal blood flow autoregulation, increased reactivity of the vasculature, intravascular volume depletion, glomerular sclerosis, and left ventricular hypertrophy are anticipated in the hypertensive patient. Effective cerebral, myocardial, and renal perfusion in patients with long-standing hypertension occurs at higher blood pressures than in normotensive patients. Hypertension alone is not clearly associated with a worsened perioperative outcome, but its consequences have the potential to complicate anesthetic management.

Cardiovascular Drugs

Alpha Agonists. The alpha agonists, clonidine and guanabenz, are centrally acting antihypertensives that decrease sympathetic outflow and blood pressure. Clonidine decreases dose requirements for general anesthetics, contributes to intraoperative hemodynamic stability in hypertensive patients, and

has found application in the management of postoperative pain.

Angiotensin-converting enzyme inhibitors (ACE inhibitors) do not alter anesthetic requirements or sensitivity to muscle relaxants. However, their synergistic action with sodium nitroprusside (SNP) may result in profound hypotension if SNP is not used in reduced doses.

Diuretics. Diuretic administration may alter the course of an anesthetic because of its effects on body fluid volume, distribution, and content. Diuretic-induced hypovolemia may predispose to hemodynamic instability and renal dysfunction. Decreased serum magnesium, potassium, and sodium concentrations may impair CNS (depression or irritability), cardiac (conduction, contractility, and rhythmicity), neuromuscular, and renal function.

Beta Adrenergic Antagonists. Cardiac and pulmonary function is modified by the balance of activity at the β_1 and β_2 adrenergic receptors. Patients with coronary artery disease may have an improved outcome from perioperative administration of beta adrenergic receptor antagonists. The negative inotropic and chronotropic effects of beta adrenergic receptor antagonists may be augmented by the reduction in sympathetic outflow, inhibition of compensatory autonomic responses, and direct myocardial depression associated with inhaled and intravenous anesthetic drugs.

Bronchiolar smooth muscle tone is influenced by beta-adrenergic receptor antagonists. Beta adrenergic receptor agonism results in increases in intracellular cAMP, which is associated with bronchodilation. The beta-adrenergic receptor antagonists, especially those that are not selective for the β_1 receptor, are associated with bronchospasm and increases in airway resistance.

Calcium Channel Antagonists. The calcium channel antagonists have effects upon the myocardium, cardiac conduction system, and peripheral vascular resistance. Verapamil is most likely to depress myocardial contractility and slow cardiac conduction, effects that are additive to those of the volatile inhalation agents, enflurane and halothane.

Pulmonary Disease

The respiratory capability of the lungs is a function of the relative quantities of alveolar ventilation (VA) and pulmonary blood flow (Q). Neurohumoral activity, neuromuscular function, and the caliber of the lower and upper airways are essential components of VA. Pulmonary vascular capacity and resistance and cardiac output are essential components of Q. Abnormalities of oxygenation and ventilation may be anticipated on the basis of a pulmonary disease's features.

When pulmonary disease is recognized before the

administration of an anesthetic, its severity and response to treatment must be assessed. Asthma, chronic bronchitis, and emphysema influence the choice of anesthetic drugs and the intensity of perioperative respiratory management. Pulmonary compromise may arise in the perioperative period in the forms of anaphylaxis, bronchospasm, pulmonary aspiration, pulmonary barotrauma, and pulmonary embolism. Foresight facilitates swift diagnosis and treatment.

Normal oxygen uptake assumes adequacy of both oxygen supply and lung function. An ambient inspired oxygen concentration of 21 per cent is sufficient for the awake person. During sleep, even normal subjects have intermittent periods of mild hypoxia. Anesthesia imposes dynamic compromises on pulmonary mechanics and respiratory control such that the minimum inspired oxygen concentration probably should be 30 per cent.

Tissue hypoxia is not produced exclusively by abnormalities of pulmonary function. Intracardiac shunts, low cardiac output states, carbon monoxide, and methemoglobinemia, can decrease arterial oxygen content independent of pulmonary function.

Hematologic Disease

Oxygen transport and delivery to the tissues are influenced by the quantity of hemoglobin and its affinity for oxygen. The ideal quantity of hemoglobin for oxygen transport is a variable function of the patient's age and condition. Hemoglobinopathies and alterations of the chemical composition of the blood influence the avidity of hemoglobin for oxygen as depicted by the oxyhemoglobin dissociation curve.

Anemia. Anemia is a sign of systemic disease, but a decreased hematocrit is not a predictor of adverse perioperative outcome. Oxygen delivery remains remarkably stable over a wide range of hematocrits. Under normal conditions, oxygen delivery is greatly in excess of tissue oxygen consumption. An increased cardiac output and decreased affinity of hemoglobin for oxygen can compensate for a decreased hematocrit. A minimum acceptable hematocrit is determined on an individual basis. Redefinition of the indications and risks of transfusion therapy has resulted in decreases in the transfusion of blood and blood products.

Erythrocytosis. An abnormally elevated hematocrit increases the amount of hemoglobin available for oxygen transport. However, the associated increase in blood viscosity impairs microcirculatory blood flow. Cerebral, coronary, and retinal sludging and thrombosis are potential complications of an increased red cell mass.

BIBLIOGRAPHY

1. Barash, P.G., Cullen, B.F., and Stoelting, R.K. (eds.): Clinical Anesthesia. Philadelphia, J.B. Lippincott Co., 1989.
2. Birmingham, P.K., Cheney, F.W., and Ward, R.J.: Esophageal intubation: A review of detection techniques. Anesth. Analg., 65:886–891, 1986.
3. Brown, D.L.: Risk and Outcome in Anesthesia. Philadelphia, J.B. Lippincott Co., 1988.
4. Cousins, M.J., and Bridenbaugh, P.O. (eds.): Neural Blockade in Clinical Anesthesia and Management of Pain, 2nd ed. Philadelphia, J.B. Lippincott Co., 1988.
5. Dorsch, J.A., and Dorsch, S.E.: Understanding Anesthesia Equipment: Construction, Care, and Complications, 2nd ed. Baltimore, Williams & Wilkins, 1984.
6. Gaba, D.M., Maxwell, M., and DeAnda, A.: Anesthetic mishaps: Breaking the chain of accident evolution. Anesthesiology, 66:670–676, 1987.
7. Greene, N.M.: Anesthesia and the development of surgery (1846-1896). Anesth. Analg., 58:5–12, 1979.
8. Nunn, J.F.: Applied Respiratory Physiology, 3rd ed. Boston, Butterworths, 1987.
9. Stanski, D.R., and Watkins, W.D. Drug Disposition in Anesthesia. Orlando, FL: Grune and Stratton, 1982.
10. Stoelting, R.K., and Miller, R.D.: Basics of Anesthesia, 2nd ed. New York, Churchill Livingstone, 1989.

30

PHARMACOLOGY OF PAIN MANAGEMENT

MICHAEL C. BRODY

Postoperative pain is a ubiquitous experience among surgical patients. It is often a primary concern when patients describe their fears of impending surgery. Despite this, opioid therapy is often withheld due to fears of masking postoperative complications or concerns about iatrogenic addiction. An understanding of the basic pharmacokinetic and pharmacodynamic principles of systemic opioids will enable the clinician to control safely and effectively the pain experienced postoperatively.

ADDICTION VERSUS HABITUATION

Addiction describes compulsive drug seeking and drug use, behavior that is associated with a high risk of relapse after detoxification. This pattern of *abuse* often persists despite the patient's recognition of recurrent social, occupational, psychological, or physical problems caused by it.

Patients may become habituated from daily narcotic exposure within a 1-or 2-week period. They may exhibit signs of sympathetic nervous system hyperexcitability (withdrawal) if the opioid is discontinued abruptly. They may also exhibit withdrawal symptoms if opioid antagonists or agonist-antagonists are co-administered.

Although patients may become physiologically dependent (i.e., habituated) to opioid analgesics, they do not develop an "addiction" from postoperative opioid use. Habituated patients may be gradually tapered from opioids and are at little risk for withdrawal symptoms or future drug-seeking behaviors.

Tolerance is simply the requirement for an increased dose of a drug to achieve an effect initially achieved at a lower dose. It is a physiologic and behavioral response that occurs in most patients exposed to prolonged opioid administration. Because pain is short-lived, clinically significant tolerance is unusual in the postoperative period. When tolerance does develop, doses may usually be safely increased to achieve analgesia because tolerance to troublesome side effects has also occurred. Tolerance to constipation (and miosis), however, is slow to occur.

NARCOTIC ANALGESICS

Morphine, codeine, and thebaine are naturally occurring alkaloids (phenanthrenes) derived from opium. Semisynthetic derivatives of these naturally occurring opioids are made by substitution into a parent molecule (Table 30–1). A second class of chemical compounds are the synthetic phenylpiperidine analgesics, such as meperidine and fentanyl, which resemble atropine in structure (Fig. 30–1). Methadone and propoxyphene are yet another distinctive chemical class with analgesic properties.

Analgesia results from both presynaptic and postsynaptic effects of opioids on receptors within the central nervous system. Four primary classes of opioid receptors have been identified: Mu, Delta, Kappa, and Sigma receptors. Each Class is associated with specific effects. Subpopulations of these primary receptors have also been identified (Table 30–2). Systemically administered opioids produce a physiologic response similar to that produced by endogenous opioids, including endorphins, enkephalins, and dynorphins. The degree of analgesia is related to the per cent saturation at these opioid receptors. In contrast, analgesic potency describes the relative dose of opioid required to produce equal analgesic effects. Since all opioids are capable of producing equal analgesic effects, the choice of opioid for the control of postoperative pain is chiefly based on the associated side effect profiles of each drug and the available routes of administration.

TABLE 30–1. STRUCTURES OF OPIOIDS AND OPIOID ANTAGONISTS CHEMICALLY RELATED TO MORPHINE

| NONPROPRIETARY NAME | CHEMICAL RADICALS AND POSITIONS | | | |
	3*	6*	17*	Other+
Morphine	–OH	–OH	–CH$_3$	–
Heroin	–OCOCH$_3$	–OCOCH$_3$	–CH$_3$	–
Hydromorphone	–OH	=O	–CH$_3$	(1)
Oxymorphone	–OH	=O	–CH$_3$	(1),(2)
Levorphanol	–OH	–H	–CH$_3$	(1),(3)
Levallorphan	–OH	–H	–CH$_2$CH=CH$_2$	(1),(3)
Codeine	–OCH$_3$	–OH	–CH$_3$	–
Hydrocodone	–OCH$_3$	=O	–CH$_3$	(1)
Oxycodone	–OCH$_3$	=O	–CH$_3$	(1),(2)
Nalorphine	–OH	–OH	–CH$_3$CH=CH$_2$	–
Naloxone	–OH	=O	–CH$_2$Ch=CH$_2$	(1),(2)
Naltrexone	–OH	=O	–CH$_2$	(1),(2)
Buprenorphine	–OH	–OCH$_3$	–CH$_2$	(1),(2),(4)
Butorphanol	–OH	–H	–CH$_2$	(2),(3)
Nalbuphine	–OH	–OH	–CH$_2$	(1),(2)

* The numbers 3, 6 and 17 refer to positions on the morphine molecule, as shown above.

+ Other changes in the morphine molecule are as follows:
  (1) Single instead of double bond between C7 and C8
  (2) OH added to C14
  (3) No oxygen between C4 and C5
  (4) *Endo*theno bridge between C6 and C14; 1-hydroxy-1,2,2-trimethylpropyl substitution on C7

Reprinted from Jaffe, F.H., and Martin W.R.: Opioid analgesics and antagonists. *In* Gilman, A.G., Goodman, L.S., Rall, T.W., and Murad, F. (eds.): Goodman and Gilman's The Pharmacological Basis of Therapeutics, 7th ed. New York, Macmillan, 1985. Table 22–2, p. 496.

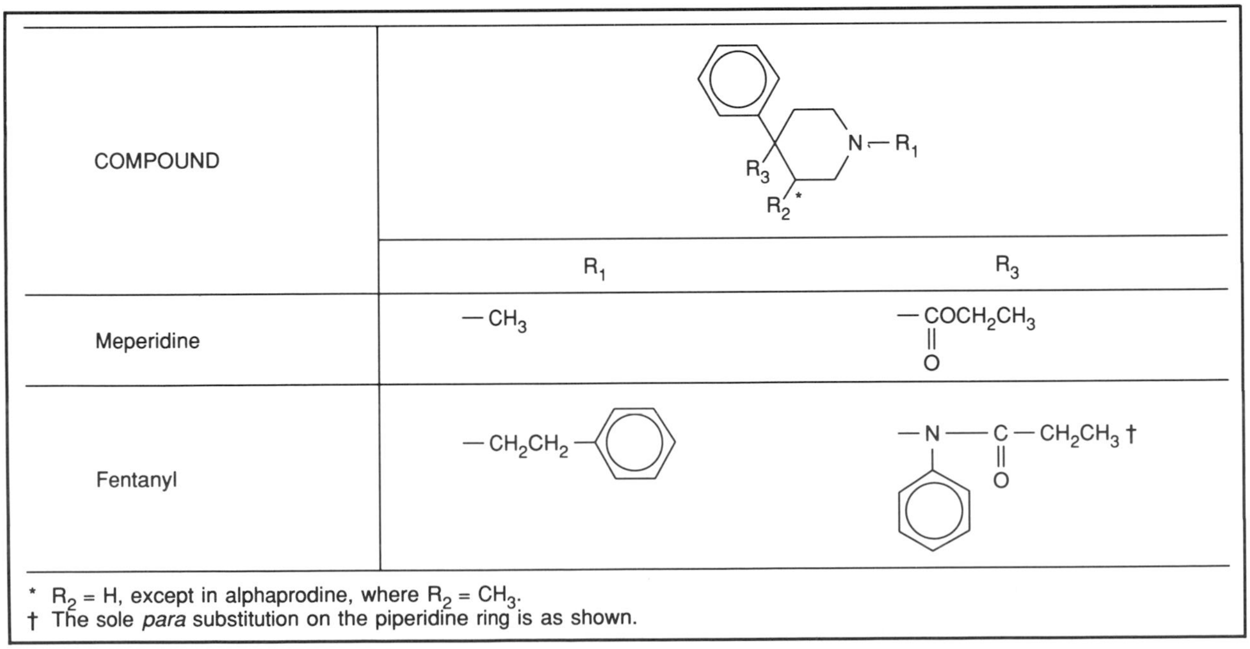

FIGURE 30–1. Chemical structures of phenylpiperidine analgesics. (Modified from Jaffe, J.H., and Martin, W.R.: Opioid analgesics and antagonists. *In* Gilman, A.G., Goodman, L.S., Rall, T.W., and Murad, F. (eds.): Goodman and Gilman's The Pharmacological Basis of Therapeutics, 7th ed. New York, Macmillan, 1985. Table 22–4, p. 513.)

TABLE 30-2.   CLASSIFICATION OF OPIOID RECEPTORS

	EFFECT	AGONIST	ANTAGONIST
Mu-1	Supraspinal analgesia	Beta-endorphin, morphine	Naloxone, pentazocine, nalbuphine
Mu-2	Depression of ventilation, decreased heart rate, physical dependence, euphoria	Meperidine, fentanyl, sulfentanil, alfentanil, leu-enkephalin	
Delta	Modulation of mu receptor activity		Naloxone, metenkephalin
Kappa	Analgesia, sedation, depression of ventilation (?), miosis	Dynorphin, pentazocine, butorphanol, nalbuphine, buprenorphine, nalorphine	Naloxone
Sigma	Dysphoria, hypertonia, tachycardia, tachypnea	Pentazocine (?), ketamine (?)	Naloxone

Reprinted from Stoelting, R.K.: Pharmacology and Physiology in Anesthetic Practice. Philadelphia, J.B. Lippincott Co., 1987. Table 3–2, p. 71.

ROUTE OF ADMINISTRATION

The most basic pharmacologic principle in prescribing opioids for postoperative pain control is to achieve therapeutic steady-state plasma levels. Effective analgesia may be achieved regardless of the route of administration as long as equal analgesic doses of opioid are administered (Table 30–3). Principles of equal analgesic dosing may be applied when converting from one route of administration to another or when changing the opioid. The increase in dosage when converting to the oral route reflects a variable absorption of drug through the GI tract, as well as differing rates of first-pass hepatic metabo-

TABLE 30-3.   ORAL AND PARENTERAL OPIOID ANALGESICS FOR MODERATE TO SEVERE PAIN

	EQUIANALGESIC			PLASMA HALF-LIFE (H)	COMMENTS
	ROUTE	DOSE*	DURATION		
Narcotic Agonists					
Morphine	im	10	4-6	2-3.5	Standard for comparison; also available in slow-release tablets and rectal suppositories
	po	60	4-7		
Codeine	im	130	4-6	3	Biotransformed to morphine; useful as initial narcotic analgesic
	po	200+	4-6		
Oxycodone	im	15		—	Short acting; available as 5 mg dose in combination with aspirin and acetaminophen
	po	30	3-5		
Hydromorphone (Dilaudid)	im	1.5	4-5	2-3	Available in high-potency injectable form (10 mg/mL) for cachetic patients and as rectal suppositories; more soluble than morphine
	po	7.5	4-6		
Meperidine (Demerol)	im	75	4-5	3-4	Contraindicated in patients with renal disease; accumulation of active toxic metabolite normeperidine; produces CNS excitation
	po	300+	4-6	normeperidine 12-16	
Methadone (Dolophine)	im	10		15-30	Good oral potency; requires careful titration of the initial dose to avoid drug accumulation
	po	20			

* Based on single-dose studies in which an intramuscular dose of each drug listed was compared with morphine to establish the relative potency. Oral doses are those recommended when changing from a parenteral to an oral route.

Modified from Foley, K.M.: Pain syndromes and pharmacologic management of pancreative cancer pain. Pain Symptom Manage. 3:1984, 1988. Table 6.

lism. Oral bioavailability of morphine varies from 35 to 75 per cent and is reflective of the variance in patient requirements to control postoperative pain.

Frequently, clinicians feel that one form of opioid provides superior analgesia compared to another opioid. However, these observed differences are likely due to differences in dosing, rather than the choice of opioid. As an example, changing from 10 mg of intramuscular morphine to 3 mg of intramuscular hydromorphine likely results in improved analgesia because of an effective 100 per cent increase in dosing (since the equianalgesic dose of hydromorphine would be 1.5 mg). Another common misconception is that the intramuscular route provides superior analgesia to the oral route. A patient whose narcotic prescription was changed from 10 mg of intramuscular morphine to 10 mg of oral oxycodone experiences increased pain not because of the difference in route of administration, but because the patient is receiving only 33 per cent of the equal analgesic dose of narcotic.

DOSING INTERVAL

To achieve steady-state plasma levels, the dosing interval must be based on the plasma half-life of the opioid chosen to control postoperative pain. If dosing intervals are prescribed that are longer than the plasma half-life, a peak-and-trough effect will result in periods of breakthrough pain. As needed administration of opioids also results in periods of subtherapeutic plasma levels. Steady-state plasma levels are best achieved by a time-contingent (by-the-clock) dosing schedule (Fig. 30–2). Dosages must be individually titrated to an effective level while avoiding accumulation from repetitive dosing, especially in patients with decreased hepatic or renal function.

METABOLISM AND CLEARANCE

Opioids are primarily metabolized in the liver. The metabolites are excreted in the urine and bile with small amounts of unchanged drug. Morphine is conjugated with glucuronic acid and eliminated primarily in the urine, with only 7 to 10 per cent undergoing biliary excretion. Meperidine undergoes demethylation to normeperidine. Of note, the plasma half-life of normeperidine is 12 to 16 hours, and it may accumulate with prolonged use, especially in patients with renal dysfunction. Normeperidine is a toxic CNS stimulant that may cause symptoms of tremulousness, myoclonus, or seizures.

SIDE EFFECTS

Comparison of side effects between different opioid analgesics is based largely on anecdotal reports. Controlled clinical studies that describe the relative side effects of various routes of administration are lacking. Side effects most commonly attributed to the use of opioid analgesics include respiratory depression, sedation, nausea and vomiting, constipation, and urinary retention.

Respiratory depression is a dose-dependent effect of opioid analgesics that results in CO_2 retention. The effects of opioid analgesics at the brainstem respiratory centers result in decreased responsiveness to carbon dioxide. In addition, depression of pontine and medullary centers results in irregular and periodic breathing. A decrease in minute ventilation is due primarily to a decreased respiratory rate, with a variable response in tidal volumes. Opioids may also produce a dose-dependent depression of ciliary activity in the bronchioles and increase airway resistance due to bronchoconstriction.

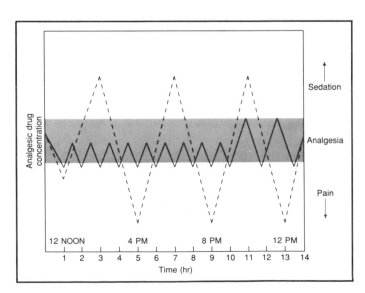

FIGURE 30–2. A time-contingent dosing schedule used to maintain steady-state plasma levels. (Reprinted from Harmer, M., Rosen, M., and Vickers, M.D. (eds.): Patient-Controlled Analgesia. St. Louis, C.V. Mosby Co., 1985, pp. 140–148.)

Sedation is primarily due to CNS depression that is reflected by a slowing of the electroencephalogram. In addition, significant hypercarbia may also contribute to sedation and mental obtundation. Extreme caution must be used when opioids are combined with other CNS depressants, such as benzodiazepines.

Opioids should be used with extreme caution in patients at risk for elevations in intracranial pressure. Although opioids do not have a direct effect on cerebral circulation, respiratory depression and subsequent hypercarbia can produce cerebral vasodilation and increases in cerebral spinal fluid pressures.

Cardiovascular side effects are uncommon with clinically used doses of opioid analgesia. Alterations in blood pressure or cardiac rate and rhythm should not be attributed to opioid therapy in euvolemic, supine patients. However, baroreceptor reflexes and sympathetic responsiveness may be blunted, resulting in orthostatic hypertension. Morphine may be associated with bradycardia secondary to increased vagal activity, as well as direct depression of the sinoatrial node and conduction delay through the atrioventricular node. Meperidine, in contrast, may be associated with an increase in heart rate due to its atropine-like structure, especially when it is administered intravenously in large doses. Meperidine has also been associated with direct myocardial depression, reducing contractility when administered in large doses.

Gastric, biliary, and pancreatic secretions are decreased with opioid administration. The direct effects of opioids within the GI tract and CNS result in decreased peristalsis and increased resting tone of GI smooth muscle. Decreased peristalsis and subsequent increased absorption of water may result in constipation, which can delay the return of normal GI function in the postoperative period. Opioids should be used with caution in patients with biliary colic because of the associated elevation in biliary pressures. Meperidine is reportedly associated with less inhibition of GI motility and lower biliary pressures. However, definitive evidence of this effect is lacking. The reported decreased spasmodic effects of meperidine may be related to its atropine-like structure.

Nausea and vomiting are primarily due to direct stimulation of the receptors located in the chemoreceptor trigger zone. An increased incidence of opioid-induced nausea and vomiting in ambulatory patients also suggests a vestibular mechanism. In addition, a delay in GI transit time may also contribute to opioid-induced nausea and vomiting.

Urinary retention results from opioid-induced increases in detrusor muscle tone and an increased tone of the internal urethral sphincter. In addition to an increase in smooth muscle tone, inhibition of spinal reflexes are likely to contribute to opioid-induced urinary retention.

Reversal of opioid-induced side effects may be achieved with the use of an opioid antagonist, such as naloxone. Naloxone, however, should be used judiciously to avoid precipitating withdrawal symptoms or analgesia reversal.

PATIENT-CONTROLLED ANALGESIA

Patient-controlled analgesia allows the patient to self-administer small, frequent doses of opioid at set intervals and thereby titrate plasma levels to therapeutic effect. It minimizes the peak-and-trough effect that occurs with intermittent bolus dosing and may reduce the incidence of side effects (Fig. 30–2). By maintaining plasma levels that more closely approximate a steady state, the patient can better achieve an optimal analgesic effect. The patient is also provided with an important element of self-control in relieving pain, which alleviates anxiety and reduces dependency on health care providers. Intramuscular injections that are painful and associated with the risks of bleeding and infection may also be avoided.

Many patients are unable to tolerate oral medications in the immediate postoperative period and therefore require parenteral administration of narcotics for pain control. Implicit in the basic construct of patient-controlled analgesia is the requirement that the patient is alert and cognitively capable of operating the infusion device. Failure to achieve adequate postoperative pain control using patient-controlled analgesia devices is most commonly due to inadequate patient training. Patients not only require instruction in the use of the patient-controlled analgesia machine but also should be offered the opportunity to discuss such concerns as perceived risks of addiction and overdosage. Poor patient selection, inadequate loading dose, and the inadequate treatment of side effects can also result in suboptimal analgesia. It should be emphasized that patient-controlled analgesia machines provide effective *maintenance* of opioid therapy, rather than loading of therapeutic plasma levels.

EPIDURAL ANALGESIA

Epidural local anesthetics produce blockade of nerve impulse conduction in axonal membranes at the nerve roots and in the long tracts of the spinal cord (Table 30–4). Although epidural local anesthetic administration results in virtual complete pain relief, it also causes blockade of sympathetic, sensory, and motor fibers. Sympathetic nervous system blockade may result in subsequent hypotension. Impaired motor function results in the inability to ambulate early in the recovery period.

TABLE 30–4. A COMPARISON OF ACTIONS AND EFFICACY OF SPINALLY APPLIED OPIOIDS AND LOCAL ANESTHETIC BLOCK

	OPIOIDS	LOCAL ANESTHETICS
ACTIONS		
Site of action	Substantial gelatinosa of dorsal horn of spinal cord*	Nerve roots (and long tracts in spinal cord)
Type of blockade	Presynaptic and (postsynaptic) inhibition of neuron cell excitation	Blockade of nerve impulse conduction in axonal membrane
Modalities blocked	"Selective" block of pain conduction	Blockade of sympathetic and pain fibers; often also loss of sensation and motor function
EFFICACY		
Surgical pain	Partial relief	Complete relief possible
Labor pain	Partial relief	Complete relief
Postoperative pain		
Early first 24 hours	Fair relief (high dose)	Complete relief
24 hours +	Good relief (low dose)	Complete relief
Chronic pain	Good relief	Impracticable (usually)

* And other sites where opioid receptors (binding sites) are present.

Reprinted from Cousins, M.J., Cherry, D., and Gourlay, G.: Acute and chronic pain: The use of spinal opioids. *In* Cousins, M.J., and Bridenbaugh, P.O. (eds.): Neural Blockage in Clinical Anesthesia and Management of Pain, 2nd ed. Philadelphia, J.B. Lippincott Co., 1988. Table 28–4, p. 959.

Recently, epidural opioid administration has been used to achieve effective postoperative analgesia through selective blockade of the pain fiber system. Epidurally administered opioids produce pre- and postsynaptic inhibition of neuronal cell exitation within the superficial layers of the dorsal horn of the spinal cord. Effective analgesia is achieved without corresponding sympathetic or motor blockade.

The physiocochemical properties of opioid analgesics and local anesthetics are similar. In general, they are weak bases of similar molecular weight. Opioids are described as either hydrophilic, such as morphine, or relatively lipophilic, such as fentanyl. Although morphine is the only FDA-approved opioid for use within the epidural space, a variety of other opioids have also proven useful. Lipophilic opioids, such as fentanyl, are associated with a rapid onset and short duration of action compared to the longer-acting but slower in onset hydrophilic opioids.

The traditional three-compartment model suggests that epidurally deposited opioid diffuses across the dural membrane, through the cerebral spinal fluid (CSF), and enters the superficial layers of the dorsal horn. It has been proposed that more lipophilic agents, such as fentanyl, may gain access to the dorsal horn not only by diffusion across the CSF but also by vascular supply via the posterior radicular artery (Fig. 30–3).

Analgesia is profound with epidurally administered opioids because of the increased opioid concentrations at the level of opioid spinal receptors. Dosages of epidural morphine equivalent to systemically administered morphine produce CSF levels that are 100 to 200 times higher than levels achieved within the plasma. This results in a increased saturation of opioid receptors and corresponding improvement in pain control when compared to systemic opioids. The prolonged duration of effect with epidural morphine is also due to the high concentrations of the drug at receptor sites.

Enhanced analgesia may result in early mobilization of the patient, as well as improved pulmonary mechanics. Significantly improved arterial oxygenation, decreased CO_2 retention, improved peak expiratory flow, and earlier mobilization may decrease postoperative morbidity.

Epidural analgesia is recommended in patients who are expected to experience severe degrees of postoperative pain, such as after knee reconstruction or thoracotomy. Patients who have compromised pulmonary mechanics due to obesity or incisional pain (abdominal, thoracic splinting) will likely also benefit from epidural analgesia.

Major side effects associated with the use of epidural analgesia include respiratory depression (less than 1 per cent), urinary retention (40 per cent), pruritus (10 per cent), nausea and vomiting (35 per cent), and catheter infection (less than 1 percent) (Table 30–5). Although significant respiratory depression is reported to occur is less than 1 per cent of patients receiving epidural analgesia, the risk is increased in patients receiving co-administration of other CNS depressants. The respiratory depression seen with epidural morphine analgesia is biphasic and is characterized by an early peak in arterial CO_2 approximately 1 hour after administration, due to systemic absorption, and another peak 6 to 12 hours after administration presumably due to rostral spread via the CSF. Bolus dosages of greater than 5 mg of preservative free morphine are not recommended because of an increased risk of respiratory depression. Respiratory depression is more common in the elderly. Therefore, dosages should be reduced accordingly.

Apnea monitors are useful to monitor patients after epidural opioid administration. In addition, frequent assessment of the patient's mental status

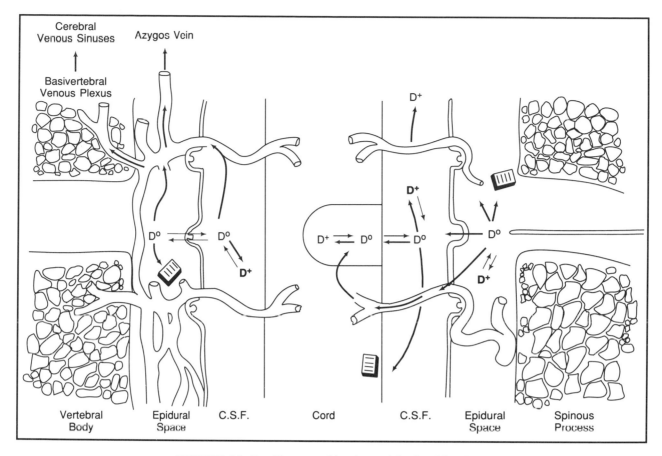

FIGURE 30–3. Pharmacokinetic model of epidural injection of a lipophilic opioid, such as meperidine or fentanyl. Note the rapid passage of un ionized species (D°) into CSF and thence to spinal opioid receptors. Thus, the amount of ionized species (D$^+$), that remains to migrate to the brain is less than that for morphine. (Reprinted from Cousins, M.J., Cherry, D., and Gourlay, G.: Acute and chronic pain: The use of spinal opioids. *In* Cousins, M.J., and Bridenbaugh, P.O. (eds.): Neural Blockade in Clinical Anesthesia and Management of Pain, 2nd ed. Philadelphia, J.B. Lippincott Co., 1988, Table 28–4, p. 959.)

TABLE 30–5.   SIDE EFFECTS POSSIBLY CAUSED BY EPIDURAL MORPHINE: RELATIONSHIP TO TYPE OF SURGERY

Type of Surgery	Urinary Retention	%	Pruritis	%	Nausea	%	Respiratory Depression	%
Hip arthroplasty	65/142	46	27/262	10	115/262	44	2/262	0.8
Major lower extremity operation	10/28	36	13/76	17	25/76	33	0/76	0
Prostatectomy	—	—	19/152	13	43/152	28	1/152	0.7
Laparotomy	48/119	40	54/539	10	176/539	33	5/539	0.9
Thoractomy	8/21	38	5/56	9	14/56	25	2/56	3.6
All	131/310 $X^2=1.54$ p = not significant	42	118/1085 $X^2=4/.17$ p = not significant	11	373/1085 $X^2=15.98$ $p < 0.01$	34	10/1085 $X^2=5.20$ p = not significant	0.9

Reprinted from Stenseth, R., Sellevold, O., and Breivil, H.: Epidural morphine for post-operative pain: Experience with 1085 patients. Acta Anaesthesiol. Scand. *29:* 153, 1984, Table 5.

using a sedation scale is essential to the detection of clinically significant respiratory depression and hypercarbia.

The urinary dynamics associated with epidural morphine administration are characterized by a decrease in detrusor muscle tone with a corresponding contraction of the external urethral sphincter. These effects are not reversed with either cholinergic, serotinergic, or a variety of adrenergic agonist and antagonist drugs. Apomorphine's effects, although improving urinary dynamics, include a high incidence of associated nausea and vomiting. Naloxone may also be used to reverse urinary retention, but may result in reversal of pain control.

The pruritus associated with epidural opioids is usually well tolerated and does not require therapy. For those patients complaining of intolerable pruritus and requesting medication, low doses of systemic naloxone (i.e., 0.1 mg) are extremely effective without reversing analgesia. Pruritis is likely due to a direct effect of the epidural opioid on the spinal cord. Antihistamines are less effective and may also produce sedation that can potentiate respiratory depressant effects of epidural opioids.

Nausea and vomiting are also common side effects of epidural opioid analgesia. Of interest, recent studies have suggested the advantages of using transdermal scopolamine as effective prophylaxis for epidural-opioid-induced nausea and vomiting. Few side effects were associated with the use of transdermal scopolamine, presumably due to the low doses delivered by the patch (5 μg/h).

SUMMARY

In addition to patient comfort, the goals of effective postoperative pain control include decreased patient morbidity and reduced health care costs. These goals can be achieved through early mobilization of patients in the recovery period, as well as enhanced pulmonary mechanics (cough, deep breathing). The method of pain relief chosen must be individualized for each patient. In patients who are at high risk for postoperative complications due to pre-existing medical conditions, such as obesity or coronary artery disease, or who are expected to experience severe postoperative pain, epidural narcotic analgesia will likely be most effective. In other patients experiencing postoperative pain, systemic opioid administration may be preferable because of the high incidence of side effects associated with epidural opioids, especially urinary retention.

If the patient is able to tolerate oral medications, then oral administration of opioids should be provided. When the patient requires a parenteral route of administration, alternative routes should always be considered, such as rectal, subcutaneous, transdermal, intramuscular, and intravenous administration. A basic understanding of the pharmacokinetic and pharmacodynamic principles of opioid administration is essential to the effective control of postoperative pain.

BIBLIOGRAPHY

1. Bromage, P.R., Camporesi, E., and Chestnut, D.: Epidural narcotics for post-operative analgesia. Anesth. Analg. *59*:475–480, 1980.
2. Camporesi, E.M., Nielsen, C.H., Bromage, P.R., and Durant, P.A.: Ventilatory CO_2 sensitivity after intravenous and epidural morphine in volunteers. Anesth. Analg. *62*: 633–40, 1983.
3. Cousins, M.J., and Bridenbaugh, P.O.: Neural Blockage in Clinical Anesthesia and Management of Pain, 2nd ed. Philadelphia, J.B. Lippincott Co., 1988.
4. Diagnostic and Statistical Manual of Mental Disorders, Third Edition—Revised. Washington, DC, American Psychiatric Association, 1983.
5. Durant, P.A., and Yaksh, T.L.: Drug effects on urinary bladder tone during spinal morphine-induced inhibition of the micturation reflex in unanesthetized rats. Anesthesiology, *68*:325–334, 1988.
6. Foley, K.M.: Pain syndromes and pharmacologic management of pancreatic cancer pain. J. Pain Symptom Manage. *3*:184, 1988.
7. Foley, K.M., and Inturrisi, C.E.: Analgesic drug therapy in cancer pain: Principles and practice. Med. Clin. North Am., *71*:207–232, 1987.
8. Gilman, A.G., Goodman, L.S., Rall, T.W., and Murad, F.: Goodman and Gilman's The Pharmacological Basis of Therapeutics, 7th ed. New York, Macmillan, 1985.
9. Harmer, M., Rosen, M., and Vickers, M.D. (eds.): Patient-Controlled Analgesia. St. Louis, C.V. Mosby Co., 1985.
10. Nordberg, G.N., Hedner, T, Mellstrand, T., and Dahlstrom, B.: Pharmacokinetic aspects of epidural morphine analgesia. Anesthesiology, *58*:545–551, 1983.
11. Rawal, N., Sjostrand, U., Christoffersson, E., Dahlstrom, B., Arvill, A., and Rydman, H.: Comparison of intramuscular and epidural morphine for post-operative analgesia in the grossly obese: Influence on post-operative ambulation and pulmonary function. Anesth. Analg., *63*:583–92, 1984.
12. Stenseth, R., Sillevold, O., and Breivik, H.: Epidural morphine for post-operative pain: Experience with 1085 patients. Acta Anaesthesiol. Scand., *29*:148–156, 1985.
13. Stoelting, R.K.: Pharmacology and Physiology in Anesthetic Practice. Philadelphia, J.B. Lippincott Co., 1987.

31

BLOOD PHYSIOLOGY AND TRANSFUSION THERAPY

GLENN RAMSEY

HEMATOPOIESIS AND RED BLOOD CELL PHYSIOLOGY

All blood cells arise from a multipotential stem cell, which at a primitive level divides into two broad lineages, lymphocytes and hematopoietic cells. Hematopoietic stem cells in turn give rise to four series of cell lines: red cells, megakarytocytes, the granulocyte-monocyte series, and the eosinophil-basophil series. It is the transfer of these primitive stem cells that is sought in bone marrow transplantation. Their differentiation to mature end-stage cells requires a host of growth factors.

The production of red cells in governed by a hormone, erythropoietin (Epo), which is produced mainly by the kidneys in response to diminished tissue oxygen supply. Epo stimulates division of all levels of erythroid precursors. Its main counterpart for granulocytes is granulocyte-monocyte colony-stimulating factor (GM-CSF). GM-CSF and other closely related factors are produced by several types of cells involved in the inflammatory response—macrophages, T cells, and endothelial cells. Megakaryocyte production involves two factors—interleukin-3 from T cells, which stimulates megakaryocyte stem-cell production (and also granulocyte-monocyte precursors), and thrombopoietin, which assists in maturation of end-stage megakaryocytic cells.

Red blood cells (RBC) mediate respiration by delivering O_2 to and removing CO_2 from the tissues. Each RBC normally circulates for 120 days, and thus about 1 per cent of them turn over each day. Normal RBC formation requires iron for hemoglobin and vitamin B_{12} and folic acid for normal DNA synthesis in rapidly dividing hematopoietic precursors.

The RBC must maintain a proper intracellular milieu for hemoglobin function. This requires transmembrane balance of the osmotic and ionic burden of the large hemoglobin molecule and generation of the needed energy from the surrounding plasma in an anucleate cell. The osmotic and ionic balance is achieved by a membrane "pump" sending Na^+ out and K^+ in, against the concentration gradients. The ATP needed for this process is generated by anaerobic glycolysis of glucose to lactate, which does not utilize the O_2 being transported. The alternate hexose monophosphate pathway, through the action of glucose-6-phosphate dehydrogenase (G6PD) and other enzymes, provides reducing agents to protect hemoglobin and other proteins from being oxidized by the oxygen being carried. Hemoglobin consists of four globin protein chains around heme, the iron-bearing organic molecule that binds O_2. O_2 binding occurs in the high O_2 concentrations of the lungs, and unloading takes place at low pH concentrations in the tissues. This dissociation process is affected by various physiologic variables. Hemoglobin's oxygen affinity is reduced by low pH and by the presence of 2,3-diphosphoglycerate (2,3-DPG). 2,3-DPG is a major glycolysis intermediate, and it maintains physiologic O_2 dissociation by changing the shape of hemoglobin and by helping shift the intracellular pH to 7.20.

Red cell disorders can be caused by problems in each of the functions described above. General categories of these problems and examples of each are outlined in Table 31–1.

Granulocytes and Monocytes

Granulocytes take part in acute inflammatory reactions to bacteria and other foreign antigens. In the broad sense, granulocytes include not only neutrophils but also basophils and eosinophils, which take part in allergic reactions. Neutrophils are the first-line phagocytic defense against pyogenic bacteria. Once released into the blood from the marrow, they circulate only briefly (half-life of 7 to 10 hours) before egressing into the tissues for another few hours.

A reserve pool is present in the marrow, and about

425

TABLE 31–1. RED CELL DISORDERS

Overproduction
Abnormal growth
 Erythropoietin from renal and other tumors
 Intrinsic—polycythemia vera, erythroleukemia
Response to an abnormal stress
 Hypoxia—lung disease, smoking
 Abnormal hemoglobin—poor O_2 release
Decreased Production
Erythropoietin deficiency
 Chronic renal failure
Nutrient deficiency
 Iron, folate, B_{12} deficiencies
Decreased use of nutrients
 Anemia of chronic disease—poor iron bioavailability
 Pernicious anemia—lack of co-factor for B_{12} uptake
Decreased hemoglobin production
 Thalassemia—genetic hemoglobin defects
Marrow disease
 Marrow-displacing tumors
 Marrow failure—toxins, infections, idiopathic marrow
  aplasia
Increased Destruction
Hemoglobin defects
 Sickle-cell anemia
Physical rupture
 Burns, RBC trauma, osmotic, microangiopathy (DIC,
  thrombotic thrombocytopenic purpura)
Metabolic enzyme deficiencies
 Glucose-6-phosphate dehydrogenase deficiency
Membrane defects
 Hereditary spherocytosis, elliptocytosis
 Paroxysmal nocturnal hemoglobinuria
RBC antibodies
 Auto- or alloimmune antibodies
Decreased Heme Synthesis
Porphyrias—toxic effects of various excess heme
 precursors

er's functions. Basophils bind IgE and release histamine and other mediators of allergic reactions. Eosinophils release histaminase, prostaglandins, and other metabolites that dampen allergic reactions. Eosinophils also are prominent in response to parasites.

Monocytes also perform phagocytosis and microbial killing via mechanisms similar to granulocytes. After their transient blood passage, they become macrophages (or histiocytes), chronic inflammatory cells residing in tissues for several weeks. They form the granulomas of intracellular infections, such as tuberculosis, listeriosis, syphilis, and parasitic conditions. They also give key assistance to both the humoral and the cellular immune systems. They present foreign antigens to T cells and, via various cytokines, both stimulate and are stimulated by T cells to assist in immune responses. Macrophages produce interleukin-1, the wide-ranging mediator of fever, acute phase reactions, and B and T lymphocyte activation. Their complex array of degradation enzymes makes them subject to several congenital "storage diseases," enzyme deficiencies in which various metabolic products accumulate in macrophages. Abnormal proliferation is seen in blood-borne acute or chronic monocytic or myelomonocytic leukemias and in localized or systemic tissue histiocytoses.

Platelet Physiology

Platelets are small circulating anuclear fragments of bone marrow megakaryocytes. The marrow's daily production is normally enough to raise the platelet count by 40,000/μL. About one third of peripheral platelets reside in the spleen and are subject to release by epinephrine in the acute phase reaction.

half of the blood neutrophils are marginated; hence, there is normally a large reservoir for rapid leukocytosis when needed. Successful antibacterial neutrophil phagocytic function requires numerous steps: (1) chemotaxis—migration in response to activated complement or kinin, or to cytokines from other white blood cells; (2) surface receptor recognition through opsonization, i.e., coating of the target pathogen with immunoglobulins, complement, or fibronectin; (3) phagocytosis; and (4) killing of pathogens by the contents of cytoplasmic granules. Bacterial killing is performed in granules by the generation of destructive hydroxyl and oxygen radicals from superoxide (O_2^-) and by degradative enzymes, such as myeloperoxidase, lysozyme, and elastase. Lactoferrin in granules both enhances hydroxyl radical formation and chelates iron necessary for baceterial growth. Granulocyte disorders are classified and illustrated in Table 31–2.

Basophils and eosinophils are derived from a common precursor, but counteract certain of each oth-

TABLE 31–2. GRANULOCYTE DISORDERS

Functional Deficiencies
Granule enzyme deficiencies—myeloperoxidase,
 lactoferrin
Granule defects—Chédiak-Higashi syndrome, May-
 Hegglin anomaly
Superoxide deficiency—chronic granulomatous disease
Suppression of phagocytosis—corticosteroids
Deficient Production
Congenital—agranulocytosis, cyclic neutropenia
Marrow-suppressive agents—drugs, toxins, radiation
Marrow failure—aplasia, metastatic tumor
Nutrient deficiencies—B_{12}, folate
Increased Destruction
Immune—peripheral or marrow antibodies
Consumptive—sepsis
Sequestrative—hypersplenism
Increased Production
Benign—leukemoid reaction to infection
Malignant—acute or chronic myelocytic leukemia

Platelets have a complex dual role in hemostasis. They plug vascular leaks, and they serve as a platform for coagulation factor activation. To accomplish these roles, platelets have several membrane receptors to anchor coagulation factors, and they carry an elaborate internal machinery for self-activation when damaged endothelium is encountered.

Formation of the platelet plug involves platelet adhesion to the site of injury, release of platelet agonists from the platelets' own granules, and aggregation of platelets to each other. Either subendothelial collagen or thrombin in the coagulation cascade can set this process in motion.

Platelets first adhere to subendothelial collagen, using von Willebrand's factor (vWF) as a bridge between the blood vessel and the vWF-binding platelet surface protein, glycoprotein Ib. Adherent platelets are then susceptible to activation by various agonists, chiefly collagen, thrombin, epinephrine, adenosine diphosphonate (ADP), and arachidonic acid. Activation increases the intracellular calcium concentration, which is necessary for the contractile action of converting the discoid platelet surface into sticky pseudopodia and for the release of platelet granules containing further activators. One major pathway for activation, whereby arachidonic acid is converted to the powerful aggregator thromboxane A_2, is blocked by aspirin.

The platelet's granules contain activators, such as ADP, and numerous coagulation-related factors, such as vWF, fibrinogen, and factor V. When released, these granule contents induce a strong positive feedback for further activation and aggregation. The activation process also induces changes in the platelet membrane configuration that favor receptor binding of clotting factors. In this fashion, fibrinogen binds to another membrane protein complex, glycoprotein IIb/IIIa, and factors V and X come together on the platelet surface to catalyze thrombin formation. The other major platelet function—to serve as a platform for coagulation factor activation—completes the formation of the platelet-fibrin plug by helping enmesh the aggregated platelets in a web of fibrin. Platelet disorders are categorized with examples in Table 31–3.

TRANSFUSION THERAPY

Red Blood Cells and Whole Blood

A unit of whole blood comprises 450 mL of blood drawn from the donor into 60 mL of anticoagulant-preservative solution. Most donations are then centrifuged to sediment the red cells and remove the plasma for further production of platelets and fresh-frozen plasma or cryoprecipitate.

TABLE 31–3. PLATELET DISORDERS

Decreased Production
Congenital—amegakaryocytosis, Wiskott-Aldrich syndrome
Acquired—infections, drug toxicity, ethanol, other marrow diseases

Increased Destruction
Immune—autoantibodies, posttransfusion purpura
Consumptive—thrombotic thrombocytopenic purpura, disseminated intravascular coagulation, giant hemangiomas
Sequestrative—hypersplenism

Decreased Function
Congenital—Bernard-Soulier (deficient glycoprotein Ib for vWF), Glanzmann's (deficient glycoprotein IIb/IIIa for fibrinogen), storage-granule deficiencies
Drugs—aspirin, penicillins, anti-inflammatory agents
Medical conditions—uremia, liver disease, myeloproliferative diseases

Increased Production
Benign—iron deficiency, acute phase reaction, idiopathic
Malignant—myeloproliferative diseases, leukemia

Two types of red blood cells (RBCs) are currently used. The traditional unit of "packed red cells" is preserved in citrate-phospate-dextrose-adenine-1 (CPDA-1) with a 300 mL volume, 75 per cent hematocrit, and 35-day shelf-life when stored at 1° to 6° C. In the newer additive-solution (AS) RBCs, 100 mL of saline with more adenine and dextrose is added to the RBCs, for a final hematocrit of 55 per cent. The additional adenine allows a longer 42-day RBC storage. CPDA-1 and AS RBCs are used interchangeably, except for some concern about AS in neonates because of the high dextrose levels and uncertainty about adenine metabolism.

One unit of whole blood or RBCs should raise the average adult's hemoglobin level by 1 gm/dL or the hematocrit by 3.

The need for perioperative RBC transfusions should be evaluated according to each patient's tolerance for anemia. At hemoglobin levels below 7 gm/dL, cardiac output sharply increases, and most acutely anemic patients require transfusion. At hemoglobin levels equal to or above 10 gm/dL, blood is rarely needed in otherwise healthy patients. However, there is no evidence that a hemoglobin level below 10 gm/dL needs to be a universal rule of thumb for transfusion. The decision to transfuse, particularly between 7 to 10 gm/dL, should take into account the rapidity of blood loss and other conditions, such as chronic anemia, impaired cardiopulmonary reserve, or cerebrovascular or peripheral circulatory disease. Hemoglobin levels in the 7 to 10 gm/dL range do not impair wound healing or promote infection, and there are little clinical data to support the common impression of faster recuperation or improved well-being after transfusion.

Platelets

Platelets are usually provided as units of 50-mL platelet concentrates made from individual whole-blood donations. Their shelf-life is either 3 days or 5 days, depending on the type of blood bag used. Physiologic function is best maintained at 20° to 24° C storage, since refrigerated platelets have poor viability. Platelets are usually selected to be ABO- and Rh-compatible.

The standard dose of platelets is one unit for each 10 kg of body weight in order to increase the patient's platelet count by an expected 50,000/μL or more. Follow-up platelet counts in the first hour and the next day after transfusion are helpful in assessing the platelets' effect. Reduced 24-hour increments are seen in splenomegaly, fever, sepsis, severe bleeding, and disseminated intravascular coagulation. Reduced 1-hour increments are typical of HLA antibody formation (see the section, "Adverse Effects of Transfusion") and should prompt consideration of HLA-matched single-donor platelets collected by apheresis. These plateletpheresis concentrates typically contain six to eight units' worth of platelets.

Patients with platelet counts below 10,000 to 20,000/μL are usually prophylactically transfused because of an increased risk of spontaneous severe hemorrhage. Platelet counts above 80,000 to 100,000/μL usually do not cause bleeding, and transfusion is not needed unless a hemostatic challenge is superimposed on platelet dysfunction caused by uremia, drugs (aspirin, nonsteroidal anti-inflammatory drugs, penicillin, carbenicillin), myeloproliferative disease, or congenital disorders (most commonly von Willebrand's disease). At levels between 20,000 and 80,000 platelets/μL, the need for platelets depends on the presence of bleeding, invasive procedures, or other disease or injury in a sensitive area. Platelets are not routinely needed for the temporary platelet dysfunction of cardiopulmonary bypass or for hemodilution when less than one to two blood volumes are transfused. However, transfusion may be indicated for unexpectedly severe bleeding or thrombocytopenia in these settings.

Fresh-Frozen Plasma

Fresh-frozen plasma (FFP) is prepared by centrifuging the cellular components of the whole blood donation and freezing the plasma within 6 hours of collection to preserve fully the labile coagulation factors V and VIII. Each unit contains 225 mL and is stored below −18°C for up to 1 year. The plasma must be ABO-identical or ABO-compatible to the patient's blood type.

Fresh-frozen plasma provides clotting factors in patients with documented deficiencies. In moderate deficiencies, a reasonable goal is to increase factor levels to 25 per cent of normal. For an average plasma volume of 40 mL/kg of body weight, this goal can be accomplished by giving 15 mL/kg of FFP or four to five units in the average adult. Normal hemostasis is achieved when the prothrombin time and partial thromboplastin time are within 2 to 3 seconds of the normal control. However, the effect may be short-lived; factors VII and VIII have the shortest half-lives, 6 hours and 12 hours, respectively.

FFP therapy is indicated when hemostasis is needed in the face of the multiple factor deficiencies of liver disease. FFP is also useful in disseminated intravascular coagulation (DIC), although supplementation by cryoprecipitate may be needed as a more concentrated source of factor VIII and fibrinogen (see below). Coumadin therapy can be reversed rapidly by FFP, if there is not time for vitamin K to act, which takes 6 to 12 hours. FFP is indicated in some massive transfusions with plasma factor dilution, but generally only when there is a documented coagulopathy. FFP should not be used as a plasma expander because there are disease-free agents for this purpose: albumin, plasma protein fraction, or synthetic colloids.

Cryoprecipitate

Cryoprecipitate is prepared in individual units of 15 mL each and is often pooled like platelets before administration. To make cryoprecipitate, fresh-frozen plasma is thawed at 1° to 6°C, whereupon factor VIII, fibrinogen, and certain other cold-insoluble proteins are precipitated. The "cryo-poor" plasma is then drawn off, and the precipitate is refrozen quickly. The frozen shelf-life is 1 year from collection. ABO compatibility with the patient's blood type is favored, although the plasma volume of the product is small.

A unit of cryoprecipitate contains 80 to 120 International Units (IU) of factor VIII (see below) and 150 mg of fibrinogen and is also enriched in von Willebrand's factor, factor XIII, and fibronectin. Its established main indications are in von Willebrand's disease and in severe DIC with factor VIII and fibrinogen consumption. Cryoprecipitate therapy in factor VIII deficiency (hemophilia A) has waned now that factor VIII concentrates are treated to inactivate HIV and hepatitis viruses. Cryoprecipitate is sometimes succcessful in reversing the platelet dysfunction of uremia and is also a source of fibronectin, which has been proposed to be of benefit in microbial opsonization.

Granulocyte Concentrates

Granulocyte concentrates are collected by a 3-hour donor leukapheresis procedure. To increase the granulocyte yield, donors are given corticosteroids several hours before the procedure to increase their circulating granulocyte count, and hydroxyethyl starch is infused during the procedure to sediment the RBCs and improve WBC separation. This procedure obtains 10^{10} granulocytes, but this amount still represents only 10 per cent of the normal daily marrow production in adults. Granulocyte concentrates also contain as many platelets as a plateletpheresis product. The granulocytes must be ABO−, Rh−, and crossmatch-compatible because they contain 50 mL of RBCs. Granulocytes can be stored at room temperature for up to 24 hours, but should be given as soon as possible for best granulocyte function.

The efficacy of granulocyte transfusions is best demonstrated in patients with persistent neutropenia (less than 500 granulocytes/μL), documented infection, and initial unresponsiveness to appropriate antibiotics.

Factors VIII and IX

Factor VIII and factor IX concentrates are used in patients with congenital deficiencies of these factors. Patients with hemophilia A (factor VIII deficiency) or hemophilia B (factor IX deficiency) are treated for ongoing hemorrhage or prophylactically treated before invasive procedures. By convention, one IU of factor per mL of plasma equals 100 per cent of the normal level; therefore, the number of IUs needed for a 100 per cent level equals the plasma volume expressed in milliliters. The desired dosage varies with the severity and critical nature of the hemorrhage; for example, 20 to 40 per cent (0.2 to 0.4 IU/mL) levels are adequate for hemarthrosis, but 100 per cent is needed for central nervous system or retroperitoneal hemorrhage.

Factor IX is also given to hemophilia A patients who develop an antibody (inhibitor) to factor VIII. Factor IX concentrate contains the other vitamin-K-dependent factors II, VII, and X. It could be given for emergency reversal of congenital or acquired (coumadin, vitamin K depletion) deficiencies of these other factors, but is usually avoided in preference to FFP because of a higher hepatitis risk. Human immunodeficiency virus (HIV) is no longer transmitted by these concentrates now that purification and sterilization measures have been developed in response to the AIDS epidemic in hemophiliacs.

BLOOD GROUPS AND BLOOD COMPATIBILITY

The ABO blood group system is of major importance in transfusion and transplantation. The four possible ABO types—O, A, B, and AB—are the phenotypic expression of two co-dominantly inherited enzymes used to construct either A or B carbohydrate structures on red cells, endothelial cells, and secretory epithelia. Group O subjects have two alleles that produce an inactive protein. The ABO carbohydrate structures are strongly immunogenic, and probably owing to universal exposure to similar naturally occurring antigens, all O, A, and B subjects normally have circulating antibodies to whichever ABO antigen(s) they do not have. These powerful complement-fixing IgM and IgG ABO antibodies can cause hemolysis of ABO-incompatible RBC transfusions (see the section, "Transfusion Reactions") and severe damage to ABO-incompatible organ transplants (see Chapter 26). About 45 per cent of American whites are group O, 40 per cent are group A, 10 per cent are group B, and 5 per cent are group AB.

The Rh-positive or Rh-negative factor in a patient's blood type refers to the presence or absence of the D RBC antigen in the Rh blood group system. The importance of the D antigen lies in its strong immunogenicity in Rh-negative people (15 per cent of whites, 7 per cent of blacks). Exposure to even less than 1 mL of Rh+ RBCs via transfusion or by fetomaternal hemorrhage in pregnant women can induce formation of strong lifelong anti-D antibodies. Anti-D causes hemolysis of subsequent Rh+ RBC transfusions, but is most feared in young women for its role in hemolytic disease of the newborn (HDN), in which fetal Rh+ RBCs are destroyed by IgG anti-D crossing the placenta. Until the 1970s, hydrops fetalis due to anti-D was a major perinatal disease. Fortunately, Rh immune globulin, one of the great modern public health advances, prevents nearly all Rh alloimmunization in Rh-negative pregnant woman bearing Rh+ children.

In addition to ABO and the Rh D antigen, hundreds of other RBC blood groups have been discovered, and several are well known to the blood bank for their hemolysis- and HDN-causing antibodies. These clinically significant blood groups include other antigens in the Rh system (C,c,E,e), and the Kell (K), Duffy (Fy), Kidd (Jk), MNSs, and other blood group systems. These antigens are much less immunogenic than the Rh D antigen, but the antibodies are seen frequently enough to be of concern for safe transfusion. About 1 per cent of hospitalized patients and 5 to 15 per cent of chronically transfused patients have clinically significant "irregular" (i.e., non-ABO) RBC antibodies.

There are also some RBC antibodies that do not usually cause hemolysis, but must be identified when present so as to rule out other significant problems. The most common of these clinically insignificant antibodies are Lewis, P_1, M, cold agglutinins, such as anti-I, and high-titer low-avidity antibodies.

A few patients present severe crossmatching difficulties because they either have multiple hemolytic RBC antibodies or one hemolytic antibody to a very high-frequency antigen that they lack. Blood from rare donors for these patients can be frozen for up to

10 years and then obtained either locally or through nationwide rare-donor networks. Once thawed, these RBCs must be given within 24 hours because of concerns about sterility when the blood bag is opened for the thawing process.

Some patients develop autoantibodies to all RBCs, including their own. The blood bank can categorize these antibodies as warm-reacting (IgG), cold-reacting (IgM), or drug-related (IgG, several mechanisms) and can perform special tests to identify any complicating alloantibodies. A direct antiglobulin test (direct Coombs' test) should be done to identify IgG or complement on the RBC surface if there is suspicion of autoimmune or alloimmune hemolysis.

Compatibility Testing

Routine RBC compatibility testing consists of patient ABO typing, a screen for non-ABO antibodies, a crossmatch of patient serum versus the intended unit of RBCs, and a check of past records for past blood typings, antibodies, or transfusion reactions. In ABO typing, the patient's RBCs are tested for hemagglutination with anti-A and anti-B antisera, and the patient's serum is checked for the expected reciprocal reactions against group A and B RBCs. The serum antibody screen (indirect Coombs' test) is performed by testing the patient's serum against two or three group O RBCs specially selected to have all the common clinically significant non-ABO antigens. The screening technique includes detection of IgG RBC antibodies, using 37°C incubation and antiglobulin antisera containing anti-IgG for detecting binding of IgG to the test RBCs. Any reactions against the screening cells are characterized with additional sets of reagent RBCs ("panels"), selected according to their phenotypes to reveal antibody specificity. The crossmatch can be either "full"—incubated like the antibody screen to show IgG binding to the RBCs—or "abbreviated," in which only a brief immediate-spin crossmatch is performed for direct IgM hemagglutination to verify the ABO compatibility of the unit of RBCs. The abbreviated crossmatch is used in some laboratories when there is no historical or current screening evidence of RBC antibodies; only one in several thousand patients have clinically significant antibodies that are missed in the screen and are then detected only by the full crossmatch.

This sensitivity of the antibody screen permits use of the "type-and-screen" and the maximum surgical blood order schedule in preoperative compatibility testing. For surgical procedures in which blood use is possible but not usually necessary, the type-and-screen confirms the blood type and, when the antibody screen is negative, allows the rapid, safe use of type-specific RBCs if blood is needed suddenly. The blood ordering schedule defines the routine number of units to be crossmatched for each common surgical procedure, based on usual local blood needs. Together, the type-and-screen and the blood ordering schedule reduce unnecessary crossmatching and tying up of blood inventory.

In life-threatening hemorrhage, uncrossmatched group O packed RBCs can be given when there is no time to obtain at least a blood type (5 minutes of laboratory time). Type-specific blood (ABO and Rh-matched) can be given when the blood type is known, but the antibody screen and crossmatch are not complete (30 to 60 minutes). However, in this case, there is a 1 per cent overall risk of the presence of significant antibodies and the potential for hemolytic transfusion reactions in a subset of that 1 per cent who would happen to receive blood from an incompatible donor. Obtaining a pretransfusion specimen for typing is vital so that there is no later confusion about the patient's blood type and so that the patient can receive type-specific blood as soon as possible.

ADVERSE EFFECTS OF TRANSFUSION

Transfusion reactions occur in 1 to 2 per cent of all transfusions. The main categories are summarized in Table 31–4. The primary cause of serious acute hemolytic transfusion reactions is the administration of ABO-incompatible blood, accidentally given through errors in sample or patient identification, laboratory testing, or records. Correct identification of samples, blood, and the patient throughout each step of the process is mandatory for transfusion safety.

HLA alloimmunization can occur after exposure to foreign leukocytes through tranfusions or pregnancies. The HLA system is a very complex array of tissue antigens. Functionally, HLA class I antigens are ubiquitous to all cells and mediate suppressor/cytotoxic T cell action. Class II antigens are on immune cells and assist in helper T cell responses. Class I antigens HLA-A and HLA-B are the most important in general transfusion therapy. Because these antigens are on platelets and WBCs, antibodies cause destruction of incompatible transfused platelets and also result in most febrile reactions to WBC-containing blood. Chronically transfused patients often develop these antibodies; therefore, when long-term platelet support is needed, prospective HLA-A and HLA-B patient typing is recommended in the event that HLA-matched plateletpheresis donors are needed. Because the HLA antigen system is so complex, usually thousands of donor HLA types must be checked to find a few donors who are HLA-matched for a given patient. Special leukocyte filters for transfused RBCs and platelets can ameliorate febrile reactions to contaminating WBCs, and these filters are also being increasingly used for the prevention of HLA alloimmunization during the course of chronic transfusions. Class I HLA-C antigens are of little

TABLE 31–4. TRANSFUSION REACTIONS

Type	Frequency*	Cause	Therapy	Prevention
Febrile	1%	Patient WBC antibodies	Antipyretics, meperidine	Recurrent: leukopoor blood, premedication, slower transfusion
Allergic—Hives	1%	Antibodies to plasma substances	Antihistamines	Recurrent: washed RBCs, minimal plasma exposure, premedication
Hemolytic—				
Acute	1:25,000	Usually ABO incompatibility	ATN-diuresis DIC - FFP, cryoprecipitate	Patient and sample identity
Delayed	1:2,500	Past RBC antibodies	Antigen-negative blood	Past blood bank records
Pulmonary	1:10,000	Donor WBC antibodies	Corticosteroids	Not predictable
Anaphylactic	1:100,000	Some IgA-deficient patients with anti-IgA	Epinephrine	Plasma-free or IgA-deficient blood

ATN = acute tubular necrosis, kidneys; DIC = disseminated intravascular coagulation.
* Data from Walker, R.H.: Special report: Transfusion risks. Am. J. Clin. Pathol., *88*:374–378, 1987.

clinical significance. Class II HLA antigens (D, DP, DQ, DR) can stimulate humoral or cellular alloimmunization via the WBCs in cellular blood transfusions, but their main clinical significance lies in immune response control, disease associations, and transplantation.

Recurrent allergic (usually urticarial) reactions to transfused plasma are usually prevented by washing RBCs and concentrating platelets. Patients known to have complete IgA deficiency (1 in 700 people) should have minimal exposure to plasma (e.g., washed or frozen-thawed RBCs) because of their risk of forming anaphylactic anti-IgA antibodies.

Several other possible immunologic effects of blood transfusions are of note. Graft-versus-host disease from transfused lymphocytes can occur in severely immunosuppressed patients and in patients receiving closely matched blood from family members. Irradiation of cellular blood products (1500 to 2500 rads) is recommended in bone marrow transplants, congenital deficiencies of cellular immunity (DiGeorge's and Wiskott-Aldrich syndromes and severe combined immune deficiency), during intensive oncologic chemotherapy in some centers, and when the blood is from a first-degree relative of the patient.

Posttransfusion purpura is a sudden severe thrombocytopenia that occurs 1 week after transfusion. It is caused by stimulation of patient platelet-specific alloantibodies (usually anti PL^{A1} specificity), which also destroy the patient's own platelets by cross-reactivity or by coating of the patient's PL^{A1}-negative platelets with soluble transfused PL^{A1} substance.

Transfusion itself has an immunosuppressive effect in the setting of kidney transplantation. Because graft survival is improved in patients who have received pretransplant transfusions, some centers perform living-related renal transplantation only after intentional transfusion of blood from the prospective donor. Suggested mechanisms of action include induction of suppressor T cells or activation of antiidiotypic antibody networks. In most studies the improved transplant results seen with cyclosporine have blunted this transfusion advantage. By analogy, reduced immune surveillance has been invoked to explain some studies that show higher cancer recurrence and infection rates after perioperative transfusions.

Massive transfusion of more than one to two blood volumes' worth of RBCs has the potential to cause several complications due to the metabolic and storage properties of banked blood. The most likely problems include (1) metabolic alkalosis due to conversion of the citrate anticoagulant to bicarbonate, (2) thrombocytopenia due to dilution, and (3) hypothermia from chilled blood. Platelet counts and body warming are recommended. Other problems caused by hemodilution are usually seen only in extreme or special circumstances. Routine use of FFP is not recommended, but dilution of clotting factors is possible after two or more blood volumes. Citrate toxicity due to chelation of calcium by the anticoagulant is seldom seen except when the liver cannot normally rapidly convert citrate to bicarbonate, such as during liver transplantation. Stored RBCs can leak free potassium, up to 8 mEq per unit by the time of outdate, but the usual alkalosis counteracts this leakage; hyperkalemia is usually a potential problem only in patients with poor renal function receiving large numbers of RBCs. After 10 to 14 days of storage, RBC 2,3-DPG levels decline, although the associated decreased off-loading of O_2 from hemoglobin is of uncertain clinical significance.

Transfusion-Transmitted Infections

A number of infections can be transmitted by transfusion. However, it was AIDS that served to focus attention on the safety of the blood supply in the 1980s. About 3 per cent of U.S. AIDS cases have been caused by blood transfusions and another 1 per cent by coagulation factor concentrates given to hemophiliacs. Currently, careful prescreening to eliminate high-risk blood donors, together with anti-HIV testing of every donation, has virtually eliminated HIV transmission, except for the rare but tragic circumstance of donor infection without detectable HIV antibodies. In the first 6 years since testing began in 1985, only 15 reported U.S. cases of AIDS were confirmed to be caused by tested blood. In 1989, estimates of the likelihood of HIV transmission were around 1 in 40,000 to 1 in 150,000 units.

Hepatitis remains the major threat from transfusion in terms of numbers of cases. In the 1970s, paid donors were virtually eliminated from the regular blood supply because of their high rate of hepatitis transmission. (The plasma now collected in paid-donor plasma centers is processed into virally sterile albumin and gamma globulin or into HIV-inactivated factor concentrates.) However, despite this, and despite universal donor testing for hepatitis B surface antigen, about 1 in 20 units of blood still transmitted hepatitis as of 1980, as defined by otherwise unexplained recipient transaminase elevations within 6 months. Ninety per cent of these cases were non-A, non-B hepatitis (NANBH).

Most cases of NANBH are initially asymptomatic, but about 20 per cent are thought to progress to chronic active hepatitis and another 10 per cent to cirrhosis. In 1986 to 1987, U.S. blood banks adopted two "surrogate" donor markers: ALT(SGPT) and antibody to hepatitis B core antigen (anti-HBc). Each of these abnormalities carried a statistically increased risk of NANBH transmission, and discarding these units was expected to reduce infection rates by two thirds. Indeed, after surrogate testing and the increased anti-AIDS measures, reported NANBH rates dropped by over half nationally. Thus, the risk of hepatitis in the late 1980s was estimated to be 1 per cent or less per unit.

In 1989 the main cause of NANBH was identified as hepatitis C virus (HCV). Since 1990, all blood donors have been screened for anti-HCV, thus further reducing the risk of NANBH to perhaps 1 to 2 per 1000 units.

Cytomegalovirus (CMV) can be transmitted in transfused leukocytes in RBCs, platelets, and granulocytes. In immunocompetent patients this transmission is not a problem. However, certain groups of immunosuppressed patients should receive CMV-antibody-negative blood to avoid the risk of severe CMV morbidity. Premature infants under 1200 gm birthweight have benefitted from CMV seronegative blood. CMV-negative bone marrow transplant recipients, particularly when their marrow donor is CMV-negative, should also receive CMV-negative blood. Some kidney, heart, and liver transplant programs also provide CMV-negative blood to CMV-negative patients.

Testing all U.S. blood donors for antibodies to another retrovirus, human T-lymphotropic virus type I (HTLV-I), was instituted in 1988 to 1989 as a public health measure. HTLV-I is associated with a rare form of T-cell leukemia and also with a chronic disabling myelopathy. The virus can be transmitted by cellular blood products, although development of transfusion-associated disease is very rare. Other blood-borne infections, such as malaria, babesiosis, syphilis, and bacterial contamination, are also rare.

Reducing Homologous Blood Transfusions

Reduction of homologous (non-self) blood transfusions in surgery lessens the risks not only of disease transmission but also of transfusion reactions and alloimmunization. This can be accomplished by autologous blood transfusion and by surgical and pharmacologic methods for reducing blood loss. The role of erythropoietin administration to stimulate RBC production in this setting is also under current investigation.

Autologous blood may be collected pre-, intra-, or postoperatively. It has been estimated in some centers that up to 10 per cent of all RBC transfusions could be autologous if all eligible patients gave presurgical autologous donations. Preoperative blood donations require iron therapy and a minimum hematocrit of 33 per cent. In most healthy patients, as many as four or five units can be obtained at weekly intervals up to 3 days before surgery. The main contraindications are unstable cardiopulmonary conditions in which the phlebotomy may pose a risk, and possible bacteremia, to avoid reinfusing contaminated blood later. Rechecking the patient's and the unit's blood types before autologous transfusion is necessary to confirm that no blood labeling error has occurred.

Intraoperative blood collections involve either hemodilution, the volume-replenished collection of one or two units immediately before surgery, or RBC salvage of shed blood aspirated from a sterile, nonmalignant surgical field. Salvage utilizes blood-washing centrifuge instruments or canister collection systems. Postoperatively, blood can also be collected from surgical drains of sterile areas.

Some patients or families may wish to obtain so-called directed blood donations from family or friends, in the hope that such blood is safer than the regular blood supply. Studies to date of anti-HIV and hepatitis marker rates in these donors have found no differences from regular volunteer donors, and concerns have been voiced that some donors recruited by the patients could feel pressured to give despite having risk factors for viral infections. However, most blood programs now provide this option for participation in the patient's care, and the overall blood donor pool is augmented because many such donors have never given before. RBCs and platelets from first-degree relatives should be irradiated to prevent graft-versus-host disease.

When bleeding can be reduced significantly, so too is the potential need for transfusions. There is no substitute for good surgical technique, and measures to reduce blood flow, such as tourniquets and relative hypotension, have long been used in some procedures. In recent years, the hemostasis-enhancing effects of several agents—desmopressin, aprotinin, and topical fibrin glue—have been investigated in several settings. Also, stimulation of the patient's own blood production is now possible.

Desmopressin, or DDAVP (1-deamino-8-D-arginine vasopressin), is a synthetic analogue of vasopressin, or antidiuretic hormone. DDAVP temporarily increases circulating levels of factor VIII and von Willebrand's factor, probably by inducing release from storage sites. DDAVP has become standard therapy for many patients with mild to moderate congenital deficiencies of these factors (5 to 15 per cent of normal). (DDAVP is contraindicated in the rare subtype IIB of von Willebrand's disease because it is ineffective and causes thrombocytopenia.) In some congenital platelet defects, the bleeding time can be temporarily corrected by DDAVP. In all of these settings, the effect is obtained within 1 hour and lasts several hours. Tachyphylaxis may occur with repeated doses over several days.

Because of its hemostatic properties, DDAVP has been investigated for various acquired platelet dysfunctions and for reducing blood loss in major surgery. Prolonged bleeding times have been shortened in uremia and liver disease and after drug-induced thrombocytopathies, such as from aspirin, although the mechanisms and the efficacy in reducing bleeding are uncertain. DDAVP has also decreased blood loss and usage in some cardiopulmonary bypass patients with large blood needs, again possibly by improving platelet dysfunction in this setting.

Another hemostatic agent of possible benefit is aprotinin, an antifibrinolytic agent that in European studies has significantly reduced blood needs in cardiac surgery.

Fibrin glue or fibrin sealant is a concentrated source of fibrinogen, applied topically along with thrombin to induce clotting. Fibrin sealant is commercially available in Europe, but because the fibrinogen is from pooled concentrates, the Food and Drug Administration has not yet licensed it in the United States. Alternatively, fibrin glue can be made from small aliquots of single-donor plasma, in a fashion similar to cryoprecipitate. It can also be prepared autologously.

Recombinant human erythropoietin (Epo) became available for clinical use in 1989. Epo is the main physiologic factor stimulating red cell differentiation, usually in response to tissue hypoxia. Ninety per cent of the body's normal production comes from the kidneys, and thus patients with the anemia of chronic renal failure were the first to benefit from Epo therapy. In addition to enabling a major reduction of transfusion needs in most of these patients, the improved hematocrit also helps correct the platelet dysfunction accompanying uremia. Epo is being studied in various other anemias and for possible augmentation of preoperative autologous blood collection. Other recombinant bone-marrow growth factors, such as GM-CSF and IL-3 (see the section, "Hematopoiesis") are being investigated for potential benefit in stimulating production of white cells and platelets.

BIBLIOGRAPHY

1. Williams, W.J., Beutler, E., Erslev, A.S., and Lichtman, M.A. (eds.): Hematology, 4th ed. New York, McGraw-Hill, 1990.
2. Petz, L.D., and Swisher, S.N. (eds.): Clinical Practice of Transfusion Medicine. New York, Churchill Livingstone, 1989.
3. Cooper, E.D. (ed.): College of American Pathologists Conference XIV on safety in transfusion practices revisited. Arch. Pathol. Lab. Med., 113:225, 1989.
4. Cumming, P.D. Wallace, E.L., Schorr, J.B., and Dodd, R.Y.: Exposure of patients to human immunodeficiency virus through the transfusion of blood components that test antibody-negative. N. Engl. J. Med., 321:941, 1989.
5. Alter, H.S., Purcell, R.H., Shih, J.W, et al.: Detection of antibody to hepatitis C virus in prospectively followed transfusion recipients with acute and chronic non-A, non-B hepatitis. N. Engl. J. Med., 321:1494, 1989.

INDEX

Note: Page numbers in *italics* refer to illustrations; page numbers followed by t refer to tables.

435